Congenital Muscular Dystrophies

Congenital Muscular Dystrophies

Edited by

Yukio Fukuyama
Makiko Osawa
Kayoko Saito
Tokyo Women's Medical College
Tokyo, Japan

1997

ELSEVIER

AMSTERDAM • LAUSANNE • NEW YORK • OXFORD • SHANNON • TOKYO

ELSEVIER SCIENCE B.V.
Sara Burgerhartstraat 25
P.O. Box 211, 1000 AE Amsterdam, The Netherlands

Library of Congress Cataloging-in-Publication Data

Congenital muscular dystrophies / edited by Yukio Fukuyama, Makiko
   Osawa, Kayoko Saito.
        p.   cm. -- (Developments in neurology ; 13)
     Includes bibliographical references and index.
     ISBN 0-444-82487-1
     1. Muscular dystrophy.   I. Fukuyama, Yukio.   II. Osawa, Makiko.
   III. Saito, Kayoko.   IV. Series.
   RC935.M7C66   1997
   616.7'48043--dc21   97-17026
                                                                     CIP

ISBN: 0 444 82487 1

Printed in The Netherlands.

Preface

The term congenital muscular dystrophy (CMD) is generally regarded as a subtype of progressive muscular dystrophy, that is, a primary progressive degenerative disorder affecting skeletal muscles which is usually of genetic origin. An actual historical review of CMD research tells us, however, that the basic concept of progressive muscular dystrophy outlined above has often been ignored in the designation of CMD not only in the early literature, but also even in recent literature.

Gordon Holmes, a pioneering advocate of the term CMD, first reported an autopsy study of a 7-day-old baby in 1908, under a confusing title in which a static condition (congenital defect of the muscular system) and an essentially progressive one (dystrophia muscularis congenita) were dealt with interchangeably.

In the majority of reported cases, the duration of clinical follow-up was inadequate to discern a slowly progressive course. Some investigators have claimed that CMD may take a static, non-progressive course, while others have accepted as CMD even cases in whom normal deep tendon reflexes were elicited and whose serum creatine kinase activity was normal. Histopathological examinations of skeletal muscles were sometimes neglected, or even when carried out, were done with a poor technique or using vague histologic diagnostic criteria for dystrophic changes. Furthermore, the absolute number of studies on CMD was small, each study dealing with quite a small number of subjects. Clinical features as well as laboratory findings varied considerably among reported cases.

Thus, it is probably safe to say that CMD had been only poorly defined during the first 50 years of what might now be called CMD research. More importantly, there are a considerable number of investigators who recongnize CMD as a group of conditions which are not compatible with the concept of progressive muscular dystrophy.

The recognition and delineation of Fukuyama type congenital muscular dystrophy (FCMD) as a distinct clinico-genetic entity, dating back to 1960, brought about a revolutionary turn in the aforementional trend in two important ways:
(1)   It clearly demonstrated that there exists a type of CMD which deserves acceptance as a genuine member of the family of progressive muscular dystrophies, based upon its characteristic clinical as well as laboratory findings.
(2)   It offered a completely new avenue to approaching the pathogenesis of progressive muscular dystrophy in general as a multi-systemic disease, rather than simply as a form of muscle pathology.

The second point perhaps is worthy of further comment. In patients with FCMD, static developmental abnormalities of the central nervous system are invariably associated with primary progressive muscular dystrophy; mental retardation of moderate to severe degree is a constant clinical feature. Neuropathologically, characteristic brain dysplasia, called cobblestone lissencephaly, have been noted without exception. These observations led the authors to advocate the term congenital cerebro-muscular dystrophy, already in 1960. Thus the recognition of FCMD presented a fresh impetus to broaden the spectrum of neuroblast migrational disorder, in turn.

Knowledge of FCMD was gradually disseminated from Japan to the rest of the world, triggering an explosion of interest, and thereby facilitating a comparative study of experiences between different institutions worldwide, which led to the re-evaluation of previously overlooked related syndromes, such as the Walker–Warburg and muscle–eye–brain syndromes, etc.

Retrospectively, however, the discovery of FCMD in 1960 was only one major milestone during the history of CMD research. The second revolution took place in 1993, when Toda and his colleagues published a report announcing the successful mapping of the candidate FCMD gene to chromosome 9q31-33. In parallel with rapid progress in molecular genetics, advances in cell biology and neuroimaging techniques were fully applied to CMD research, and ultimately, merosin deficient CMD, an essentially homogeneous clinico-genetic entity, was first identified in 1994. As a consequence, the third major group of CMD patients, although apparently heterogeneous, was excluded. This group constitutes merosin positive non-Fukuyama type CMD.

Thus, recent progress in CMD research has been rapid, and the pace continues to accelerate. This remarkable progress raises challenges for anyone attempting to closely follow the breakthroughs which are taking place daily in various corners of the world. To promote further progress in this research, however, quick acquisition of up-to-date information is of vital importance.

In this sense, the International Symposium on Congenital Muscular Dystrophies which was held in Tokyo, July 7–8, 1994, was an extremely significant event. In this Symposium, a large volume of new data on various aspects of CMD was presented and discussed. By attending the speech presentations and participating in the free discussions for 2 full days, the participants had many worthwhile experiences; correcting, modifying and/or reconfirming their own knowledge of CMD, as well as the intellectual excitement of gaining new knowledge. There is no doubt that all participants were satisfied with the Symposium, thanks to the exposure to and the opportunity to acquire a broad and comprehensive perspective on the current status of the vanguard of research into this hitherto mysterious, and still controversial, subject of CMD.

There can be no doubt that the present book, a product of this highly significant Symposium, constitutes a memorable monument in the history of CMD research, and will, as an essential reference book, continuously serve and stimulate those engaged in future research on CMD.

Before closing, the editors would like to express their heartfelt appreciation to all contributors including those who generously attended the Symposium in Tokyo in 1994, and those who made the enormous commitment to submit manuscripts of the highest quality to this volume.

Yukio Fukuyama, MD, PhD
Makiko Osawa, MD, PhD
Kayoko Saito, MD, PhD

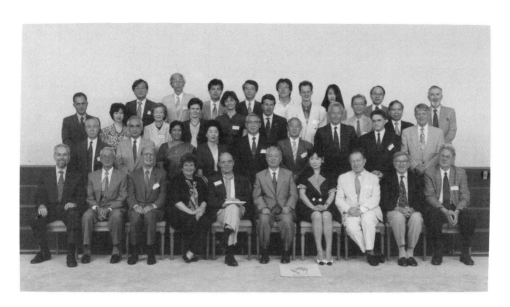

Speakers and chairperson at the International Symposium on Congenital Muscular Dystrophies, Tokyo, July 7–8, 1994.

Front row (from left to right): D. Stumpf (Chicago), M. Gomez (Rochester), G. Serratrice (Marseille), L. Dubowitz (London), J. Aicardi (Paris), Y. Fukuyama (Tokyo), M. OSawa (TWMC), M. Fardeau (Paris), V. Dubowitz (London), H. Goebel (Mainz).

Second row (from left to right): Y. Suzuki (Tokyo), M. Segawa (Tokyo), V. Karla (New Delhi), M. Yoshioka (Kobe), J. Tanaka (Tokyo), S. Miyoshino (Beppu), H.G. Lenard (Düsseldorf), B.F. Reitter (Mainz), O. Eeg-Olofsson (Uppsala).

Third row (from left to right): H. Topaloglu (Ankara), K. Saito (Tokyo), Wu Xi-Ru (Beijing), H. Pihko (Helsinki), A. Berardinelli (Pavia), E. Parano (Catania), V. Straub (Düsseldorf), I. Nonaka (Kodairo), K. Kumagai (Atsugi), R. Ouvrier (Sydney).

Fourth row (from left to right): S. Takashima (Kodaira), T. Abe (Tokyo), T. Toda (Tokyo), T. Miike (Kumamoto), K. Matsumura (Tokyo), E. Kondo (Tokyo), K. Hashimoto (Kawasaki).

List of contributors

M. ALBANI — Department of Paediatrics, Municipal Hospital, Wiesbaden, Germany

L. ANDERSON — Muscular Dystrophy Group Research Laboratories, Regional Neurosciences Centre, Newcastle General Hospital, Newcastle-upon-Tyne, NE4 6BE, UK

C. ANGELINI — Neurological Institute, University of Padua, Padua, Italy

K. ARAHATA — Department of Neuromuscular Research, National Institute of Neuroscience, NCNP, Tokyo, Japan

Y. ARAI — Department of Pediatrics, Tokyo Women's Medical College, Shinjuku-ku, Tokyo, Japan

E. ARIKAWA-HIRASAWA — Department of Neuromuscular Research, National Institute of Neuroscience, NCNP, Tokyo, Japan and Department of Neurology, Juntendo University School of Medicine, Tokyo, Japan

A. BERARDINELLI — Department of Child Neuropsychiatry IRCCS "C. Mondino", University of Pavia, Pavia, Italy

R. BITTNER — Institute of Anatomy, Department 3, University of Vienna, Waehringer Straße 13, A-1090 Vienna, Austria

A. BORNEMANN — Department of Neuropathology, University of Mainz Medical Center, Mainz, Germany

K.P. CAMPBELL — Howard Hughes Medical Institute and Department of Physiology & Biophysics, University of Iowa College of Medicine, Iowa City, USA

C. CAROLLO — Neurological Institute, University of Padua, Padua, Italy

C.W. CHOW — Department of Anatomical Pathology, Royal Children's Hospital, Melbourne, Australia

W.B. DOBYNS — Department of Neurology and Pediatrics, University of Minnesota, Minneapolis, MN, USA

P. DRIGO — Department of Paediatrics, University of Padua, Padua, Italy

V. DUBOWITZ — Department of Paediatrics and Neonatal Medicine, Royal Postgraduate Medical School, Hammersmith Hospital, London W12 ONN, UK

K.E. EEG-OLOFSSON — Department of Clinical Neurophysiology, University Hospital, Uppsala, Sweden

O. EEG-OLOFSSON — Department of Pediatrics, University Hospital, Uppsala, Sweden

T. EVANGELISTA — INSERM U153 and CNRS ERS 064, Paris, France

R. FALSAPERLA — Pediatric Clinic, University of Catania, Catania, Italy

M. FANIN	Neurological Institute, University of Padua, Padua, Italy
M. FARDEAU	Research Group on Development, Pathology and Regeneration of the Neuromuscular System, INSERM U.153, Institut de Myologie, Hôpital de la Salpêtrière, 47, boulevard de l'Hôpital, FR-75651, Paris Cédex 13, France
E. FAZZI	Department of Child Neuropsychiatry, IRCCS "C. Mondino", University of Pavia, Pavia, Italy
A. FIUMARA	Pediatric Clinic, University of Catania, Catania, Italy
S. FUJITA	Department of Neurology and Neuroscience, Teikyo University School of Medicine, Tokyo, Japan
H. FUKUTA-OHI	Department of Neurology and Neuroscience, Teikyo University School of Medicine, Tokyo, Japan
Y. FUKUYAMA	Department of Pediatrics, Tokyo Women's Medical College, Shinjuku-ku, Tokyo, Japan
H.H. GOEBEL	Department of Neuropathology, University of Mainz Medical Center, Mainz, Germany
M. GOTO	Department of Neurology, Chiba Children's Hospital, Chiba, Japan
S. GÖĞÜS	Departments of Pediatrics, Neurology and Pathology, Hacettepe Children's Hospital, Ankara, Turkey
T. HAYASHI	Department of Pediatrics, Yamaguchi University, Ube, Yamaguchi, Japan
Y.K. HAYASHI	Department of Neuromuscular Research, National Institute of Neuroscience, NCNP, Tokyo, Japan and Department of Neurology, Juntendo University School of Medicine, Tokyo, Japan
R. HERRMANN	Department of Paediatrics, University of Essen, Hufelandstr. 55, D-45122 Essen, Germany
S. IKEGAWA	Institute of Medical Science, University of Tokyo, Tokyo, Japan
H. IKENAKA	Department of Pediatrics, Tokyo Women's Medical College, Shinjuku-ku, Tokyo, Japan
H. ISHII	Tokyo Metropolitan Higashiyamato Medical Center for Disabilities, Tokyo, Japan
T. JIMI	Division of Neurology, Department of Medicine, Showa University, Fujigaoka Hospital, Yokohama, Japan
I. KANAZAWA	Department of Neurology, University of Tokyo, Tokyo, Japan
S. KIMURA	Department of Pediatrics, Urafune Hospital of Yokohama City University, Yokohama, Japan
T. KOBAYASHI	Department of Pediatrics, Urafune Hospital of Yokohama City University, Yokohama, Japan and Division of Pathology, Kanagawa Children's Medical Center, Yokohama, Japan
M. KOBAYASHI	Department of Pathology, Tokyo Women's Medical College, Tokyo, Japan

O. KOBAYASHI	National Center of Neurology and Psychiatry, Kodaira, Tokyo, Japan
R. KOGA	National Institute of Neuroscience, NCNP, Tokyo, Japan
E. KONDO	Department of Pediatrics, Tokyo Women's Medical College, Tokyo, Japan
T. KUMAGAI	Division of Pediatric Neurology, Central Hospital, Aichi Prefectural Colony, Kasugai, Japan
S. KUROKI	Department of Pediatrics, Kobe General Hospital, 4-6 Minatojima-Nakamachi, Chuo-ku, Kobe 650, Japan
G. LANZI	Department of Child Neuropsychiatry, IRCCS "C. Mondino", University of Pavia, Pavia, Italy
A.M. LAVERDA	Department of Paediatrics, University of Padua, Padua, Italy
J.J. LÉGER	INSERM, Unité 300, Faculté de Pharmacie, Avenue Charles Flahaut, F-3400 Montpellier, France
F. MARTINELLO	Neurological Institute, University of Padua, Padua, Italy
T. MATSUISHI	Department of Pediatrics, Kurume University Medical School, Kurume, Japan
K. MATSUMURA	Department of Neurology and Neuroscience, Teikyo University School of Medicine, Tokyo, Japan
T. MATSUZAKI	National Institute of Neuroscience, NCNP, Tokyo, Japan
T. MIIKE	Department of Child Development, Kumamoto University School of Medicine, Kumamoto, Japan
M. MINAMITANI	Division of Neuropathology, Institute of Neuroscience, The Jikei University School of Medicine, Tokyo, Japan
N. MISUGI	Department of Orthopedics, Kanagawa Children's Medical Center, Yokohama, Japan
S. MIYAKE	Department of Neurology, Kanagawa Children's Medical Center, Yokohama, Japan
M. MIYAKE	Department of Human Genetics, University of Tokyo, Tokyo, Japan
M. MIZUGUCHI	Department of Mental Retardation and Birth Defect Research, National Institute of Neuroscience, NCNP, Kodaira, Tokyo, Japan
Y. MIZUNO	Department of Neuromuscular Research, National Institute of Neuroscience, NCNP, Tokyo, Japan and Department of Neurology, Juntendo University School of Medicine, Tokyo, Japan
M.L. MOSTACCIUOLO	Department of Biology, University of Padua, Padua, Italy
M. MURAHASHI	Division of Neurology, Department of Medicine, Showa University, Fujigaoka Hospital, Yokohama, Japan
H. MURASUGI	Department of Pediatrics, Tokyo Women's Medical College, Shinjuku-ku, Tokyo, Japan
T. MUTOH	Second Internal Medicine, Fukui Medical School, Fukui, Japan
Y. NAKAGOME	Department of Human Genetics, University of Tokyo, Tokyo, Japan

Y. NAKAHORI	Department of Human Genetics, University of Tokyo, Tokyo, Japan
Y. NAKAMURA	Institute of Medical Science, University of Tokyo, Tokyo, Japan
Y. NOMURA	Segawa Neurological Clinic for Children, Tokyo, Japan
I. NONAKA	Department of Neuromuscular Research, National Institute of Neuroscience, NCNP, Tokyo, Japan
J. OHTA	Department of Child Development, University School of Medicine, Kumamoto, Japan
Y. OKAWA	Department of Rehabilitation Medicine, Teikyo University Ichihara Hospital, Ichihara, Chiba, Japan
Y. OLSSON	Department of Neuropathology, University Hospital, Uppsala, Sweden
H. ONIKI	Electron Microscopic Laboratory, Showa University Fujigaoka Hospital, Yokohama, Japan
S.-I. OSARI	National Center of Neurology and Psychiatry, Kodaira, Tokyo, Japan
M. OSAWA	Department of Pediatrics, Tokyo Women's Medical College, Shinjuku-ku, Tokyo, Japan
E. OZAWA	National Center of Neurology and Psychiatry, Kodaira, Tokyo, Japan
E. PARANO	Pediatric Clinic, University of Catania, Catania, Italy
L. PAVONE	Pediatric Clinic, University of Catania, Catania, Italy
J.-F. PELLISSIER	Professeur de Neuropathologie Service d'Anatomie Pathologique et de Neuropathologie, Timone, Marseille, France
P. PERINI	Neurological Institute, University of Padua, Padua, Italy
H. PIHKO	Department of Pediatrics and Child Neurology, Children's Hospital, University of Helsinki, Helsinki, Finland
B. REITTER	Department of Paediatrics, University of Mainz Medical Center, Mainz, Germany
R. ROETTGER	Department of Pathology, Municipal Hospital Braunschweig, Germany
K. SAITO	Department of Pediatrics, Tokyo Women's Medical College, Shinjuku-ku, Tokyo, Japan
P. SANTAVUORI	Department of Pediatrics and Child Neurology, Children's Hospital, University of Helsinki, Helsinki, Finland
Y. SASAKI	Division of Pathology, Kanagawa Children's Medical Center, Yokohama, Japan
M. SEGAWA	Segawa Neurological Clinic for Children, Tokyo, Japan
G. SERRATRICE	Professeur de Neurologie, Clinique des Maladies du Système Nerveux et de l'Appareil Locomoteur, Timone, Marseille, France
S. SHIBUYA	Division of Neurology, Department of Medicine, Showa University, Fujigaoka Hospital, Yokohama, Japan
T. SHIMIZU	Department of Neurology and Neuroscience, Teikyo University School of Medicine, Tokyo, Japan

K. SHISHIKURA	Department of Pediatrics, Tokyo Women's Medical College, Shinjuku-ku, Tokyo, Japan
V. STRAUB	Department of Pediatrics, University of Düsseldorf, Moorenstrasse 5, D-40225 Düsseldorf, Germany
S. SUGINO	Department of Child Development, Kumamoto University School of Medicine, Kumamoto, Japan
S. SUMIDA	Department of Pediatrics, Tokyo Women's Medical College, Shinjuku-ku, Tokyo, Japan
N. SUZUKI	Department of Pediatrics, Tokyo Women's Medical College, Shinjuku-ku, Tokyo, Japan
H. SUZUKI	Department of Pediatrics, Tokyo Women's Medical College, Shinjuku-ku, Tokyo, Japan
K. TAKADA	Department of Clinical Neuropathology, Tokyo Metropolitan Institute for Neuroscience, Fuchu, Japan
S. TAKASHIMA	Department of Mental Retardation and Birth Defect Research, National Institute of Neuroscience, NCNP, Kodaira, Tokyo, Japan
Y. TANABE	Department of Neurology, Chiba Children's Hospital, Chiba, Japan
H. TANAKA	Department of Neurology, Brain Research Institute, Niigata University, Niigata, Japan
J. TANAKA	Division of Neuropathology, Institute of Neuroscience, The Jikei University School of Medicine, Tokyo, Japan
T. TANAKA	Saitama Red Cross Blood Center, Yono, Japan
T. TODA	Department of Human Genetics, University of Tokyo, Tokyo, Japan
F.M.S. TOMÉ	INSERM U.153 and CNRS ERS 064, Paris, France
H. TOPALOĞLU	Departments of Pediatrics, Neurology and Pathology, Hacettepe Children's Hospital, Ankara, Turkey
A.P. TORMENE	Institute of Ophthalmology,University of Padua, Padua, Italy
C.P. TREVISAN	Neurological Institute, University of Padua, Padua, Italy
S. TSUJI	Department of Neurology, Brain Research Institute, Niigata University, Niigata, Japan
S. UEDA	Department of Rehabilitation Medicine, Teikyo University Ichihara Hospital, Ichihara, Chiba, Japan
C. UGGETTI	Neuroradiological Department, IRCCS "C. Mondino", University of Pavia, Pavia, Italy
P. VEGGIOTTI	Department of Child Neuropsychiatry, IRCCS "C. Mondino", University of Pavia, Pavia, Italy
T. VOIT	Department of Paediatrics, University of Essen, Hufelandstr. 55, D-45122 Essen, Germany
Y. WAKAYAMA	Division of Neurology, Department of Medicine, Showa University, Fujigaoka Hospital, Yokohama, Japan
K. YALAZ	Departments of Pediatrics, Neurology and Pathology, Hacettepe Children's Hospital, Ankara, Turkey

H. YAMADA — Department of Neurology and Neuroscience, Teikyo University School of Medicine, Tokyo, Japan

E. YAMAGUCHI — Department of Pediatrics, Yamaguchi University, Ube, Yamaguchi, Japan

T. YAMAMOTO — Department of Pathology, Tokyo Women's Medical College, Tokyo, Japan

S. YAMASHITA — Department of Neurology, Kanagawa Children's Medical Center, Yokohama, Japan

Y. YAMASHITA — Department of Pediatrics, Kurume University Medical School, Kurume, Japan

M. YOSHIOKA — Department of Pediatrics, Kobe General Hospital, 4-6 Minatojima-Nakamachi, Chuo-ku, Kobe 650, Japan

J.-E. ZHAO — Department of Child Development, Kumamoto University School of Medicine, Kumamoto, Japan

Contents

1. Nosological establishment of congenital muscular dystrophies in the history of medicine 1
    Y. Fukuyama

2. Exciting new developments in congenital muscular dystrophy 21
    V. Dubowitz

3. Fukuyama type congenital progressive muscular dystrophy 31
    M. Osawa, S. Sumida, N. Suzuki, Y. Arai, H. Ikenaka, H. Murasugi,
    K. Shishikura, H. Suzuki, K. Saito and Y. Fukuyama

4. Classical (occidental) congenital muscular dystrophy: clinical and pathologic reevaluation 69
    I. Nonaka, O. Kobayashi, S.-I. Osari, Y. Yamashita, T. Matsuishi, M. Goto,
    Y. Tanabe, Y. Hayashi, K. Arahata and E. Ozawa

5. Clinical and immunocytochemical evidence of heterogeneity in classical (occidental) congenital muscular dystrophy 79
    M. Fardeau and F.M.S. Tomé

6. Walker–Warburg and other cobblestone lissencephaly syndromes: 1995 update 89
    W.B. Dobyns

7. Muscle-eye-brain (MEB) disease – a review 99
    H. Pihko and P. Santavuori

8. The clinical spectrum and genetic studies of Fukuyama congenital muscular dystrophy 105
    M. Yoshioka, T. Toda and S. Kuroki

9. Characteristics of muscle involvement evaluated by computerized tomography scanning in early stages of progressive muscular dystrophy: comparison between Duchenne and Fukuyama types 119
    Y. Arai, M. Osawa and Y. Fukuyama

10. Longitudinal evaluation of leukoencephalopathy in congenital muscular dystrophy: data on a heterogeneous series of Western cases 137
    C.P. Trevisan, F. Martinello, M. Fanin, C. Carollo, P. Perini, C. Angelini,
    P. Drigo, A.M. Laverda, M.L. Mostacciuolo, A. P. Tormene, M. Fardeau and
    F.M.S. Tomé

11. Congenital muscular dystrophy: clinical variability in Sicilian patients 147
    E. Parano, L. Pavone, A. Fiumara, R. Falsaperla and W.B. Dobyns

12. Merosin and clinical characteristics of congenital muscular dystrophy in an unselected group of Turkish patients 153
    H. Topaloğlu, T. Evangelista, S. Göğüs, K. Yalaz and F.M.S. Tomé

13. Rehabilitation of children with Fukuyama congenital muscular dystrophy 159
    Y. Okawa and S. Ueda

14. Congenital muscular dystrophies: myo- and neuropathological studies 171
    H.H. Goebel, B. Reitter, M. Albani, A. Bornemann, R. Roettger and C.W. Chow

15. Brain pathology in Fukuyama type congenital muscular dystrophy with special reference to the cortical dysplasia and the occurrence of neurofibrillary tangles 189
    J. Tanaka, M. Minamitani and K. Takada

16. Cytoarchitectonic alterations of the cerebral cortex in Fukuyama-type congenital muscular dystrophy and other cortical dysplasia syndrome 199
    S. Takashima and M. Mizuguchi

17. Neuronal and vascular involvement in Fukuyama type congenital muscular dystrophy 207
    T. Miike, J. Ohta, S. Sugino, J.-E. Zhao and T. Mutoh

18. Ultrastructural alterations of the muscle plasma membrane and related structures in Fukuyama muscular dystrophy: comparative study with other types of muscular dystrophies 213
    Y. Wakayama, S. Shibuya, T. Kumagai, T. Kobayashi, S. Yamashita, N. Misugi, S. Miyake, M. Murahashi, T. Jimi and H. Oniki

19. Walker–Warburg syndrome in Japan: a comparative study with Fukuyama type congenital muscular dystrophy 231
    S. Kimura, Y. Sasaki, S. Miyake, N. Misugi, T. Kobayashi, E. Yamaguchi and T. Hayashi

20. Membrane abnormality in Fukuyama congenital muscular dystrophy 253
    E. Arikawa-Hirasawa, Y.K. Hayashi, Y. Mizuno, I. Nonaka and K. Arahata

21. Laminin $\alpha 2$ (or M) chain abnormality in congenital muscular dystrophy 259
    Y.K. Hayashi, I. Nonaka and K. Arahata

22. Peripheral nerve dystroglycan: its function and potential role in the molecular pathogenesis of neuromuscular diseases 267
    K. Matsumura, H. Yamada, S. Fujita, H. Fukuta-Ohi, T. Tanaka, K.P. Campbell and T. Shimizu

23. Distribution and organization of utrophin and the laminin $\alpha 2$ chain in normal and dystrophic skeletal muscle fibers 275
    V. Straub, R. Herrmann, R. Bittner, L. Anderson, J.J. Léger and T. Voit

24. Laminin in animal models for muscular dystrophy: deficiency of the laminin $\alpha 2$ chain in the homozygous dystrophic *dy/dy* mouse 291
    K. Arahata, Y.K. Hayashi, R. Koga, H. Ishii and T. Matsuzaki

25. Toward identification of the Fukuyama type congenital muscular dystrophy gene 301
    T. Toda, M. Miyake, Y. Nakahori, M. Segawa, Y. Nomura, I. Nonaka,
    S. Ikegawa, E. Kondo, K. Saito, M. Osawa, Y. Fukuyama, M. Yoshioka,
    T. Shimizu, I. Kanazawa, Y. Nakamura and Y. Nakagome

26. Reconfirmation of the Fukuyama congenital muscular dystrophy (FCMD) gene locus at chromosome 9q31, and a successful prenatal diagnosis of FCMD in two families 309
    E. Kondo, K. Saito, T. Toda, M. Osawa, H. Tanaka, S. Tsuji, T. Yamamoto,
    M. Kobayashi, Y. Nakamura and Y. Fukuyama

27. Tubular aggregates myopathy 321
    G. Serratrice and J.-F. Pellissier

28. Cerebral cortical gyration abnormality and denervation muscular atrophy: a case report 329
    G. Lanzi, A. Berardinelli, E. Fazzi, C. Uggetti and P. Veggiotti

29. Congenital muscular dystrophy and brain malformation in two sibs: a pathological and neuroradiological comparison 337
    K.E. Eeg-Olofsson, O. Eeg-Olofsson and Y. Olsson

30. A milder form of Walker–Warburg syndrome 345
    K. Saito, H. Suzuki, K. Shishikura, M. Osawa and Y. Fukuyama

Bibliography of congenital muscular dystrophies: the up-dated, second edition (February, 1997) 355
    Compiled by Y. Fukuyama

Subject Index 437

Y. Fukuyama, M. Osawa and K. Saito (Eds.), *Congenital Muscular Dystrophies*

1

Nosological establishment of congenital muscular dystrophies in the history of medicine

YUKIO FUKUYAMA

Department of Pediatrics, Tokyo Women's Medical College, Tokyo, Japan

Introduction

It has long been claimed that Dr. Frederick E. Batten [1–5] was the first who described a condition which appeared to mimic what is now known as congenital muscular dystrophy (CMD), while a pioneering advocate of the term CMD was Dr. Russel Howard [6].

Batten first reported 3 cases of infantile type myopathy, aged 6, 7 and 6 years, in a short note of only 2 pages [1]. Batten published a critical review article on the classification and nosological problems pertaining to myopathies or muscular dystrophies [2]. This review included an extensive literature search with regards to the relation of myatonia congenita to the myopathies, especially in cases which showed recovery or arrest of disease progression. He tried to introduce a new subtype of progressive muscular dystrophy called "simple atrophic type" to replace the term of myatonia congenita. He subsequently reported another case (a 6-year-old boy) with the simple atrophic type of myopathy [3], the diagnosis being given purely on clinical grounds. He believed this disease to be congenital or to manifest in early infancy. It was characterized by smallness, weakness, and global loss of muscle tone throughout the body, without localized atrophy or hypertrophy of individual muscles or group of muscles. The condition was slowly progressive: the child might learn to sit up or possibly stand with support. In later stages, contractures usually appeared. The intellect was unimpaired. Some cases were familial. Later, some authors gave to this group of patients the designation "congenital or early infantile muscular dystrophy of Batten", or "Batten-Turner type" muscular dystrophy, in honor of Dr. Batten. However, neither muscle biopsy nor necropsy studies were documented in a series of Batten's articles. Thus, there is nowadays no appropriate means of ascertaining the type of disease from which Batten's patients had suffered, in view of the current knowledge. Contrary to Greenfield et al. [7], who acknowledged Batten's cases as examples of CMD, I am quite dubious about the authenticity of the diagnosis, as criticized in a leading article in Lancet [11]. It may be reasonable to consider these cases as having a form of myopathy, but there is no convincing evidence for muscular dystrophy. In my view, the clinical descriptions in Batten's papers were far less detailed than those of other authors in the early days, such as Howard [6], Schlivek [12] or Haushalter's case 3 [13].

A question thus arises as to which cases reported in the classic literature would most fit to authentic CMD. This is an interesting challenging question and it is difficult to find a definitive answer. Pertaining to this problem, there are a number of modern articles which have critically reviewed such classic reports from the nosological viewpoint. Maintaining rather strict myopathological criteria, Greenfield et al. [7] recognized Haushalter's 3 cases [13], the family reported by Turner [14,15], Brandt's 3 cases [16], and a case described by Richter and Humphrey [17], as examples of CMD. They also expressed an affirmative opinion on the cases reported by Silvestri [18], but were uncertain about Dubois's case [19], and clearly rejected the cases reported by Spiller [20], Collier and Holmes [21], Lereboullet and Baudouin [22], Councilman and Dunn [23] and de Lange [24].

Short [25] reported an autopsied CMD case together with a review of 7 cases in which the diagnosis of CMD was thought to have been confirmed. The list included one case each from Lereboullet and Baudouin [22] and Councilman and Dunn [23], both of which had been excluded by Greenfield et al. [7]. The others on Short's list included one case each from Haushalter [13], Turner [14,15], and the Children's Medical Center, Boston [26], and two cases described by Banker et al. [27]. Lereboullet and Baudouin's case was recognized as having severe CMD by Zellweger et al. [28].

Review of classic literature (1900–1969)

A more extensive review of 17 potential CMD patients reported in the old literature was presented in tabular form by Vassella et al. [29] and was subsequently further expanded by Rotthauwe et al. [30] to demonstrate the individual profile of 52 cases. The same type of review work was continuously being carried out by the author. He gathered 42 articles, including 80 potential CMD patients, from literature published before 1970 [1,3,4,7–10,12, 14–17,21–30,35–51], in addition to his own article in 1960 [31] (Table 1). To compare with Rotthauwe's review, this expanded collection includes 4 new Japanese articles [31–34], several cases of unusual CDM forms such as the Ullrich type and CMD with selective diaphragmatic involvement [45]. Cases 1 and 2 in the paper by Rotthauwe et al. [30] were both excluded from the table, because these patients were the same subjects as cases 1 and 2 in the paper by Gött and Josten [40]. It should be noted that the profiles of 15 patients in that landmark publication were described collectively, but not individually, in Table 1, so they have not been included in the total count.

It is evident from Table 1 that the study on CMD has long been inactive, and there have been only 38 articles during the 70 year period, if 4 articles from Japan are excluded. They become more scanty if we limit the time to the year 1960 or earlier: only 23 papers were found during the earlier 60 year period. Furthermore, the majority of the articles dealt with one or two cases each. The scarcity of study reports concerning CMD in the first half of the 20th century may be related partly to the actual low incidence of CMD patients among the western population, as well as to the virtual absence of established medical knowledge of the condition, but it is also likely that another factor mentioned below would have hampered the progress of CMD study. That is, most investigators at that time might have devoted their major interests to the nosological problem of amyotonia congenita Oppenheim in relation to infantile spinal muscular atrophy Werdnig–Hoffmann. Since 1900, a hot debate on the latter topic prevailed in the medical society for more than 50 years.

A complicated, confusing state of investigations in those days was clearly demonstrated and critically analyzed by Brandt in 1950 [16]. After a detailed clinical and pathological study on a huge number of patients, as well as an exhaustive review of literature, Brandt

Table 1
Review of Classic Literatures (1900–1969)

Author	Case	Sex	Family history	Fetal movement	Joint contracture at birth	Hypotonia	Hypokinesia	Sit up (age[a])	Walk (age[a])	Age at first consultation[a]	Intelligence[b]	Body part with weakness[c]	DTR	EMG[d]	Muscle dystrophy on biopsy	Course[a,e]	Comments[a]
Batten (1903) [1]	1	M	–	?	?	?	+	+	–	6y	N	T, L > U	–	Ne	Ne	Static ?	Description too simple
	2	M	–	?	?	?	+	+	–	7y	?	T, E	–	Ne	Ne	Static ?	Ditto
	3	F	–	?	?	?	+	+	–	6y	N	T, L > U	–	Ne	Ne	Static	Ditto
Howard (1908) [6]	1	M	?	?	+	?	?	?	?	7d	?	T	?	Ne	+	Died (7d)	CNS normal
Collier and Holmes (1909) [21]	2	M	–	?	–	+	+	–	–	3y6m	N	T, L > U	–	Ne	+	Sl prog	Diag suspicious (Greenfield et al.)
Lereboullet and Baudouin (1909) [22]	1	M	–	?	–	+	+	–	–	11m	?	T, neck L > U	(+)	Ne	+	Died (11m)	Spinal cord intact, diag suspicious (Greenfield et al.)
Schlivek (1910) [12]	1	F	–	?	+	+	+	+	1y10m	2y3m	N	T, E proximal	+	Ne	Ne	Sl improv ?	Description too simple
Batten (1915) [3]	1	M	–	?	–	+	+	+	–	6y	N	T	+	Ne	Ne	Sl improv	Description too simple
Councilman and Dunn (1911) [23]	1	M	–	N	–	+	+	–	–	6w	N	G	–	Ne	+ (autopsy)	Prog, died (6m)	CNS, spinal cord intact, diag suspicious (Greenfield et al.)
Batten (1915) [4]	1	F	+	?	?	+	+	+	–	5y	N	G	?	Ne	Ne	Improv	Description too simple, hard to make diagnosis
Haushalter (1920) [15]	2	F	+	?	?	+	+	–	+	2y	?	G	?	Ne	Ne	Improv	Ditto
	3	F	+	?	–	+	+	–	–	2y5m	N	G, L > U	?	Ne	+	Relat static, died (14y)	Spinal cord intact

Author	Case	Sex	Family history	Fetal move-ment	Joint contrac-ture at birth	Hypo-tonia	Hypo-kinesia	Sit up (age)[a]	Walk (age)[a]	Age at first con-sulta-tion[a]	Intelli-gence[b]	Body part with weak-ness[c]	DTR	EMG[d]	Muscle dystro-phy on biopsy	Course[a,e]	Comments[a]
Silberberg (1923) [35]	1	?	?	?	?	+	+	?	?	4m	?	G	?	Ne		Died (4m)	CNS, spinal cord, PNS intact
Ullrich (1930) [36]	2	M	–	+	+	+	+	?	?	9m	?	G	+	Ne	+	Died (10m)	Parents consan-guineous
Menges (1931) [37]	1	F	–	?	?	+	+	?	?	6m	?	T, E	?	Ne	+	Died (6m)	
Middleton (1934) [38]	7	?	?	?	+	?	+	?	?	2y	?	E	?	Ne	+	Died (8m)	
de Lange (1938) [24]	1	M	+	?	–	+	+	?	?	2y6m	N	G	(+)	Ne	+	Died (2y6m)	CNS intact, dia-phragm involved, 2 sisters, 3 cous-ins affected
Turner (1940) [14], Turner and Lee (1962) [39]	10	F	+	+	(+)	+	+	1y	2y	4y	N	Shoulder	+	Ne	+	Static, died (21y)	2 sisters, 1 brother affected, aged 40–50
Brandt (1950) [16]	54	F	–	?	–	+	+	?	?	4y	?	G	?	Ne	+	Static	
	60	M	–	?	–	±	+	?	+	2y	?	G	?	Ne	?	Prog	
Gött and Josten (1954) [14]	1	M	+	?	+	+	+	1y	?	15m	N	T, E	(+)	Ne	+	SI prog	Sibship
	2	F	+	?	+	+	+	6m	2y		N	T, E	+	Ne	Ne	Static	
Richter and Humphreys (1955) [17]	1	F	?	?	–	+	–	+	16m		N	Pelvic, neck		Ne	Ne	Static	
Levesque et al. (1956) [41]	2	M	+	?	–	+	+			13d	?	G	+	M	+	Died (2y6m)	Brother and sister, died 2m, 7.5m respectively
Banker et al. (1957) [27]	1	M	+	?	+	?	+	?	?	5.5m	N		–	M	+	Died (5.8m)	CNS intact
	2	M	+	?	–	+		?	?	1h					+	Died (1.5h)	Brother of case 1, scoliosis

										Age	IQ	Distribution				Course	Notes
Faber and Craig (1958) [26]	1	F	-	-	-	-	+	-	-	6m	?	T, E	-	?	+	Died (6m)	Sister had same muscle pathology
Greenfield et al. (1958) [7]	1	F	+	+	+	+	+	-	-	2y6m		F, T, E proximal	-	M	+	Static (mild improv)	Sibship
Joseph et al. (1958) [42]	2	M	+	?	+	?	+	-	-	2y		F, T, E	(+)	N	+	Static 2y, unknown thereafter	Sibship
Fukuyama et al. (1960) [31]	2'	F	+	?	+	+	+	+	-	1m		Ptosis	?	Ne	+	Died (1y)	Consanguinity in 6: fraternal affliction in 2 pairs
	15 cases	M6, F9	+	+	-	+	+	+	+:2, -:13	3m to 12m	IQ 62 ↓↓	G, F proximal	-	M	+	Sl prog	
Watanabe (1961) [32]	1	F	+	+	-	+	+	+ 2y	-	8y		G, F	-	M	-	Sl prog	Sibship
	2	F	+	+	-	+	+	-	-	6m		G, F	-	M	+	Sl prog	
Lelong et al. (1962) [43]	1	F	-	+	-	+	+	?	3y	9y	N	T, E, F	(+)	?	±	Static or sl prog	2 cousins: LCC
O'Brien (1962) [44]	1	M	-	?	-	+	+	7m	5y	2y	N	T, E, F	-	(N)	+	Prog, died (8y7m)	CNS intact
Lewis and Besant (1962) [45]	1	M	Sib	-	-	+	+	-	-	11d		G, diaphragm	?	Ne	Diaphragm +	Died (2.5m)	Respiratory failure due to diaphragmatic muscle dystrophy
	2	F	Sib	→	-	+	+	-	-	At birth		G, diaphragm	+	Ne	Diaphragm +, other m -	Died (6w)	Ditto, CNS intact
Pearson and Fowler (1963) [46]	1	M	+	?	+	+	+	?	2y6m	6y5m	N	G, U > L	(+)		+	Prog to 7y, then static for 2y	Sibship
	2	F	+	?	+	+	+	N				F, T, U > L	(+)		+	Static or s1 prog	
Short (1963) [25]	1	M	+	+	-	+	+	?			?	T, E	(+)	?	+	Contracture since 3m, died (6m)	CNS intact, a brother died of a myotonia congenita (11d)
Lamy et al. (1965) [47]	1	F	-	?	+	+	+		-	10d		T, E Ptosis	-	Not clear	+	Improv, died (16m)	Spinal cord intact
Wharton (1965) [48]	1	F	+	?	-	+	+	?	-			T, E	+	N/M	+	Prog, died (1y)	A sister affected

Author	Case	Sex	Family history	Fetal move-ment	Joint contrac-ture at birth	Hypo-tonia	Hypo-kinesia	Sit up (age)[a]	Walk (age)[a]	Age at first con-sulta-tion[a]	Intelli-gence[b]	Body part with weak-ness[c]	DTR	EMG[d]	Muscle dystro-phy on biopsy	Course[a,e]	Comments[a]
Fontaine et al. (1965) [49]	1	M	–	?	?	+	+	6m	16m	6y6m	N	G	+	N	+	No prog	
	2	F	–	+	?	+	+			10m	N	G	(+)	N/M	+	Static, contract ↑	
Gubbay et al. (1966) [8]	1	F	–	+	?	+	?	5y6m	–	1y	N	T, E, F prox > dist	?	M	+	Sl improv	
Fenichel and Bazelon (1966) [50]	1	M	–	+	(+)	+	?	N	14m	4y	N	G	(+)	M	+	Non-prog	
Yamagata (1967) [33]	1	M	+	?	–	+	+	–	–	9m	?	G, E	–	Ne	Ne	Sl prog	A sister affected, died (9y)
Vassella et al. (1967) [29]	1	F	+	–	+	+	+			5m	N	T, E	(+)	M	+	Prog con-tracture ↑	A sister affected, died (2y)
	2	M	+	?	+	+	+			7.5m	N	T, E, F	–	M	+	Unable to judge	Mother is a cousin of case 1
	3	F	–	–	?	+	+		20m	7y6m	IQ 60–70	T, E, F (?)	+	?	+	Static (?)	
	4	M	–	?	+	+	+		14m	2y0m	N	T, E prox > dist	+	+	+	Static or sl improv	
	5	M	–	–	+	+	+	9m		4y9m	N	T, E, F	+	+	+	Con-tracture ↑	
	6	F	–	–	+	+	+	13m	4y	5y	N	T, E	(+)	+	+	Knee con-tracture ↑ after 3y	
	7	M	–	+	–	+	+	10m		3w		T, E	(+)	Ne	+	Unable to judge	
	8	M	–	+	+	+	+			3w		T, E	?	+	+	Unable to judge	
Engel (1967) [51]	Fig. 8	F								22m		G	?	?	+	Prog	
	Fig 9	F								10y		G prox > dist	?	?	+	Static	

Reference	No.	Sex					Age 1	Age 2	Age 3	CK	Muscle				Course	Remarks
Zellweger et al. (1967) [10]	1	M	–	–	+	+	10m	14m	13y	N	Hip prox > dist	+	+	+	Static	Dyslexia
	2	M	–	–	+	+	?	?	15y	N	Hip, neck, F	(+)	+	+	Static	MR, stuttering in maternal relatives
	3	M	–	?	±	+	?	2y	15y	N	Hip, neck, F	(+) ~++	+	+	Sl improv	Dizygotic twin
Zellweger et al. (1967) [28]	1	F	+	+	–	+	2y6m	3y		N	T, E, F	–	+	+	Sl improv contract ↑	A sister: dystrophic arthrogryoposis, died (3m)
	2	F	–	?	–	+	3y6m		6m	N	T, E, F	–	+	+	Sl improv contract ↑	
	3	F	–	–	?	+	4y		4y5m	53–66	T, E, F	+ to –	+	+	Sl prog	
Ueda et al. (1968) [34]	1	F	–	–	+	+	–		5m		G, F	–	M	+	?	Convulsion (+), retinal pigmentary degeneration, pseudohypertrophy
	2	M	–	–	+	+	–		1y	→	G, F	–	M	+	?	Megacolon pseudohypertrophy
	3	M	–	–	+	+	1y2m	–	1y7m	→	G, F	–	M	+		Difficult delivery convulsion (+) pseudohypertrophy
	4	F	–	–	+	+	1y2m	–	1y8m	→	G, F	–	M	+	Contracture	Recurrent convulsions pseudohypertrophy
	5	F	–	–	+	+	10m	–	2y10m	→	G	–	M	+	Contract ↑	Pseudohypertrophy
	6	M	+	+	+	+	–	–	3y	→	G	–	M	+	Died (3y6m)	Febrile convulsions, spina bifida occulta, pseudohypertrophy
	7	F	–	–	+	+	+	–	3y	→	G	–		+		Pseudohypertrophy

Author	Case	Sex	Family history	Fetal movement	Joint contracture at birth	Hypotonia	Hypokinesia	Sit up (age)[a]	Walk (age)[a]	Age at first consultation[a]	Intelligence[b]	Body part with weakness[c]	DTR	EMG[d]	Muscle dystrophy on biopsy[c]	Course[a,e]	Comments[a]
	8	F	-	-	-	+	+	1y	-	3y	→	G	-	M	+	Sl prog	Pseudohypertrophy convulsions (+)
	9	M	-	-	-	+	+	12m	-	6y	→	G	-	M	+	Sl prog	Convulsions (+)
	10	F	-	+	-	+	+	7m	-	7y	→	G	-	M	+	Sl prog	Salivation
	11	F	+	-	-	+	+	4y	-	10y	→	G	-	M	+	Sl prog	Pelvic delivery, sister of case 13
	12	M	-	-	-	+	+	2y	-	11y	→	G	-	M	+	Sl prog	Pseudohypertrophy, brother of case 11
	13	M	-	-	-	-	+	+	2y6m	5y3m	?	Shoulder, hip	-	M	+	Static	
Rotthauwe et al. (1969) [30]	3	M	-	+	+	+	+	10m	2y	2y4m	N	G, F	(+)	Ne	+	Sl prog	Hip dysplasia
	4	F	-	+	+	+	+	10m	-	1y10m	N	G	-	Ne	+	Prog	Hip dysplasia
	5	F	-	+	-	+	+			1y6m	N	G	-	Ne	+	Rapid prog, died (2y9m)	Hip dysplasia
	6	M	-	-	++	-	+		1d			G		Ne	+	Unable to judge	AMC type
	7	M	-	-	++	-	+		5w			G		Ne	+	Unable to judge	AMC type
	8	M	-	-	-	-	+	10m	2y6m	2m	N	G	-	Ne	+	Improved	2 maternal uncles had neuromuscular disorder

[a] y, years; d, days; m, months; w, weeks
[b] N, normal
[c] T, trunk; L, lower extremity; U, upper extremity; E, extremity; G, generalized; F, face
[d] Ne, not examined; M, myogenic
[e] sl, slightly; prog, progressive; improv, improving; relat, relatively

concluded that Werdnig–Hoffmann disease stands as an independent anatomo-clinical entity, and that the identity of Oppenheim disease could not be substantiated any more. With Brandt's monumental monograph, a long-held nosological dispute between Werdnig–Hoffmann and Oppenheim diseases ended.

However, there was another problem left unsolved after Brandt, that is, the problem of floppy infants. For a few years after Brandt's monograph, an extensive study was carried out by Walton [52–56] to better delineate the concept of floppy infants, or limp child, or the amyotonia congenita syndrome. As a result, a new term of benign congenital hypotonia was introduced to designate a group of patients which was considerably purified on clinical grounds. At that time, however, diagnostic laboratory tools were still quite limited, so that certain ambiguity could not be cleared-up fully. In Walton's series of cases which were regarded as examples of benign congenital hypotonia, half the patients recovered completely, while half, although improving up to a point, had smallness and weakness of some muscles throughout life. So, Greenfield et al. [7] suggested that those of Walton's cases which recovered incompletely should properly be regarded as examples of muscular dystrophy, even though the weakness was not progressive and muscle-biopsy specimens in several showed no abnormality. Although I cannot agree with Greenfield's comment in full, it is still undeniable that there is a difficulty in understanding the essential nature of benign congenital hypotonia, especially in cases with incomplete recovery.

Discovery of Fukuyama type congenital muscular dystrophy (FCMD)

In the late 1950s, a number of powerful laboratory examinations for the diagnosis of neuromuscular diseases, such as electromyography, muscle biopsy with modified Gomori and other various histochemical staining techniques, and serum creatine kinase (CK) activity measurement was successively explored and rapidly incorporated into clinical practice. In our clinic, a battery of EMG, muscle biopsy and serum CK determination were applied rather routinely to many infants and children with neuromuscular problems, and proved to be extremely useful in finding out clues for, or confirmation of clinical diagnosis [57]. We have developed a strong staff team for neuromuscular disorders within a pediatric department of the University Hospital. All procedures involved in the above examinations, including electrodiagnostics, surgical biopsy, histopathological processing and the CK activity measurement, were carried out by someone from our team, with close cooperation with each other. Our child neurologists had an advantage in carrying out this kind of clinical research because we are well acquainted with peculiarities of infants and young children. The author proudly recalls each member of his neuromuscular team at the University of Tokyo at that time, all of whom greatly contributed to the discovery of FCMD. It might also be significant to note that our special clinic was already established in the late 1950s, comparatively early in view of the world standard.

The first report on 15 cases of FCMD was delivered orally at a Tokyo district meeting of the Japan Pediatric Society on December 12, 1959, and then a short English paper entitled "A Peculiar Form of Congenital Progressive Muscular Dystrophy" [31], and two other Japanese papers in more detail [58,59], were published in 1960 and 1961 (Table 2). Most of the patients reported at that time had been treated under the wrong diagnosis of cerebral palsy or multiply neurologically handicapped at other institutions. What prompted the

Table 2

Clinical characteristics of Fukuyama type congenital muscular dystrophy according to its original description in 1960 [12]

1.	Early onset, usually before 9 months
2.	Hypotonia and weakness in early infancy
3.	Later development of muscle wasting and joint contractures
4.	Involvement is diffuse and extensive, but most prominent proximally
5.	Myopathic facies in nearly all cases, pseudohypertrophy present in half of cases
6.	Mental and speech retardation in nearly all cases, febrile or afebrile convulsions in half of cases
7.	EMG, CK and muscle biopsy findings characteristic of muscular dystrophy
8.	Course is either slowly progressive or stationary
9.	Autosomal recessive inheritance

author to explore another diagnosis in these patients? Firstly, there was no sign of spasticity or increased muscle tone in these patients. Deep tendon reflexes were either absent or reduced, without exceptions. Muscle resistance against passive movement was always reduced. All these signs were against the diagnosis of cerebral palsy. Patients were therefore submitted to our battery of examinations which clearly demonstrated the fact that skeletal muscles in these patients are suffering from progressive muscular dystrophy.

At any rate, our original report on FCMD was well accepted by many Japanese investigators from the beginning, and numerous supportive reports followed. The clinical spectrum as well as laboratory findings, including high CK levels, EMG and muscle histology, are so unique, and more or less pathognomonic, that the condition was easily recognizable to any attentive clinician. A rather high prevalence rate of the condition in Japan also facilitated the propagation of knowledge on this newly described condition among medical staff throughout the country. Consequently, there was no one in Japan who doubted the existence of CMD as a disease entity. Futhermore, most Japanese physicians once tended to believe that all CMD patients were of the so-called Fukuyama type (FCMD). Currently, of course, most Japanese physicians well understand that that is not true; there are CMD children who do not belong to the Fukuyama type. Thus, a subclassification of CMD patients into FCMD and non-FCMD is now widely accepted in Japan.

Propagation of knowledge and position of FCMD in the world

Turning to the rest of the world, a similar system of subclassifying CMD into FCMD and non-FCMD was also adopted in principle by the ICD-10 NA of WHO in 1991 [60], which contains two groups of CMD in the category of muscular dystrophy (G71.0); that is, G 71.084-CMD with CNS abnormalities (Fukuyama) and G71.085-CMD without CNS abnormalities (Table 3). The WFN Research Committee on Neuromuscular Diseases also supported a similar subdivision of CMD in 1991 (Table 4) [61].

It is probably not an over-exaggeration to state that the history of CMD research in the world actually started with the discovery and establishment of the entity of FCMD. The original work of the author's team was quickly and fully appreciated inside Japan, but was not recognized for many years outside of Japan. The ignorance and confusion which surrounded CMD in the international arena until the end of the 1970s is well illustrated in the famous textbook by Raymond D. Adams, Diseases of Muscle, 3rd edition, published in 1975 [62], which read that congenital muscular dystrophies consist of two groups: (1)

Table 3

Classification of muscular dystrophy in ICD-10NA (draft) [60]

G71.0	*Muscular dystrophy*	
	G71.00	Benign Becker-type muscular dystrophy
	G71.01	Benign scapuloperoneal muscular dystrophy with early contractures(Emery-Dreifuss)
	G71.02	Facioscapulohumeral muscular dystrophy (Landouzy-Dejerine)
	G71.03	Limb-girdle muscular dystrophy (Erb)
	G71.04	Ocular muscular dystrophy
	G71.05	Oculopharyngeal muscular dystrophy
	G71.06	Scapuloperoneal muscular dystrophy
	G71.07	Severe Duchenne-type muscular dystrophy
	G71.08	Other specified muscular dystrophy
		G71.080 Autosomal recessive muscular dystrophy, childhood type, resembling Duchenne/Becker
		G71.081 Distal muscular dystrophy and distal myopathy
		G71.082 Humeroperoneal muscular dystrophy with early contractures
		G71.083 Muscular dystrophy with excessive autophagy
		G71.084 Congenital muscular dystrophy with central nervous system abnormalities (Fukuyama)
		G71.085 Congenital muscular dystrophy without central nervous system abnormalities
	Excludes:	congenital muscular dystrophy, NOS (G71.2), with specific morphological abnormalities of the muscle fiber (G71.2)

established progressive muscular dystrophy at birth or infancy; and (2) congenital myopathy (? dystrophy) of unidentified type. The former group conforms with the strict definition of progressive muscular dystrophy and includes Duchenne muscular dystrophy, the facioscapulohumeral type of Landouzy–Dejerine and the myotonic dystrophy of Steinert. In contrast, the latter group includes variable conditions which do not necessarily fit with the definition. Thus, there is no trace of the knowledge we now have concerning CMD in the 3rd edition of Adams' book. In 1979, Lazaro and his colleagues [63] wrote in their article on CMD that this disorder is a vanishing category or a simple misnomer.

To enlighten western investigators, except German-speaking areas where CMD became a target of bigger studies since earlier days [64,65,66], it took about 20 years or even longer. The first paper by the Fukuyama group appeared in an unpopular local journal, and in fact the prevalence of FCMD in foreign countries is extrmely low. A considerable time was necessary to disseminate the knowledge in the international sphere, but there were several momentous activities which merit specific mention: These include the publications of good papers by Kamoshita et al. [67], Nonaka and Chou [68] and Fukuyama et al. [69] in either an influential journal or an internationally popular handbook. A number of free papers on FCMD were impressively presented at the First International Congress of Child Neurology (ICCN) in Toronto, in October of 1975. The author presented a lecture on FCMD in a symposium at the 2nd ICCN, in Sydney, in November of 1979. Moreover, the author also gave lectures on FCMD at various institutions and societies worldwide, by invitation, 38 times from 1977 through 1994, Through these unwavering activities, knowledge of FCMD spread worldwide, gradually at first and then explosively in recent years. Finally, FCMD was first registered under the number M 253800 in the 7th edition of McKusick's Mendelian Inheritance in Man in 1986. Subsequently, it was first included formally as an independent subtype of muscular dystrophy in the 10th revision of the Neurological Adaptation of the Inter-

Table 4

Classification of muscular dystrophy according to the Research Group on Neuromuscular Diseases, World Federation of Neurology Research Committee, 1991[61].

G71–74	Disorders of muscle
I	Congenital muscular dystrophies[a]
	Congenital muscular dystrophy
	Congenital muscular dystrophy with central nervous system involvement (Fukuyama type)
II	Morphologically defined congenital myopathy
	Central core disease
	Multicore disease
	Nemaline myopathy
	Myotubular(centronuclear) myopathy
	Fiber-type disproportion
	Other types
III.	Muscular dystrophies
	Duchenne type
	Becker type
	Emery-Dreifuss type
	Scapuloperoneal muscular dystrophy
	Fascioscapulohumeral type
	Limb-girdle muscular dystrophy
	Scapulohumeral type
	Pelvifemoral type
	Autosomal recessive childhood dystrophy resembling Duchenne/Becker
	Ocular type
	Oculopharyngeal type
	Distal type
	Other types
IV–XI.[b]	

[a]Note that CMD was put independently outside the frame of muscular dystrophies in this classification.
[b]Descriptions were omitted by the author.

national Classification of Diseases [60] in 1991, as mentioned above. Fig. 1 in the Introduction to the Bibliography shows the chronological trend in world publications or original articles specifically focusing on CMD (including both FCMD and non-FCMD), illustrating well the dramatic globalization of research on CMD-associated issues.

As shown in Table 5, 1103 infants and children with various neuromuscular disorders were treated at the specialized clinic of the Department of Pediatrics, Tokyo Women's Medical College (TWMC), during the last 23 years 2 months period (January 1971–February 1994). The majority of the patients comprised those with muscle disorders (710 out of 1103 patients, 64.4%). The breakdown of the latter by disorder is shown in Table 6. Special attention may be called upon the unusually large proportion of CMD patients among the population of progressive muscular dystrophy (PMD), that is, 117 CMD among 337 PMD patients (34.7%). CMD was the second largest subtype of PMD, only after Duchenne muscular dystrophy (DMD), and the relative ratio between FCMD and DMD was 1.00:1.44 at the TWMC Hospital. This high figure for FCMD in our hospital is clearly skewed from the average, reflecting the nature of our tertiary referral special clinic, but still it will be helpful to understand how often Japanese physicians encounter FCMD patients.

Genetic identity of FCMD established

Despite numerous attempts, over many years, to locate the chromosomal region harboring the gene responsible for causing FCMD, neither positive data, nor even a hint as to the location, were obtained until recently. In 1993, however, a dramatic breakthrough took place when Toda et al. [70] succeeded in mapping the FCMD gene to chromosome 9q31-33 by means of genetic linkage analyses with 6 polymorphic microsatellite markers, involving 21 Japanese families, in 13 of which the parental marriage was consanguineous. A hint as to which location to probe was provided by a FCMD patient from a consanguineous family which was also affected with group A xeroderma pigmentosum (XP), which has been localized to chromosome 9q34.1. As no other siblings were affected with either FCMD or XP, Toda et al. [70] assumed the co-existence of FCMD and group A XP to be attributable to homozygosity by descent in this individual. In this first report from Toda's group, the most probable location of the FCMD gene was said to lie within a 7.7 cM interval between D9S58 and D9S59.

Subsequently, in 1994, Toda et al. [71] further narrowed the locus to a region of −5 cM

Table 5

Patients with neuromuscular disorders seen at the Department of Pediatrics, Tokyo Women's Medical College, during the period from January 1971 through February 1994.

			No.	Total	(%)
I.	Motor neuron diseases			103	(9.3)
	A.	Spinal muscular atrophies			
		a. Werdnig–Hoffmann I, II, III.	66		
		b. Kugelberg–Welander	13		
		c. Fazio–Londe	1		
	B.	Amyotrophic lateral sclerosis	6		
	C.	Spino-cerebellar degeneration	10		
	D.	Hereditary spastic paraplegia	4		
	E.	Cord injury due to birth trauma	2		
	F.	Others	1		
II.	Peripheral neuropathies			45	(4.1)
	A.	Charcot-Marie-Tooth	14		
	B.	Guillain-Barré syndrome	14		
	C.	Mono/poly-neuritis	9		
	D.	Others	8		
III.	Disorders of N–M junction			109	(9.9)
	A.	Myasthenia gravis			
		a. Ocular type	82		
		b. Generalized type	27		
	B.	Others	0		
IV.	Disorders of muscle			710	(64.48)
V.	CNS disorders			136	(12.38)
	A.	Cerebral hypotonia	87		
	B.	Cerebral palsy (hypotonic type)	8		
	C.	Down syndrome	19		
	D.	Prader–Willi syndrome	22		
Total cases with neuromuscular disorders				1103	(1.3)
Grand total of out-patients				82385	

Table 6

Patients with disorders of muscle seen at the Department of Pediatrics, Tokyo Women's Medical College, during the period from January 1971 through February 1994

		No.	Total	(%)
Cases with neuromuscular disorders:			1103	
Cases with disorders of muscle:			710	(64.4)
A.	Progressive muscular dystrophy		337	(47.5)
	a. Duchenne	169		
	b. Becker	15		
	c. Limb-girdle	16		
	d. Facioscapulohumeral	9		
	e. Scapuloperoneal	3		
	f. Autosomal recessive in childhood	6		
	g. Congenital	117		
	h. Symptomatic Duchenne carrier	2		
B.	Myotonias		21	(3.0)
	a. Myotonic dystrophy	16		
	b. Myotonia congenita	5		
C.	Inflammatory disorders		49	(6.9)
	a. Viral myositis	24		
	b. Dermatomyositis	16		
	c. Polymyositis	9		
D.	Congenital myopathies		29	(4.1)
	a. Nemaline	4		
	b. Central core	4		
	c. Minicore	3		
	d. Myotubular	2		
	e. Congenital fiber type disproportion	4		
	f. Others (unclassifiable)	12		
E.	Metabolic myopathies		127	(17.9)
	a. Mitochondrial			
	CCO deficiency	14		
	PDH deficiency	4		
	MELAS (unknown origin)	3		
	Kearns-Sayre syndrome	2		
	Others (with lactic acidosis)	69		
	b. Lipid storage myopathy	16		
	c. Glycogen storage disease	9		
	d. Others			
	OTC deficiency	1		
	Methylmalonic aciduria	1		
	Thyrotoxic myopathy	2		
	Malignant hyperthermia	5		
	Hoffmann syndrome	1		
F.	Periodic paralysis		4	(0.6)
G.	Benign congenital hypotonia (Walton)		24	(3.6)
H.	Floppy infant syndrome, unclassifiable		88	(12.4)
I.	Arthrogryposis multiplex congenita		5	(0.7)
J.	Rigid spine syndrome		2	(0.3)
K.	Others (hyper CKemia)		24	(3.4)

between loci D9S127 and CA246 by homozygosity mapping in patients born to consanguineous parents and by recombination analysis in other families. They also found strong evidence of linkage disequilibrium between the FCMD gene and a polymorphic microsatellite marker, mfd220, and suggested that the FCMD gene could lie within a few hundred kilobases of the mfd220 gene.

More recently, Toda et al. [72] developed 5 new CA repeat markers from YAC contigs containing mfd220, and demonstrated that the FCMD gene could lie within a region of less than 100 kb containing J12. (The distance between the FCMD gene and marker J12 is presumed to be 30 kb).

By using polymorphism analysis with 9 microsatellite CA repeat markers flanking the FCMD locus, Kondo and her colleagues successfully carried out a reliable prenatal diagnosis in 2 families [73].

It can be said that, in view of these developments in molecular genetic information on FCMD in recent years, an aforementioned empirical subdivision of CMD into 2 groups, FCMD and non-FCMD, have now found a very sound basis.

Characteristics of non-Japanese cases with CMD

A detailed review of the literature also indicates the fact that intellectual development has been considered to be normal in the vast majority of western cases, except for 2 cases only which were reported to be retarded, that is, case 3 of Vassella et al. [29] and case 3 of Zellweger et al. [28]. As to the former case, the authors themselves admitted that some doubts exist concerning the diagnosis. This 7 year, 3-month-old girl started to walk at 20 months of age, and at the time of reporting, she could go up and down the staircase unsupported, and stand up from the floor in a "climbing up herself" fashion. Weakness was more prominent in proximal than in distal muscles, and more in hip than in shoulder girdles. IQ was estimated to be between 60 and 70. Atypical findings which are not well consistent with the diagnosis of CMD in this case included well-retained deep tendon reflexes, normal serum CK levels, and only mildly abnormal histology of biopsied muscle. In contrast, case 3 of Zellweger et al. [28] was well studied and described in detail. This 6 year, 6-month-old girl could neither stand nor walk, but moved around while sitting on the buttocks. She had a flat, expressionless face, and could not close her eyes or mouth, as shown in Fig. 5 of the paper. These clinical features, together with muscle histology and other laboratory findings, are all quite consistent with those in typical FCMD patients. IQs (Stanford–Binet) at 4 and 5 years of age in this case were reported to be 53 and 66, respectively, which are also compatible with that of FCMD, although Zellweger et al. commented that mental subnormality was in part due to familial mental retardation and cultural deprivation. Nothing was mentioned as to her ethnic origin; however, she does not look like a Japanese girl, judging from the photo attached in the paper, at least.

Exempting intellectual impairment, clinical signs and symptoms suggestive for central nervous system (CNS) involvement had scarcely been referred to in any western CMD patients reported in the 1960s or before, although seizure episodes or EEG findings had been briefly touched on only occasionally. It is highly probable, thus, that the great majority of CMD patients in western countries in the past had not been complicated with CNS abnormality, confining the main lesion to skeletal muscles. This is a characteristic feature of western patients persistently notable in most contemporary papers, also.

In connection with the above, the following observation might be of some interest. The author is convinced that 2 sibling cases reported by Fowler and Manson at the 2nd International Congress of Muscle Diseases, Perth, in 1971 [74] probably represent a rare sample of typical FCMD among Caucasians. To tell the truth, there are a few odd descriptions in their paper, such as "knee and ankle jerks are very brisk and bilateral ankle cloni are positive", but an overall clinical feature and course, and particularly, widespread pachygyria and micropolygyria of the brain are well compatible with critical characteristics of typical FCMD. The author will refrain from extending the discussion further on the legitimacy of diagnosis in other presumed FCMD cases reported in recent literature, but just one comment that molecular analysis of DNA from preserved brain tissue will provide a definite answer to this argument.

Expansion and classification of CMD families

As FCMD was better delineated over time, it became clear that there are other forms of CMD which do not fit well clinically with FCMD. At first, a major difference as a distinguishing hallmark was recognized in terms of intellectual development. Contrary to FCMD which is always accompanied by mental retardation, the vast majority of European CMD cases presents age-corresponding normal mental development as written previously, and they were called by some as the classical or pure or occidental form of CMD. It has recently become clear that more than 40% of European CMD patients have a laminin $\alpha2$-chain (alpha 2 subunit of laminin-2 or merosin) deficiency, and the disease is now referred to as merosin-negative or merosin-deficient CMD [75–77].

Clinically, merosin-negative CMD shows rather homogeneous features with a marked elevation of serum CK levels, severe neonatal hypotonia and delayed motor milestones, respiratory insufficiency and abnormal brain MRI/CT scans, but normal intellectual development in most cases [78]. Neuroimaging abnormality in the merosin-deficient CMD is characteristically localized to white matter, which diffusely shows an abnormal, increased signal intensity on T_2-weighted MRI, but no abnormal gyral pattern, heterotopia or other migration abnormalities are noticeable [79].

On the other hand, the merosin-positive CMD is considered by Fardeau et al. [79] as a heterogeneous group of CMDs which is only poorly delineated but usually affected clinically to a milder degree in comparison to the merosin-negative CMD patients. Nonaka et al. [80], however, pointed out the possibility that the merosin-positive CMD may constitute a single disease, because of its clinico-pathological uniformity.

The Walker–Warburg syndrome (WWS) is an another extreme of CMDs, with severest brain malformation, eye involvement and a very short life span. There are many common clinico-pathological features between FCMD and WWS, as do the difference as well. A report appeared claiming the genetic identity of both conditions [81], but other reports on many other cases do not support the claim [82].

The nosological relation of WWS with muscle-eye-brain (MEB) syndrome advocated by Santavuori et al. [83] is still controversial, but most investigators momentarily agree to leave the 2 conditions as an independent entity to each other until more definite evidence becomes available [84].

Based upon the information currently available, the author proposes to subclassify CMD into 5 subtypes as shown in Table 7, although there will be rare cases which are elusive.

Table 7

Classification of congenital muscular dystrophies

Subtype	Mental retardation	Muscle dystrophy	PNS abnormality	CNS anomalies			Eye anomalies	Gene locus
				WM	GM	CV		
Pure form	–	+	–	–	–	–	–	?
Merosin deficiency	–	++	+	++	–	–	–	6q2
FCMD	+	++	–	+	++	±	±	9q31
MEB	++	+	–	+	++ (Giant VEP)	++	++	?
WWS	++	+	–	++	++	++	++	?

FCMD, Fukuyama type congenital muscular dystrophy; MEB, muscle-eye-brain syndrome; WWS, Walker–Warburg syndrome; PNS, peripheral nervous system; CNS, central nervous system; WM, white matter; GM, gray matter; CV, cerebeller vermis; VEP, visual evoked potential.

Conclusion

It is amazing to observe a dramatic advance of medical knowledge on a single disease or syndrome like CMD which occurred in the last decade or so. Detailed clinical observations coupled with an application of cell biology/molecular genetics techniques greatly contributed to the establishment of the current realms of CMD [85], although there are undoubtedly so many things still to be done. It is anticipated, however, that the progress in research will be further accelerated and bring out a solution of elucidating the pathogenesis and a substantial measure for curing the disease and preventing its occurrence in the near future.

References

1. Batten FE. Three cases of myopathy, infantile type. Brain 1903; 26: 147–148.
2. Batten FE. The myopathies or muscular dystrophies (critical review). Q J Med 1909/1910; 3: 313–328.
3. Batten FE. Simple atrophic type of myopathy: so-called "myatonia congenita" or "amyotonia congenita". Proc R Soc Med 1911; 4: 100–103.
4. Batten FE. Myopathy, simple atrophic type. Proc R Soc Med (Neurol) 1915; 8: 69–70.
5. Batten FE. Case of amyotonia congenita. Proc R Soc Med (Neurol) 1917; 10: 47.
6. Howard R. A case of congenital defect of the muscular system (dystrophia muscularis congenita) and its association with congenital talipes equinovarus. Proc R Soc Med (Pathol) 1908; 1: 157–166.
7. Greenfield JG, Cornman T, Shy GM. The prognostic value of the muscle biopsy in the "floppy infant". Brain 1958; 81: 461–484.
8. Gubbay SS, Walton JN, Pearce GW. Clinical and pathological study of a case of congenital muscular dystrophy. J Neurol Neurosurg Psychiatry 1966; 29: 500–508.
9. Becker PE. Handbuch der Humangenetik. Band III/1. Stuttgart: Thieme 1954.
10. Zellweger H, Afifi A, McCormick WF, Mergner W. Benign congenital muscular dystrophy; a special form of congenital hypotonia. Clin Pediatr 1967; 6: 655–663.
11. (Leading article). The "floppy" infant. Lancet 1959; i: 294–295.
12. Schlivek K. Report of a case of congenital muscular dystrophy. Arch Pediatr 1910; 27: 34–36.
13. Haushalter P. Sur la myatonie congénitale (maladie d'Oppenheim). Arch Med Enfants 1920; 23: 133–144.

18

14. Turner JWA. The relationship between amyotonia congenita and congenital myopathy. Brain 1940; 63: 163–177.
15. Turner JWA. On amyotonia congenita. Brain 1949; 72: 25–34.
16. Brandt S. Werdnig-Hoffmann's infantile progressive muscular atrophy. Clinical aspects, pathology, heredity and relation to Oppenheim's amyotonia congenita and other morbid conditions with laxity of joints or muscles in infants. Copenhagen: Munksgaard, 1950.
17. Richter RB, Humphreys EM. Unusual myopathy: presentation of two cases with muscle biopsies. AMA Arch Neurol Psychiatry 1955; 73: 574–575.
18. Silvestri T. Contributo allo studio della "myatonia congenita' (Malatteo di Oppenheim). Gazz Osp Clin 1909; 30: 577.
19. Dubois R, Graffar M, Ley R. Forme précoce de myopathie infantile simulant la maladie de Werdnig-Hoffmann. Acta Paediatr Belg 1946; 1: 1–8.
20. Spiller WG. General or localized hypotonia of the muscles in childhood (Myatonia congenita). Univ Pennsylvania Med Bull 1904/1905; 17: 342.
21. Collier J, Holmes G. The pathological examination of two cases of amyotonia congenita with the clinical description of a fresh case. Brain 1909; 32: 269–284.
22. Lereboullet P, Baudouin A. Un cas de myatonia congenitale avec autopsie. Bull Soc Med Hop Paris 1909; 27: 1162.
23. Councilman WT, Dunn CH. Myatonia congenita: a report of a case with autopsy. Am J Dis Child 1911; 2: 340–355.
24. de Lange, C. Studien über angeborene Lähmungen bzw angeborene Hypotonie. II Über die angeborene oder frühinfantile Form der Dystrophia musculorum progressiva (Erb). Acta Paediatr (Uppsala) 1938; 20 (Suppl 33): 1–51.
25. Short JK. Congenital muscular dystrophy. A case report with autopsy findings. Neurology 1963; 13: 526–530.
26. Farber S, Craig JM, eds. Clinical pathological conference. The Children's Medical Center, Boston, MA. (Muscular dystrophy of the congenital type). J Pediatr 1959; 53: 744–750.
27. Banker BQ, Victor M, Adams RD. Arthrogryposis multiplex due to congenital muscular dystrophy. Brain 1957; 80: 319–334.
28. Zellweger H, Afifi A, McCormick WF, Mergner W. Severe congenital muscular dystrophy. Am J Dis Child 1967; 114: 591–602.
29. Vassella F, Mumenthaler M, Rossi E, Moser H, Wiesmann U. Die kongenitale Muskeldystrophie. Dtsch Z Nervenheilk 1967; 190: 349–374.
30. Rotthauwe HW, Kowalewski S. Mumenthaler M. Kongenitale Muskeldystrophie. Z Kinderheilk 1969; 106: 131–162.
31. Fukuyama Y, Kawazura M, Haruna H. A peculiar form of congenital progressive muscular dystrophy. Report of fifteen cases. Paediatr Univ Tokyo 1960; 4: 5–8.
32. Watanabe T. Congenital muscular dystrophy in two siblings (in Japanese). Shonika Shinryo (J Pediatr Pract) (Tokyo) 1961; 24: 1620–1629.
33. Yamagata Y. A case of congenital muscular dystrophy (in Japanese). Shonika Shinryo (J Pediatr Pract) (Tokyo) 1976; 30: 792–795.
34. Ueda K, Ito T, Matsumoto K, et al. Hypotonic infant. Nihon Rinsho (Jpn J Clin Med) (Osaka) 1968; 26: 3231–3256.
35. Silberberg M. Über die pathologische Anatomie der Myatonia congenita und die Muskeldystrophie im allgemeinen. Arch Pathol Anat Physiol 1923; 242: 42–57.
36. Ullrich O. Kongenitale, atonisch- sklerotische Muskeldystrophie. Monatsschr Kinderheilk 1930; 47: 502–510.
37. Menges O. Ein Beitrag zur Pathologie der Myatonia congenita. Dtsch Z Nervenheilk 1931; 121: 240–254.
38. Middleton DS. Studies on prenatal lesions of striated muscle as a cause of congenital deformity. I. Congenital tibial kyphosis. II. Congenital high shoulder. III. Myodystrophia foetalis deformans. Edinburgh Med J 1934; 41: 401–442.
39. Turner JWA, Lee F. Congenital myopathy, a fifty-year follow-up. Brain 1962; 85: 733–740.
40. Gött H, Josten EA. Beitrag zur kongeni atonisch-sklerotischen Muskeldystrophie (Typ Ullrich). Z Kinderheilk 1954; 75: 105–118.

41. Levesque J, Lepage F, Boeswillwald M, Grüner J. Deux cas de dystrophie musculaire familiale congénitale simulant une maladie de Werdnig–Hoffmann–Oppenheim. Arch Fr Pédiatr 1956; 13: 202–207.

42. Joseph R. Pellerin D, Job JC. L'arthrogrypose multiple congénitale. Sem Hop Paris 1958; 34: 525–536.

43. Lelong M, Canlorbe P, Le Tan-Vinh, Cobbin JG, Vassal J. Myopathie chez une fille de 9 ans révélée à la naissance par une hypotonie musculaire généralisée. Arch Fr Pédiatr 1962; 19: 581–596.

44. O'Brien MD. An infantile muscular dystrophy: report of a case with autopsy findings. Guy's Hosp Rep 1962; 111: 98–106.

45. Lewis AJ, Besant DF. Muscular dystrophy in infancy. Report of 2 cases in siblings with diaphragmatic weakness. J Pediatr 1962; 60: 376–384.

46. Pearson CM, Fowler WG Jr. Hereditary non-progressive muscular dystrophy inducing arthrogryposis syndrome. Brain 1963; 86: 75–88.

47. Lamy M, Jammet MI, Ajjan N. Arthrogrypose ou syndrome arthrogryposique? A propos de dix observations. Ann Pediat (Paris) 1965; 12: 591–602.

48. Wharton BA. An unusual variety of muscular dystrophy. Lancet 1965; i: 248–249.

49. Fontaine J-L, Graveleau D, Houllemare L, Laplane R. Les myopathies congénitales. A propos de 2 observations. Ann Pédiatr (Paris) 1965; 12: 1563–1568.

50. Fenichel GM, Bazelon M. Myopathies in search of a name; benign congenital forms. Dev Med Child Neurol 1966; 8: 532–548.

51. Engel WK. Muscle biopsies in neuromuscular diseases. Pediatr Clin North Am 1967; 14: 963.

52. Walton JN, Nattrass FJ. On the classification, natural history and treatment of the myopathies. Brain 1954; 77: 169–231.

53. Walton JN. Amyotonia congenita: a follow-up study. Lancet 1956; i: 1023–1027.

54. Walton JN, Geschwind N, Simpson JA. Benign congenital myopathy with myasthenic features. J Neurol Neurosurg Psychiatry 1956; 19: 224–231.

55. Walton JN. "The limp child". J Neurol Neurosurg Psychiatry 1957; 29: 144–154.

56. Walton JN. The amyotonia congenita syndrome. Proc R Soc Med 1957; 50: 301–308.

57. Fukuyama Y, Shima N, Kawazura M, Sugita H. On the value of the determination of serum enzyme activities in the differential diagnosis of various neuromuscular diseases in children. Its correlation with clinical, electromyographic, histologic and metabolic findings. No To Shinkei (Brain Nerve) (Tokyo) 1960; 12: 783–795.

58. Fukuyama Y. Progressive muscular dystrophy and related disorders. Naika (Intern Med) (Tokyo) 1960; 5: 1082–1089.

59. Fukuyama Y. Pediatric muscle diseases. Rinsho Shinkeigaku (Clin Neurol) (Tokyo) 1961; 1: 409–416.

60. The neurological adaptation of the international classification of diseases, draft for 10th rev. Geneva: World Health Organization, 1991.

61. Walton J. Revised classification of neuromuscular diseases. Neuro-Muscular Diseases News Bull 1991; March: 9–10.

62. Adams RD. Diseases of muscle: a study in pathology, 3rd edn. Hagerstown: Harper and Row, 1975: 245.

63. Lazaro RP, Fenichel GM, Kilroy AW. Congenital muscular dystrophy: case reports and reappraisal. Muscle Nerve 1979; 2: 349–355.

64. Otto HF, Lücking T. Congenitale Muskeldystrophie. Licht- und elekronenmikroskopische Befunde. Virchows Arch Abt A Pathol Anat 1971; 352: 324–339.

65. Lücking T, Otto HF. Kongenitale Muskeldystrophie. Z Kinderheilk 1971; 110: 59–73.

66. Ketelsen UP, Freund-Mölbert E, Beckmann R. Klinische und ultrastrukturelle Befunde bei kongenitaler Muskeldystrophie. Msch Kinderheilk 1971; 119: 586–592.

67. Kamoshita S, Konishi Y, Segawa M, Fukuyama Y. Congenital muscular dystrophy as a disease of the central nervous system. Arch Neurol 1975; 33: 513–516.

68. Nonaka I, Chou SM. Congenital muscular dystrophy. In: Vinken PJ, Bruyn GW, eds. Handbook of clinical neurology, Vol 41. Amsterdam: North Holland, 1979: 27–50.

69. Fukuyama Y, Osawa M, Suzuki H. Congenital progressive muscular dystrophy of the Fukuyama type. Clinical, genetic and pathological considerations. Brain Dev (Tokyo) 1981; 3: 1–29.

70. Toda T, Segawa M, Nomura Y, et al. Localization of a gene for Fukuyama type congenital muscular dystrophy to chromosome 9q31-33. Nat Genet 1993; 5: 283–286.

71. Toda T, Ikegawa S, Okui K, et al. Refined mapping of a gene responsible for Fukuyama-type congenital muscular dystrophy: evidence for strong linkage disequilibrium. Am J Hum Genet 1994; 55: 946–955.

20

72. Toda T, Miyake M, Mizuno K, Nakagome Y, Nakahori Y. Linkage disequilibrium of a gene for Fukuyama-type congenital muscular dystrophy (abstract). Jpn J Hum Genet (Tokyo) 1996; 41: 41.
73. Kondo E, Saito K, Toda T, Osawa M, Fukuyama Y. Prenatal diagnosis in Fukuyama type congenital muscular dystrophy by polymorphism analysis. Am J Med. Genet 1996; 66: 169–174.
74. Fowler M, Manson JI. Congenital muscular dystrophy with malformation of the central nervous system. In: Kakulas BA, ed. Clinical studies in myology. Amsterdam: Excerpta Medica, 1973: 192–197.
75. Tomé FMS, Evangelista T, Leclerc A, et al. Congenital muscular dystrophy with merosin deficiency. C R Acad Sci Paris (III) 1994; 317: 351–357.
76. Hillaire D, Leclerc A, Fauré S, et al. Localization of merosin-negative congenital muscular dystrophy to chromosome 6q2 by homozygosity mapping. Hum Mol Genet 1994; 3: 1657–1661.
77. Dubowitz V, Fardeau M. Workshop report; proceedings of the 27th ENMC sponsored workshop on congenital muscular dystrophy. Neuromusc Disord 1995; 5. 253–258.
78. Philpot J, Sewry C, Pennock J, Dubowitz V. Clinical phenotype in congenital muscular dystrophy: correlation with expression of merosin in skeletal muscle. Neuromusc Disord 1995; 5: 301–305.
79. Fardeau M, Tomé FMS, Helbling-Leclerc A, et al. Dystrophie musculaire congénitale avec déficience en mérosin: analyse clinique, histopathologique, immunocytochimique et génétique. Rev Neurol 1996; 252: 11–19.
80. Nonaka I, Kobayashi O, Osari S. Clinico-genetic analysis on non-Fukuyama (classical) form of congenital muscular dystrophy (abstract). Jpn J Hum Genet (Tokyo) 1996; 41: 26.
81. Toda T, Yoshioka M, Nakahori Y, Kanazawa I, Nakamura Y, Nakagome Y. Genetic identity of Fukuyama type congenital muscular dystrophy and Walker–Warburg syndrome. Ann Neurol 1995; 37: 99–101.
82. Ranta S, Pihko H, Santavuori P, Takvanainen E, de la Chapelle A. Muscle-eye-brain disease and Fukuyama type congenital muscular dystrophy are not allelic. Neuromusc Disord 1995; 5: 221–225.
83. Santavuori P, Leisti J, Kruus S. Muscle, eye and brain disease: a new syndrome. Neuropaediatrie 1977; 8(Suppl): 553–558.
84. Dobyns WB, Truwit CL. Lissencephaly and other malformations of cortical development: 1995 update. Neuropediatrics 1995; 26: 132–147.
85. Arahata K, Ishii H, Hayashi YK. Congenital muscular dystrophies. Curr Opin Neurol 1995; 8: 385–390.

Fukuyama, M. Osawa and K. Saito (Eds.), *Congenital Muscular Dystrophies*
1997 Elsevier Science B.V. All rights reserved

CHAPTER 2

Exciting new developments in congenital muscular dystrophy

VICTOR DUBOWITZ

*Department of Paediatrics and Neonatal Medicine, Royal Postgraduate Medical School,
Hammersmith Hospital, London W12 ONN, UK*

I am extremely honoured and privileged and also very pleased to have this unique opportunity of giving the introductory lecture in this special symposium on Congenital Muscular Dystrophy and also take the opportunity of honouring Professor Fukuyama and wishing him well for his future career on the occasion of his retirement. By way of introduction I would first like to give a historical overview on the subject, and although time is somewhat limited, I feel one needs to go back to the "dark ages", when there was still no congenital muscular dystrophy. In fact we do not have to go back all that far; in the 1960s many people were not recognising the existence of congenital muscular dystrophy or in fact actively denying that it existed at all and the main publications in the world literature were mainly still isolated single case reports.

I have drawn up a list of the faithful to the subject (Table 1) who in the 1960s started writing about congenital muscular dystrophy, trying to delineate its clinical phenotype and also drawing attention to its marked variability in presentation and clinical features and also variability in prognosis [1–7]. Zellweger tried to subdivide it into a more severe and less severe form, although not clearly delineating the boundary between them. You will note that Fukuyama headed that list and in fact it was in 1960 that he wrote his seminal paper on "An unusual type of congenital muscular dystrophy in 15 patients" and if you have an opportunity of looking at the very nice updated bibliography of World Publications on Congenital Muscular Dystrophy that he has prepared for us as a handout at this meeting, you will note not only the inclusion of this 1960 paper under the alphabetical section "FU", but those of you who are fluent in Japanese will also realise that there have been a steady flow of papers emanating from his group on the subject.

Table 1

CMD: the faithful

Fukuyama
Zellweger
Vassella
Rotthauwe
Dubowitz
Donner

Disciples

Fukuyama has been well known in European circles since the 1960s and has participated on many occasions in the meetings of our collective European Child Neurology Societies, which were initially established by Ronnie MacKeith in the 1960s. I wonder why no-one had thought of making him an Honorary European citizen in view of his extensive contributions.

I have pulled out one picture of historical interest which was taken at a meeting of our European Neurological Society hosted in Finland in 1987 (Fig. 1) and which features Fukuyama with Santavuori, our hostess at that meeting, who has of course also made a major contribution to the CMD field herself, with her muscle-eye-brain disease.

The next illustration (Fig. 1b) is also of some historical interest. As you will note it is an almost identical picture to the first one, except for the occupant of Fukuyama's chair. It illustrates the prowess of Fukuyama as a photographer.

With the clear-cut definition of the Fukuyama type of muscular dystrophy, with its associated brain malformation and mental retardation, efforts were also made to define more clearly the non-Fukuyama congenital muscular dystrophy, the classical or "pure" form, without brain malformation or mental retardation. The terminology got somewhat into a twist and additional terms were introduced for this group such as "occidental". As this implies a geographical distribution, in contrast to "oriental", it raised an additional problem of trying to define exactly what occidental is and whether it refers to all zones west of Samarkand, or possibly west of Japan and what do we do about the case of non-Fukuyama dystrophy that arises in the Orient itself?

I consulted the Oxford English dictionary but was still unable to resolve this semantic conundrum. I must confess that I personally am still quite content with the concept of "Fukuyama muscular dystrophy" and "non-Fukuyama muscular dystrophy" and at least it gives us a simple and clear-cut definition, and certainly for the purposes of this meeting and particularly this special occasion, I feel it quite appropriate. As a latent, and somewhat frustrated, botanist, I am in fact also quite happy with this approach. I have had a longstanding interest in flowers but have always had some difficulty recognising individual species, and managed to resolve this quite adequately some years ago by dividing all flowers into daffodils and non-daffodils; since then I have never on any single occasion got things wrong!

A little more than a year ago I convened our first international workshop on congenital muscular dystrophy [8], supported by the European Neuromuscular Centre (ENMC) (a brainchild of the original European Alliance of Muscular Dystrophy Associations, genetically engineered by Alan Emery), which has been promoting the collaborative study of different neuromuscular disorders and encouraging people to convene workshop meetings in order to achieve the two main goals of trying to define specific clinical phenotypes and in parallel with this to set up collaborative studies for gene location and identification.

Although the main participants at that meeting (which due to financial constraints had to be limited to around 20) were European, we did in fact also have some of the main international key figures in the field such as Fukuyama himself, Santavuori (Finland) who had made a major contribution in defining the muscle-eye-brain disease and also Dobyns (USA) who had contributed extensively on another syndrome, the Walker–Warburg syndrome. The main purpose of this first workshop was to try and define the main clinical phenotypes and to get some consensus on how many different syndromes there were and to sort out the nomenclature.

As one might have expected from any group of primates from the animal kingdom, arguments and battles raged amongst the individual protagonists of the individual syndromes

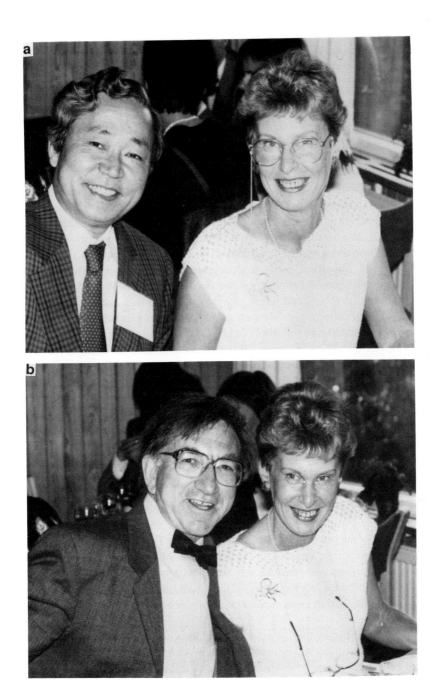

Fig. 1. (a) Dr Y. Fukuyama (left) and Dr P. Santavuori (right). (b) Dr V. Dubowitz (left) and Dr P. Santavuori (right). Both photos were taken on the occasion of the meeting of European Federation of Child Neurology Societies, Hyvinkää, Finland, 1987.

Table 2

Clinical syndromes in relation to congenital muscular dystrophy

1.	"Pure" congenital muscular dystrophy
	With normal intellect and no structural changes in the brain
	With or without imaging changes on CT or MRI
2.	Fukuyama congenital muscular dystrophy
	CMD with associated brain malformation and intellectual retardation
3.	Muscle-eye-brain disease (Santavuori)
	CMD with associated brain malformation, major ocular abnormalities and mental retardation
4.	Walker–Warburg syndrome
	CMD with associated brain malformations and less significant ocular changes

to demarcate the boundaries of their own syndromes, and to resist being absorbed into someone else's syndrome, a behaviour somewhat reminiscent of the canine world demarcating their individual territory. We ended up with a consensus of defining four basic syndromes (Table 2): the pure CMD, having no structural brain abnormality, and normal intellect; the other three associated with structural brain abnormalities plus mental retardation. We considered this important, partly from a practical clinical point of view, and also as a basis for looking for gene location in relation to what might well be four totally separate conditions, but on the other hand might prove to be allelic with each other either individually or perhaps even collectively. We were still at a stage of blissful ignorance in relation to the molecular genetic basis of the whole field.

The first major breakthrough came a few months later with the discovery of the gene locus for the Fukuyama-type muscular dystrophy on chromosome 9q by a remarkable bit of serendipity [9]. In a prospective study of some 20 potentially informative Japanese families, with either consanguinity or multiplex cases, there was one single child with a combination of Fukuyama-type congenital muscular dystrophy as well as a relatively rare skin disorder, xeroderma pigmentosum. As the family was also consanguineous and no other individuals were affected with either disorder, the astute clinicians argued that this might represent an instance of homozygosity by descent, and if one single grandparent was heterozygous for the mutant genes for both Fukuyama dystrophy and for xeroderma pigmentosum, a grandchild as a result of consanguinity between his heterozygote parents could become homozygous for both mutant genes and thus express both diseases. This would only be likely if the genes were closely associated with each other (Fig. 2). They accordingly went straight for the locus of xeroderma pigmentosum and discovered the Fukuyama gene to be there as well.

This gave an immediate impetus for the European collaborative study. The collaboration which Professor Fardeau and I had already set up with our respective groups, together with Dr Topaloglu, who had a large number of potentially informative, consanguineous and/or multiplex families in Turkey, was expanded at our workshop to also include other centres of interest.

Through the facilities of the Genethon laboratories in Paris we now had the opportunity in our potentially informative European families to at least establish whether the non-Fukuyama congenital muscular dystrophy was non-linked to chromosome 9q and therefore represented a separate entity or not. Another major development was the parallel interest from a biochemical and immunocytochemical point of view in proteins of potential interest in relation to congenital muscular dystrophy. This was of course inspired by the remarkable advances in earlier years in relation to Duchenne dystrophy and the recognition of the pro-

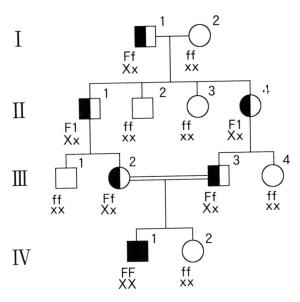

Fig. 2. Stylized illustration of homozygosity by descent showing co-segregation of the genes for Fukuyama muscular dystrophy and xeroderma pigmentosum in one grandparent (I,1) and in heterozygotes in the next two generations (II,1 and II,4; III,2 and III,3) and finally resulting after a consanguineous marriage between III,2 and III,3 in an individual (IV,1) homozygous for both genes. F, gene for Fukuyama congenital muscular dystrophy; x, gene for xeroderma pigmentosum; half-filled squares and circles, heterozygous for the two closely linked mutant genes (Ff, Xx); filled squares, homozygous for the two mutant genes (FF, XX); ρ=l, consanguineous mating. (Reprinted from Dubowitz V, Muscle disorders in childhood, 2nd edn., with the permission of the publishers).

tein, dystrophin, whose gene is abnormal in Duchenne and Becker dystrophy and also the subsequent definition of a series of transmembrane, dystrophin-associated glycoproteins (DAGs), which link dystrophin on the inner side of the sarcolemma membrane to the extracellular matrix protein, laminin, outside the membrane.

In a study of the laminins by Arahata's group in Japan, some abnormality was found in relation to Fukuyama congenital muscular dystrophy, with a deficiency of one of the forms of laminin, laminin-M (merosin), in the muscle membrane [10]. However, this was not consistently present in all cases and did not consistently affect all muscle fibres and was thought to be a secondary phenomenon rather than representing the primary gene locus. This was subsequently borne out by the fact that the gene for merosin does not lie on chromosome 9.

Parallel studies in Europe led to the discovery by Tomé and his associates of the deficiency of merosin in a large proportion (approximately half) of cases of classical congenital muscular dystrophy [11]. This now provided a biochemical basis for subdividing the families with congenital muscular dystrophy into merosin-negative (deficient) or merosin-positive cases. The next part of the jigsaw to be resolved was to show that the merosin-negative cases did not link to the Fukuyama muscular dystrophy locus on chromosome 9, but in fact did show linkage to the locus for the human merosin gene on chromosome 6q, suggesting that the merosin gene was a potential candidate for the classical congenital muscular dystrophy [12].

Further studies of the merosin-positive families showed that this form of CMD was not linked to either chromosome 9 or chromosome 6, thus confirming the genetic heterogeneity of the classical congenital muscular dystrophy, with the implication that there must be at least one more locus for this form of congenital muscular dystrophy [12].

Work has also been going on over the past 10 years or so in relation to imaging changes in the white matter of the brain in the classical congenital muscular dystrophy, without intellectual retardation, and several contributions on this were made at our first ENMC workshop meeting [8]. One of the interesting aspects raised by Dobyns at that meeting was the possibility of studying siblings to see if there was concordance in relation to the central nervous system changes. It was quite remarkable that, in spite of the large number of individual cases studied, how very few siblings had been studied. The few cases mentioned at the meeting suggested that there might be concordance. We accordingly undertook a prospective study of four sibling pairs under our care and were able to establish that there was complete concordance and almost identical imaging changes in the two families where there were marked changes in the white matter and also in the two families where the siblings both had normal brain scans [13]. Similar observations were made in three pairs of siblings by Dr Topaloglu [13].

The question now arose as to whether one could possibly define a separate clinical phenotype for the merosin-negative and the merosin-positive cases. We have analysed in detail the clinical phenotype in relation to a series of 24 cases of congenital muscular dystrophy fulfilling the criteria for clinical acceptance of the diagnosis of our international consortium [14]. Of these, 13 turned out to be merosin-positive and 11 merosin-negative. When we looked at the pathology, there did not seem to be any recognisable difference in the type or extent of pathological change in the muscle that would help us to distinguish one form from the other.

At a clinical level, the early onset and presenting features such as hypotonia or associated contractures seemed very similar in the two groups. In the merosin-positive group (Table 3) 11 of the 13 cases were able to walk without support and of the remaining two, one was walking with callipers (case 10), the other only able to sit unsupported (case 6). In contrast, in the merosin-negative group (Table 3), no single case had achieved independent standing or walking. Nine of the 11 were able to stand with support and only two to walk with support. This gave the distinct impression that the merosin-negative group were more severe overall in their muscle weakness and motor dysfunction than the merosin-positive group. It was also striking that the CK levels in the merosin-negative group seemed consistently much higher; 9 of the 11 cases had levels above 2000 IU/l and a further case was above 1000 IU/l whereas in the merosin-positive group there was only one patient above 1000 IU/l (case 6, the only child who was also unable to stand unsupported).

Another striking difference emerged in relation to the brain imaging. Of the cases in this particular series that had their merosin status established and had also had magnetic resonance imaging of the brain, all eight cases who were merosin-positive had normal brain scans, whereas all seven merosin-negative had moderate or severe changes in the white matter of the brain (Fig. 3a,b).

We recently convened the second meeting of our consortium on congenital muscular dystrophy [15] and many of these advances, which were still in the pipeline, were presented at that meeting. Work was also in progress in order to try and establish whether muscle–eye–brain disease and Walker–Warburg syndrome were allelic with the Fukuyama congenital muscular dystrophy or not, and I would anticipate that by the end of this Fu-

Table 3

Clinical details and brain magnetic resonance imaging in merosin-deficient and merosin-positive congenital muscular dystrophy patients

Case (age last seen)	Merosin	Age of onset (months)	Sit (months)	Stand	Walk	Maximum motor ability	Creatine kinase (normal <190 IU l^{-1})	MRI (white matter)
1 (7 years, 9 months)	Positive	0–3	10	16 months	18 months	Walk	215	Normal
2 (14 years, 3 months)	Positive	3–6	8	3 years	4 years	Walk	245	Normal
3 (12 years, 4 months)	Positive	3–6	8	2 years	2 years	Walk	455	Normal
4 (9 years, 8 months)	Positive	3–6	6	14 months	2 years	Walk	470	Normal
5 (7 years, 5 months)	Positive	3–6	8	12 months	15 months	Walk	455	Normal
6 (1 years, 6 months)	Positive	0–3	7	Not able	Not able	Sit	2478	Not done
7 (18 years, 9 months)	Positive	Birth	8	12 months	15 months	Walk	800	Not done
8 (10 years)	Positive	3–6	4	3 years	3.5 years	Walk	102	Not done
9 (14 years, 3 months)	Positive	Birth	8	12 months	14 months	Walk	460	Normal
10 (4 years, 10 months)	Positive	3–6	7	18 months	Not able	Walk with support	510	Normal
11 (14 years, 5 months)	Positive	Birth	10	16 months	18 months	Walk	695	Not done
12 (7 years)	Positive	Birth	9	17 months	2 years	Walk	Not done	Not done
13 (12 years)	Positive	Birth	8	12 months	4.5 years	Walk	325	Normal
14 (7 years, 3 months)	Deficient	Birth	8	Not able	Not able	Stand with support	4050	Abnormal
15 (5 years)	Deficient	3–6	16	Not able	Not able	Stand with support	1745	Abnormal
16 (5 years, 3 months)	Deficient	0–3	15	Not able	Not able	Stand with support	2309	Abnormal
17 (4 years, 6 months)	Deficient	Birth	10	Not able	Not able	Stand with support	3139	Not done
18 (10 years)	Deficient	3–6	36	Not able	Not able	Stand with support	2675	Not done
19 (died) (7 years)	Deficient	Birth	18	Not able	Not able	Stand with support	10250	Not done
20 (6 years, 3 months)	Abnormal	Birth	27	Not able	Not able	Walk with support	15260	Abnormal
21 (died) (12 years)	Deficient	Birth	12	Not able	Not able	Stand with support	574	Not done
22 (10 years, 9 months)	Deficient	3–6	30	Not able	Not able	Stand with support	3420	Abnormal
23 (9 years)	Deficient	Birth	8	Not able	Not able	Stand with support	2562	Abnormal
24 (9 years)	Deficient	Birth	18	Not able	Not able	Walk with support	2760	Abnormal

Reproduced from Ref. [14] with the permission of the authors and Pergamon Press.

28

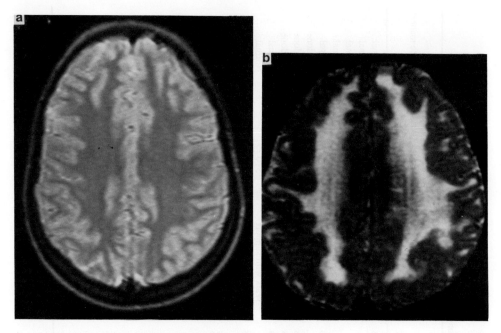

Fig. 3. Magnetic resonance imaging of the brain at the level of the centrum semiovale in (a) a child with a merosin-positive muscle showing a normal pattern on the T_2 weighted image, and (b) a merosin-negative case showing marked changes in the white matter.

kuyama festschrift meeting, we will probably have some of the answers to that question as well.

I think we are passing through a historic moment in relation to congenital muscular dystrophy with the rapid resolution not only of the Fukuyama type and the classical type from a molecular genetic point of view, but also of the other major syndromes. With the very active interest now in trying to identify other proteins linked to the dystrophin/glycoprotein/laminin complex in relation to merosin-positive cases, the scene seems well set for major new exciting developments within the months and years ahead and hopefully a complete understanding of this intriguing disorder.

A parallel exciting development has recently occurred in relation to the dy/dy mouse, a popular (autosomal recessive) model for muscular dystrophy, extensively studied in the 1960s and early 1970s, which fell by the wayside following the discovery of some dysmyelination changes in the ventral roots, and the suggestion that this was no longer a dystrophy but a neuropathy [16,17]. We now know better, and it is of course still a dystrophy, with an associated neuropathy. The recent observations of Arahata and his group [18] and also Campbell and his group [19] that there is a deficiency of merosin in the dy mouse fully explains the disorder, since merosin is expressed not only in the membrane of skeletal muscle but also in Schwann cells and myelin. The dy/dy mouse has thus been catapulted back into prominence and is a superbly good animal model of congenital muscular dystrophy because, unlike the mdx mouse in relation to Duchenne dystrophy, which has a normal clinical phenotype, the dy mouse is severely paralysed and has a comparable clinical phenotype as well as a molecular and biochemical one. Moreover, the gene for the dy mouse has previously been located on chromosome 10, which is also the locus for the merosin gene. As mouse chromosome 10 is homologous with human chromosome 6 and the locus for merosin has already been located on human chromosome 6, the circle has now been completed, with the linkage established of a series of merosin-negative CMD families to chromosome 6q [12]. This makes the merosin gene a likely candidate for this form of CMD and studies are now underway to try and identify mutations in the laminin-M (merosin) gene.

It is perhaps particularly satisfying for Fukuyama to see an almost complete history of congenital muscular dystrophy unfolding during his academic lifetime, with his personal involvement at the beginning with the recognition of one key form of the disease and now being able to witness, at the time of his "official" retirement, the almost total resolution of the problem. I cannot imagine him leaving the ranks completely, and I am sure that he will continue to maintain his active interest and to provide his active inspiration in relation to this important disease in the years to come.

References

1. Fukuyama Y, Kawazura M, Haruna H. A peculiar form of congenital progressive muscular dystrophy. Report of fifteen cases. Pediatria Universitatis Tokyo (Tokyo) 1960; 4: 5–8.
2. Zellweger H, Afifi A, McCormick WF, Mergner W. Benign congenital muscular dystrophy: a special form of congenital hypotonia. Clin Pediatr (Philadelphia) 1967; 6: 655–663.
3. Zellweger H, Afifi A, McCormick WF, Mergner W. Severe congenital muscular dystrophy. Am J Dis Child 1967; 114: 591–602.
4. Vassella F, Mumenthaler M, Rossi E, Moser H, Wiesmann U. Die kongenitale Muskeldystrophie. Dtsch Z Nervenheilk 1967; 190: 349–374.
5. Rotthauwe HW, Kowalewski S, Mumenthaler M. Kongenitale Muskeldystrophie. Z. Kinderheilk 1969; 106: 131–162.
6. Dubowitz V. The floppy infant. Clinics in developmental medicine, 31. London: Spastics International/Heinemann, 1969.
7. Donner M, Rapola J, Somer H. Congenital muscular dystrophy: a clinico-pathological and follow-up study of 15 patients. Neuropaediatrie 1975; 6: 239–258.
8. Dubowitz V. Workshop report: 22nd ENMC sponsored workshop on congenital muscular dystrophy, Baarn, The Netherlands, 1993. Neuromusc Disord 1994; 4: 75–81.
9. Toda T, Segawa M, Nomura Y, et al. Localisation of a gene for Fukuyama type congenital muscular dystrophy to chromosome 9q31-33. Nat Genet 1993; 5: 283–286.
10. Hayashi YK, Engvall E, Arikawa-Hirasawa E, et al. Abnormal localisation of laminin subunits in muscular dystrophies. J Neurol Sci 1993; 119: 53–64.
11. Tomé FMS, Evangelista T, Leclerc A, et al. Congenital muscular dystrophy with merosin deficiency. C R Acad Sci Paris, Sciences de la vie/Life Sciences 1994; 317: 351–357.
12. Hillaire D, Leclerc A, Fauré S, et al. Localisation of merosin-negative congenital muscular dystrophy to chromosome 6q2 by homozygosity mapping. Hum Mol Genet 1994; 3: 1657–1661.
13. Philpot J, Topaloglu H, Pennock J, Dubowitz V. Familial concordance of brain magnetic resonance imaging changes in congenital muscular dystrophy. Neuromusc Disord 1994; 4: 301–305.
14. Philpot J, Sewry C, Pennock J, Dubowitz V. Clinical phenotype in congenital muscular dystrophy: correlation with expression of merosin in skeletal muscle. Neuromusc Disord 1995, 5: 301–305.
15. Dubowitz V, Fardeau M. Proceedings of the 27th ENMC sponsored workshop on congenital muscular dystrophy, The Netherlands, 1994. Neuromusc Disord 1995; 5: 253–258.
16. Bradley WG, Jenkison, M. Abnormalities of peripheral nerves in murine muscular dystrophy. J Neurol Sci 1973; 18: 1276–1280.
17. Madrid RE, Jaros E, Cullen MJ, et al. Genetically determined defect of Schwann basement membrane in dystrophic mouse. Nature 1975; 257: 319–321.

18. Arahata K, Hayashi YK, Koga R, et al. Laminin in animal models for muscular dystrophy: defect of laminin M in skeletal and cardiac muscles and peripheral nerve of the homozygous dystrophic dy/dy mice. Proc Jpn Acad (Tokyo) 1993; 69 Ser B: 259–264.

19. Sunada Y, Bernier SM, Kozak CA, Yamada Y, Campbell KP. Deficiency of merosin in dystrophic dy mice and genetic linkage of laminin M chain gene to dy locus. J Biol Chem 1994; 269: 13729–13732.

Y. Fukuyama, M. Osawa and K. Saito (Eds.), *Congenital Muscular Dystrophies*

31

CHAPTER 3

Fukuyama type congenital progressive muscular dystrophy

MAKIKO OSAWA, SAWAKO SUMIDA, NORIKO SUZUKI, YUMI ARAI,
HARUMI IKENAKA, HIROKO MURASUGI, KEIKO SHISHIKURA,
HARUKO SUZUKI, KAYOKO SAITO and YUKIO FUKUYAMA

Department of Pediatrics, Tokyo Women's Medical College, Shinjuku-ku, Tokyo, Japan

Introduction

Fukuyama type congenital muscular dystrophy (FCMD) [1–4], the second most common progressive muscular dystrophy (PMD) in Japan, is rarely described outside of Japan [5]. It is an autosomal recessive disorder [6,7] characterized by congenital progressive muscular dystrophy (CMD) with facial muscle involvement and central nervous system (CNS) dysgenesis. Two other disorders, Walker–Warburg syndrome (WWS) [8] and Santavuori disease (muscle-eye-brain disease; MEB) [9], also present with a combination of brain malformation and CMD. Several avenues of research have aimed at elucidating the relationships among these 3 disorders.

The identification of CNS involvement even in so-called "pure" CMD with normal mentality, has led many researchers to conclude that the combination of CMD and CNS involvement is not an uncommon phenomenon [10–13]. Among reported cases with this combination, there are a few, such as case 3 of Egger et al. [11], the case described by Koga et al. [12], and case 8 of Trevisan et al. [13], who were neither mentally retarded nor showed any clinical symptoms and signs suggesting cortical dysplasia, although cerebral or cerebellar dysgenesis, specifically focal micropolygyria or pachygyria, was identified at autopsy. The relationship between these cases and FCMD should also be resolved in the future.

Herein, we present a review of the clinical features of FCMD with numerous illustrations. Our aim is to give the reader an understanding of the actual clinical course of FCMD and thereby to provide a more vivid image of FCMD.

The concept of FCMD and the global impression of its clinical course

Though all agree that delayed psychomotor development due to CMD with facial muscle involvement and cerebral dysgenesis since infancy are the salient features of FCMD, our long-term observations of motor abilities revealed that the clinical course can follow 3 general patterns. The chronological courses of motor function changes in these 3 types of CMD are shown, along with the courses typical of Duchenne type muscular dystrophy (DMD) and normal motor development, in Fig. 1.

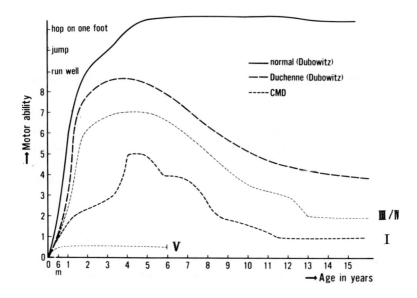

Fig. 1. Schematic drawing of chronological changes of the motor function levels in FCMD patients as compared with those in normal subjects and Duchenne PMD patients (Dubowitz). The abscissa indicates motor function level, as follows: Level 1, head control; 2, maintain sitting posture; 3, able to turn while sitting; 4, sliding on the buttocks while sitting by extending and flexing the knees with hip rotation; 5, maintain standing posture with support, crawl; 6, maintain standing posture; 7, ambulant; 8, walk up stairs. The 3 lower dotted lines indicate the 3 courses into which FCMD can be broadly divided. As shown by the 3 courses of motor function, benign cases can learn to walk without support (CMD III/IV), average cases generally do not ever acquire the ability to walk but may crawl or slide on the buttocks while sitting (CMD I), and severe cases are invariably bedridden for the duration of their lives.

Peak motor function is observed between the ages of 2 and 8 years [2,3]. The functional levels, initially devised by Ueda [2,3], a standard means of describing motor function in FCMD, were attained significantly earlier in CMD III/IV of Fukuyama et al. [3,4], than in CMD I of Fukuyama et al. [3,4] (Table 1). We have never experienced a case in which motor function improved after age 6 years. Generally, the peak motor function is achieved by age 6 years and maintained until 6–8 years of age in CMD I, while the peak is reached by age 4 years and maintained until 4–6 years in CMD III/IV (Table 2).

Several cases never achieve the capacity to hold their heads completely upright despite being able to maintain a sitting position with limited support provided by a special chair (severe FCMD, compatible with CMD V as described by Fukuyama et al. [3]). The majority of patients attain the peak function of turning while sitting or sliding on the buttocks, extending and flexing the knees with hip rotation while sitting (previously termed "shuffling") or crawling (typical FCMD, termed CMD I by Fukuyama et al. [3]), and a minority actually become ambulant (benign FCMD, CMD III/IV of Fukuyama et al. [3,4]). It is difficult, however, to divide these cases into definite categories because some cases take a course which is intermediate between 2 patterns. Cases belonging to the second subgroup (CMD I, typical FCMD) show pseudohypertrophy of the cheeks, forearms and calves, at some stage in their clinical course, are moderately to severely mentally retarded, and have a very limited vocabulary, rarely more than 20 words. Most cases with the first clinical pattern (CMD V, severe FCMD) are profoundly retarded, never learn any meaningful words, some can not

Table 1

Average age at attainment of each motor function level

Motor function level	Subtype			
	Typical FCMD (CMD I)		Benign FCMD(III/IV)	
	Number of cases	Average age at attainment (months ± SD)	Number of cases	Average age at attainment (months ± SD)
1[a]	70	6.56 ± 4.38	11	4.00 ± 1.67
2[a]	67	16.68 ± 13.99	11	8.64 ± 2.57
3	21	34.95 ± 14.98		
4	38	39.87 ± 18.30	1	9.00
5[a]	12	44.25 ± 12.58	5	16.00 ± 5.15
6[a]	2	67.00 ± 7.07	8	23.50 ± 6.59
7	0		10	34.40 ± 11.23
8	0		4	48.00 ± 11.43

Motor function levels are the same as those indicated numerically in Fig. 1.
[a]Significant difference was observed between typical FCMD and benign FCMD ($P < 0.05$).

even recognize their mother, and there is pseudohypertrophy of the cheeks and calves at some point in their clinical course. Those cases whose clinical course is consistent with the third clinical pattern show diffuse (including the cheeks) marked pseudohypertrophy at some stage, have relatively good mentality and generally learn to speak in short phrases, some can even learn to write figures of the syllabic Japanese alphabet ("Hiragana" or "Katakana") and a few very simple Chinese characters ("Kanji").

In 1980, we proposed a subclassification system based on mental deficiency, the ability to walk and pseudohypertrophy [2,3]. The latter finding was the basis for distinguishing CMD III from CMD IV (benign FCMD). Our long-term follow-up results [4], published in

Table 2

Average age at loss of each motor function level

Motor function level	Subtype			
	Typical FCMD (CMD I)		Benign FCMD(III/IV)	
	Number of cases	Average age at loss (months ± SD)	Number of cases	Average age at loss (months ± SD)
1	2	57.00 ± 4.24	0	
2	9	127.00 ± 25.31	2	150.00 ± 15.56
3	4	90.00 ± 25.35	1	156.00
4	9	100.67 ± 24.69	4	151.75 ± 19.81
5	5	81.20 ± 15.53	4	105.00 ± 24.47
6	1	108.00	7	103.71 ± 18.14
7	0		6	87.67 ± 10.75
8	0		3	78.67 ± 15.95

Motor function levels are the same as those indicated numerically in Fig. 1.
[a]Significant difference was observed between typical FCMD and benign FCMD ($P < 0.05$).

1991, prompted us to classify types III and IV as benign CMD, because we found pseudo-hypertrophy in cases subclassified as CMD III. CMD V was subclassified based on histo-pathological findings of numerous regenerative fibers, although all of the biopsy specimens were obtained before 1 year of age. Most of these children had been brought to a hospital earlier because of hypotonia and delayed motor development, apparent in the neonatal period. Those rare cases in whom improved motor function was observed, showed widely distributed pachygyria with poor development of the operculum. Recently, the separation of types CMD I and V has generated considerable discussion in light of similar histopathological features being identified, simply at different ages, in these 2 groups of patients. CMD V (severe FCMD) may represent an earlier onset and more severe course of the typical form of FCMD (CMD I).

The aforementioned observations illustrate how classifying patients into different subtypes of FCMD has been complicated by the variable severities of the clinical, as well as neuropathologic, features which can vary markedly, even among individuals from the same family. We expect further modifications in the subclassification of FCMD. Specifically, whether the different types are due to the same genetic defect or are phenocopies of different genes, awaits clarification. At present, we regard all of these cases as FCMD.

Etiology and pathophysiology

The relationship between FCMD and other forms of CMD has been discussed in terms of whether WWS and MEB are clinical entities belonging to the same disease spectrum. The differentiation of WWS from severe FCMD, especially with extensive pachygyria, and poor development of the operculum, can be difficult in the presence of hydrocephalus.

Recent advances in molecular genetics showed that MEB and WWS are not at the same gene locus as FCMD. Toda et al. [14] mapped the gene related to FCMD to the long arm of chromosome No 9 (9q31-33). Subsequently, further localization to 9q31-32 [15], made prenatal diagnosis, using the mfd220 locus, a reality [16]. Dobyns et al. [17] and Pihko et al. [18] have demonstrated that the gene locus for WWS and MEB is not at 9q31-33.

At the same time, however, Toda and Yoshioka et al. [19,20] proposed that the genes for WWS and FCMD are at the same locus based on genetic analysis of 1 family in which the first son had typical FCMD with retinal detachment, the second pregnancy resulted in an encephalic infant and the third in CMD with pachygyria, hydrocephalus, encephalocele and retinal detachment, which was considered by them to be consistent with WWS.

Epidemiological aspects of CMD

A nationwide FCMD survey was conducted in 1976, utilizing a questionnaire sent to university and training hospital pediatric departments, and revealed a CMD to DMD ratio of 1:2.1 or 2.36. The gene frequency in Shimane prefecture [21], based on a population study, was estimated to be 7.5×10^{-3}. The incidence of CMD was thus 5.6×10^{-5}. The gene frequency [6,7], estimated from the consanguinity rate, is $5.2-9.7 \times 10^{-3}$. This value yielded an estimated CMD I incidence of $6.2-11.9 \times 10^{-5}$. In Okinawa [22,23], in 1988, the prevalence of FCMD was 1 per 100 000 people. Eighty percent of CMD cases were FCMD, for a prevalence of 0.8. Only 3 cases in the Okinawan study had type III/IV. At the Tokyo

Table 3

Results of nationwide questionnaire survey

Pre-1989[a]		Newly diagnosed, annually										Total	
		1989		1990[b]		1991[c]		1992[d]				1989–1992	
F	N	F	N	F	N	F	N	F	N			F	N
418	85	24	6	55	17	51	20	42	22			172	65

[a]Including all cases currently under observation.
Not including Saitama[b], Niigata (Neurol)[c], Iwaki[d] and Shimoshizu[d] National Sanatoria.
F, Fukuyama type congenital muscular dystrophy; N, non-Fukuyama type congenital muscular dystrophy.

Women's Medical College Hospital, we experienced 83 FCMD (CMD I/V), but only 14 benign FCMD (CMD III/IV), during the 1972–1993 period. Hirayama et al. [24] carried out a survey of CMD focused on children enrolled in special schools for the handicapped, in the Tokyo area, and identified 26 FCMD cases. The estimated prevalence of FCMD, based on their data, is 2.1×10^{-5}.

Another nationwide survey [25], the results of which are shown in Table 3, was carried out in 1993. All 54 institutions with which the members of the PMD research group, sponsored by the Japanese Ministry of Health and Welfare, were affiliated, responded. Two-thirds (36/54; 67%) reported having some clinical experience with CMD patients. Questionnaires were also sent to 238 university hospital pediatric departments and institutions, with which the councilors of the Japan Society of Child Neurologists were affiliated. The response rate was 63% (149/238). Fewer than half (94/238; 39%) had seen patients, 55 (23%) had no experience with CMD and 89 (37%) did not return the questionnaire. During the period from 1989 through 1992, FCMD cases outnumbered N-FCMD (non-Fukuyama type CMD including all forms of CMD other than FCMD) by nearly 3 to 1 (Table 3). The annual incidences of FCMD and N-FCMD, per 100 000 population, for the years 1974 through 1978, and 1989 through 1992, are shown in Table 4. The apparent increases in the incidences of both forms of CMD are attributable to heightened awareness of the diagnosis, as well as the marked decline in the consanguinity rate in modern Japanese society.

Clinical features

Initial symptoms and signs

When parents bring a FCMD patient to our clinic for the first time, the infant is invariably floppy. The parents generally describe motor developmental delay, and weak fetal movement had been recognized on occasion. Poor sucking and a mildly weak cry during the neonatal period, which can be overlooked in a newborn, had been noticed in about half of the cases. It is rather rare, however, to observe feeding difficulty or respiratory distress of sufficient severity to necessitate specialized care in a NICU for an extended period of time after birth. This is in contrast to other more severe forms of congenital myopathy. According to our experience with a FCMD case who was diagnosed shortly after birth because her elder sister had been affected with typical FCMD, muscle tone is mildly to moderately hypotonic

Table 4

Estimated annual incidences (per 10^5) of CMDs in Japan

Birth year	All live-newborns in Japan	FCMD		NFCMD		Total	
		Cases	Incidence	Cases	Incidence	Cases	Incidence
1974	2029989	22	1.08	9	0.44	31	1.53
1975	1901440	22	1.16	4	0.21	26	1.37
1976	1832617	17	0.93	7	0.38	24	1.31
1977	1755100	22	1.25	3	0.17	25	1.42
1978	1708643	19	1.11	9	0.53	28	1.64
Total	9227789	102	1.11	32	0.35	134	1.45
1989	1246802	24	1.92	6	0.48	30	2.41
1990[a]	1221585	41	3.36	15	1.23	56	4.48
1991[b]	1223245	45	3.68	19	1.55	64	5.23
1992[c]	1208977	32	2.65	19	1.57	51	4.22
Total	4900609	142	2.89	49	0.99	200	4.08

[a]The 1990 data do not include Saitama National Sanatorium.
[b]The 1991 data do not include Niigata National Sanatorium Neurology Department.
[c]The 1992 data do not include Iwaki and Shimoshizu National Sanatoria.

and spontaneous movement is decreased. Limitations of joint movement at the hips and ankles were also observed in this case. Some patients have initially been pointed out to have poor weight gain at the 1 month perinatal check up. In some, limitations of hip abduction are recognized at the 3 month check-up. Although facial muscle involvement is not a chief complaint, when asked how the patients close their eyes during sleep or when crying, the parents report that these childrens' eyes are slightly open during sleep. Upon reflection, most parents realize that the patients can not close their eyes tightly.

Symptoms and signs on physical examination (Figs. 2–5)

Diffuse but variable muscle weakness is generally found on physical examination, even at the first visit. Relatively proximal muscles of the upper body, i.e. the shoulder girdle and upper arm, are involved while relatively distal muscles tend to be affected in the lower body, specifically the calf muscles. Patients can lift their lower extremities with flexion of the hips and knees against gravity while in the supine position (Fig. 3c).

Hyperextensibility of the joints is evident in the shoulders (scarf sign, loose shoulder sign), wrists (window sign), elbows, and trunk (double folding). Limitations of hip extension and abduction, as well as ankle extension are also recognized. Even infants older than 5 months of age do not exhibit a positive supporting reaction.

Muscle consistency is not necessarily soft and may even be rather hard, having a somewhat fibrous feeling.

Pseudohypertrophy of the cheeks becomes evident in infancy, in the calves and forearms by early childhood and is prominent after patients have begun to use the affected muscles. Muscle atrophy is unremarkable in infancy but becomes increasingly evident after age 3 years, initially manifesting in the chest area.

Deep tendon reflexes can not be elicited except in very early infancy, before 3 months of age, at which point knee joint contractures have not yet developed. Long tract signs are not usually identified, although some primitive reflexes remain longer in rare cases. Plagiocephalic deformity and a tendency to turn the head to one side are frequently observed (Fig. 5).

Pale optic discs and strabismus are occasionally recognized. Likewise, ptosis is only

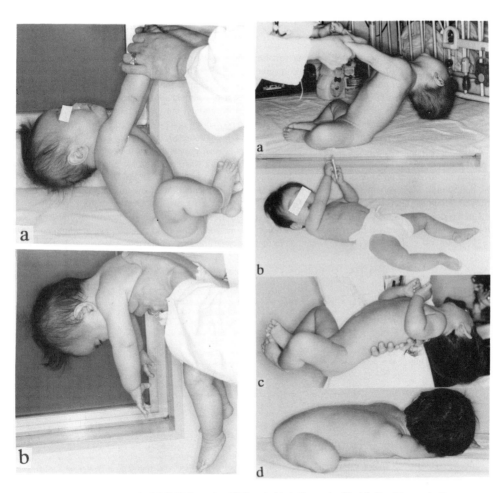

Fig. 2. Clinical features of typical FCMD in early childhood. (a) A 5-month-old girl. Head lag and elbow extension were evident with traction. She was able to flex her hip against gravity. Babinskis were also elicited bilaterally. (b) The same patient as in (a). The extremities could not be raised against gravity. The Landau reaction was not elicited but the trunk arched when the baby was held at chest level.

Fig. 3. Clinical features of typical FCMD in early childhood. (a) An 8-month-old boy. Head lag and elbow extension were more evident with traction than in the girl shown in Fig. 2. His hips remained in an abducted position with flexed knees. (b) The same patient as in Fig. 2a,b at 10 months old. She was able lift her upper arms to reach for a toy and to use both hands to play with the toy. Lower extremities show the so-called pithed frog position with abducted hip joints and knee flexion. (c) A 1 year 3 month old girl. She was able to lift her lower extremities with flexion of the hips and knees against gravity. (d) A 2 year 4 month old girl showing double folding.

38

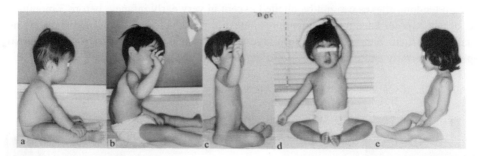

Fig. 4. Patients in the sitting position showing variable trunk muscle power at the same age (b,c,d). (a) The girl shown in Fig. 2a,b at 10 months of age, could maintain a sitting posture, though with a rounded back, by supporting herself with her arms. No remarkable muscle atrophy is present at this age. (b) A 2 year 4 month old boy trying to sit cross-legged fashion. Trunk muscles are inadequate to maintain a sitting posture and the back is rounded. He can flex his elbows and raise his forearms against gravity, but cannot raise his upper arms against gravity higher than shoulder level. (c) A 2 year 4 month old boy sitting in a cross-legged position. Trunk muscles are adequate to maintain a fully upright posture and the back is not rounded. He can flex his elbows and raise his forearms against gravity, but can not raise his upper arms against gravity higher than shoulder level. (d) The 2 year 4 month old girl shown is trying to remove a towel which was placed on her head. She showed motor function improvement up to level 5, and was able to form sentence fragments, despite having "round lesions" in the optic fundi. Most patients with "round lesions" are severely mentally retarded and show markedly delayed motor development. In contrast, this patient was able to sit upright at 1 year and learned to crawl. (e) A 3-year-old girl in the sitting position. Mild muscle atrophy was noted in the shoulder and upper chest on examination. Skin in the patellar area appears shiny. This finding is especially marked in the distal patellar area, at which no sweating was observed, and had initially become apparent around this age.

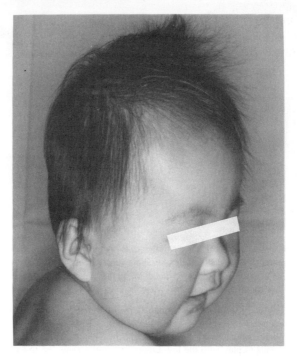

Fig. 5. This 9-month-old girl is a typical FCMD case. Note the plagiocephalic deformity and rounded cheeks suggesting pseudohypertrophy and rather poor development of the temporal muscles.

rarely observed. Facial muscle involvement tends to be distinct but no other signs of cranial nerve abnormality are present.

Development of joint contractures

Joint contractures are not marked at birth. Hip, knee and ankle contractures generally appear before age 1 year, in typical FCMD (Fig. 6). From early infancy, proximal interphalangeal (PIP) and distal interphalangeal (DIP) joints of the fingers can be passively extended and held straight when the wrist is in an intermediate position but when the wrist is extended the finger joints flex, probably due to shortening of the musculus flexor digitorum superficialis (Fig. 7). By age 10 years all affected joints, except the shoulder, have developed striking progressive contractures (Figs. 6,8). Limited anterior flexion of the neck, due to shortening of the trapezius muscle (Fig. 8c), is noticeable at age 2 years or thereafter.

In contrast, pes equinovarus appears between 5 and 8 years as the initial contracture in benign FCMD (Figs. 9–12).

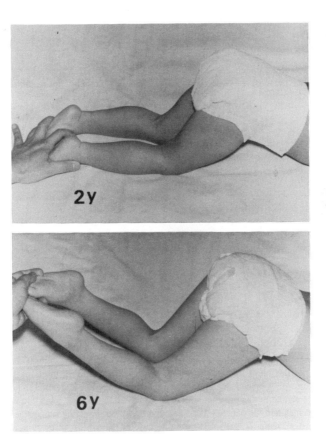

Fig. 6. Joint contractures are progressive. Limitations of passive hip and knee extension and ankle dorsiflexion can easily be observed with the patient in the prone position. These pictures were taken of 2 sisters. Note the limited hip, knee and ankle extension which are more severe in the older sister.

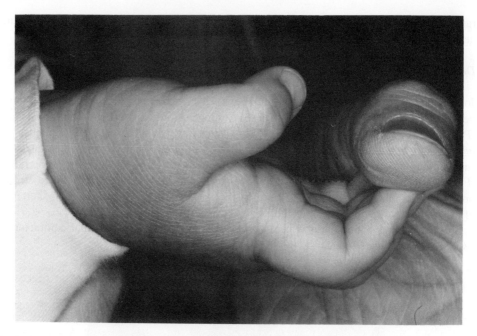

Fig. 7. PIP and DIP joints of the fingers can be passively extended and held straight when the wrist is in an intermediate position but when the wrist is extended, the finger joints flex, probably due to shortening of the musculus flexor digitorum superficialis. These findings are present in infancy.

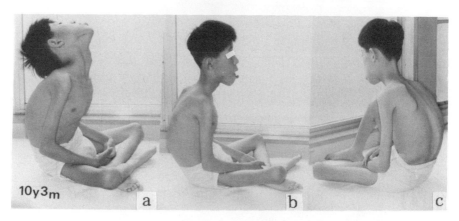

Fig. 8. Typical FCMD case at 10 years 3 months. This patient could maintain his trunk in an upright posture while sitting cross-legged despite his back being kyphotic. He could hold his head upright by keeping the weight slightly forward. Anterior flexion of the neck was limited due to shortening of the trapezius muscle (visible in (c)), such that muscle strength was inadequate for head control and the neck was prone to posterior flexion. Most patients around this age can sit in this position with the chin up while the neck joints are slightly extended. The caretaker must strive to maintain the patient's head in a good position providing support at the back of the neck. This is especially important while the patient is eating because of the risk of suffocation. Jaw articulation problems are common, and most patients can not close their mouths. Even at this point the patient can hold one leg in a middle upright position with his hip and knee flexed. Diffuse marked muscle atrophy and joint contractures (limitations in anterior neck flexion, and extension of the elbows, hips and knees) are apparent. There is no limitation of passive movement at the shoulder joint.

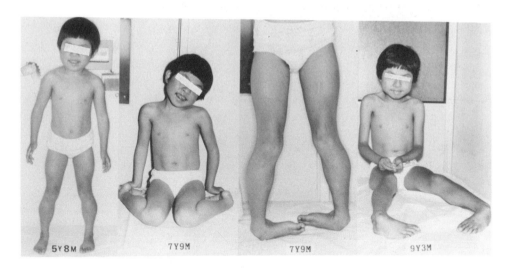

Fig. 9. These photographs illustrate the course of a benign FCMD (CMD III/IV) case. She visited our hospital at 3 years 3 months of age. She had started to walk with support at 2 years of age, and without support at 3 years 6 months. At 5 years 8 months, the patient was ambulant though pseudohypertrophy was apparent in the cheeks, forearms, thighs and calves. By 7 years 9 months, she had lost the ability to walk due to pes equinovarus. She could no longer stand without support. By 9 years 3 months, joint contractures affected the elbows, wrists, fingers, hips and knees. Anterior flexion of the neck was limited due to trapezius shortening.

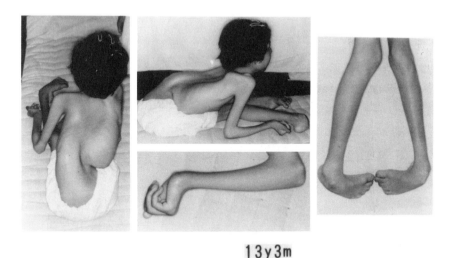

13y3m

Fig. 10. By 13 years 3 months (the same case as shown in Fig. 9), remarkable scoliosis had developed due largely to the patient's preference for maintaining a sitting posture despite having lost the ability to sit upright. Attempts were made to introduce braces, for maintaining upright posture of the torso, but were rejected by the patient as these devices limited her activities. At this point in her course, severe flexion contractures were apparent in all joints of the hands and feet.

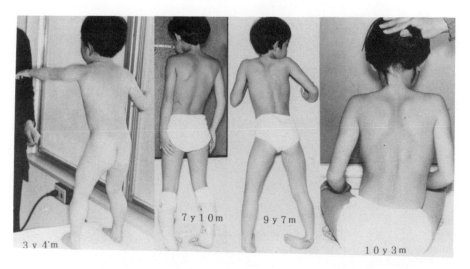

Fig. 11. These photographs illustrate the course of another benign FCMD (CMD III/IV of Fukuyama) case. She visited our hospital at 3 years 4 months old. She had started to walk with support at 1 year 5 months, and without support at 2 years 1 month. At 3 years 4 months, she was ambulant though pseudohypertrophy was apparent in the cheeks, forearms, thighs and calves (a). By 7 years 10 months, she had lost the ability to walk without short braces due to pes equinovarus (b). By 9 years 7 months she could no longer walk without long braces (c). She could no longer stand without support by 10 years 3 months and showed mild right sided concave scoliosis (d).

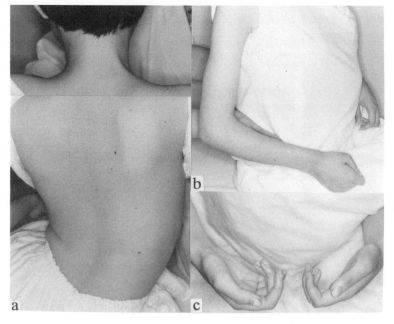

Fig. 12. By 20 years 3 months (the same case as shown in Fig. 11), joint contracture affected the elbows, wrists, fingers, hips and knees. Anterior flexion of the neck was limited due to trapezius shortening. Scoliosis had developed but was not as severe as that of the case shown in Fig. 10. Progression of scoliosis was partially prevented by applying a chest brace to maintain an upright torso posture.

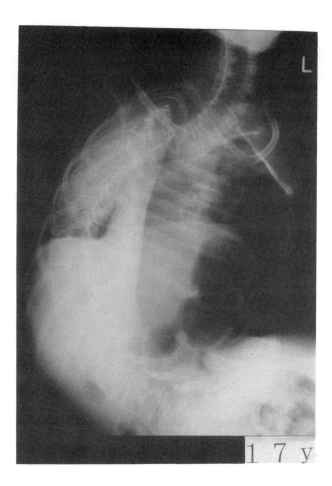

Fig. 13. Chest and abdominal X-ray from a 17-year-old female (CMD I) with remarkable scoliosis. The curvature of the spine, which was obviously to the right, had begun at age 9 years and slowly progressed thereafter. Despite having a typical FCMD course, this patient had relatively good mental development. She had limited abilities to draw, read and write and enjoyed doing various crafts while sitting in her wheelchair. She rejected a brace designed to maintain an upright trunk posture, as well as suggestions that she remain recumbent most of the time, as these interventions limited her activities. Aggressive therapy may well have slowed the progression of scoliosis in this patient but would also have meant a significant reduction in her quality of life.

Those cases who engage in hobbies while in a sitting position develop marked scoliosis upon losing the ability to maintain a proper sitting position after age 9 years (Fig. 13).

Clinical course of facial muscle involvement

Facial muscle involvement tends to result in characteristic changes in appearance with aging. Figs. 14 and 15 illustrate the progressive changes observed in a typical case from 1 to 6 years, and in a severe case from the neonatal period to 10 years of age, respectively. Before age 3 years, the cheeks are rounded, hypertrophic and the overlying skin appears to be shiny. The cheeks are smooth and very firm to the touch but subsequently become atrophic. Prognathism also develops. A tendency for the mouth to remain partially open is apparent

44

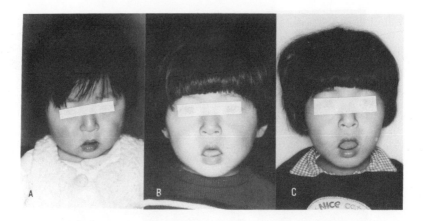

Fig. 14. Changes in facial appearance in a typical FCMD patient at 1 year 7 months (A), 3 years 3 months (B) and 6 years 5 months (C). The cheeks were rounded at 1 year 7 months (A), but gradually thinned along with an increasingly marked tendency to keep the mouth open with the tongue resting in a somewhat forward position on the lower teeth and lip (B). Myopathic facial involvement is prominent in the cheek muscles, the mouth is open, and macroglossia and an everted lower lip are evident (C). This patient died at age 6 years 6 months. His mother reported that he had died in his sleep. The preceding day, he had been seen by a neighborhood physician and was diagnosed as having had a "common cold", and was considered to have been nearly recovered from a febrile illness of a few days duration.

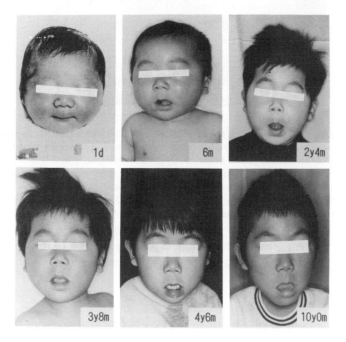

Fig. 15. Age-related progression of myopathic facial changes in a boy with severe FCMD who showed round lesions in the optic fundi, and whose peak motor function level was 2. He had shown a tendency to keep his mouth open since 6 months of age, the cheeks were also rounded at 6 months and had become atrophic by 3 years 8 months. Prognathism was discernible around age 3 years and is quite evident in the photo taken at 4 years 6 months. He died at age 17 years.

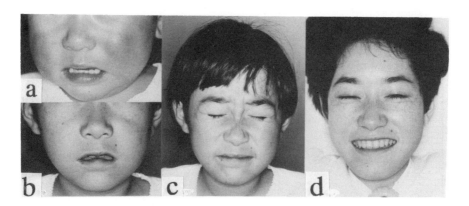

Fig. 16. Age-related progression of myopathic facial changes in a girl with benign FCMD (the same case as shown in Figs. 11 and 12) whose peak motor function level was 8. She visited our hospital at age 3 years 4 months, at which time the tendency to keep the mouth open was noted but was unremarkable as compared to typical FCMD cases. The cheeks were rounded with shiny skin and were hard to the touch at 3 years 4 months (a). The cheek pseudohypertrophy was not particularly marked at 3 years or at 10 years 3 months. She could not envelop her eye-lashes with her eyelids while closing her eyes as tightly as possible at 10 years 3 months. Cheek atrophy is not evident in the picture taken at 20 years 10 months. Prognathism and macroglossia were discernible around age 3 years and are quite evident in the photo taken at 4 years 6 months.

from infancy. The upper lip forms an inverted V while the lower is everted, making it appear rather thick. The course of facial involvement is similar, though slower, in benign FCMD (CMD III/IV) (Fig. 16).

Mental retardation suggesting involvement of the central nervous system

Mental development is consistently subnormal even in benign FCMD (CMD III/IV) [2,3]. There is, however, no remarkable regression in mentality with aging. Social development such as eye contact, smiling, some communication with others (supplemented with eye and neck movement) can be achieved despite a very small vocabulary and delayed speech, in all benign and many typical FCMD. Covering the ears with the hands, probably due to heightened sensitivity to sound, and spontaneous verbalization not in response to the environment, are noted in very rare cases. Even in severe FCMD (CMD V) with a poor prognosis, recognition of the mother and vocalization to express demands can be attained but are delayed. Most typical FCMD (CMD I) cases can learn to speak up to a few dozen words.

Seizures [26]

Ninety seven children with FCMD (CMD I in 83 cases, type III/IV in 14) were assessed for febrile and afebrile seizures (Fig. 17). Prevalences of seizures were 58.3% in CMD I and 66.7% in CMD III/IV. In this study, we regarded seizures associated with a fever above 37.5°C as febrile seizures. The median age of seizure onset was 1 year in both types. In nearly 80% of children with seizures, clinical seizure disorders manifested during the period from 1 to 3 years or after age 6 years. Sixty-seven percent of cases with febrile seizures before age 1 year (6 cases) developed afebrile seizures while 18% of those with febrile seizures initially occurring between ages 1 and 3 years (28 cases) developed afebrile seizures.

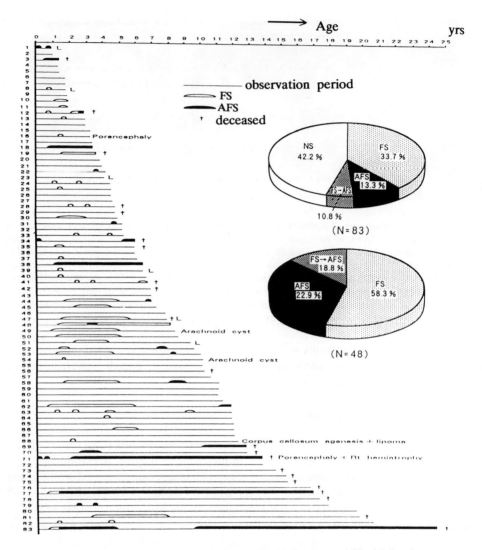

Fig. 17. Seizure courses of 83 cases of CMD I. FS, febrile seizures; AFS, afebrile seizures.

Cases with febrile seizures before age 1 year were likely to subsequently develop afebrile seizures. The most common seizure type observed was a generalized tonic clonic seizure. Half of the type I cases and one third of the type III/IV cases showed epileptic discharges. The prevalence of focal epileptic discharges on EEG was higher than that of diffuse epileptic discharges. In 5 CMD I cases, and 1 CMD III/IV case, seizures were triggered by hot water bathing. Seven CMD I cases had died due to status epilepticus, and one CMD III/IV case had experienced status convulsivus which lasted more than 30 min. Febrile seizures in FCMD tended to more often be associated with low grade fever, frequent seizure recurrence, longer durations of each seizure episode and seizure clustering in a 24 h period, in comparison to benign febrile seizures. In those with epileptic discharges on EEG, status epilepticus, or seizures triggered by hot water bathing, we evaluate the indications for anti-convulsant therapy on an individual basis.

Ophthalmological findings and relationships of FCMD to Santavuori disease (MEB) and Walker–Warburg syndrome (WWS)

As mentioned above, the observation that the cardinal lesions of WWS [8,27] and MEB [9,28] commonly affect muscle and brain, as well as ocular tissues, has generated consider-able research interest in the possible nosological relationship between these two conditions and FCMD.

Thirty-two CMDI/V and 6 CMD III/IV cases underwent detailed ophthalmologic exami-nations conducted by experienced pediatric ophthalmologists at our TWMC hospital [29,31]. Ocular abnormalities identified in this study are shown in Fig. 18, for comparison with those of MEB and WWS. The most remarkable ocular findings in FCMD were "round lesions" at the retinal periphery [5,32] (Fig. 19) and abnormal eye movements [4,32]. Find-ings were negative in the 2 patients who underwent fluorescent angiography. Similar find-ings have also been reported as "uneven and grayish mottling of the retina" in CMD I [32,33] and as "sharply defined ring atrophic patches" in CMD III/IV [34]. The clinical findings of those cases showing round lesions or abnormal eye movements were compared with those of cases without such specific ophthalmological findings, as shown in Table 5. No significant differences were recognized between the 2 groups. None of our FCMD cases had glaucoma. Furthermore, the characteristic ocular features of WWS [27], such as corneal opacities, abnormalities of the iris or anterior chamber, and microphthalmos, were not pres-ent in FCMD.

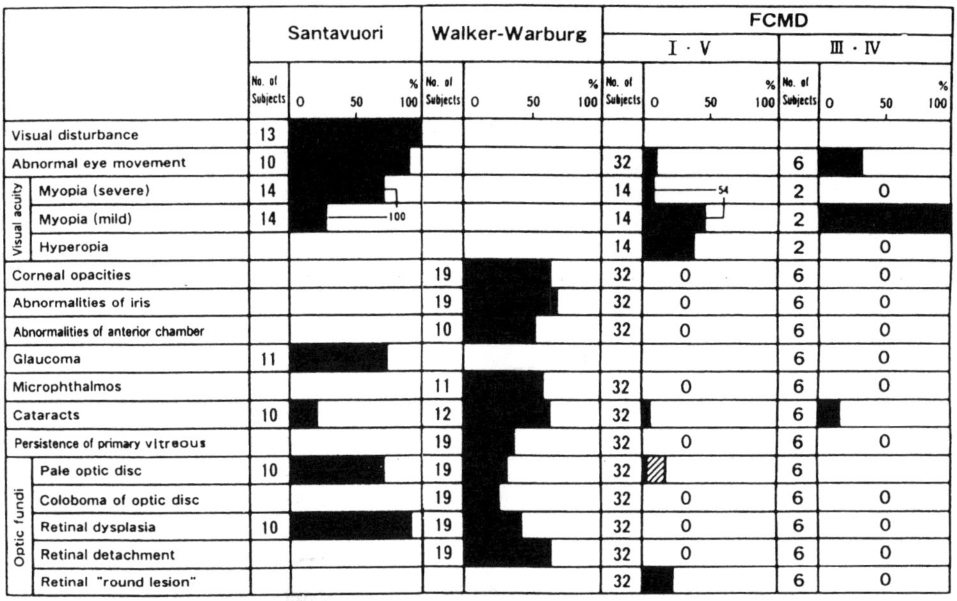

| | Santavuori | | | Walker-Warburg | | | FCMD | | | | | |
| | | | | | | | I · V | | | III · IV | | |
	No. of Subjects	0 50	% 100	No. of Subjects	0 50	% 100	No. of Subjects	0 50	% 100	No. of Subjects	0 50	% 100
Visual disturbance	13											
Abnormal eye movement	10						32			6		
Myopia (severe)	14						14	54		2	0	
Myopia (mild)	14	100					14			2		
Hyperopia							14			2	0	
Corneal opacities				19			32	0		6	0	
Abnormalities of iris				19			32	0		6	0	
Abnormalities of anterior chamber				10			32	0		6	0	
Glaucoma	11									6	0	
Microphthalmos				11			32	0		6	0	
Cataracts	10			12			32			6		
Persistence of primary vitreous				19			32	0		6	0	
Pale optic disc	10			19			32			6		
Coloboma of optic disc				19			32	0		6	0	
Retinal dysplasia	10			19			32	0		6	0	
Retinal detachment				19			32	0		6	0	
Retinal "round lesion"							32			6	0	

Fig. 18. Ophthalmological findings in FCMD compared with those in Santavuori disease [28] and Walker–Warburg syndrome [27].

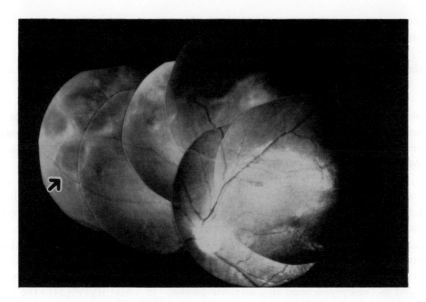

Fig. 19. An optic fundus picture from a patient with FCMD. Several "round lesions"(arrow), approximately the same size as the papilla and surrounded by a whitish color, are evident at the periphery of the optic fundus.

Table 5

Comparison of clinical features of FCMD with and without "round lesions" of the retina and abnormal eye movements

Clinical features	Type			
	With eye symptoms		Without eye symptoms	
	"Round lesions"	AEM[a]	I,V	III,IV
Consanguinity	0/5	0/3	2/24	1/6
Affected siblings	0/4	0/0	3/12	0/4
Abnormalities during pregnancy	3/5	1/3	7/24	4/6
History of abortion				
Spontaneous	1/5	1/3	5/24	1/5
Artificial	1/5	1/3	2/24	3/6
MRI/CT				
WM hyperlucency	5/5	2/3	12/23	2/3
Dilated ventricles	5/5	3/3	16/23	3/6
Opercular dysplasia	3/5	2/3	1/23	0/6
DQ	46.9	57.0	42.3	53.3
Average age (months) at acquisition of motor function level[b]				
Level 1	11.1 ± 11.6	6.0 ± 2.2	5.5 ± 2.3	3.4 ± 1.33
Level 2	29.5 ± 24.1	17.5 ± 13.4	13.6 ± 6.2	8.8 ± 2.0
Level 3	28		29.5 ± 16.3	
Level 4	34		39.4 ± 25.1	
Level 5		18.0		18.8 ± 5.0

[a]Abnormal eye movements.
[b]The CMD motor function level described by Ueda.

Growth

An investigation of growth patterns in 75 typical FCMD (CMD I) and 14 benign FCMD (CMD III/IV), followed for 1–17 years, revealed that growth was more severely affected in typical FCMD. Serially collected data demonstrated reduced growth parameters, in the following order of severity: chest circumference, head circumference, height and weight. Longitudinally based height and weight velocity curves for 8 children, all of whom had either typical or benign FCMD, showed a small growth spurt, earlier than normal, especially in typical FCMD. The maximum rate of height increase was more severely reduced than that of weight, as compared with data from normal children.

Skin changes

In addition to the rather rough, dry skin characteristic of FCMD, we have also found that the subcutaneous tissue becomes increasingly firm to the touch with disease progression. This firmness is especially marked in the calves. The skin eventually becomes so adherent to underlying structures that it is no longer possible to test its elasticity by pinching a small area of skin. The skin appears shiny in the distal patellar area, at which no sweating is observed, and this is initially seen around 3 years of age.

Non-neurologic congenital anomalies

The prevalences of minor anomalies were determined in 72 typical FCMD and 12 benign FCMD cases [36]. One benign FCMD case had a diaphragmatic hernia. Another typical FCMD case had syndactyly, in addition to partial agenesis of the corpus callosum with lipoma (Fig. 20). Congenital heart defects [37–39], atresia ani [40] and cleft palates [41]

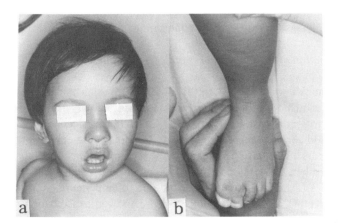

Fig. 20. A 1 year 9 month old girl with FCMD and agenesis of the corpus callosum. Hypertelorism and a high, wide nasal bridge are apparent. She also suffered from syndactyly of the first and second left toes, which was surgically corrected in infancy.

have also been reported. More than half of patients have dysmorphic features such as brachycephalus, high arched palate, café-au-lait spot, hypertrichosis, heel protrusion and dermatoglyphic abnormalities [42].

Cardiac involvement

As we have already reported in detail [43], those patients who live more than 10 years tend to develop fibrosis of the myocardium, as evidenced by postmortem findings. In a review of the Japanese literature, although the autopsy studies demonstrated a high incidence of cardiac muscle involvement, clinical manifestations of cardiac impairment intra vitam are rather rare [44–50]. Slowly progressive cardiac involvement is, nonetheless, thought to be characteristic of FCMD.

In a study on arterial pH, pCO_2 and pO_2 in 15 FCMD cases [44] ranging in age from 7 to 27 years (average 15 ± 5 years), blood gas values were revealed to be significantly better than in DMD cases of the same age. These investigators also reported one 15-year-old FCMD patient who died of cardiac insufficiency. This patient showed severe cardiac deterioration while intercostal muscle degeneration was relatively mild, indicating that there is a significant risk of developing cardiac insufficiency in FCMD [44]. The authors thus recommended that these patients be monitored for cardiac involvement.

Yoshikawa et al. [50] reported a FCMD case presenting with rapidly progressive heart failure. This 15-year-old boy was diagnosed as having FCMD at 8 months of age, based on the pathological findings of biopsied muscle and clinical symptoms. At 15 years 4 months, dyspnea, oliguria and edema developed. A chest X-ray film and echocardiogram disclosed marked cardiomegaly and a decreased left ventricular ejection fraction. His heart failure subsequently worsened. At 15 years 7 months, he experienced cardiac arrest induced by infection, and was successfully resuscitated. At 15 years 9 months, he developed pneumonia which exacerbated the heart failure, thereby leading to death. An autopsy examination revealed heart muscle involvement including hypertrophy, degeneration and fibrosis, predominantly in the right ventricle. The authors found no other reports of FCMD presenting with such a rapid progression of heart failure, and concluded that their case suggests the possibility of various forms of cardiac involvement in FCMD. Again, the observations should prompt clinicians to closely monitor the cardiac functions of FCMD patients.

Transient exacerbation of muscle weakness after febrile illness

Approximately one fifth of CMD I/V and III/IV cases experience transient exacerbations of muscle weakness which are probably attributable to acute myolysis manifesting as CK elevation, generally triggered by a viral infection. Analyzing the records of 82 typical FCMD cases, we found a history of such episodes in 16 of them. These episodes occurred between 3 months and 9 years 1 month of age, mainly in the summer time; 8 in July, 2 each in June, August and September, and 1 case each in December and January. Muscle weakness was noticed at 3–9 days (average 4.4 days) after the initial temperature elevation and was concomitant with a decline in motor function. No case showed exacerbation of muscle weakness on the day on which the fever peaked. Two cases required artificial ventilation because of transient respiratory muscle weakness. All 16 cases started to show signs of recovery after 5–36 days (average 12.7 days) and subsequently returned to nearly their peak motor function level. Viral titers were examined in 6 cases, 2 of whom showed elevation of the complement fixation test for coxsackie virus. Serum CK levels were examined immediately after these episodes and were found to be 2–6 times higher than usual.

Laboratory findings

Serum enzyme activities

In CMD I and III/IV, the serum CK level was 10–50 times higher than normal but subsequently decreased after age 7 years. We studied the relations between patient age and serum GOT, GPT, LDH and CK activities in CMD I (68 cases, aged from 4 months to 17 years), II (2 cases, 4 months to 17 years) and III/IV (11 cases, 6 months to 21 years 6 months) [52]. Enzyme activity was found to generally be higher in benign FCMD. One member of our group (Ikenaka [52]) demonstrated negative correlations between enzyme values and age. In CMD I: GOT = 93.41–$4.82 \times$ age (years), $r = -0.459$; GPT = 64.86–$2.80 \times$ age, $r = -0.30$; LDH = 902.29–$36.83 \times$ age, $r = -0.364$; CK = 3723.55–$232.19 \times$ age, $r = -0.470$ ($P <$ 0.0001); and in CMD III/IV: GOT = 123.28–$5.73 \times$ age, $r = -0.369$; GPT = 107.40–$4.74 \times$ age, $r = -0.598$; LDH = 1260.43–$55.26 \times$ age, $r = -0.691$; CK = 5602.02–$302.98 \times$ age, $r = -0.606$ ($P < 0.0001$). The relation between GOT and GPT, one of which predominates in each age group (0–5, 5–10 and >10 years), was also evaluated. GOT levels exceeded those of GPT in 94, 80 and 100% of CMD I, and 76, 38 and 78% of CMD III/IV cases, respectively. In contrast, GPT levels were higher than those of GOT in 36, 55 and 59% of DMD cases, respectively [53].

Skeletal muscle CT scanning

Cross sectional muscle CT scans obtained at the mid-calf, mid-thigh and L3 trunk levels, were compared with those of DMD [54,55]. In CMD I, mid-calf changes preceded those at the other 2 levels. Changes in CMD III/IV were milder and there was no tendency for early mid-calf change. There was a negative correlation between the average CT number and age, unrelated to the motor function level, in every muscle except m. quadratum lumborum and m. gracilis. In all muscles, though most markedly at calf level, the CT number in CMD I was lower than that in DMD even before 1 year of age. Precise data are presented in another portion of this text [56].

Skeletal muscle histopathology

Histochemical studies [57] were conducted on biopsied quadriceps muscle specimens, from 26 typical FCMD (CMD I), 9 benign FCMD (CMD III/IV) and 3 FCMD with a poor prognosis (CMD V). There were no signs of inflammatory or neurogenic change. In typical FCMD, increased endo-, peri- and epimysial connective and fatty tissues, loss of basic muscle architecture, and marked decreases in muscle fiber numbers were documented. Findings suggesting degenerative change were common. In benign FCMD, fiber size varied markedly, with hypertrophic fibers (>100 μm) being more abundant than in CMD I. In infants under 2 years, changes were milder than in older cases but phagocytosis and regenerating fibers were present. There were also occasional clusters of small fibers. Takada et al. [58], in one of only 2 reports to date on aborted fetuses (23 weeks), found all fibers to be IIc, but no dystrophic changes, degenerating or necrotic fibers, were seen. It was therefore assumed that the degenerative process had not yet begun at this stage of gestation.

Nonaka et al. [59], Miike et al. [60] and Wakayama et al. [61] describe precise histological findings in other portions of this text. The results of a study on the expression of dystrophin [62] and merosin are also presented in detail in another portion of this text [63,64]. The authors of the dystrophin study concluded that FCMD muscle may have a secondary dystrophin defect, which remains to be characterized, in the surface membrane dystrophin arrangement.

Takemitsu et al. [65] reported strongly positive immunoreactivity to dystrophin-related protein at the neuromuscular junction in FCMD. Matsumura et al. [66] have also detailed their findings of a dystrophin-associated protein, which was expressed at abnormally low levels in FCMD.

Neuroradiological findings

Basic knowledge of brain malformations in FCMD
Autopsy reports have revealed micropolygyria ('pachygyric-micropolygyria' as described by Ogasawara et al. [67]) in the cerebrum and cerebellum, hemispheric fusion, hypoplastic pyramidal tracts and mild to moderate ventricular dilatation, but no evidence of the CNS exerting a direct influence on skeletal muscle. These abnormalities are most likely attributable to early embryonic developmental defects [2,3]. A significant contribution to this field was made by Takada et al. [68,69] who reported 5 FCMD cases in which cerebral cortical dysplasia was not uniform, even within the same brain. These authors categorized the dysplasia into 3 major patterns, each with a predictable topography despite individual variations, and discussed the features of cortical dysplasia in FCMD. A limited resemblance to the cortical dysplasia of Walker's lissencephaly was noted. Tanaka et al. [70] and Takashima et al. [71] present detailed findings in other portions of this text.

Our postmortem examinations [72] of one severe (bedridden), one typical and one benign FCMD case revealed micropolygyria, agyria and pyramidal tract dysgenesis. The severe FCMD case had extensive agyria and polymicrogyria, while the typical FCMD case had extensive polymicrogyria and the benign FCMD case had only the latter and in the cerebrum rather than the cerebellum. A correlation between the severity of clinical symptoms and pathological findings was also recognized. The severity of brain anomalies correlated strongly with both maximal motor function and mentality. Our review of 24 autopsied cases, from the Japanese literature, demonstrated similar correlations [72].

Neuroimaging of brain malformations
We examined brain malformations in 51 cases with either severe or typical FCMD, using neuroradiological techniques. Broad gyri with a thick cortex and poor development of the operculum, as well as pachygyria, were visualized on brain MRI (Fig. 21). Most cases showed pachygyria which can be detected relatively easily in the frontal regions on axial slices and in parietal and temporal regions on coronal slices but is difficult to visualize in the occipital region. Six cases (11.8%) showed extensive pachygyria with poor development of the operculum (Fig. 22). In assessing these findings in terms of Dobyns' criteria [73] for lissencephaly, we found that all 6 cases showed 1 point each for the cerebral surface, lamination, ventricles, and posterior fossa, for a maximum point total of no more than 4. These children had never learned any meaningful words, and all showed a clinical course compati-

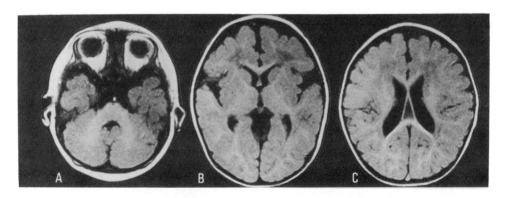

Fig. 21. A T_1-weighted MRI of the brain of a 1-year-old boy with typical FCMD. The findings of pachygyria, including a thickened cortex, poor GM/WM differentiation (note the relative paucity of sulci in the superior, middle and inferior frontal regions and in the superior and middle temporal regions with abnormally wide gyri giving the surface of the brain a smooth appearance) and wide Sylvian fissures, are typical of FCMD. (A) Image obtained at pons level; (B) image obtained at pineal body level; (C), image obtained at corpus callosum level.

ble with severe FCMD (Table 6). Five of the 6 were bedridden and one, who had undergone a shunt operation for hydrocephalus [74] (case 4, Table 6), had attained the ability to maintain a sitting posture while in a special chair which provided adequate support.

Rare brain anomalies (Fig. 23), observed in FCMD on MRI, include arachnoid cyst in the temporal fossa in 2 cases (Fig. 23A,B), porencephaly in 2 cases (Fig. 23C) and partial agenesis of the corpus callosum with lipoma at the genu in 1 case. One of the cases who showed porencephaly had a history of neonatel meningitis and West syndrome.

Evaluating the relationships among clinical features and brain CT/MRI findings revealed that mental disability and peak motor function were more closely related to the degree and extent of brain malformation than to muscle degeneration, supporting the results of our pathological study [72].

Diffuse white matter hyperlucency on CT
Hyperlucency in the periventricular white matter (WM) is frequently identified in infancy in FCMD patients. Mild to moderate ventricular dilatation is known to be associated with this WM hyperlucency, which resembles the periventricular lucency of hydrocephalus. Thus, it was initially suggested that the WM hyperlucency reflected hydrocephalic involvement in the pathogenesis of brain dysplasia. However, the absence of contrast enhancement on CT subsequently ruled out a hydrocephalic process. RI cisternography [75] has also been done in CMD patients, and although the results suggested some abnormalities of cerebrospinal fluid circulation, the precise nature and significance of such abnormalities remain to be clarified.

Two FCMD cases in our series had hydrocephalus with intracranial hypertension. One, a 15-month-old male diagnosed as FCMD at 4 months, manifested progressive head enlargement [75]. MRI, shown in Fig. 22, revealed a thickened cortex and poor development of the operculum with a dilated ventricular system and subarachnoid space. Intracranial pressure and CSF dynamics monitoring revealed high intracranial pressure and high CSF outflow resistance, indicating a high pressure hydrocephalus. V–P shunt produced not only sympto-

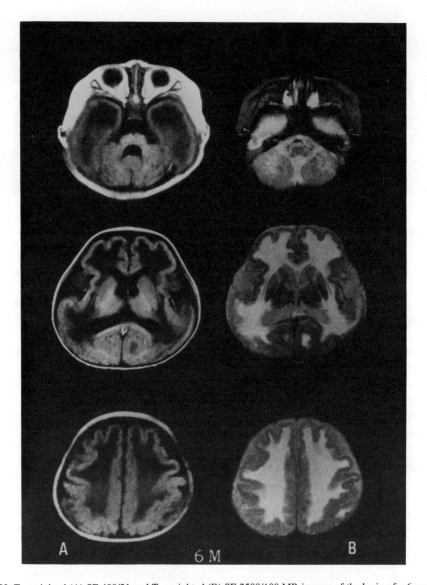

Fig. 22. T_1-weighted (A) SE 400/21 and T_2-weighted (B) SE 2500/100 MR images of the brain of a 6-month-old patient with severe FCMD. This patient is presently 6 years of age and can only briefly maintain a sitting posture (Case 4, Table 6). The upper, middle, and lower pairs of images were obtained at the levels of the pons, pineal body and above the corpus callosum, respectively. The WM is hyperintense in T_2-weighted and hypointense in T_1-weighted images. Approximately 10% of FCMD patients show this combination of remarkable pachygyria, a very thickened cortex and poor opercular development.

matic improvement, but also marked physiologic changes including increased cerebral blood flow and decreases in both intracranial pressure and CSF outflow resistance.

In a study [76] conducted in 1990, we found that the WM hyperlucency was remarkable in 13 out of 17 (76%) CMD I. The hyperlucency was bilaterally symmetrical in most cases. Delayed myelination was recognized in 3 out of 4 who underwent MRI using G-50 [76].

Table 6

Clinical features of cases with marked pachygyria and poor development of the operculum

Case	1	2	3	4	5	6
Age at most recent exam (years:months)	0:9	3:5	6:0	6:6	7:8	9:2
Maximum motor function level	0	0	2	0	0	0
Seizures						
Age at onset (years:months)[a]	0:4	0:10	Not experienced	1:6	1:11	2:11
Relationship c̄ fever[a]	s̄ fever	c̄ fever		c̄ fever	c̄ fever	c fever
Seizure types	Infantile spasms	CPS to a secondary GTCS	−	CPS	GTCS	GTCS
Seizure courses	Relapsed at 9 months	Clustering formation	−	×1	×9 Clustering formation	Total ×10 (last attack at 4 years)
EEG						
Paroxysmal discharge	Hypsarrhythmia	Spikes at rt mT (11 months)	Sharp waves at lt and rt pT, F, O while awake, diffuse sharp waves and poly-spikes during sleep (6 years)	Spikes at lt mT and pT, diffuse spikes by photic stimulation (2 years)	Sharp waves at lt C (8 months), rt O spikes and poly-spikes (3 years)	(−) (4 years)
Background activities			Dysrhythmia only (1 year 11 months), extreme spindles (1 year 11 months, 6 years)			
Ophthalmological findings	Not examined	"Round lesion"	Strabismus	"Round lesion"	"Round lesion"	Not examined
Others			Shunting operation for hydrocephalus		Deceased (7 years 8 months)	
Therapy	Clonazepam ACTH	PB (3 years)		(−)	PB, PHT (1 year)	PB (4 years)

CPS, complex partial seizure; GTCS, generalized tonic clonic convulsion; lt, left; rt, right; C, central; F, frontal; mT, mid-temporal; O, occipital; pT, posterior temporal; PB, phenobarbital; PHT, phenytoin; ACTH, adrenocorticotropic hormone.
[a]Above 37.5°C.

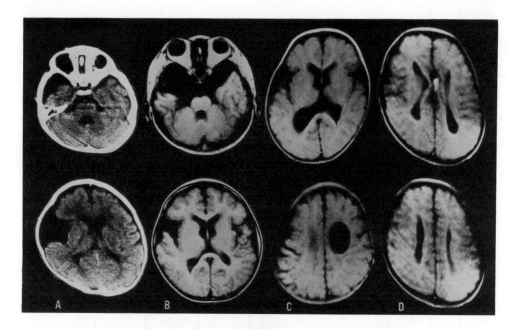

Fig. 23. Rare brain anomalies observed by CT (A) and MRI (B–D). Each pair of images in the upper and lower rows, are from the same patient, respectively. Arachnoid cyst in the middle cerebral fossa (A,B), porencephaly (C), partial agenesis of the corpus callosum with lipoma at the genu (D).

The frequency of WM hyperlucency, observed on CT in the frontal and occipital regions of several FCMD patients, clearly diminished with advancing age. Around age 4 years or earlier, the prevalence of remarkable, bilateral hyperlucency is higher in the frontal than in the occipital regions. We recognized myelin pallor in 2 autopsied cases, one with severe and the other with typical FCMD [72]. The former had diffuse WM hyperlucency, associated with marked ventricular dilatation on CT at 1 year, which had diminished by age 5 years with no change in the ventricles. This case also showed poor axonal development though lack of gliosis and lipid-laden macrophages indicated that a destructive process was unlikely. Comparisons of brain lipid composition between an age-matched normal control and a FCMD case revealed the FCMD to have normal lipid compositions of cerebral WM but an unusual ganglioside pattern in the gray matter [77]. A DMD patient was examined in the same study and no such abnormality was recognized.

When does the WM abnormality manifest? It is noteworthy that Takada et al. [58], examining a 23 week FCMD fetus, found no WM abnormalities. Cases in whom brain CT showed no abnormalities, except for mild ventricular dilatation in the neonatal period, have been reported (Mori et al. [78], Takanashi et al. [79] and Osawa et al., unpublished). However, WM hyperlucency was seen on CT, or an abnormal signal intensity was demonstrated by the IR method on MRI, in these cases at ages 3 months, 50 days and 9 months, respectively. Delayed myelination, as demonstrated by MRI, suggests WM hyperlucency to be a reflection of dysmyelination resulting from a developmental defect. This speculation cannot, however, explain the appearance of WM hyperlucency between days 3 and 50. At present, we do not know the precise nature of this WM abnormality.

The WM hyperlucency in FCMD, in whom hyperlucency is present in early infancy, gradually diminishes with aging and finally disappears after age 3 years. This contrasts with "pure" CMD cases in whom the WM hyperlucency shows no tendency to regress with aging.

The corpus callosum [80]

The corpus callosum (CC) was studied in 24 FCMD patients using mid-sagittal MRI and the results were compared with those of 20 age-matched controls. The measurements included the thickness of the genu, body and splenium; the length, height and 5 specific angles of the CC. The cephalic index was also measured on axial MRI. The correlations among CC length, CC height, the 5 angles and the cephalic index were evaluated. One FCMD case was found to have CC agenesis, as shown in Fig. 24. The thickness of the genu, body, and splenium, as well as CC length, were significantly reduced in FCMD, while the CC height was increased, the angle α was greater and the angle δ reduced. Furthermore, the CC configuration was more rounded, showing a high arch on imaging (Fig. 24). No significant correlations among CC length, CC height, the 5 specific angles and the cephalic index were recognized from any of the FCMD data. These observations demonstrate that CC development in

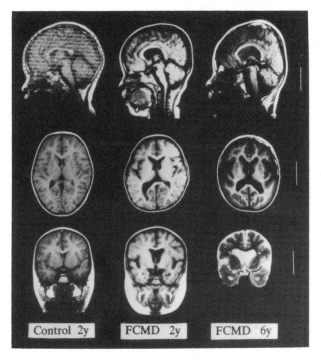

Control 2y   FCMD 2y   FCMD 6y

Fig. 24. Mid-sagittal, axial and coronal T_1-weighted MRI sections from a FCMD case in comparison with those of a normal control. A small, thin, but morphologically complete, corpus callosum was seen in most of the FCMD cases. Significant differences between normal controls and FCMD in the thickness of the genu, body and splenium were identified. All 3 structures were obviously thinner in FCMD. The length of the CC was significantly shorter in FCMD than in controls. There was, however, no apparent difference in the ratio of the CC length to the maximal cranial length. A deformed CC was evident in FCMD, in that the CC was significantly more rounded than in control corpora, showing a high arch on imaging and a dome-like configuration.

58

FCMD is uniquely abnormal, and that the abnormal CC configuration does not correlate with altered cephalic indices.

Cerebellar abnormalities

Aida et al. [81] reviewed brain MR images of 25 patients with FCMD and examined the autopsy specimen of a 23-month-old girl to determine the pathologic nature of the MR findings. MR studies revealed 2 characteristic cerebellar abnormalities: (1) disorganized cerebellar folia (16 cases) recognizable as unusual distortions of the cortex; and (2) clusters of intraparenchymal cysts (23 cases). They found that the two aforementioned-lesions were located close to each other, and, in milder cases, tended to affect only the superior semilunar lobule. At the same time, the autopsied brain revealed small cerebellar cysts, which consisted of dilated subarachnoid spaces buried beneath the malformed cortex. It was speculated that the disorganized folia represent cerebellar polymicrogyria, and that the presence of cerebellar cysts is related to the polymicrogyria. According to their studies, these two MR changes were often present in FCMD and are distinct enough to suggest the radiologic diagnosis. We have not yet studied these clusters of intraparenchymal cysts in any of our typical FCMD cases although such clusters were observed in one of our benign FCMD cases (Fig. 25).

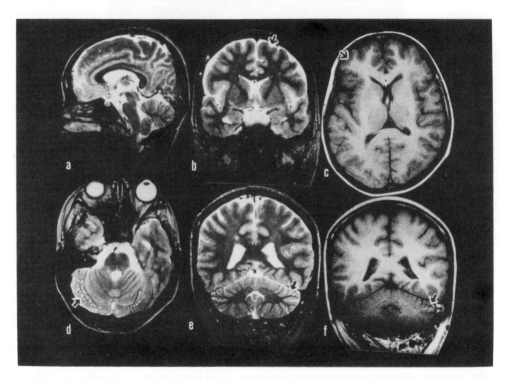

Fig. 25. T_1-weighted (c,f) SE 400/21 and T_2-weighted (a,b,d,e) SE 2500/100 MR images of the brain of a 20-year-old woman with benign FCMD (CMD III/IV of Fukuyama). Pachygyria is recognizable in the left frontal region. The corpus callosum shape is normal. Cerebellar abnormalities, e.g., disorganized cerebellar folia, recognized as unusual distortions of the cortex and clusters of intraparenchymal cysts, can be seen.

Prognosis and cause of death

The most common cause of death in FCMD has long been thought to be pulmonary insufficiency [82].

As shown in Fig. 17, 22 of the 83 typical FCMD cases in our series and 4 of our 14 benign FCMD cases have died. One case died at 1 year, 2 each at the ages of 3, 5 and 6 years, 1 case each at 7, 10 and 11 years, 2 cases each at 12 and 14 years, 1 case at 15 years, 2 at 16 years, and 1 each at 17, 19 and 21 years. In 4 of the 10 cases who died before age 7 years, death was sudden and occurred during sleep. All had been seen by a neighborhood physician, had been diagnosed as having had a "common cold", and were considered to have been nearly recovered from a febrile illness of a few days duration. Other reported causes of death, seen in 1 case each, were suffocation due to difficulty expectorating, status convulsivus, sudden death during sleep, drowning in a deep bath tub due to the mother's inattention, and unknown. Death during sleep, upon recovering from a febrile illness of a few days duration, might be due to respiratory insufficiency caused by the aforementioned transient exacerbation of muscle weakness which follows a febrile illness. Five of the 12 cases who died after age 10 years succumbed to respiratory insufficiency with pneumonia, 1 case to cardiac insufficiency and 1 case to suffocation after a seizure. The causes of death were unknown in the remaining 5 cases.

Mukoyama et al. [82] conducted a study on the prognosis of FCMD using the medical records of autopsied cases, which included clinical data and pathological findings, obtained from 10 national hospitals and 2 other institutes in Japan. The records of 24 patients who died between 1978 and 1991 were collected and analyzed for this study. The ages at death ranged from 2 to 27 years with a mean of 14.29 ± 6.18 years and represented a nearly unimodal distribution. In the 12 patients who died before 1983 the ages at death ranged from 2 to 21 years and the average was 11.58 ± 5.11 years, whereas the 12 patients who died after 1984 ranged in age from 3 to 27 years of age with an average of 17.00 ± 6.44 years. The latter group lived significantly longer than the former ($P < 0.05$). Pulmonary infection was a more frequent cause of death in the group of patients who died before 1983 than in those who died after 1984 (83.3% versus 25.0%). On the other hand, cardiac failure was a more common cause of death in the latter group (8.3% versus 50.0%). The author concluded that these data on the life spans and causes of death in FCMD were similar to those observed in studies of DMD.

Intrafamilial variability

Several FCMD families have been reported in which the clinical pictures of affected siblings differed because of variable disease severity [83–85]. A long time ago, one of the authors, Fukuyama, experienced a family in which two sibs were affected with FCMD while the third sib presented moderate mental retardation without muscle involvement. This is a rather exceptional case; in general, the incidence of neurodevelopmental disorders such as mental retardation among first relatives of FCMD patients is not increased (unpublished data). Intrafamilial variability is further discussed below, in the section on genetic counseling.

60

Management

Principles of management

Unfortunately, no specific treatment for FCMD has yet been developed. As such, treatment of symptoms, appropriate management of complications and psychosocial support for patients and their parents are essential. FCMD patients are prone to certain problems: Dental carries, mild frostbite of the extremities in the winter time due to poor circulation, malnutrition due to limitations in mastication, stemming primarily from jaw muscle involvement, and constipation due to weak abdominal muscle pressure and inadequate exercise. In addition, swallowing difficulty, due to macroglossia, generally develops around 5–6 years.

Respiratory care

FCMD patients have difficulty expectorating, due to weakness of the chest and laryngeal muscles, and are therefore susceptible to pneumonia. It is advisable to prescribe expectorants to clear sputum from the airways and to frequently change the patient's position, especially when bedridden, to prevent the prolonged accumulation of sputum at one anatomical site.

Support and education for patients and their families

Patients show mental retardation and delayed speech. As closing the mouth is eventually impossible, in most cases, it is difficult for patients to pronounce sounds requiring use of the lips, e.g., pa, pi, pu, pe, po, ma, mi, mu, me and mo. Some patients attempt to use the tongue instead of the lower lip. For example, they vocalize "na" in place of "ma" (Fig. 26). These

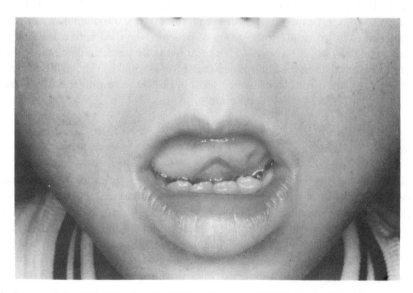

Fig. 26. A close-up of the mouth of a 10-year-old boy with severe FCMD is shown. The patient had to use his tongue, due to marked eversion and thickening of the low lip, to pronounce certain sounds. As a consequence, he could not say "ma", and would instead pronounce the syllable "na".

pronounciation difficulties should prompt the clinician and family members to pay close attention when communicating with patients.

Most patients are shy but they are not autistic. In our experience, the lives of these children have been enriched by joining an ordinary nursery school. Although attending a special school for disabled children is the most appropriate means of educating FCMD patients, most enjoy and benefit from some interaction with healthy children.

As discussed previously, patients generally attain their best motor function level in early childhood. This period provides an opportunity to enhance motor function by introducing toys with wheels and, when necessary, postural supports. We often recommend the use of a slightly inclined board to promote sliding on the buttocks. Infancy is also the period in which parents should be encouraged to actively apply physical therapy aimed at slowing the development of contractures. As the patient ages, and muscle weakness becomes increasingly severe, the risk of pressure sores due to prolonged periods in one position increases. The patient must be actively moved to prevent this complication. Encouraging the parents to maximize the patient's quality of life, by presenting a stimulating and appropriately challenging environment, is also very important (Fig. 27).

Social support systems, provided by the government, for disabled children should be introduced to the family.

Genetic counseling

As FCMD shows an autosomal recessive inheritance pattern, there is a 25% chance of each subsequent offspring having FCMD. Recently, it has become possible to offer reliable prenatal diagnosis, using linkage analysis, to parents requesting this service in our laboratory [16]. In offering genetic counseling, an accurate diagnosis is essential, particularly when dealing with an atypical case.

As an example, we experienced a family with a boy who had been diagnosed as having severe DMD, because he was mentally retarded and had lost the ability to walk without support at age 7 years. During his lifetime, a younger sister was born under the presumption that she was at no genetic risk of muscular dystrophy. The brother died at 14 years due to acute cardiac failure. Polymicrogyria was revealed at autopsy, raising a strong suspicion of CMD. The parents had sought genetic counseling in 1982 as they were concerned about having a similarly afflicted child in the future. No reliable diagnostic technique was available at that time such that without a positive family history and a normal maternal CK value, genetic counseling was offered under a probable but not definite diagnosis of DMD with the possibility of mutation. Two healthy younger sisters were subsequently born. However, a third younger sister, born 6 months before the proband's death, was a floppy infant. This youngest sister was considered to have CMD based on muscle biopsy findings compatible with dystrophic change, dystrophin positivity and pachygyria of the brain by MRI, though the diagnosis is still in question as she has milder facial muscle involvement, milder mental retardation, and less severe involvement of all muscles, than typical FCMD. There were no deletions in the brother's dystrophin DNA. Immunocytochemical staining was performed using 4 dystrophin staining panels. In the brother, dystrophin was positive in muscle cell membranes, suggesting CMD rather than DMD. However, although dystrophin staining was positive with N-terminal antibodies, many membranes showed weak or absent staining with rod domain and C-terminal antibodies. Precise data obtained from this family will be described in another report.

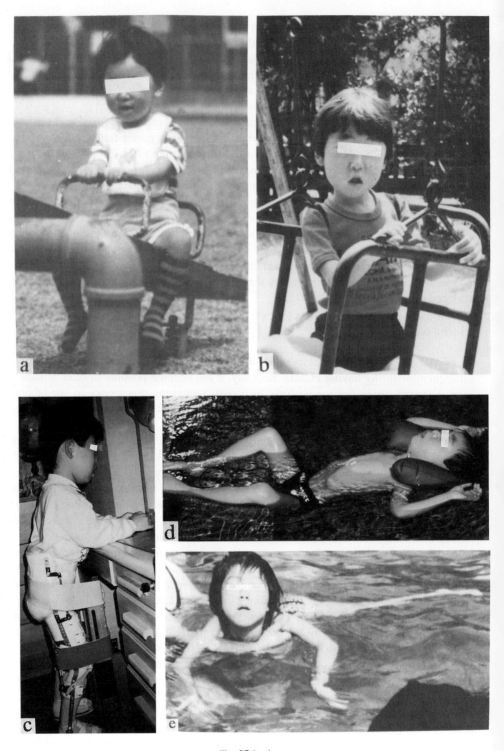

Fig. 27 (a-e).

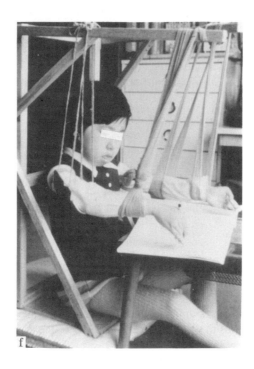

Fig. 27. Enriching the lives of CMD patients. A patient is pictured enjoying a see-saw at age 3 years (a) and a swing at age 4 years (b). A 6 year 10 month old boy with FCMD is able to maintain a standing position by using a long brace, up to hip level, which allows him a wider view than would be possible in the sitting position (c). A 6 year 10 month old boy with FCMD is able to float in a swimming pool, using an air pillow to support his back and compensate for limited anterior flexion of the neck. Note the joint contractures at the hips, knees and ankles (d). A 9 year 6 month old girl with FCMD is able to float in a pool, with assistance from her mother. She has no difficulty holding her head up, due to the tendency for the neck to be extended, and her weight is partially supported by her mother (e). A 10 year 10 month old girl with benign FCMD is shown drawing, with the aid of a special table and arm supports developed by her father. This support system was designed to compensate for the patient's inability to raise either her upper arm or her forearm against gravity (f).

Discussion and summary

It has become increasingly clear that the congenital muscular dystrophies constitute a complex of heterogeneous disease entities. There are forms of CMD with no CNS involvement and, at the same time, it has been demonstrated that some of the congenital muscular dystrophies which do show CNS involvement are associated with mental retardation while others are not. It is also clear that FCMD predominates in Japan, MEB is found mainly in Finland, and WWS is common in other Caucasian populations. We propose the classification of CMDs shown in Table 7. The relationship between CMDs with mental retardation has generated considerable discussion. Dobyns [8] came to the conclusion that MEB and WWS are the same disease while FCMD is a distinct clinical entity. Dobyns et al. [17] and Phiko et al. [18] have demonstrated that the gene locus for WWS and MEB is not at the 9q31-33 locus, though Toda et al. [20] and Yoshioka et al. [19] proposed that the gene locus for WWS and FCMD are the same based on genetic analysis of one family, as discussed above. A com-

64

Table 7

Classification of congenital muscular dystrophies (CMD)

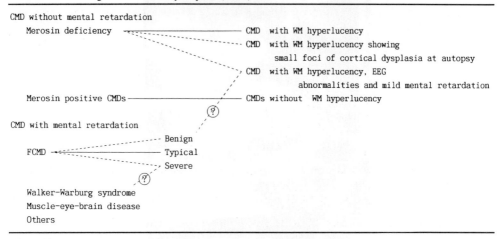

```
CMD without mental retardation
   Merosin deficiency                               CMD  with WM hyperlucency
                                                    CMD  with WM hyperlucency showing
                                                             small foci of cortical dysplasia at autopsy
                                                    CMD  with WM hyperlucency, EEG
                                                             abnormalities and mild mental retardation
   Merosin positive CMDs                            CMDs without  WM hyperlucency
                                              (?)
CMD with mental retardation
                                       Benign
   FCMD                                Typical
                                       Severe
                             (?)
   Walker-Warburg syndrome
   Muscle-eye-brain disease
   Others
```

WM, white matter.

parison of the range of ocular findings in these 3 disorders, some of which overlap, may point to a spectrum analogous to that of Becker and DMD or the acute and chronic forms of Werdnig–Hoffmann disease. In other words, some cases showing an MEB, WWS or FCMD phenotype may represent different defects at the same gene locus. Why these disorders are concentrated in different populations is a question that must be answered by further research. The observation that MEB and WWS tend to have clinicopathological features at the opposite end of the spectrum from FCMD, also remains to be clarified. We speculate that a single defective gene, producing a metabolic error, leads to developmental defects in the CNS and ocular systems, as well as to muscle fragility which leads to the progressive muscle degeneration characteristic of FCMD.

The so-called "pure" form of CMD, which predominates in western countries, and is not associated with mental retardation but does show WM hyperlucency, is probably related to a recently-identified merosin deficiency.

There are some cases which can not easily be diagnosed as belonging to a specific type of CMD. The relationship between severe FCMD and mild WWS (Dobyns), and that between benign FCMD and "pure" CMD with cortical dysplasia at autopsy or ventricular dilatation [12], must be clarified in the future.

Recent advances in genetic analysis, diagnostic imaging modalities and biochemical markers may allow us to elucidate the relationships, or lack thereof, among the various forms of CMD which have been reported to date. Detailed evaluation of each case and an active exchange of information are expected to contribute to further breakthroughs in this field.

Acknowledgments

The authors would like to thank Mrs Masako Hirano and Ms Masami Yamauchi for typing the manuscript. This study was supported by a Research Grant (5A-3 and 8A-3) for Nervous and Mental Disorders from the Ministry of Health and Welfare.

References

1. Fukuyama Y, Kawazura M, Haruna H. A peculiar form of congenital muscular dystrophy. Paediatr Univ Tokyo (Tokyo) 1960; 4: 5–8.

2. Osawa M, Suzuki H, Fukuyama Y. Congenital muscular dystrophy (in Japanese). Shinkei Kenkyu no Shinpo (Tokyo) 1980; 24: 702–717.

3. Fukuyama Y, Osawa M, Suzuki H. Congenital progressive muscular dystrophy of the Fukuyama type – clinical, genetic and pathological considerations. Brain Dev (Tokyo) 1981; 3: 1–29.

4. Osawa M, Arai M, Ikenaka H, et al. Fukuyama type congenital progressive muscular dystrophy. Acta Paediatr Jpn (Tokyo) 1991; 33: 261–269.

5. Huh J, Kim KJ, Ko TS, Kim DW, Hwang SH, Hwang YS. A case of Fukuyama congenital muscular dystrophy (in Korean). Korean J Neurol 1992; 10: 388–394.

6. Osawa M. A genetical and epidemiological study on congenital progressive muscular dystrophy (Fukuyama type) (in Japanese). Tokyo Joshi Ikadaigaku Zasshi (Tokyo) 1978; 48: 204–241.

7. Fukuyama Y, Osawa M. A genetic study of the Fukuyama type congenital muscular dystrophy. Brain Dev (Tokyo) 1984; 6: 373–390.

8. Dobyns WB, Pagon RA, Armstrong D, et al. Diagnostic criteria for Walker–Warburg syndrome. Am J Med Genet 1989; 32: 195–210.

9. Santavuori P, Somer H, Sainio K, et al. Muscle-eye-brain disease (MEB). Brain Dev (Tokyo) 1989; 11: 147–153.

10. Bernier J-P, Brooke MH, Naidich TP, Carroll JE. Myoencephalopathy: cerebral hypomyelination revealed by CT scan of the head in a muscle disease. Trans Am Neurol Assoc 1979; 104: 244–246.

11. Egger J, Kendall BE, Erdohazi M, Lake BD, Wilson J, Brett EM. Involvement of the central nervous system in congenital muscular dystrophies. Dev Med Child Neurol 1983; 25: 32–42.

12. Koga M, Abe M, Tateishi J, Antoku Y, Iwashita H, Miyoshino S. Two autopsy cases of congenital muscular dystrophy of Fukuyama type – a typical and an atypical case (in Japanese). No To Shinkei (Tokyo) 1984; 36: 1103–1108.

13. Trevisan CPT, Carollo C, Segalla P, Angelini C, Drigo P, Giordano D. Congenital muscular dystrophy: brain alterations in an unselected series of Western patients. J Neurol Neurosurg Psychiatry 1991; 54: 330–334.

14. Toda T, Segawa M, Nomura Y, et al. Localization of gene responsible for Fukuyama type congenital muscular dystrophy (FCMD) to chromosome 9q31-33 by linkage analysis. Nat Genet 1993; 5: 283–286.

15. Toda T, Ikegawa S, Okui K, et al. Refined mapping of a gene responsible for Fukuyama-type congenital muscular dystrophy: evidence for strong linkage disequilibrium. Am J Hum Genet 1994; 55: 946–950.

16. Kondo E, Saito K, Toda T, et al. Prenatal diagnosis in two Fukuyama type congenital muscular dystrophy families by polymorphism analysis (in Japanese). Igaku No Ayumi (Tokyo) 1995; 173: 889–890.

17. Dobyns WB. Gene mapping studies in Walker–Warburg syndrome. In: Abstracts for the International Symposium on Congenital Muscular Dystrophies (Satellite Symposium of the VIII International Congress on Neuromuscular Diseases, Kyoto), 1994: 13.

18. Pihko H. Gene mapping studies in muscle-eye-brain disease. In: Abstracts for the International Symposium on Congenital Muscular Dystrophies (Satellite Symposium of the VIII International Congress on Neuromuscular Diseases, Kyoto), 1994: 14.

19. Yoshioka M, Kuroki S, Nigami H, Kawai T, Nakamura H. Clinical variation within sibsip in Fukuyama-type congenital muscular dystrophy. Brain Dev (Tokyo) 1992; 14: 334–337.

20. Toda T, Yoshioka M, Nakahori Y, Kanazawa I, Nakamura Y, Nakagome Y. Genetic identity of Fukuyama-type congenital muscular dystrophy and Walker–Warburg syndrome. Ann Neurol 1995; 37: 99–101.

21. Takeshita K, Yoshino K, Kitahara T, Nakashima T, Kato N. Survey of Duchenne type and congenital type muscular dystrophy in Shimane, Japan. Jpn J Hum Genet (Tokyo) 1977; 22: 43–47.

22. Nakagawa M, Nakamura A, Kubota T, Isashiki Y. Epidemiology of progressive muscular dystrophy in Okinawa, Japan. A study on epidemiology and with emphasis on congenital muscular dystrophy (in Japanese). Kokuryo Okinawa Byoin Igaku Zasshi (Naha) 1989; 10: 45–49.

23. Nakagawa M, Nakahara K, Yoshidome H, et al. Epidemiology of progressive muscular dystrophy in Okinawa, Japan. Classification with molecular biological techniques. Neuroepidemiology 1991; 10: 185–191.

24. Hirayama Y, Suzuki H, Arima M. Survey of Fukuyama type congenital muscular dystrophy in Tokyo (in Japanese). No To Hattatsu (Tokyo) 1992; 24: 27–31.

25. Osawa M, Saito K, Suzuki N, et al. Congenital muscular dystrophy (in Japanese). In: Takahashi K, ed. The 1993 annual report of the research committee on clinics, genetic counseling and epidemiology of progressive muscular dystrophy, sponsored by the Ministry of Health and Welfare of Japan. Hyogo, 1994: 179–184.

26. Sumida S, Osawa M, Arai Y, et al. Clinical and electroencephalographic study on seizure in congenital muscular dystrophy (in Japanese). Tokyo Joshi Ikadaigaku Zasshi (Tokyo) 1993; 63 (extra edn): 36–42.

27. Bordarier C, Aicardi J, Goutières F. Congenital hydrocephalus and eye abnormalities with severe developmental brain defects: Warburg's syndrome. Ann Neurol 1984; 16: 61–65.

28. Raitta C, Lamminen M, Santavuori P, Leisti J. Ophthalmological findings in a new syndrome with muscle, eye and brain involvement. Acta Ophthalmol 1978; 56: 465–472.

29. Fukuyama Y, Osawa M, Okada N, et al. Eye findings in our personal cases with the Fukuyama type congenital muscular dystrophy (in Japanese). In: Nishitani H, ed. The 1985 annual report of the research committee on epidemiology, pathogenesis and therapeutic exploration of progressive muscular dystrophy, sponsored by the Ministry of Health and Welfare of Japan. Kyoto, 1986: 74–79.

30. Osawa M, Okada N, Sugama M, et al. Ophthalmological findings in the patients with Fukuyama type congenital muscular dystrophy. Abstracts for the XXIInd Canadian Congress of Neurological Sciences, Vancouver, 1987: 36–37.

31. Tsutsumi A, Uchida Y, Osawa M, Fukuyama Y. Ocular findings in Fukuyama type congenital muscular dystrophy. Brain Dev (Tokyo) 1989; 11: 413–419.

32. Chijiiwa T, Nishimura M, Inomata EI, Yamana J, Narazaki O, Kurokawa T. Ocular manifestations of congenital muscular dystrophy (Fukuyama type). Ann Ophthalmol 1983; 15: 921–928.

33. Honda K, Yoshioka M. Eye findings in muscular dystrophies (in Japanese). Ganka Rinsho Iho (Tokyo) 1978; 72: 1483–1485.

34. Mishima H, Hirata H, Ono H, Choshi K, Nishi Y, Fukuda K. A Fukuyama type congenital muscular dystrophy associated with atypical gyrate atrophy of the choroid and retina: a case report. Acta Ophthalmol 1985; 63: 155–159.

35. Okada N, Osawa M, Jong Y-J, et al. Physical growth of patients with Fukuyama type congenital muscular dystrophy (in Japanese). Tokyo Joshi Ikadaigaku Zasshi (Tokyo) 1987; 57 (extra edn): 532–539.

36. Fukuyama Y, Osawa M, Sumida S, et al. Teratogenic factors in congenital muscular dystrophy (CMD) – elements of congenital anomalies in congenital muscular dystrophy. Report I. On physical minor anomalies (in Japanese). In: Nishitani H, ed. The 1990 annual report of the research committee on genetics, epidemiology, clinics and treatment of progressive muscular dystrophy, sponsored by the Ministry of Health and Welfare of Japan. Hyogo, 1990: 227–230.

37. Konishi Y, Aoyama M, Segawa M, Kamoshita S. An autopsy case of congenital muscular dystrophy (in Japanese). No To Hattatsu (Tokyo) 1974; 6: 320–327.

38. Nihei K, Naito H, Koizumi N, Suzuki S. Three cases of congenital muscular dystrophy associated with congenital heart malformations. Brain Dev (Tokyo) 1981; 3: 241.

39. Horikawa H, Konishi T, Konagaya M, Mano Y, Takayanagi T. A case of Fukuyama type congenital muscular dystrophy with tetralogy of Fallot (in Japanese). Shinkei Naika (Tokyo) 1986; 24: 99.

40. Ogihara Y, Yagi Y, Sawai N, et al. A case of Fukuyama type congenital muscular dystrophy associated with congenital anal atresia (in Japanese). No To Hattatsu (Tokyo) 1989; 21: 392–393.

41. Miura K, Shirasawa H. Congenital muscular dystrophy of the Fukuyama type (FCMD) with severe myocardial fibrosis; a case report with post-mortem angiography. Acta Pathol Jpn (Tokyo) 1987; 37: 1823–1835.

42. Sumida S, Osawa M, Ikenaka H, et al. Dermatoglyphic findings in children with congenital muscular dystrophy (in Japanese). Tokyo Joshi Ikadaigaku Zasshi (Tokyo) 1992; 62: 1197–1202.

43. Osawa M, Suzuki N, Arai Y, et al. Fukuyama type congenital progressive muscular dystrophy (FCMD) – special comment on the relationship between the case reported by Nakayama et al. and FCMD. Neuropathology (Tokyo) 1993; 13: 259–268.

44. Ishihara T, Yoshitake S, Aoyagi T, Nonaka I, Sugita H. Causes of death in Fukuyama congenital muscular dystrophy. Rinsho Shinkei-gaku (Tokyo) 1984; 24: 968–974.

45. Natsume K, Mizutani A. Long-term observation of two institutionalized cases of Fukuyama type congenital muscular dystrophy (in Japanese). Shoni Naika (Tokyo) 1983; 15: 573–579.

46. Ohtani T, Ozeki E, Ishikawa N, Awaya A, Hashizume Y. An autopsy case of Fukuyama type congenital muscular dystrophy expired at the age of 20 years (in Japanese). No To Hattatsu (Tokyo) 1988; 20: S220.

47. Wada M, Masuda K, Hiraki Y, et al. The 1979 survey of autopsy registry for progressive muscular dystrophy. Particularly on cardiac findings in congenital muscular dystrophy (Fukuyama type) (in Japanese). In: Sobue I, ed. The 1979 annual report of the research committee on clinics, epidemiology and management of progressive muscular dystrophy, sponsored by the Ministry of Health and Welfare of Japan. Nagoya, 1980: 317–322.

48. Tsukagosi H, Toyokura Y, Iwata M, Sugita H, Murakami S. An autopsy case of Fukuyama type congenital muscular dystrophy. In: Okinaka S, ed. Cumulative articles of the research committee on progressive muscular dystrophy, sponsored by the Ministry of Health and Welfare of Japan (II). Tokyo, 1974: 25–30.

49. Fukuyama Y, Ashida E, Osawa M, et al. An evaluation of a study on cardiac function in congenital and Duchenne muscular dystrophies (in Japanese). In: Sobue I, ed. The 1982 annual report of the research committee on epidemiology, clinics and treatment of progressive muscular dystrophy, sponsored by the Ministry of Health and Welfare of Japan. Nagoya, 1983: 160–165.

50. Yoshikawa H, Hirayama Y, Kurokawa T, Houdo S. A case of Fukuyama type congenital muscular dystrophy presenting with rapidly progressive heart failure (in Japanese). Iryo (Tokyo) 1991; 45: 898–902.

51. Osawa M, Ikenaka H. Takeuchi M, et al. Transient exacerbation of muscle weakness induced by febrile illness in patients with Fukuyama type muscular dystrophy (in Japanese). In: Takahashi K, ed. The 1993 annual report of the research committee on clinics, genetic counseling and epidemiology of progressive muscular dystrophy, sponsored by the Ministry of Health and Welfare of Japan. Hyogo, 1994: 191–194.

52. Ikenaka H. Serum enzyme activities in progressive muscular dystrophies. Part 2. Serial changes of serum GOT, GPT, LDH and CK activities in congenital muscular dystrophy (in Japanese). Tokyo Joshi Ikadaigaku Zasshi (Tokyo) 1992; 62: 1185–1196.

53. Ikenaka H. Serum enzyme activities in progressive muscular dystrophies. Part 1. Serial changes of serum GOT, GPT, LDH and CK activities and correlation between GOT and GPT in Duchenne muscular dystrophy (in Japanese). Tokyo Joshi Ikadaigaku Zasshi (Tokyo) 1992; 62: 1175–1184.

54. Sumida S, Osawa M, Okada N, et al. A study of muscle CT findings in patients with Fukuyama type congenital muscular dystrophy (in Japanese). Nihon Shonika Gakkai Zasshi (Tokyo) 1988; 92: 2389–2397.

55. Arai Y, Osawa M, Sumida S, et al. Skeletal muscle CT scannings in early stages of progressive muscular dystrophy: comparison between Duchenne type and Fukuyama type. Brain Dev (Tokyo) 1990; 12 (Suppl): 698.

56. Arai Y, Osawa M, Fukuyama Y. Characteristics of muscle involvement evaluated by computed tomography scanning in early stages of progressive muscular dystrophy: comparison between Duchenne and Fukuyama types. In: Fukuyama Y, Osawa M, Saito K, eds. Congenital muscular dystrophies. Amsterdam: Elsevier, 1997: 119–136.

57. Suzuki H, Osawa M, Shishikura K, et al. Histological changes of skeletal muscles in Fukuyama type congenital muscular dystrophy (in Japanese). Nihon Shonika Gakkai Zasshi (Tokyo) 1984; 88: 1763–1774.

58. Takada K, Nakamura H, Suzumori K, Ishikawa T, Sugiyama N. Cortical dysplasia in a 23-week fetus with Fukuyama congenital muscular dystrophy (FCMD). Acta Neuropathol (Berlin) 1987; 74: 300–306.

59. Nonaka I, Kobayashi O, Osari S, et al. Classical (occidental) congenital muscular dystrophy: clinical and pathologic reevaluation. In: Fukuyama Y, Osawa M, Saito K, eds. Congenital muscular dystrophies. Amsterdam: Elsevier, 1997: 69–77.

60. Miike T, Sugino S, Ohta J, Zhao J, Mutoh T. Neuronal and vascular involvement in Fukuyama type congenital muscular dystrophy. In: Fukuyama Y, Osawa M, Saito K, eds. Congenital muscular dystrophies. Amsterdam: Elsevier, 1997: 207–211.

61. Wakayama Y, Shibuya S, Kumagai T, et al. Ultrastructural alterations of the muscle plasma membrane and related structures in Fukuyama muscular dystrophy: comparative study with other types of muscular dystrophies. In: Fukuyama Y, Osawa M, Saito K, eds. Congenital muscular dystrophies. Amsterdam: Elsevier, 1997: 213–230.

62. Arikawa E, Ishihara T, Nonaka I, Sugita H, Arahata K. Immunocytochemical analysis of dystrophin in congenital muscular dystrophy. J Neurol Sci 1991; 105: 79–87.

63. Arikawa-Hirasawa E, Hayashi Y, Mizuno Y, Nonaka I, Arahata K. Membrane abnormality in Fukuyama congenital muscular dystrophy. In: Fukuyama Y, Osawa M, Saito K, eds. Congenital muscular dystrophies. Amsterdam: Elsevier, 1997: 253–258.

64. Hayashi Y, Nonaka I, Arahata K. Laminin $\alpha2$ (or M) chain abnormality in congenital muscular dystrophy. In: Fukuyama Y, Osawa M, Saito K, eds. Congenital muscular dystrophies. Amsterdam: Elsevier, 1997: 259–265.

68

65. Takemitsu M, Nonaka I, Sugita H. Dystrophin-related protein in skeletal muscles in neuromuscular disorders: immunohistochemical study. Acta Neuropathol (Berlin) 1993; 85: 256–259.

66. Matsumura K, Nonaka I, Campbell KP. Abnormal expression of dystrophin-associated protein in Fukuyama-type congenital muscular dystrophy. Lancet 1993; 27: 521–522.

67. Ogasawara Y, Ito K, Murofushi K. Neuropathological studies on two cases of congenital muscular dystrophy, with special reference to morphological characteristics of micropolygyria found in the cerebral and cerebellar cortex (in Japanese). No to Shinkei (Tokyo) 1976; 28: 451–457.

68. Takada K, Nakamura H, Suzumori K, Tanaka J. Cortical dysplasia in congenital muscular dystrophy with central nervous system involvement (Fukuyama type). J Neuropathol Exp Neurol 1984; 43: 395–407.

69. Takada K, Kasaki S, Rin YS, Nakamura H. Fukuyama type congenital muscular dystrophy; neurofibrillary changes in the locus ceruleus and nucleus basalis of Meynert in a patient with long survival (in Japanese). Shinkei-Naika (Tokyo) 1986; 25: 418–420.

70. Tanaka J, Minamitani M, Takada K. Brain pathology in Fukuyama type congenital muscular dystrophy with special reference to the cortical dysplasia and the occurrence of neurofibrillary tangles. In: Fukuyama Y, Osawa M, Saito K, eds. Congenital muscular dystrophies. Amsterdam: Elsevier, 1997: 189–197.

71. Takashima S, Mizuguchi M. Cytoarchitectonic alterations of the cerebral cortex in FCMD and other cortical dysplasia syndromes. In: Fukuyama Y, Osawa M, Saito K, eds. Congenital muscular dystrophies. Amsterdam: Elsevier, 1997: 199–206.

72. Shishikura K, Osawa M, Suzuki H, et al. Clinicopathologic study of congenital progressive muscular dystrophy (Fukuyama type) (in Japanese). Nihon Shonika Gakkai Zasshi (Tokyo) 1988; 92: 215–224.

73. Dobyns WB, McCluggage CW. Computed tomographic appearance of lissencephaly syndromes. Am J Neuroradiol 1985; 6: 545–550.

74. Okudaira Y, Bandoh K, Wachi A, et al. A case of congenital muscular dystrophy associated with hydrocephalus – CSF dynamics and surgical treatment (in Japanese). No To Hattatsu (Tokyo) 1994; 26: 57–62.

75. Fukuyama Y, Mitsuishi Y, Osawa M, et al. Evaluation of apparently hydrocephalic CT findings in Fukuyama type congenital muscular dystrophy with RI cisternography and serial CT findings (in Japanese). In: Matsumoto S, ed. The 1986 annual report of the research committee on intractable hydrocephalus, sponsored by the Ministry of Health and Welfare of Japan. Kobe, 1987: 111–118.

76. Murasugi H. Neuroimaging study of Fukuyama type congenital muscular dystrophy (in Japanese). Tokyo Joshi Ikadaigaku Zasshi (Tokyo) 1992; 62: 1155–1174.

77. Eda I, Takashima S, Ohno K, Takeshita K. Lipid composition of the cerebral gray and white matter in a case with Fukuyama type congenital muscular dystrophy. Brain Dev (Tokyo) 1985, 7: 523–525.

78. Mori K, Saijo T, Hamaguchi H, et al. A case of Fukuyama type congenital muscular dystrophy with progressive changes of brain CT scanning (in Japanese). No To Hattatsu (Tokyo) 1988; 20: 418–422.

79. Takanashi J, Uetaki K, Iai M, Sugita K, Tanabe Y. A case of Fukuyama type congenital muscular dystrophy; cranial MRI findings prior to the onset of neuromuscular signs (in Japanese). No To Hattatsu (Tokyo) 1989; 21: 588–589.

80. Wang Z-P, Osawa M, Fukuyama Y. Morphometric study of the corpus callosum in Fukuyama type congenital muscular dystrophy by magnetic resonance imaging. Brain Dev (Tokyo) 1995; 17: 104–110.

81. Aida N, Yagishita A, Takada K, Katsumata Y. Cerebellar MR in Fukuyama congenital muscular dystrophy: polymicrogyria with cystic lesions. Am J Neuroradiol 1994; 15: 1755–1759.

82. Mukoyama M, Hizawa K, Kagawa, et al. The life spans, cause of death and pathological findings of Fukuyama type congenital muscular dystrophy – analysis of 24 autopsy cases (in Japanese). Rinsho Shinkeigaku (Tokyo) 1993; 33 (11): 1154–1156.

83. Osawa M, Fukuyama Y. Sumida S, et al. Genetic counseling for muscular dystrophy – problems and dilemma: a practical proposal for problem solving (in Japanese). Tokyo Joshi Ikadaigaku Zasshi (Tokyo) 1992; 62 (11): 1118–1136.

84. Fukuyama Y, Osawa M, Ikeya K, et al. A muscular dystrophy case diagnosed as severe Duchenne muscular dystrophy who showed polymicrogyria on autopsy and positive immunoreactive staining with antidystrophin antibody (in Japanese). In: Takahashi K, ed. The 1992 annual report of the research committee on clinics, genetic counseling and epidemiology of progressive muscular dystrophy, sponsored by the Ministry of Health and Welfare of Japan. Hyogo, 1993: 247–251.

85. Kondo E, Saito K, Ikeya K, et al. Immunocytochemical analysis of dystrophin in muscle specimens in a brother with in intra vitam diagnosis of Duchenne muscular dystrophy and in his sister with congenital muscular dystrophy (in Japanese). Tokyo Joshi Ikadaigaku Zasshi (Tokyo) 1993; 63 (Suppl): E60–E69.

Y. Fukuyama, M. Osawa and K. Saito (Eds.), *Congenital Muscular Dystrophies*
© 1997 Elsevier Science B.V. All rights reserved

Classical (occidental) congenital muscular dystrophy: clinical and pathologic reevaluation

IKUYA NONAKA[1], OSAMU KOBAYASHI[1], SHIN-ICHI OSARI[1],
YUSHIRO YAMASHITA[2], TOYOJIRO MATSUISHI[2], MICHIYO GOTO[3],
YUZO TANABE[3], YUKIKO HAYASHI[1],
KIICHI ARAHATA[1] and EIJIRO OZAWA[1]

[1]*National Center of Neurology and Psychiatry, Kodaira, Tokyo, Japan,*
[2]*Department of Pediatrics, Kurume University Medical School, Kurume, Japan and*
[3]*Department of Neurology, Chiba Children's Hospital, Chiba, Japan*

Introduction

Congenital muscular dystrophy (CMD) has been classified into two major categories, the classical (occidental) form, and Fukuyama type CMD (FCMD) with significant central nervous system (CNS) involvement. Recently, the classical form was further divided into merosin (laminin $\alpha2$)-positive and -negative forms [1]. Patients with the merosin-negative form have relatively severe clinical symptoms, including a marked delay in developmental milestones, marked muscle weakness and hypotonia from early infancy. They exhibit no apparent CNS symptoms but frequent white matter lucency on brain CT-MRI, suggesting delayed myelination [2]. The disease is linked to chromosome 6q22-23 in the merosin-coding region, representing a single disease entity [3]. Patients with the merosin-positive form seem to have milder symptoms with slower progression, but detailed information on large numbers of patients is not available.

In this study, we analyzed the clinical and pathological features of 52 patients with classical (occidental) CMD who fulfilled the following diagnostic criteria: (1) muscle weakness and hypotonia responsible for delayed developmental milestones from early infancy, or apparent muscle weakness on starting to walk; (2) no significant CNS symptoms except for mild mental retardation; (3) no brain CT-MRI abnormalities except for white matter lucency; (4) a muscle pathology with evidence of a necrotic and regenerating process; and (5) normal immunohistochemistry and immunoblotting with anti-dystrophin and anti-dystrophin-associated glycoprotein antibodies. We also applied an anti-merosin antibody [4] to differentiate the merosin-positive and -negative forms.

Patients and methods

From among a total of 4434 patients who had undergone muscle biopsies from 1978 to 1993, we selected those who fulfilled the diagnostic criteria for the classical form of CMD. Questionnaires were sent to the attending physicians regarding the present status and laboratory findings, or we examined patients ourselves at the time of muscle biopsy.

70

Muscle specimens were taken from the biceps brachii muscle in most patients and the quadriceps femoris in some, at ages from 1 month to 19 years. The biopsied muscle was fixed in isopentane cooled with liquid nitrogen, and then serial sections were stained with H&E, modified Gomori trichrome, NADH tetrazolium reductase, succinate dehydrogenase, ATPase with alkaline and acid preincubations, non-specific esterase, cytochrome c oxidase, and acid and alkaline phosphatase stains. Immunohistochemical examinations with monoclonal anti-dystrophin, and anti-dystrophin-associated glycoproteins (DAGs) antibodies of 50 kDa and 43 kDa subunits [4,5] were performed for all muscle biopsies, as described previously.

Results

Incidence of congenital muscular dystrophies

Of 4434 muscle biopsy specimens, 838 revealed progressive muscular dystrophies, i.e. 324 Duchenne (38.7%), 113 Becker (13.5%), 113 limb-girdle (13.5%), 48 facioscapulohumeral (5.7%), and 168 congenital (20.0%), and 72 miscellaneous dystrophies (8.6%). The CMD cases comprised 112 with FCMD, 50 (22 male and 28 female) with merosin-positive CMD (MPCMD), 2 with merosin-negative CMD (MNCMD), and 4 with Ullrich muscular dystrophy. The incidence of MPCMD was approximately half that of FCMD, and 1/6 that of

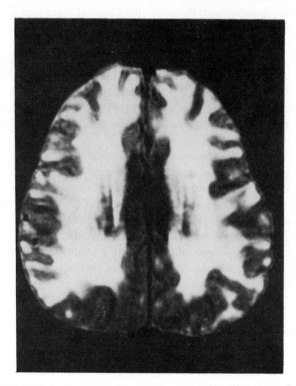

Fig. 1. T2-weighted brain MRI of patient 1 with the merosin-negative form. Note the marked high intensity in the white matter mimicking leukodystrophy.

DMD. Since the incidence of FCMD was estimated to be one in 18 000 youths in Shimane, Japan [6], the incidence of the classical form of CMD may be around 1 in 37 000.

Merosin-negative CMD (MNCMD)

Two patients, one male (patient 1) and one female (patient 2), had similar symptoms. Both patients had no family history. They had marked muscle weakness and hypotonia from birth, with a significant delay in developmental milestones. They were bed-ridden and had not obtained head control by the age of 12 months. They had generalized muscle weakness, with facial muscle involvement and a high-arched palate. Both patients exhibited normal mental development with no central nervous system symptoms. Patient 1 was still wheelchair-bound when last examined at 13 years of age. Patient 2 died at 16 months of age from pneumonia.

The creatine kinase (CK) level was elevated, being 2769 and 1214, respectively. EMG showed a myopathic pattern. Strikingly, both patients exhibited diffuse white matter lucency on CT and T1-weighted MRI, and high intensity on T2-weighted MRI (Fig. 1). Muscle biopsy specimens obtained at 15 months and 23 months, respectively, showed marked variation in fiber size, with scattered necrotic and regenerating fibers, and dense fibrosis (Fig. 2). Intramuscular peripheral nerves were well-myelinated. On immunostaining with a merosin (laminin α2) antibody (Chemicon), no fibers were stained positively (Fig. 3). On electron microscopy, the basal lamina was occasionally observed to be blurred and disrupted (Fig. 4).

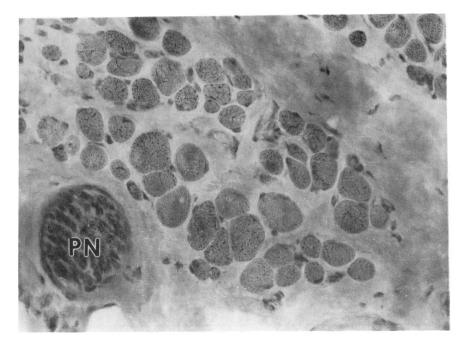

Fig. 2. In addition to marked variation in fiber size, there is dense interstitial fibrosis. A peripheral nerve bundle (PN) is well myelinated. Patient 2 with the merosin-negative form. Modified Gomori trichrome, ×500.

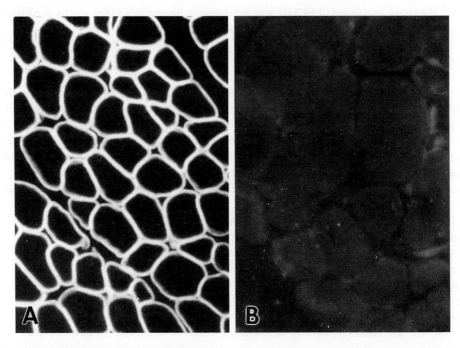

Fig. 3. Immunohistochemical staining with an anti-merosin (laminin $\alpha2$) antibody. Although all muscle fibers in a normal control exhibit positive reactivity (A), no fibers are stained positively in a patient with the merosin-negative form (B). A, ×300; B, ×600.

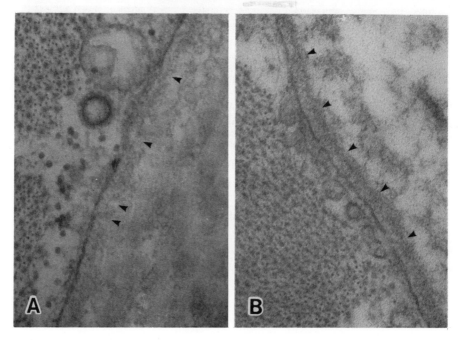

Fig. 4. While most of fibers have blurred basal lamina (arrowheads) in the merosin-negative form (both patients 1 and 2) (A), all have clearly identifiable lamina in the merosin-positive form (B). A,B, ×60 000.

Merosin-positive CMD (MPCMD)

Of the 50 patients with MPCMD, none were familial except for one pair of siblings with similar symptoms. One parent was a first cousin.

During pregnancy, 7 mothers (14%) noticed decreased fetal movements. At birth, 27 patients (54%) were noted to be abnormal, including notable muscle weakness and hypotonia, poor sucking and respiratory difficulty. One patient died of respiratory failure at 3 months of age. Forty-three patients (86%) had delayed developmental milestones; the ages on obtaining head control, rolling over, sitting, standing and walking alone were delayed, averaging 5.0, 9.5, 10.8, 19.0 and 23.9 months, respectively. None started to walk after 4 years of age. Of 38 patients followed for over 4 years of age, 35 (92%) learned to walk alone, and 6 became non-ambulant at 4, 6, 8, 10, 12, 13 and 19 years, respectively. Two patients died before they obtained head control. As shown in Fig. 5, most patients followed up did not exhibit rapid progression. Five patients died of respiratory failure between 3 months and 12 years of age. All 6 patients above 20 years of age had remarkable muscle weakness, suggesting that the disease was progressive.

All patients had proximal dominant or generalized muscle weakness. Mild facial muscle involvement was noted in 26/47 (55%) patients. Two patients had difficulty in swallowing. One patient was on mechanical ventilation during sleep because of respiratory muscle weakness. Joint contractures were noted in 27 (54%) patients, involving the knee, ankle and hip joints, and spine deformity was noted in 16 (32%) patients. A high-arched palate was noted in 13 (26%) patients. Four patients were moderately and 3 mildly mentally retarded.

Of 38 patients who underwent cranial CT and/or MRI, cerebral atrophy was noted in 9 (24%) and white matter lucency in 4 (11%). The CK level was elevated in 27 (54%) patients, averaging 715 (normal range 30–200). Twenty-five of the 30 (83%) patients aged above 5 years had normal CK levels.

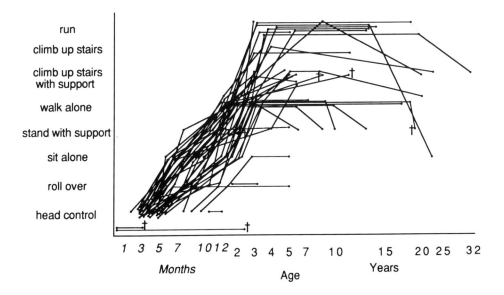

Fig. 5. A follow-up study of 50 patients with the merosin-positive form.

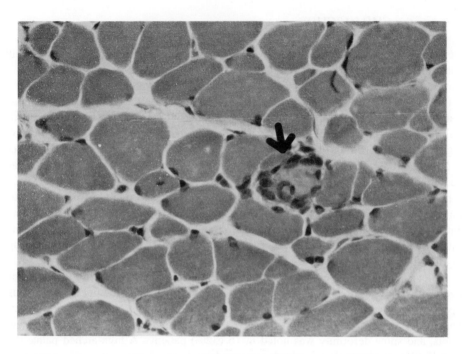

Fig. 6. Representative muscle histology in patients with the merosin-positive form. In addition to mild variation in fiber size, there are necrotic (arrow) and regenerating fibers showing dystrophic changes. Interstitial fibrosis is minimal. HE, ×500.

In all muscle biopsy specimens, there was a myopathic change, with evidence of a necrotic and regenerating process. Among the 30 patients of less than 5 years of age, necrotic fibers were seen in 24 (80%), with minimal to moderate fibrosis (Fig. 6). The muscle pathology in 22 patients aged over 5 years showed more advanced myopathic changes, with moderate to marked variation in fiber size, cytoarchitectural changes with lobulated fibers, fiber splitting and a moth-eaten appearance. Necrotic fibers were seen in only 13 (59%) biopsy specimens. Marked fat replacement was noted in patients above 10 years of age. An abnormal fiber type distribution, including fiber type grouping, type 1 fiber predominance and type 2B fiber deficiency was predominantly seen in older children. All biopsy specimens showed normal immunohistochemical expression as to dystrophin, 50DAG, 43 DAG and merosin antibodies. The pathologic findings are summarized in Fig. 7.

Discussion

Congenital muscular dystrophy comprises a group of heterogeneous disorders with variable clinical expressions and pathological findings. Among them, FCMD is a distinct clinical entity characterized by early onset of muscle weakness, notable mental retardation, peculiar brain anomalies and advanced dystrophic muscle changes from early infancy [7]. Recently, the gene locus in FCMD was proved to be linked to chromosome 9q31–33 [8]. Since Tomé et al. [1] identified patients with a merosin-negative form of CMD, non-FCMD is now di-

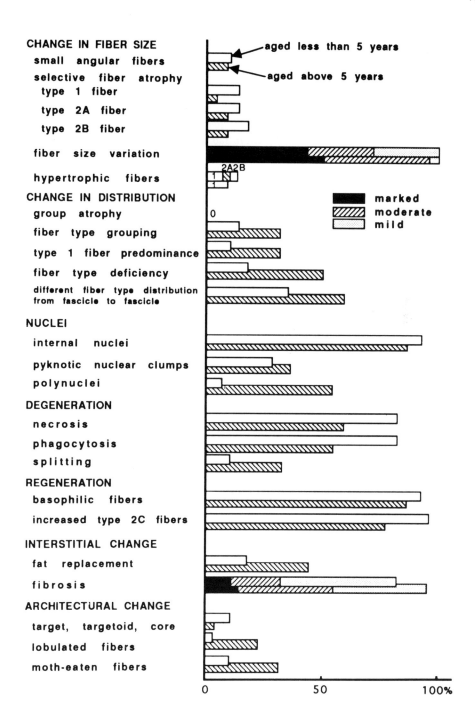

Fig. 7. Histologic and histochemical summary of the 50 patients with the merosin-positive form.

vided into two types, the merosin-negative (MNCMD) and -positive forms (MPCMD). In European countries, the ratio of MNCMD to MPCMD patients is approximately 1 to 1 [9].

In MNCMD, patients have relatively homogeneous clinical features, i.e. marked muscle weakness since early infancy and delayed motor milestones, a normal intelligence, an increased serum CK level, and white matter lucency on CT and MRI [2]. The white matter abnormality in CMD may be a crucial finding for understanding the pathogenetic mechanism of the disease process. Most patients remained bed-ridden and died from respiratory problems. MNCMD is probably less frequent in Japan, because only two patients have been identified in our laboratory. They had similar symptoms to those described by Tomé et al. [1].

The incidence of MPCMD is estimated to be 1/37 000 under 20 years of age in Japan, based on the incidence of FCMD described in the literature [6], although there might be an institutional difference. Since there were no patients with MPCMD inherited as an autosomal dominant trait and all but a pair of siblings did not have a positive family history, the disease may be inherited as an autosomal recessive trait. Since 14% of the patients were noted to have decreased fetal movements, and approximately half the patients were hypotonic, with muscle weakness and frequent joint contractures at birth, the disease probably starts from the fetal stage. In FCMD, decreased fetal movements are recognized in 6% of pregnancies [10], and about half the patients have muscle symptoms at birth [7]. Although the muscle weakness appears at relatively early infancy, MPCMD cases are benign as to clinical symptoms. Ninety-two percent of patients with MPCMD learn to walk by 4 years of age. On the other hand, ambulatory patients with FCMD and MNCMD are quite exceptional [7,9].

MPCMD is a slowly progressive disease: patients over 10 years apparently show more marked muscle weakness and abnormal muscle pathology. The CK levels in MPCMD are not as high as those in DMD [11,12], BMD [12,13], FCMD [7], and MNCMD [9], reflecting the less necrotic process in MPCMD. The overall histopathological findings in MPCMD are milder than those in FCMD, in parallel with the disease severity. In FCMD, there is a prominent necrotic and regenerating process, with dense fibrosis from early infancy [14,15]. As seen in chronic progressive muscular dystrophies such as the limb girdle and Becker muscular dystrophies, there is an abnormal fiber type distribution in MPCMD, showing fiber type grouping and fiber type predominance, which becomes more prominent as the disease progresses. In a patient who had undergone a muscle biopsy twice, at ages 1 and 4 years, the fiber type variation, lobulated fibers and a moth-eaten appearance were observed in the second biopsy specimen, reflecting the pathologic progression of dystrophic changes. Accordingly, the fiber type variation may have been caused by modification of innervation after repeated fiber necrosis and regeneration. There was no distinct correlation between the histopathological findings and the prognosis.

References

1. Tomé FMS, Evangelista T, Leclerc A, et al. Congenital muscular dystrophy with merosin deficiency. C R Acad Sci (Paris) 1994; 317: 351–357.
2. Fardeau MP, Tomé FMS, Dubowitz V, Hillaire D. Lifting the lid on congenital muscular dystrophy. Presented at the 8th International Congress on Neuromuscular Disease, Kyoto, 1994.
3. Leivo I, Engvall E. Merosin, a tissue specific for basement membranes of Schwann cells, striated muscle, and trophoblasts, is expressed late in nerve and muscle development. Proc Natl Acad Sci USA 1988; 85: 1544–1548.

4. Yamamoto H, Hagiwara Y, Mizuno Y, Yoshida M, Ozawa E. Heterogeneity of dystrophin-associated proteins. J Biochem 1993; 114: 132–139.
5. Mizuno Y, Yoshida M, Nonaka I, Hirai S, Ozawa E. Expression of utrophin (dystrophin-related protein) and dystrophin-associated glycoproteins in muscles from patients with Duchenne muscular dystrophy. Muscle Nerve 1994; 17: 206–216.
6. Takeshita K, Yoshino K, Kitahara T, Nakashima T, Kato N. Survey of Duchenne type and congenital muscular dystrophy in Shimane, Japan. Jpn J Hum Genet (Tokyo) 1977; 22: 43–47.
7. Fukuyama Y, Osawa M, Suzuki H. Congenital progressive muscular dystrophy of the Fukuyama type - Clinical, genetic and pathological considerations. Brain Dev (Tokyo) 1981; 3: 1–29.
8. Toda T, Segawa M, Nomura Y, et al. Localization of a gene for Fukuyama type congenital muscular dystrophy to chromosome 9q31–33. Nat Genet 1993; 5: 283–286.
9. Dubowitz V. Exciting new developments in CMD. In: Fukuyama Y, Osawa M, Saito K, eds. Congenital musular dystrophies. Amsterdam: Elsevier, 1997: 21–30.
10. Segawa M. Clinical studies of congenital muscular dystrophy (in Japanese). No to Hattatsu (Tokyo) 1970; 2: 439–451.
11. Brooke MH, Fenichel GM, Griggs RC, et al. Clinical investigation in Duchenne dystrophy: 2. Determination of the "power" of therapeutic trials based on the natural history. Muscle Nerve 1983; 6: 91–103.
12. Zellweger H, Durnin R, Simpson J. The diagnostic significance of serum enzymes and electrocardiograms in various muscular dystrophies. Acta Neurol Scand 1972; 48: 87–101.
13. Bushby KMD, Gardner-Medwin D. The clinical, genetic and dystrophin characteristics of Becker muscular dystrophy. J Neurol 1993; 240: 98–104.
14. Nonaka I, Chou SM. Congenital muscular dystrophy. In: Vinken PJ, Bruyn GW, eds. Handbook of clinical neurology, Vol 41. Amsterdam: North-Holland, 1979: 27–50.
15. Nonaka I, Sugita H, Takada K, Kumagai K. Muscle histochemistry in congenital muscular dystrophy with central nervous system involvement. Muscle Nerve 1982; 5: 102–106.
16. Nonaka I, Takagi A, Sugita H. The significance of type 2C fibers in Duchenne muscular dystrophy. Muscle Nerve 1981; 4: 326–333.

Addendum

Since submission of this manuscript, we have published 4 papers on classical congenital muscular dystrophy.

1. Hayashi YK, Koga R, Tsukahara T, et al. Deficiency of laminin $\alpha2$-chain mRNA in muscle in a patient with merosin-negative congenital muscular dystrophy. Muscle Nerve 1995; 18: 1027–1030.
2. Osari S, Kobayashi O, Yamashita T, et al. Basement membrane abnormality in merosin-negative congenital muscular dystrophy. Acta Neuropathol 1996; 91: 332–336.
3. Kobayashi O, Hayashi Y, Arahata K, et al. Congenital muscular dystrophy: clinical and pathological study of 50 patients with the classical (occidental) merosin-positive form. Neurology 1996; 46: 815–818.
4. Nonaka I, Kobayashi O, Osari S. Non-dystrophinopathic muscular dystrophies including myotonic dystrophy. Sem Pediatr Neurol 1996; 3: 110–121.

Y. Fukuyama, M. Osawa and K. Saito (Eds.), *Congenital Muscular Dystrophies*

CHAPTER 5

Clinical and immunocytochemical evidence of heterogeneity in classical (occidental) congenital muscular dystrophy

MICHEL FARDEAU and FERNANDO M.S. TOMÉ

Research Group on Development, Pathology and Regeneration of the Neuromuscular System, INSERM U.153, Institut de Myologie, Hôpital de la Salpêtrière, 47, boulevard de l'Hôpital, FR-75651 Paris Cédex 13, France

Introduction

The term, "congenital muscular dystrophy" (CMD), comprises a heterogeneous group of very disabling, hereditary muscle diseases. In Western countries, they are described as [1] "pure" muscular disorders with a very early clinical onset, multiple contractures and joint deformities [2], and a myopathic or "dystrophic" histopathological pattern [3,4]. An autosomal recessive mode of inheritance has generally been postulated. The clinical presentation of this "occidental" form is in contrast with that of the peculiar form identified in Japan by Fukuyama et al. [5], usually referred to as Fukuyama congenital muscular dystrophy (FCMD), associated with severe developmental defects of the central nervous system, and with the entity reported in Finland with severe brain and eye abnormalities [6].

However, series of anatomical and radiological observations made in Western countries showed that white matter changes may also be present in certain cases of CMD [7–11], but without any marked intellectual retardation or cortical malformations. Furthermore, the relationship between CMD and other syndromes sharing similar histopathological changes in muscle biopsy specimens, such as in Ullrich's congenital atonic sclerotic syndrome [12] or cases of the rigid spine syndrome [13], raised difficult nosological questions.

The marked increase in endomysial connective tissue observed in muscle biopsy specimens from CMD patients led to the idea that the primum movens of these dystrophies could be located in the extracellular matrix, but early studies [14,15] failed to reveal any qualitative abnormalities in extracellular matrix components. The discovery of a large oligomeric complex of sarcolemmal glycoproteins associated with dystrophin, providing a link between the subsarcolemmal cytoskeleton and laminin [16], led to investigation of whether or not a laminin variant could be involved in these dystrophies. Laminin is a heterotrimer made up of three chains, which are arranged in various combinations in different basement membranes. The laminin variant in the muscle and nerve basement membranes is merosin made up of M (α2), B1 (β1) and B2 (γ1) chains (see [17] for a review). The laminin M chain was found to be partially deficient in FCMD [18]. In the classic, occidental type of CMD, we have demonstrated that merosin is markedly deficient or absent, by both immunocytochemical and immunoblot techniques, in a series of cases, but not in all [19]. This study suggested that the laminin M chain gene could cause the disease, and as this gene had been localized to chromosome 6q22-q23 [20], a genetic study involving homozygosity mapping and linkage analysis was undertaken on a panel of consanguineous families living in France and

Turkey. This allowed localization of the merosin-negative CMD locus to a 16 cM region of chromosome 6q2 [21]. Interestingly, in merosin-positive families it was not mapped to either chromosome 6q2 or chromosome 9q31-33, on which the FCMD gene was localized [22]. These findings led to clinical reevaluation of the two CMD groups, defined according to the presence or absence of merosin. Initial evaluation suggested that these two groups could be distinguished by their clinical patterns and their severity.

Material and methods

Two series of 15 patients were analyzed. All of them fulfilled the inclusion criteria defined by the International Consortium on Congenital Muscular Dystrophies [23]. Hypotonia, contractures, motor development and respiratory insufficiency were graded according a 4-grade scale: 0 (absent), + (benign), ++ (moderate), +++ (severe). Mental development was considered normal (N), subnormal (subN) or evidently delayed (D). Brain imaging was performed in 10/30 cases. Serum creatine kinase (CK) was graded as normal, or up to 3 times (+), up to 10 times (++) or more than 10 times (+++) the normal values (Tables 1 and 2).

Biopsy specimens were obtained from the deltoid muscle in 29 patients (one affected child, the sister of a patient, was not biopsied). The biopsy samples were frozen in isopentane cooled in liquid nitrogen and then stored at −80°C. All specimens were studied by conventional histology, histochemistry and immunocytochemistry, on frozen cryostat sections. Indirect immunofluorescence, using monoclonal antibodies against dystrophin (DYS2 and DYS3, Novocastra), laminin M-chain (Chemicon), and laminin chains A(4C7), B1(4E10) and B2(2E80) (Gibco BRL), was performed on cryosections of skeletal muscle biopsy specimens from the patients, as previously described [19]. For comparison, cryosections from normal controls and patients with other muscle diseases (Duchenne, Becker, severe childhood autosomal recessive with adhalin deficiency, limb girdle linked to chromosome 15, facioscapulohumeral, myotonic and oculopharyngeal muscular dystrophies) were processed identically. The sections were examined under a Zeiss Axioplan fluorescence microscope. Photographs were taken under identical conditions with the same exposure time.

Results and discussion

The immunocytochemical studies showed a merosin (laminin M chain) deficiency in the muscle biopsy specimens from 15 patients ("merosin-negative") and the normal presence of this protein in 14 other patients ("merosin-positive"). The affected child who was not biopsied was a sister of a patient with normal expression of merosin. In 13 merosin-negative cases, the merosin deficiency was complete (Fig. 1a), not only in the basement membrane of muscle fibers but also in those of peripheral nerves and neuromuscular junctions. In two merosin-negative cases, there was a trace of this protein; faint staining of varying intensity was observed around most muscle fibers. In all 15 merosin-negative cases there was overexpression, to varying degrees, of the laminin A chain (Fig. 1b) in the basement membrane of muscle fibers. In muscle biopsy specimens from normal controls, with the antibodies against this protein, labelling was almost exclusively confined to the blood vessel basement membrane. In most merosin-positive cases there was no overexpression of laminin A. However, in several of these cases, there was overexpression of this protein around a few muscle

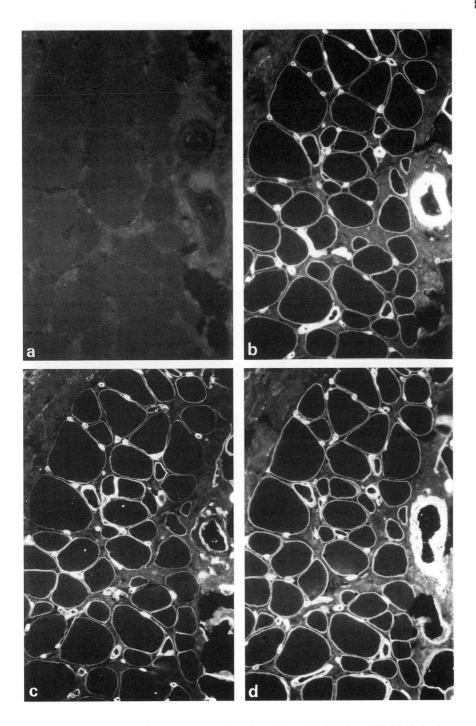

Fig. 1. Immunocytochemical analysis of merosin (a), and laminin A (b), B1 (c) and B2 (d) chains in a muscle biopsy specimen from a 10-year-old male patient (case 4 in the "merosin-negative" group). Shown is the absence of merosin (a) and the overexpression of the chain laminin A (b) around muscle fibers. There is no significant change in the expression of either the laminin B1 (c) or B2 (d) chain. Magnification ×155.

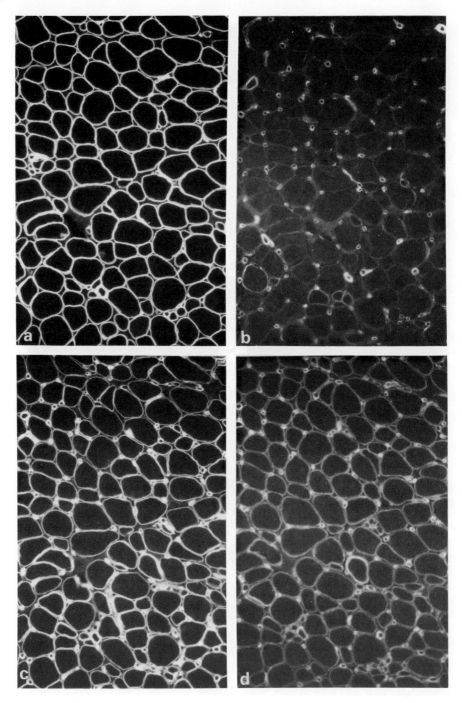

Fig. 2. Immunocytochemical analysis of merosin (a), and laminin A (b), B1 (c) and B2 (d) chains in a muscle biopsy specimen from a 7-year-old patient (case 13 in the "merosin-positive" group). Shown is the normal expression of merosin (a) and the moderate overexpression of the laminin A chain around a few muscle fibers (b). In this case, the labelling with the antibody against the laminin B1 chain (c) is stronger than that with the antibody against the laminin B2 chain (d). Magnification ×155.

Table 1
Merosin-negative CMD group

No.	Age at biopsy (years)	Sex	Hypotonia	Contractures	Delayed motor development	Respiratory insufficiency	Mental development	Brain abnormalities	Serum CK	Observations
1	3.3	F	+++	+++	++	++	N	+	n.d	Fam.
2	0.5	M	+++	+++	+++	+++	N (?)	n.d.	++	Died at 7 months
3	3	M	++	+++	+	0	N	N	+++	
4	10	M	+ (?)	++	++	n.d.	N	n.d.	n.d.	
5	2.3	F	+	++	++	+	N	n.d.	+	
6	0.25	M	+	+	+	+	N (?)	+	+++	
7	0.9	F	++	++	+++	++	N	+	+++	
8	3	F	+	++	++	n.d.	N	n.d.	n.d.	
9	0.8	M	+++	++	++(+)	+++	Sub N (?)	n.d.	++	Died at 5 years
10	0.1	F	+++	++	+++	+++	N	n.d.	+++	Died at 2 years
11	5	M	++	+++	++	+	N	+	++	
12	0.7	M	++	++	++	+(+)	Sub N (?)	+	+++	
13	0.7	M	++	++	+	+	N	n.d.	++	
14	0.2	M	+++	++	+++	++	N	+	+++	
15	4.5	F	++	+++	++	+++	n.d.	n.d.	+	Died at 6 years

84

Table 2
Merosin-positive CMD group

No.	Age at biopsy (years)	Sex	Hypotonia	Contractures	Delayed motor development	Respiratory insufficiency	Mental development	Brain abnormalities	Serum CK	Observations
1	8	M	+	+	++	n.d.	n.d.	n.d.	N	Ullrich's syndrome
2	16	F	++	+	+++	0	D	n.d.	+++	
3	20	M	+	++	N	n.d.	n.d.	n.d.	+	m. hypertrophy
4	7	F	++	+	N(?)	++	N	n.d.	+++	
5	6	M	?	±	+	n.d.	N	n.d.	n.d.	
6	11	F	+(?)	+	+	0	N	n.d.	N	
7	0.5	F	+	+	+++	+	N	n.d.	+++	
8	–	F	+	+	+	+++	N	N	+++	
9	2.3	M	+	+	+	0	N	n.d.	++	
10	5	M	+	++	+	n.d.	N	N	n.d.	
11	4	F	+	+	N	+	N	N	+	
12	8	F	+	+++	+	n.d.	D	N	N	
13	7	M	+(?)	+	N	0	N	n.d.	+	
14	9.5	M	+	+++	+	0	N	n.d.	N	Ullrich's syndrome
15	4	F	++	++	+	++	N	n.d.	++	

fibers (Fig. 2b). The anti-laminin B1 and anti-laminin B2 chain antibodies showed some variation in the intensity of the labelling in both groups of patients. Similar variation was seen in patients with other pathologies, and until now such changes were not considered as being of definite pathological significance. The anti-dystrophin antibodies did not show significant changes in either the merosin-negative or merosin-positive cases.

The clinical data allowed clear differentiation of the two series of merosin-negative and merosin-positive CMD cases. The merosin-negative cases (Table 1) formed a fairly homogeneous group: neonatal hypotonia was constant, most often marked or severe (11/15). Contractures were constant, multiple, and most often considered to be severe (14/15). Motor development was markedly delayed (12/15), and only some children were able to sit without support or to stand (3/15). Respiratory insufficiency was present in 8/13 (not determined in two cases). Mental development was generally considered normal (10/15), being doubtful in four cases. Epileptic seizures were present in one case (no. 7). In this series, seven patients underwent brain CT scanning or MRI: white matter abnormalities were present in six of them. Serum CK was markedly increased in 10/12 cases (not determined in three cases). Finally, the severity of the disease was reflected by the fact that four (out of 15) died before the age of 6 years.

In contrast, the merosin-positive cases (Table 2) formed a more heterogeneous group, generally with less severity. Neonatal hypotonia was rarely marked (3/15); contractures were constant, but rarely severe (2/15), and often delayed. Motor development was rarely severely delayed (3/15). Respiratory insufficiency was clearly noticed in only 3/15. Mental development was generally considered to be normal (10/12). Of three cases who underwent brain imaging, none showed any abnormality. Serum CK was increased in most cases (9/13). None of the children in this series were reported to have died. Furthermore, it should be noted that the group of merosin-positive patients was also heterogeneous on clinical examination. Most of the cases were considered to have classical "CMD", but two were reported to have possible Ullrich's syndrome (case nos. 1 and 14), and one case was remarkable in the presence of marked hypertrophy of the scapular, trunk and pelvic muscles before the wasting process started (case no. 4).

The differences between merosin-negative and merosin-positive CMD cases should be analyzed in a more precise and quantitative way. However, it should be noted that similar differences were found in the series of cases reported by Philpot et al. [24] and by Topaloglu et al. [25]. Taken together, these results suggest that merosin-negative CMD forms an

Table 3

Merosin-negative CMD		Merosin-positive CMD
Frequently marked	Hypotonia	Generally benign
Generally severe	Contractures	Rarely severe, often delayed
Markedly delayed	Motor development	Delayed
Marked and stable	Muscular weakness	Slowly progressive
Often severe	Respiratory involvement	Rarely severe
Generally normal	Mental development	Generally normal
Frequent	Brain imaging changes	Absent (?)
Markedly increased	Serum creatine kinase	Increased
↑		↑
HOMOGENEOUS GROUP		HETEROGENEOUS GROUP

homogeneous entity (Table 3). This is supported by the linkage to the merosin gene locus on chromosome 6q2 found in a series of merosin-negative CMD cases from France and Turkey [21]. Two familial cases in our series (nos. 7 and 8) belong to this informative group.

By contrast, the group of merosin-positive cases is clinically heterogeneous (Table 3), and should be analyzed in more detail, as several subsets seem to coexist within this group. As reported elsewhere [21], no linkage was found in this merosin-positive CMD group with either the chromosome 6q2 locus or the chromosome 9q31-33 locus. Separate panels of clinically/phenotypically similar familial cases should be analyzed in the future to precisely define their genetic and nosological situation.

Acknowledgements

This work would not have been possible without the cooperation of A. Barois, B. Estournet and all clinicians who referred the patients or provided the muscle biopsy specimens, T. Evangelista, E. Manole, M. Chevallay and H. Collin, who contributed to the study of the muscle biopsy specimens, Y. Sunada and K.P. Campbell, who collaborated in this study, and D. Hillaire, A. Leclerc and P. Guicheney, who performed the molecular genetic work.

References

1. Howard R. A case of congenital defect of the muscular system (dystrophia muscularis congenita) and its association with congenital talipes equino-varus. Proc R Soc Med 1908; 1 (Pathol): 157–166.
2. Banker BQ, Victor M, Adams RD. Arthogryposis multiplex due to congenital muscular dystrophy. Brain 1957; 80: 319–334.
3. Gubbay SS, Walton JN, Pearce GW. Clinical and pathological study of a case of congenital muscular dystrophy. J Neurol Neurosurg Psychiatry 1966; 29: 500–508.
4. Afifi A, Zellweger H, McCormick WF, Mergner W. Congenital muscular dystrophy: light and electron microscopic observations. J Neurol Neurosurg Psychiatry 1969; 32: 273–280.
5. Fukuyama Y, Kawazura M, Haruna H. A peculiar form of congenital progressive muscular dystrophy. Report of fifteen cases. Pediatr Univ Tokyo 1960; 4: 5–8.
6. Santavuori P, Leisti J, Kruus S. Muscle, eye and brain disease: a new syndrome. Neuropaediatries 1977; 8 (suppl 8): 553 (Abstract).
7. Egger J, Kendall BE, Erduhazi M, Lake BD, Wilson J, Brett EM. Involvement of the central nervous system in congenital muscular dystrophies. Dev Med Child Neurol 1983; 25: 32–42.
8. Echenne B, Arthuis M, Billard C et al. Congenital muscular dystrophy and cerebral CT scan anomalies. Results of a collaborative study of the "Société de Neurologie Infantile". J Neurol Sci 1986; 75: 7–22.
9. Leyten QH, Gabreëls FJM, Reiner WO, ter Laak HJ, Sengers RCA, Mullaart RA. Congenital muscular dystrophy. J Pediatr 1989; 115: 214–221.
10. Trevisan C, Carollo CP, Segalla P, Angelini C, Drigo P, Giordanor R. Congenital muscular dystrophy: brain alterations in an unselected series of Western patients. J Neurol Neurosurg Psychiatry 1991; 54: 330–334.
11. Topaloglu H, Yalaz K, Renda Y, et al. Occidental type cerebromuscular dystrophy. A report of eleven cases. J Neurol Neurosurg Psychiatry 1991; 54: 226–229.
12. Ullrich O. Kongenitale, atonisch-sklerotische Muskeldystrophie, ein weiterer Typus der heredodegenerativen Erkankungen des neuromuskularen Systems. Z ges Neurol Psychiatr. 1930; 126: 171–201.
13. Dubowitz V. Rigid spine syndrome: a muscle syndrome in search of a name. Proc R Soc Med 1973; 66: 219–220.
14. Duance VC, Stephens HR, Dunn M, Bailey AJ, Dubowitz V. A role for collagen in the pathogenesis of muscular dystrophy? Nature 1980; 284: 470–472.

15. Hantaï D, Labat-Robert J, Grimaud JA, Fardeau M. Fibronectin, laminin, type I, III & IV collagen in Duchenne's muscular dystrophy, congenital muscular dystrophies and congenital myopathies: an immunocytochemical study. Connect Tissue Res 1985; 13: 273–281.

16. Ibraghimov-Beskrovnaya O, Ervasti JM, Leveille CJ, Slaughter CA, Sernett SW, Campbell KP. Primary structure of dystrophin-associated glycoproteins linking dystrophin to extracellular matrix. Nature 1992; 355: 696–702.

17. Yurchenko PD, O'Rear JJ. Basal lamina assembly. Curr Opin Cell Biol 1994; 6: 674–681.

18. Arikawa E, Ishihara T, Nonaka I, Sugita H, Arahata K. Immunocytochemical analysis of dystrophin in congenital muscular dystrophy. J Neurol Sci 1991; 105; 79–87.

19. Tomé FMS, Evangelista T, Leclerc A, et al. Congenital muscular dystrophy with merosin deficiency. CR Acad Sci Paris 1994; 317: 351–357.

20. Vuolteenahno R, Nissinen M, Sainio K, et al. Human laminin M chain (merosin): complete primary structure, chromosomal assignment, and expression of the M and A chain in human fetal tissues. J Cell Biol 1994; 124: 381–394.

21. Hillaire D, Leclerc A, Fauré S, et al. Localization of merosin-negative congenital muscular dystrophy to chromosome 6q2 by homozygosity mapping. Hum Mol Genet 1994; 3: 1657–1661.

22. Toda T, Segawa M, Nomura Y, et al. Localization of a gene for Fukuyama type congenital muscular dystrophy to chromosome 9q31-33. Nature Genet 1993; 5: 283–286.

23. Dubowitz V. 22nd ENMC sponsored workshop on Congenital Muscular Dystrophy, Baarn, The Netherlands, 1993. Neuromusc Disord 1994; 4: 75–81.

24. Philpot J, Sewry C, Pennock J, Dubowitz V. Clinical phenotype in congenital muscular dystrophy: correlation with expression of merosin in skeletal muscle. Neuromusc Disord 1995; 5: 301–305.

25. Topaloglu H, Evangelista T, Gögüs S, Yalaz K, Tomé F. Merosin and clinical characteristics of congenital muscular dystrophy in an unselected group of Turkish patients. See this volume.

Y. Fukuyama, M. Osawa and K. Saito (Eds.), *Congenital Muscular Dystrophies*

CHAPTER 6

Walker–Warburg and other cobblestone lissencephaly syndromes: 1995 update

WILLIAM B. DOBYNS

Departments of Neurology and Pediatrics, University of Minnesota Medical School, Minneapolis, MN, USA

Introduction

Walker-Warburg syndrome (WWS) is a rare autosomal recessive multiple congenital anomaly/mental retardation syndrome in which unusual brain and eye malformations are combined with congenital muscular dystrophy (CMD) or myopathy [1–3]. The phenotype has substantial overlap with Finnish muscle-eye-brain disease (MEB) [4] and Fukuyama congenital muscular dystrophy (FCMD) [5,6].

The brain changes consist of an unusual malformation of neuronal migration known as cobblestone (previously type II) lissencephaly, while the eye changes always involve the retina. The characteristic brain and eye abnormalities of WWS were first described in 1942 [7], but the genetic basis was not recognized until 1975 [8], and the consistent association with CMD not until 1989 [1]. Many different descriptive names and eponyms have been used over the years (Table 1). In this review, the clinical and pathological manifestations of WWS are reviewed and compared with several related syndromes.

Methods and results

This update is based on review of 40 patients with WWS and three patients with a new syndrome or variant of MEB consisting of cobblestone lissencephaly with normal eyes and muscle. Twelve patients were examined personally, while the remainder were evaluated by

Table 1

The names have changed, but ...

	Reference
Lissencephaly	[7]
Congenital encephalo-ophthalmic dysplasia	[9]
Muscle, eye and brain disease	[10]
HARD±E syndrome	[11]
Warburg syndrome	[12]
Cerebro-oculo-muscular syndrome	[13]
Walker-Warburg syndrome	[14]
Cerebro-ocular dysgenesis	[15]
Cerebro-ocular dysplasia – muscular dystrophy	[16]

Table 2

Manifestations of Walker–Warburg syndrome

Major manifestations

Cobblestone lissencephaly	40/40
Retinal abnormality or microphthalmia	32/32
Anterior chamber abnormalities	29/38
Myopathy or CMD	31/34[a]

All manifestations

Cobblestone lissencephaly		Retinal abnormality	
Cobblestone cortex	38/38	Microphthalmia	15/36
Agyria predominate	24/33	Retinal dysplasia	10/23
PCH/PMG predominate	09/33	Retinal hypoplasia (or abnormal ERG)	11/23
White matter changes	20/25	Optic nerve hypoplasia	20/21
Ventriculomegaly	36/37	Colobomas	03/28
Hydrocephalus	35/39	Anterior chamber abnormalities	
Brainstem hypoplasia	24/24	High myopia	03/05
Cerebellar hypoplasia	29/32	Buphthalmos/glaucoma	13/26
Dandy–Walker malformation	18/31	Angle abnormality	16/26
Head size (at birth)		Cornea-iris-lens abnormalities	16/30
Macrocephaly	16/30	Cataract	16/28
Microcephaly	02/30	Pupil abnormalities	14/24
Other structures		Persistent vessels	
Arhinencephaly	08/10	Pupil, iris or lens	07/13
Absent septi pellucidi	16/24	Hyaloid artery or PHPV	12/15
Absent corpus callosum	12/22	Other abnormalities[b]	
Cephalocele	12/39	Adrenal hypoplasia	05/20
Myopathy		Cleft lip/palate	04/40
Serum CK increased	24/24	GU anomalies males	07/20
Dystrophy on biopsy	07/20	Hearing loss	02/40
Myopathy on biopsy	05/20	Renal dysplasia/hypoplasia	04/20
Contractures	09/21		

Abbreviations: PCH, pachygyria; PMG, polymicrogyria; ERG, electroretinogram; PHPV, persistent hyperplastic primary vitreous.
[a]All 3 patients with normal muscle were infants.
[b]The true frequency of the other abnormalities is unknown as records or testing were often incomplete. Additional abnormalities observed in one or a few patients include ear malformations, midline tongue defect, atrial septal defect, endocardial fibroelastosis, esophageal atresia, intestinal malrotation, anorectal malformation, testicular dysplasia, hemivertebrae, and scoliosis.

review of records, scans and photographs. The frequencies of the most important manifestations in the 40 WWS patients are summarized in Table 2. A detailed comparison of patients with WWS and Finnish MEB was made in conjunction with the second ENMC-sponsored workshop on CMD held in The Netherlands in April 1994 [3].

Discussion

WWS has been observed in many population groups with a worldwide distribution [2]. In contrast, both FCMD and MEB show striking founder effects. The typical form of FCMD occurs only in Japan while MEB has been reported primarily from Finland. All, or most, non-Japanese patients reported to have FCMD probably have MEB or WWS. While recent linkage studies show that MEB and FCMD are caused by mutations of different genes [3], WWS and MEB are so similar that they are probably allelic, that is they are probably caused by different mutations of the same gene. The same may be true of several other rare cobblestone lissencephaly syndromes including cobblestone lissencephaly only, and craniosynostosis with cobblestone lissencephaly.

Walker–Warburg syndrome

Previous diagnostic criteria for WWS

The diagnostic criteria previously used for WWS consist of type II lissencephaly, cerebellar malformation, retinal abnormality and CMD [1]. While useful, these criteria are rather broad and do not define the specific types of malformations observed. The term "type II" lissencephaly was first proposed in 1984 to differentiate this complex malformation from the classical form of lissencephaly which is often caused by deletions of the LIS1 gene on chromosome 17 [17]. But it is not very descriptive. At the first ENMC-sponsored Workshop on CMD held in May 1993 [2], Haltia suggested the term "cobblestone cortex" for the unusual cortical and leptomeningeal malformation observed in FCMD, MEB and WWS. In this review, the term "cobblestone lissencephaly" replaces the term "type II lissencephaly", and will be used to refer to the cobblestone cortex and *all* associated brain abnormalities including the cerebellar malformation.

Clinical course of WWS

Most children with WWS have profound mental retardation and hypotonia, mild distal spasticity and poor vision. Children with less severe gyral malformations still have moderate to severe mental retardation. The median survival is only 4 months, although some patients may survive more than 5 years. Those with longer survival have seizures, feeding problems and susceptibility to pneumonia. Many have a dysmorphic facial appearance but none of the anomalies are specific except for visible abnormalities of the eyes. Typical abnormalities include macrocephaly or microcephaly, puffy face, low-set and malformed ears, epicanthal folds and small jaw.

Cobblestone lissencephaly in WWS

Cobblestone lissencephaly consists of five major abnormalities including the striking cobblestone cortex, white matter dysmyelination or cystic changes, ventriculomegaly, brainstem hypoplasia and cerebellar hypoplasia (Fig. 1). The cobblestone cortex and brainstem hypoplasia occur in all WWS patients, while the other anomalies occur in a large majority of WWS patients. The clinical presentation may differ greatly between patients, even though the pathological changes are always similar. Some children present with macrocephaly and severe progressive hydrocephalus, while others have microcephaly and sometimes occipital cephaloceles.

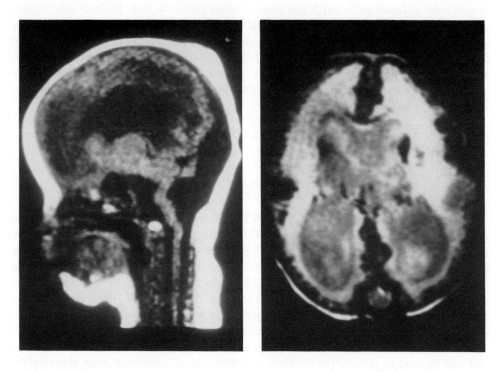

Fig. 1. MRI of patient WWS-32 shows typical changes of cobblestone lissencephaly. Sagittal T1-weighted image shows diffuse agyria with a pebbled surface, absent corpus callosum, severe hypoplasia of the brainstem and cerebellum, and Dandy–Walker malformation. Axial proton density image shows diffuse agyria with superimposed polymicrogyria, narrowing of the anterior interhemispheric fissure, diffuse increased signal of the white matter, and hydrocephalus.

Cobblestone cortex

The cobblestone cortex, observed in all 38 patients evaluated, consists of combined cortical and leptomeningeal abnormalities. In most children, the gyral malformation consists of widespread agyria with some areas of pachygyria and polymicrogyria. In others, pachygyria is observed over the frontal region and polymicrogyria posteriorly with only small areas of agyria. The brain surface has a pebbled or granular texture, and fine fibrous strands may cross the interhemispheric fissure. Sometimes the interhemispheric fissure is obliterated by fibrous tissue, especially in the frontal region, fusing the hemispheres. A thick glial rind covers most of the brain, especially the undersurface of the cerebrum and the brainstem.

Microscopic changes are striking. The cortex is thick and totally disorganized with no discernible horizontal layers, neurons which lie at irregular angles, and abnormal vascular channels and fibroglial bands. The latter divide the cortex into sheets which again lie at irregular angles. Occasionally this results in the appearance of a laminar heterotopia. The subarachnoid space is partly obliterated by glial and neuronal heterotopia which merge with the disorganized cortex [1,16].

White matter changes
The striking white matter changes of WWS consist of diffuse radiolucency on CT scan, abnormal bright signal on T2-weighted MRI images, and dysmyelination, edema and cystic changes on pathological examination [1,16]. Diffuse and severe white matter changes were seen in all but a few infants in the first several months of life (20/25 patients overall).

Ventriculomegaly
The ventricles are enlarged in almost all WWS patients as a consistent part of the malformation. The only child in this series without ventriculomegaly had a very unusual malformation which included a large occipital encephalocele [1]. Most children also have progressive hydrocephalus which may be treated with a shunt. The ependyma is thick and has a granular texture similar to the brain surface.

Brainstem
The brainstem is always hypoplastic with absent or very small corticospinal tracts, hypoplasia of other structures such as the inferior olives, and frequently aqueductal stenosis or occlusion.

Cerebellum
The cerebellar hemispheres and vermis are hypoplastic in a large majority of WWS patients (29 of 32 in this series), but have appeared normal in a few patients by CT or MRI. None were normal on pathological examination. Dandy–Walker malformation or Dandy–Walker variant was observed in just over half of the patients in this series. The foliar pattern is abnormal with areas of cerebellar polymicrogyria and severely distorted cytoarchitecture [1,16].

Other brain abnormalities
The most typical associated malformations are arhinencephaly, absent septi pellucidi, absent corpus callosum, and occipital cephaloceles. The cepaloceles are most often small meningoceles which communicate through a small bony defect in the occipital bone with a retrocerebellar or Dandy–Walker cyst. But some are true encephaloceles which may contain cerebellar or occipital lobe tissue, or both.

Eye abnormalities in WWS

A wide spectrum of eye abnormalities have been observed in WWS, but retinal abnormalities are most important as they occur in all or almost all patients, including all 32 patients evaluated in this series. This total includes patients with observed retinal changes and other patients with microphthalmia in whom an adequate retinal examination was not possible as all microphthalmic eyes have retinal abnormalities. Associated eye abnormalities include microphthalmia (15/36), colobomas (3/28), high myopia, many different anterior chamber abnormalities and persistent embryonic blood vessels.

Specific retinal changes consist of retinal detachment or more often non-attachment, retinal dysplasia with rosettes, retinal or choroidal hypoplasia which may be diffuse or occur in waves, optic nerve hypoplasia and optic nerve pallor. Electroretinograms (ERG) and visual evoked potential (VEP) studies have often been abnormal, but serial studies have not been reported so it is not known whether the abnormalities are progressive.

Typical anterior chamber malformations (29/38) include congenital glaucoma with an abnormal angle, enlarged eye or buphthalmos associated with the glaucoma, adhesions between the cornea, iris and lens especially Peter anomaly, cataracts, iris hypoplasia and cloudy corneas. A few have persistent embryonic vascular structures such as persistent pupillary membrane, tunica vasculosa lentis, persistent hyaloid artery or persistent hyperplastic primary vitreous.

Myopathy in WWS

Muscle abnormalities consist of elevated serum creatine kinase (CK) and biopsy changes of congenital muscular dystrophy. In some patients, the muscle changes are less severe and are classified as an unspecific myopathy. In this series, 31/34 patients had evidence of muscle disease. All of the children with normal serum creatine kinase and muscle biopsies were infants in the first year of life. The variation in the muscle changes has not been emphasized in previous reports. Some patients also have congenital or postnatal contractures.

Other abnormalities in WWS

Many other congenital anomalies have been reported in WWS patients. The most common of these are congenital contractures and genital anomalies in males, especially undescended testes. Other rare anomalies observed in this series or reported in the literature are listed in Table 2.

Muscle-eye-brain disease

MEB consists of cobblestone lissencephaly, retinal hypoplasia with reduced or absent responses on ERG, and congenital muscular dystrophy [2–4,10]. Most children develop very high amplitude responses on VEP by 2 years of age. Affected children have moderate or severe mental retardation, hypotonia, mild distal spasticity, weakness and poor vision. Although several have died in childhood, most survive 10–30 years and a few are still older.

The cortical malformation in MEB consists of cobblestone cortex with pachygyria over the frontal region and polymicrogyria posteriorly. The white matter has patchy areas of increased T2 signal in about half of the MEB patients, and is normal in the remainder. In contrast, most WWS patients have more severe gyral changes, although some non-Finnish WWS patients do have changes identical to MEB. All WWS patients beyond the first few months of life have diffuse white matter changes which are much more extensive than in most MEB patients. Progressive hydrocephalus, absent septum pellucidum and absent corpus callosum occur in both.

Eye abnormalities in MEB consist of high myopia, choroidal hypoplasia, optic nerve pallor, congenital or infantile glaucoma associated with angle abnormalities, iris hypoplasia, cataracts and colobomas, all of which have also been observed in WWS. Microphthalmia, typical retinal dysplasia and corneal opacities have not been observed in MEB while they are common in WWS. During early infancy ERG may be normal, but after age 1 year responses are absent or severely attenuated. VEP are also normal during infancy, but usually change to unusual giant potentials after age 1–2 years.

MEB and WWS

MEB and WWS are usually classified separately because typical WWS is more severe than MEB, and because progressive changes on ERG and VEP have been reported in MEB but not WWS. But these differences are more apparent than real. Many non-Finnish patients with less severe brain abnormalities have been reported. ERG and VEP have been performed in only a few WWS patients. MEB and WWS thus differ primarily because of severity, which is not a reliable way to separate genetic syndromes. These two disorders were recently compared in detail as part of a series of workshops on congenital muscular dystrophy [2,3].

Cobblestone lissencephaly only (Dobyns–Stratton–Patton)

Cobblestone lissencephaly without eye or muscle abnormalities has been observed in three children from two families of Middle Eastern descent [18]. All three had moderate to severe mental retardation, nystagmus, mild hypotonia and mild spasticity. CT or MRI scans showed cobblestone lissencephaly with pachygyria and polymicrogyria similar to mild WWS or Finnish MEB. Eye examinations were normal as were ERG and VEP in one of the three. Serum CK was normal in all three at ages 4–11 years, and muscle biopsy was normal in one at 4 years. Several sibs from another family may have the same disorder [19].

This syndrome may be simply another allelic variant of MEB and WWS. However, given the continuing controversy regarding classification of MEB and WWS, it should be considered a separate syndrome for linkage studies.

Craniosynostosis with cobblestone lissencephaly

A syndrome described as craniotelencephalic dysplasia, consisting of craniosynostosis with cobblestone lissencephaly, was reported in two sisters [20]. Both children had severe hypotonia, seizures, multiple craniosynostoses and a bony protrusion in the region of the open metopic suture which had a central soft area suggesting a cephalocele. Brain abnormalities were typical of cobblestone lissencephaly. Eye abnormalities consisted of bilateral microphthalmia and severe optic nerve hypoplasia. The brain and eye changes meet the current diagnostic criteria for cobblestone lissencephaly, suggesting a close relationship to WWS.

Fukuyama congenital muscular dystrophy

Typical FCMD as observed in most affected Japanese children consists of severe CMD with progressive weakness, joint contractures, elevated serum CK, mental retardation with IQ usually below 50, and cobblestone lissencephaly which is less severe than in MEB or WWS [2,5,6]. The cobblestone cortex consists of pachygyria and polymicrogyria with partial obstruction of the subarachnoid space and hemispheric fusion. A few areas of more normal gyral pattern are often present. Other abnormalities include white matter changes which often improve with age (80%), mildly enlarged ventricules, mild cerebellar polymicrogyria usually without cerebellar hypoplasia, and hypoplasia of pyramidal tracts.

About half of patients with typical FCMD have minor eye anomalies such as strabismus, abnormal eye movements or mild myopia. A few have severe myopia, cataracts, optic disc pallor or unusual round lesions of the retinal periphery. The muscle disease results in delayed motor development evident by 6 months, progressive facial and generalized muscle weakness, limited improvement in motor function which peaks between 2 and 8 years then declines, congenital and progressive joint contractures and elevated serum CK (10–50 times normal). Some patients have other minor congenital anomalies such as brachycephaly, high arched palate, hypertrichosis, and protruding heels.

Several patients have had more severe brain or eye malformations such as progressive hydrocephalus, cerebellar hypoplasia, retinal detachment or optic atrophy, or other birth defects such as cleft lip and palate, anal atresia or congenital heart disease. It appears possible and perhaps probable that some if not all of these patients had MEB or WWS rather than typical FCMD as WWS has been reported from Japan. Most non-Japanese patients diagnosed to have FCMD have had more severe anomalies typical of MEB or WWS, or less severe anomalies consistent with CMD with mental retardation.

Table 3

Research diagnostic criteria for MEB syndromes

I. Diagnosis of cobblestone lissencephaly
    A. The patient must have *ALL FIVE* of the following abnormalities,
        1. Cobblestone cortex
        2. White matter abnormalities
        3. Enlarged ventricles
        4. Brainstem hypoplasia
        5. Cerebellar especially vermis hypoplasia
    B. *OR*, the patient must have CMD and at least one of the following abnormalities.
        1. Cobblestone cortex
        2. Severe, progressive hydrocephalus
II. Diagnosis of MEB subtypes
    A. Finnish MEB
        1. Cobblestone lissencephaly with
          a. Primarily pachygyria and polymicrogyria
          b. Absent or patchy white matter changes
         2. High myopia
        3. Retinal hypoplasia with
          a. Reduced or absent ERG
          b. Very high amplitude responses on VEP (in about 75%)
        4. CMD by age 1 year
    B. Walker–Warburg syndrome
        1. Cobblestone lissencephaly with
          a. Variable gyral malformation
          b. Diffuse white matter abnormality
         2. Retinal abnormality
        3. CMD by age 1 year
    C. Cobblestone lissencephaly with normal eyes and muscle (Dobyns–Stratton–Patton)
        1. Cobblestone lissencephaly
        2. Eyes normal
        3. Muscle normal after age 1 year

Linkage studies

The gene responsible for typical FCMD was recently mapped to chromosome 9q31-33 [21]. Linkage studies in ten Finnish families with MEB excluded the MEB gene from this region [22]. Preliminary linkage data in the two families with cobblestone lissencephaly only have also excluded this disorder from the region of the FCMD gene in chromosome 9q31-33 [18].

New diagnostic criteria (research)

Because of continued controversy regarding classification and diagnostic criteria for the cobblestone lissencephaly syndromes especially MEB and WWS, new diagnostic criteria for research studies were developed in collaboration with Finnish investigators (Table 3), and presented at a recent CMD workshop [3].

Acknowledgments

This review is dedicated to Dr. Yukio Fukuyama, whose continued interest in these syndromes has led to greater understanding of all CMD syndromes, especially the cobblestone lissencephaly syndromes.

References

1. Dobyns WB, Pagon RA, Armstrong D, et al. Diagnostic criteria for Walker–Warburg syndrome. Am J Med Genet 1989; 32: 195–210.
2. Dubowitz V. Workshop Report: 22nd ENMC sponsored Workshop on Congenital Muscular Dystrophy, Baarn, The Netherlands, 14–16 May 1993. Neuromusc Disord 1994; 4: 75–81.
3. Dubowitz V, Fardeau M. Proceedings of the 27th ENMC sponsored workshop on congenital muscular dystrophy, April 1994. The Netherlands (workshop report). Neuromusc Disord 1995; 5(3): 253–258.
4. Santavuori P, Somer H, Sainio K, et al. Muscle-eye-brain disease (MEB). Brain Dev (Tokyo) 1989; 11: 147–153.
5. Fukuyama Y, Osawa M, Suzuki H. Congenital progressive muscular dystrophy of the Fukuyama type – clinical, genetic and pathological considerations. Brain Dev (Tokyo) 1981; 3: 1–29.
6. Osawa M, Arai Y, Ikenaka H, et al. Fukuyama type congenital progressive muscular dystrophy. Acta Paediatr Jpn (Tokyo) 1991; 33: 261–269.
7. Walker AE. Lissencephaly. Arch Neurol Psychiatry 1942; 48: 13–29.
8. Chemke J, Czernobilsky B, Mundel G, Barishak YR. A familial syndrome of central nervous system and ocular malformations. Clin Genet 1975; 7: 1–7.
9. Krause AC. Congenital encephalo-ophthalmic dysplasia. Arch Ophthalmol 1946; 36: 387–414.
10. Santavuori P, Leisti J, Kruus S. Muscle, eye and brain disease: a new syndrome. Neuropädiatrie (suppl) 1977; 8: 553–558.
11. Pagon RA, Chandler JW, Collie WR, et al. Hydrocephalus, agyria, retinal dysplasia, encephalocele (HARD ±E) syndrome: an autosomal recessive condition. Birth Defects 1978; 14: 232–241.
12. Pagon RA, Clarren SK. HARD ± E syndrome: Warburg's syndrome. Arch Neurol 1981; 38: 66.
13. Dambska M, Wisniewski K, Sher J, Solish G. Cerebro-oculo-muscular syndrome: a variant of Fukuyama congenital cerebro-muscular dystrophy. Clin Neuropathol 1982; 1: 93–98.
14. Dobyns WB, Stratton RF, Greenberg F. Syndromes with lissencephaly. I: Miller–Dieker and Norman–Roberts syndromes and isolated lissencephaly. Am J Med Genet 1984; 18: 509–526.

15. Williams RS, Swisher CN, Jennings M, Ambler M, Caviness VS, Jr. Cerebro-ocular dysgenesis (Walker–Warburg syndrome): neuropathologic and etiologic analysis. Neurology 1984; 34: 1531–1541.
16. Towfighi J, Sassani JW, Suzuki K, Ladda RL. Cerebro-ocular dysplasia – muscular dystrophy (COD-MD) syndrome. Acta Neuropathol 1984; 65: 110–123.
17. Dobyns WB, Reiner O, Carrozzo R, Ledbetter DH. Lissencephaly: a human brain malformation associated with deletion of the LIS1 gene located at chromosome 17p13. J Am Med Assoc 1993; 270: 2838–2842.
18. Dobyns WB, Patton MA, Stratton RF, Mastrobattista JM, Blanton SH, Northrup H. Cobblestone lissencephaly with normal eyes and muscle. Neuropediatrics 1996; 27: 70–75.
19. Hourihane JO'B, Bennett CP, Chaudhuri R, Robb SA, Martin NDT. A sibship with a neuronal migration defect, cerebellar hypoplasia and lymphedema. Neuropediatrics 1993; 24: 43–46.
20. Hughes HE, Harwood-Nash DC, Becker LE. Craniotelencephalic dysplasia in sisters: further delineation of a possible syndrome. Am J Med Genet 1983; 14: 557–565.
21. Toda T, Segawa M, Nomura Y, et al. Localization of a gene for Fukuyama type congenital muscular dystrophy to chromosome 9q31-33. Nat. Genet 1993; 5: 283–286.
22. Ranta S, Pihko H, Santavuori P, Tahvanainen E, de la Chapelle A. Muscle-eye-brain disease and Fukuyama type congenital muscular dystrophy are not allelic. Neuromusc Disord 1995; 5: 221–225.

Y. Fukuyama, M. Osawa and K. Saito (Eds.), *Congenital Muscular Dystrophies*

9.

CHAPTER 7

Muscle-eye-brain (MEB) disease – a review

HELENA PIHKO and PIRKKO SANTAVUORI

Department of Pediatrics and Child Neurology, Children's Hospital, University of Helsinki, Helsinki, Finland

Introduction

The coexistence of congenital muscular dystrophy (CMD) and brain malformation was discovered by Fukuyama and his colleagues [1,2] in Japanese patients. Muscle-eye-brain (MEB) disease, first described in Finnish patients [3,4], is another recessively inherited disease with CMD and a polymicrogyria-pachygyria type neuronal migration disorder of the brain [5,6]. The main difference between Fukuyama type CMD (FCMD) and MEB is the presence of ocular changes including severe myopia, retinal degeneration and optic atrophy in MEB [7,8]. A third clinical entity with similar features was introduced by Williams and co-workers [9], when they reported CMD in patients with the Walker–Warburg syndrome (WWS), a disease with lissencephaly and ocular malformation [10–12].

In addition to the groups already mentioned, an increasing number of CMD patients with a high degree of clinical and morphological variability have been published [13]. Cerebral findings in the form of hypodensity of the white matter have been reported in a large number of CMD patients and recent MRI studies have revealed a neuronal migration disorder in some individuals with the 'classical' CMD [13], originally thought to be a pure muscle disease. These findings have further obscured the boundaries between different types of CMD.

Molecular genetic studies have been helpful in defining some of the subgroups of CMD. The gene of FCMD has been localised to 9q31-33 [14] and MEB has been excluded from this site [15]. The discovery of CMD patients with absent merosin [16], a protein localised to chromosome 6 [17], has defined yet another subgroup. Because careful clinical description of patients and delineation of criteria used in the selection of patients for further molecular genetic studies is of crucial importance, we present a review of the clinical findings of 24 MEB patients diagnosed in our hospital between 1972 and 1993.

Patients and methods

Our series consists of 24 patients from 19 families, two of which are consanguineous. There is a male predominance with 16 male and 8 female patients. Five patients have died between 6 and 36 years of age. The present age of the patients ranges from 2 to 63 years.

ıtation

.. 2 patients presented as floppy infants with absent visual fixation. The 2 oldest patients were diagnosed at adult age after MEB was discovered in a relative. Their clinical presentation was less severe than that of the others in all aspects, including degree of mental retardation, ocular and magnetic resonance imaging (MRI) findings. All other patients were severely mentally retarded with limited ability to move. Only 3 patients could take steps unsupported. If myopia was corrected with glasses early, the patients could fix and follow large colourful objects. Five patients learned to speak a few words. Epileptic seizures were common, fits were often provoked by infection. The frequency of the seizures increased with age. Death was caused by epileptic seizures in 3 cases and ileus was discovered as the cause of death in 2 patients.

Original diagnostic criteria

The diagnosis of MEB was originally based on the presence of the following findings: severe mental retardation, ocular changes including myopia more than –1 diopter, muscle symptoms in the form of hypotonia, weakness and myopathic/dystrophic changes in muscle biopsy, myopathic electromyogram (EMG) and/or elevated serum CK values. The symptoms were present from birth or the first months of life.

Present diagnostic criteria

After the delineation of the MRI findings [4], presence of a cortical neuronal migration disorder, midline anomalies, abnormally thin brainstem and absent inferior cerebellar vermis have been included in the criteria. Typical ocular symptoms, in addition to progressive myopia, include pale retina with low or isoelectric electroretinogram (ERG), optic atrophy and delayed and giant (<50 μV) visual evoked potentials (VEP). The VEP finding, if present, strongly supports the diagnosis of MEB, but is not mandatory, especially in the young children.

Results

Muscle findings

All infants were floppy with generalised muscle weakness, including facial and neck muscles, from birth. Only 3 patients learned to take steps unsupported, all the others were bedridden. Because the patients were unable to move independently, contractures of large joints, deformities of the spine and thorax developed with age.

The CK values were elevated, up to 10 times normal values in some cases, but normal values could occasionally be seen during the first year of life. Muscle biopsies showed great variability, most constant findings were presence of central nuclei, variation of fibre size and regeneration. Increase of connective tissue and necrotic fibers were seen in later biopsies. The EMG showed a typical myopathic pattern. Respiratory muscle weakness was not the cause of death in any of our patients.

Ocular changes

Ocular findings in MEB patients have been described in detail [6–8]. Myopia was diagnosed in all patients at the first visit, even at the age of a few days. Progression of the myopia, –6 to –27 diopters, was seen in all patients in whom refractive data were available. If myopia was corrected with glasses in infancy, the patients could fix and follow large colourful objects. Visual acuity could not be measured in the majority of the patients because of mental retardation.

On MRI the eyes were elongated with posterior staphyloma in 2 patients. One patient with a myopia of –27 D, had a funnel shaped detachment of the retina at the age of 15. Five patients had congenital glaucoma and were operated on. The anterior chamber angle appeared normal in 1 patient in gonioscopy, another had a shallow angle with anterior synechiae.

Congenital cataracts were not present in any patient, but developed in 9 patients after the age of 4 years.

The optic disks were pale and the retina appeared hypopigmented. The ERG was low in the 3 youngest patients and unrecordable in all other patients, except the two mildly affected siblings. A progression from a normal to unrecordable ERG was seen in 4 cases. Flash VEPs showed a high (>50 μV) P100–N125 peak to peak amplitude and the latencies were delayed in 11 patients (Fig. 1). Two patients showed no response and two had an abnormal response. A progression of the VEP from normal to abnormal was seen in 5 cases.

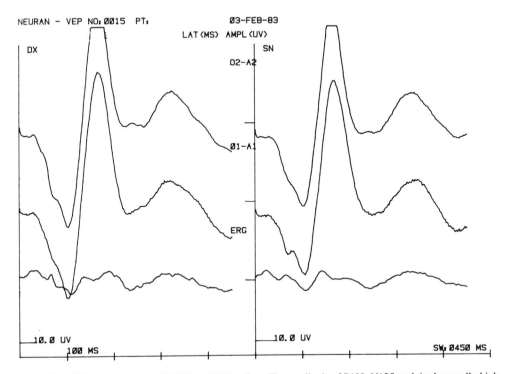

Fig. 1. Flash VEP and non-corneal ERG in a MEB patient. The amplitude of P100–N125 peak is abnormally high and the response is delayed. ERG was unrecordable. (Reproduced from Santavuori et al. [4] with permission).

Loss of ganglion cells in the retina and an atrophic optic nerve were seen in ophthalmo-pathological examination of 2 autopsy cases. The trabecular meshwork was coarse but the anterior chamber angle was normal. The internal limiting membrane was discontinuous and the glial cells, migrating through the membrane, formed a thick preretinal membrane [6].

The brain

MRI findings have been reported in detail [5]. A uniform pattern of a pachygyria-polymicrogyria type cortical neuronal migration disorder, a flat brainstem and cerebellar hypoplasia with absent inferior vermis was found in 7 of the 10 patients studied (Fig. 2). The lateral ventricles were enlarged in 5 patients and 3 patients had received a ventriculop-eritoneal shunt because of hydrocephalus. Midline anomalies consisted of an absent inter-ventricular septum and abnormal corpus callosum. The rostral parts of the corpus callosum

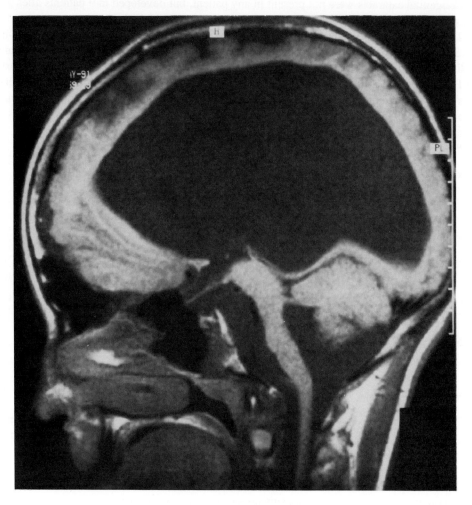

Fig. 2. Sagittal MR image of a MEB patient. There is a cortical neuronal migration disorder with abnormal gyri, enlarged lateral ventricles with absent septum pellucidum, flat brainstem and absent inferior cerebellar vermis.

were thin in the patients with enlarged ventricles and the splenium was dysplastic in 4 and absent in 2 patients. White matter changes were not prominent; 5 patients had small patchy periventricular hyperintensity and three had white matter changes subcortically. The bony posterior fossa was small and inferior vermis was absent. The surface of the cerebellum showed multiple small cyst-like lesions.

The neuropathological findings [6] showed abnormal, coarse gyri with nodular surface as well as agyric areas. Microscopically the cortex was disorganised without horizontal lamination. The pial-cortical border was irregular and there was a thick, adherent pia-arachnoid. The cerebellar cortex was disorganised.

Electroencephalogram (EEG) became progressively abnormal after the first year of life. The background activity was slow, irregular with posterior attenuation and excess of beta-activity. Irritative activity was common.

Genetic studies

Presence of siblings with MEB and consanguinity in 2 families suggests that MEB is recessively inherited. The male predominance (16/24) of our patients may be due to small number of patients.

Recently the gene for FCMD was localised to chromosome 9q31-33 [14]. A linkage study of 7 Finnish MEB families with 12 affected patients using markers D9S53, D9S58, D9S59 and HXB showed that the MEB phenotype was not linked to any of the markers [15].

Discussion

We have reviewed the data from the past 20 years of our MEB patients in order to delineate the typical clinical findings and variation of the clinical phenotype. Contrary to other views, we have claimed that the clinical features of MEB are distinct from WWS and FCMD [18]. Patients with WWS rarely survive infancy [12], while most FCMD and MEB patients live to adulthood. The ocular symptoms, largely absent in FCMD [19], are caused by a developmental malformation in WWS [12], while in MEB they can be explained by a structural weakness of the eye leading to glaucoma or progressive myopia [7]. An additional difference between MEB and WWS (and FCMD) is the occurrence of giant VEP in many MEB patients [4]. Although there is a pachygyria-polymicrogyria type neuronal migration disorder in all three, the neuropathological and neuroradiological details are distinct in each syndrome. The typical neuropathological findings in WWS-midline fusion, callosal agenesis and cystic enlargement of the posterior fossa [12], were absent in MEB patients [5,6]. The neuronal migration disorder in FCMD and MEB are very similar [20,6], but large confluent white matter changes, typical of FCMD [21], were not seen in MEB patients [5]. Since the MEB phenotype does not link to the FCMD locus, these two diseases are not allelic. The relationship of MEB to WWS and other CMD syndromes remains to be defined by molecular genetic studies.

Acknowledgements

This study has been supported by the Scandinavian-Sasakawa Foundation.

104

References

1. Fukuyama Y, Kawazura M, Haruna H. A peculiar form of congenital progressive muscular dystrophy. Report of 15 cases. Paediatr Univ Tokyo (Tokyo) 1960; 4: 5–8.
2. Fukuyama Y, Osawa M, Suzuki H. Congenital progressive muscular dystrophy of the Fukuyama type – clinical, genetic and pathological considerations. Brain Dev (Tokyo) 1981; 3: 1-29.
3. Santavuori P, Leisti J, Kruus S. Muscle, eye and brain disease: a new syndrome. Neuropädiatrie 1977; 8(Suppl.): 553–558.
4. Santavuori P, Somer H, Sainio K, et al. Muscle-eye-brain disease (MEB). Brain Dev (Tokyo) 1989; 11: 147–153.
5. Valanne L, Pihko H, Katevuo K, Karttunen P, Somer H, Santavuori P. MRI of the brain in muscle-eye-brain (MEB) disease. Neuroradiology 1994; 36: 473–476.
6. Haltia M, Leivo I, Paetau A, et al. Muscle-eye-brain (MEB) disease – a neuropathological study. Ann Neurol 1996; 40: 103–110.
7. Raitta C, Lamminen M, Santavuori P, Leisti J. Ophthalmological findings in a new syndrome with muscle, eye and brain involvement. Acta Ophthalmol 1978; 56: 465–472.
8. Pihko H, Lappi M, Raitta C, Sainio K, Somer H, Santavuori P. Ocular changes in muscle-eye-brain (MEB) disease. Brain Dev 1995; 17: 57–61.
9. Williams R, Swisher C, Jennings M, Ambler M, Caviness V. Cerebro-ocular dysgenesis (Walker-Warburg syndrome): neuropathologic and aetiologic analysis. Neurology 1984; 34: 1531–1541.
10. Walker AE. Lissencephaly. Arch Neurol Psychiatry 1942; 48: 13–20.
11. Warburg M. The heterogeneity of microphthalmia in the mentally retarded. Birth Defects 1972; 7: 136–154.
12. Dobyns W, Pagon R, Armstrong D, et al. Diagnostic criteria for Walker-Warburg syndrome. Am J Med Genet 1989; 32: 195–210.
13. Dubowitz V. Workshop report. 22nd ENMC sponsored workshop on congenital muscular dystrophy, Baarn, The Netherlands, 14–16 May 1993. Neuromusc Disord 1994; 4: 75–81.
14. Toda T, Segawa M, Nomura Y, et al. Localization of a gene for Fukuyama type congenital muscular dystrophy to chromosome 9q31-33. Nature Genet 1993; 5: 283–286.
15. Ranta S, Pihko H, Santavuori P, Tahvanainen E, de la Chapelle A. Muscle-eye-brain disease and Fukuyama type congenital muscular dystrophy are not allelic. Neuromusc Disord 1995; 5: 221–225.
16. Tomé FMS, Evangelista T, Leclerc A, et al. Congenital muscular dystrophy with merosin deficiency. CR Acad Sci (Paris)/Life Sci 1994; 317: 351–357.
17. Vuolteenaho R, Nissinen M, Sainio K, et al. Human laminin M chain (merosin): complete primary structure, chromosomal assignment and expression of the M and A chains in human fetal tissue. J Cell Biol 1994; 124: 381–394.
18. Santavuori P, Pihko H, Sainio K, et al. Muscle-eye-brain disease and Walker-Warburg syndrome. Am J Med Genet 1990; 36: 371–372.
19. Yoshioka M, Kuroki S, Kondo T. Ocular manifestations in Fukuyama type congenital muscular dystrophy. Brain Dev (Tokyo) 1990; 12: 423–426.
20. Takada K, Nakamura H, Tanaka J. Cortical dysplasia in congenital muscular dystrophy with central nervous system involvement (Fukuyama-type). J Neuropathol Exp Neurol 1984; 43: 395–407.
21. Yoshioka M, Saiwai S. Congenital muscular dystrophy (Fukuyama type)-changes in the white matter low density on CT. Am J Neuroradiol 1988; 12: 63–65.

Y. Fukuyama, M. Osawa and K. Saito (Eds.), *Congenital Muscular Dystrophies*
© 1997 Elsevier Science B.V. All rights reserved

The clinical spectrum and genetic studies of Fukuyama congenital muscular dystrophy

MIEKO YOSHIOKA[1], TATSUSHI TODA[2] and SHIGEKAZU KUROKI[1]

[1]*Department of Pediatrics, Kobe General Hospital, 4-6 Minatojima-Nakamachi, Chuo-ku, Kobe 650, Japan*
[2]*Department of Human Genetics, University of Tokyo, Tokyo, Japan*

Introduction

Congenital muscular dystrophy (CMD) is a rare and ill-defined muscular disorder characterized by generalized weakness at birth, joint contractures, delayed motor development, and muscle biopsy changes of dystrophy. Different forms of CMD have commonly been distinguished on clinico-pathological grounds (Fig. 1). The association of CMD with type II lissencephaly and eye anomalies is found in Fukuyama CMD (FCMD) [1], muscle, eye, and brain disease (MEBD) [2], and the Walker-Warburg syndrome (WWS) [3]. Autosomal recessive inheritance is suspected in all of these entities. WWS has been found in many different nationalities and races, whereas FCMD is particularly frequent in Japan and MEBD has been observed mainly in Finland. The classification of these disorders remains controver-

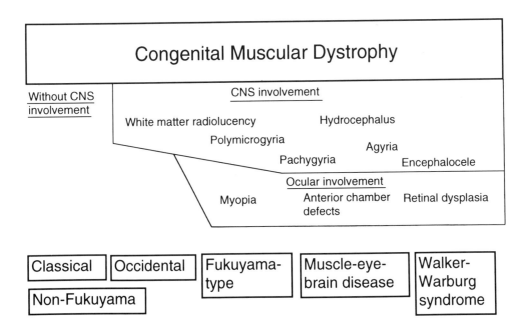

Fig. 1. Classification of congenital muscular dystrophy.

cerebellar malformations in MEBD and FCMD are milder than those in WWS. The ﬁndings in MEBD seem to be progressive in nature, while ocular anomalies are rare in FCMD.

We performed clinical and genetic studies in 41 families with FCMD-affected members with particular reference to clinical differences found among or between siblings [4]. In addition, three of the 41 families were studied using linkage analysis with polymorphic microsatellite markers flanking the FCMD locus on chromosome 9q [5]. We also reviewed the clinical findings for FCMD described in the literature.

Materials and methods

Our study included 41 families with FCMD examined by us between 1972 and 1992 (Table 1). Nine families (22%) had several affected children ('familial' FCMD). Unfortunately, two siblings in these nine families had already died at the time of examination, and detailed clinical data other than their clinical diagnosis and life spans were therefore not available. Thirty-two other families had only one affected child ('sporadic' FCMD). Parental consanguinity was documented in five sporadic FCMD families and in none of the familial cases. Twenty-two of the patients were boys and 28 were girls. The diagnosis in these patients was established according to standard criteria [1].

Clinical evaluations included assessment of maximum motor ability, mental and convulsion states, and electroencephalogram (EEG) and ophthalmological examination. The survival rate of the 50 patients was also assessed. Congenital anomalies other than those involving the muscle, eye and brain were reviewed in our patients and also in 91 families with FCMD-affected members previously reported in the literature [6–11]. Radiological studies were performed using cranial CT or magnetic resonance imaging (MRI) [12–14]. Recently, Toda and colleagues localized the FCMD locus at chromosome 9q, using linkage analysis with microsatellite polymorphisms [5]. We also conducted analysis in three of our families using the markers reported by them [15].

Results

Clinical spectrum of FCMD

The results of comparison of sibling pairs and between familial and sporadic cases in maxi-

Table 1

Patients with Fukuyama congenital muscular dystrophy (FCMD)

	Total	Familial	Sporadic
Number of families	41	9	32
Consanguineous marriage	5	0	5
Number of patients	50	18	32
Male/female	22:28	5:13	17:15

Reproduced from Yoshioka and Kuroki [4] with permission.

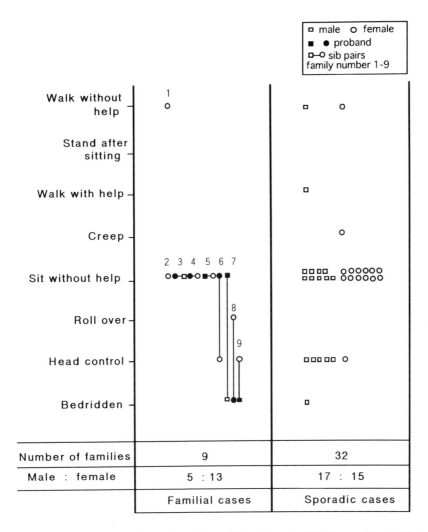

Fig. 2. Maximum motor ability in sibling pairs and in familial and sporadic FCMD cases. The familial cases are numbered from 1 to 9. The members of each sibling pair are connected by a line. In two families (#1 and 2) probands had already died at the time of examination and detailed clinical data other than their clinical diagnosis and life spans were therefore not available. (Reproduced from Yoshioka and Kuroki [4] with permission).

mum motor ability are shown in Fig. 2. Three sibling pairs with familial FCMD showed the same maximum motor ability, whereas in four other families a difference between the siblings in motor ability was apparent. In addition, three patients in the familial group but only one in the sporadic group showed no head control, but a few ambulatory patients were seen in both groups. In most patients in both groups, the maximum motor ability consisted of sitting without help.

To assess mental status, we evaluated the ability to speak meaningful words or sentences consisting of two or three words (Fig. 3). A difference between siblings in this ability was found in two pairs, but there was no marked difference between the familial and sporadic FCMD patients.

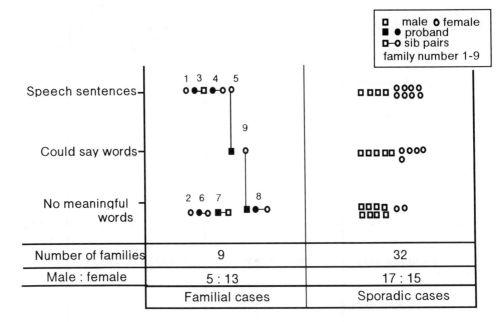

Fig. 3. Speech ability in sibling pairs and in familial and sporadic FCMD cases. Familial cases are numbered from 1 to 9, and the members of each sibling pair are connected by a line. (Reproduced from Yoshioka and Kuroki [4] with permission).

As for convulsion states, about half of the patients had afebrile or febrile convulsions in both familial and sporadic groups (Table 2). The convulsion state in seven sibling pairs is shown in Table 3. The convulsion state in the related siblings was the same; both siblings in three families had afebrile or febrile convulsions, while in the four other families neither had convulsions. EEG showed paroxysmal discharges in three sibling pairs with convulsions, while in two of the four other sibling pairs without convulsion a difference between siblings in EEG findings was apparent.

The ophthalmological findings were described in detail in 35 patients (Table 4). Myopia, weakness of the orbicularis oculi, and optic nerve atrophy were common findings. Nine (26%) of the 35 patients had no eye abnormalities. In one family (#7), both siblings showed marked ophthalmological findings including retinal detachment and severe myopia in addition to optic atrophy [16]. This family is described in detail below.

The survival rate in the 50 patients is shown in Fig. 4. The ages at death ranged from

Table 2

Convulsion states in FCMD

Convulsions	Familial (%)	Sporadic (%)	Total (%)
Afebrile	7 (43)	12 (38)	19 (40)
Febrile	1 (6)	9 (21)	10 (20)
None	8 (50)	11 (34)	19 (40)
Total	16	32	48

Table 3

Clinical variation within sibships in Fukuyama congenital muscular dystrophy

	Concordant		Discordant
	+	−	
Convulsion state			
afebrile or febrile convulsions	3	4	0
EEG			
paroxysmal discharges	3	2	2

Reproduced from Yoshioka and Kuroki [4] with permission.

1 year 11 months to 30 years with an average of 16 years. Pulmonary infection or respiratory insufficiency was the most frequent cause of death, followed by cardiac failure. The congenital anomalies other than those of the muscle, eye and brain in our 48 FCMD patients and in 91 families reported in the literature are summarized in Table 5. Various anomalies involving many systems were found [6–11], but cleft lip/palate and cryptorchidism were the most common.

Radiological studies of FCMD

The typical CT findings presented in most patients were cortical atrophy, mild to moderate dilatation of the lateral ventricles, and a low density area in the cerebral white matter [12]. Follow-up CT scans revealed change of the white matter low density areas as the patient's age increased [13]. Delayed myelination was suspected as the pathogenesis of the low density areas. Our serial MR studies demonstrated that myelination was delayed, but continued to follow the stages in an orderly and predictable manner (Fig. 5) [14]. Although the abnormal signal in the frontal lobes did not disappear completely as the child grew older, it became smaller. These areas are thought to represent the last areas of myelination, as are the

Table 4

Ophthalmological findings in FCMD

Myopia	10 (28.6)
Weakness of orbicularis oculi	15 (42.9)
Nystagmus	4 (11.4)
Strabismus	1 (2.9)
Cataracts	2 (5.7)
Hypoplasia of iris	1 (29)
Optic nerve atrophy	13 (37.1)
Diagnosis established	6 (17.1)
Suspected	7 (20.0)
Hypoplasia of macula	1 (2.9)
Retinal detachment	2 (5.7)
Duane syndrome (suspected)	1 (2.9)
Total number	35 cases
Male/female	16:19

Percentages are in parentheses.

110

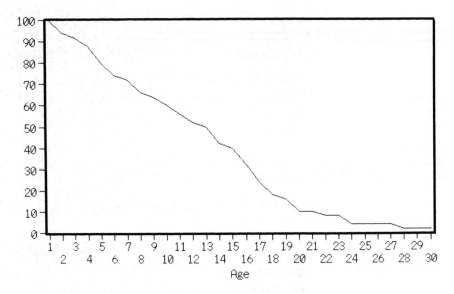

Fig. 4. Survival rate of our 50 FCMD patients assessed between 1972 and 1992.

'terminal zones' or the pathway of unmyelinated fibers in these dystrophic patients. These observations might suggest that the low-density areas found in FCMD on CT scanning are mainly due to a delay in myelination rather than to a demyelination or a dysmyelination process. Another characteristic finding revealed by MR study was the presence of pachygyria, which was noted in all three patients studied. Previous reports of neuropathologic stud-

Table 5

Other Congenital anomalies than muscle, eye and brain in Fukuyama-type congenital muscular dystrophy

Abnormalities of facial appearance	
Cleft lip/palate	2
Genital anomalies	
Cryptorchidism	4
Micropenis	1
Bicornuate uterus and double vagina	1
Cystic ovary	1
Renal anomalies	
Polycystic kidney	1
Alimentary tract malformations	
Imperforate anus	1
Megacolon	1
Diaphragmatic hernia	1
Cardiac malformations	
Ventricular septal defect (VSD)	1
Tetralogy of Fallot	1
VSD + pulmonary stenosis	1
Patent foramen ovale	1
Skeletal anomalies	
Spina bifida	1
Syndactyly	1

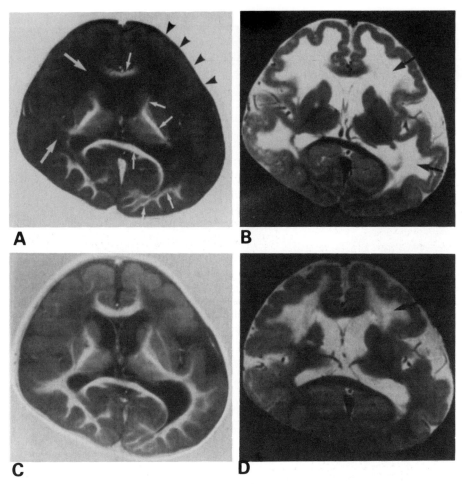

Fig. 5. Serial MR studies of the brain in a case of FCMD (the younger sister in Family #8). MRI was performed on a 1.5 T imaging system (Siemens, Erlangen, Germany). (A–D) MR images at age 11 months (A,B) and at age 18 months (C,D). (A,C) Inversion recovery sequences (3000/400/22/1); (B,D) T2-weighted spin-echo sequences (3000/90/1). (A) Myelination is present in the internal capsule, corpus callosum, and occipital region (small arrows). The temporoparietal and frontal white matter show an absence of myelination and symmetric low intensity (large arrows). Pachygyria is also apparent (arrow heads). (C) Progression of myelination from posterior to anterior is shown, but the frontal white matter remains less myelinated. This is a grossly immature pattern for 18 months of age. (B,D) Unmyelinated white matter demonstrates high intensity (arrows). (Reproduced from Yoshioka et al. [14] with permission).

ies have described pachygyria and polymicrogyria as the findings most consistently encountered in FCMD [17].

Representative cranial CT scans in one sibling pair (#8) are shown in Fig. 6. Most sibling pairs, including this pair, showed concordant CT findings. However, in one pair (#7), the CT findings were discordant (Fig. 7) [16]. While the elder brother presented the typical CT findings of FCMD, the younger brother showed marked dilatation of the lateral ventricles and an occipital encephalocele at birth. MRI in the younger brother after operation revealed aqueductal stenosis and pachygyria (Fig. 8). Table 6 is a summary of the abnormalities in this pair. Pachygyria and white matter lucency were found in both siblings, while en-

112

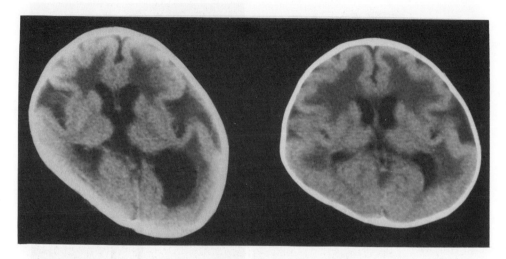

Fig. 6. Representative cranial CT scans in one sibling pair (#8). The scan on the left was obtained in the elder sister at the age of 14 months, and that on the right in the younger sister at the age of 12 months. Both show the same CT findings, e.g. pachygyria of the temporoparietal regions, moderate dilatation of the lateral ventricles, especially posteriorly (colpocephalic) and a low density area in the cerebral white matter. (Reproduced from Yoshioka and Kuroki [4] with permission).

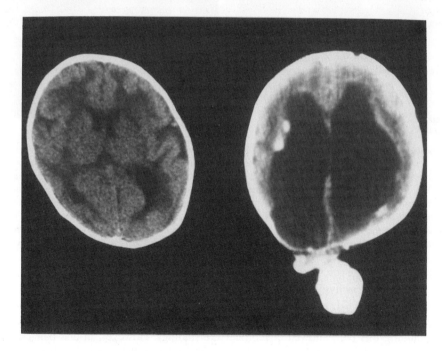

Fig. 7. Cranial CT scans in another pair (#7): the left scan was obtained in the elder brother at the age of 5 months, and the right scan in the younger brother at birth. This pair demonstrates dissimilar findings: while the elder brother shows the typical CT findings as shown in Fig. 6, the younger brother exhibits non-communicating hydrocephalus and a parieto-occipital encephalocele. (Reproduced from Yoshioka and Kuroki [4] with permission).

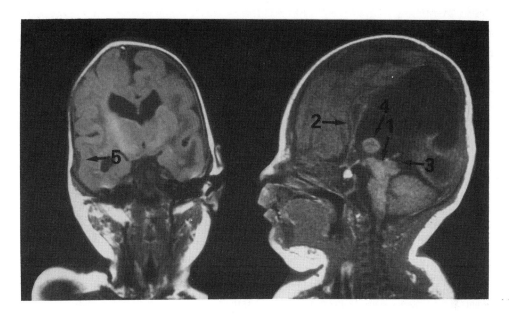

Fig. 8. MR images in the younger brother in Family #7 at 1 month of age (after the operation), demonstrating aqueductal stenosis (arrow 1), agenesis of the corpus callosum (arrow 2), tectal beaking (arrow 3), large massa intermedia (arrow 4), and pachygyria of the temporal lobe (arrow 5). (Reproduced from Yoshioka et al. [16] with permission).

cephalocele was seen only in the younger brother. In addition, retinal detachment was present in the younger brother at birth, whereas in the elder brother it developed at 3 years. From these observations, we consider that the younger brother exhibited features which were more consistent with WWS than FCMD.

Linkage analysis using microsatellite markers

Three families (#7–9) were studied using linkage analysis with polymorphic microsatellite markers flanking the FCMD locus on chromosome 9q. Among them, Family #7 showed an interesting result (Fig. 9). This family has already been reported elsewhere [16]. Briefly, both parents were healthy and non-consanguineous. There was no family history of neuromuscular disorders or anomalies. The elder brother (Patient 1) was diagnosed as having FCMD because he showed severe hypotonia with dystrophic findings on a muscle biopsy in addition to pachygyria on CT. The second pregnancy resulted in a male infant (Patient 2) who survived for 5 min. He had been diagnosed as having anencephaly at the seventh gestational month. Chromosome study revealed normal karyotype as in the other brothers. The third sibling (Patient 3) exhibited at birth such characteristic features as pachygyria, cephalocele, hydrocephalus, retinal detachment in both eyes, elevated serum creatine kinase activity, and arthrogryposis multiplex congenita, which were consistent with WWS. Since anencephaly may in some cases be associated with eye signs identical to retinal dysplasia [18], Patient 2 was regarded as having WWS with extreme brain abnormality.

The allele types of flanking markers on 9q31–33 in both parents and two affected siblings are presented in Fig. 9. We defined the FCMD locus within a region of approximately

Table 6

Comparison of two brothers (Family #7)

Abnormality	Patient 1	Patient 3
Type II lissencephaly		
Pachygyria	+	+
Predominate agyria	–	–
Predominate polymicrogyria	?	?
White matter lucency	+	+
Cerebellar malformation		
Cortical dysplasia	?	?
Vermis hypoplasia	–	–
Dandy-Walker malformation	–	–
Posterior cephalocele	–	+
Ocular malformation		
Retinal detachment	at 3 years	at birth
Optic nerve pallor	+	+
Other retinal abnormality	–	–
Microphthalmia	–	–
Anterior chamber malformation	–	–
Muscle disease		
Serum CK level (normal range, 25-188 IU/l)	6510	5280
Calf pseudohypertrophy	+	±
Associated abnormalities		
Ventricular dilatation	±	+
Hypoplastic corpus callosum	–	+
Congenital macrocephalus	–	+
Congenital microcephalus	–	–

5 cM between loci D9S127 and CA246, in which the mfd220 locus is included; mfd220 is the closest marker which showed no recombination, a high lod score of 17.49, and strong linkage disequilibrium with FCMD. We suspect that the FCMD gene lies within a few hundred kilo base pairs of mfd220 [19]. It is noteworthy that both Patient 1, with FCMD, and Patient 3, with WWS, share exactly the same haplotype at seven marker loci spanning 16 cM and surrounding the FCMD locus [15]. This suggests that both affected siblings carry the same combination of FCMD alleles, each with a mutation.

Discussion

The clinical spectrum of FCMD is much broader than we had previously suspected. The maximum motor ability differed in four sibling pairs. There have also been three reported families of FCMD in which the probands could only sit without help, whereas their siblings were ambulatory [20–22]. These ambulatory patients had been considered as having other types of muscular dystrophy, such as Duchenne type or autosomal recessive childhood muscular dystrophy, before their siblings were diagnosed with FCMD. We emphasize that ambulatory patients, even those with sporadic FCMD, should be considered to have FCMD when other clinical and laboratory data are consistent with FCMD. Furthermore, these ambulatory patients lost the ability to walk between the ages of 8 and 11 years. Our sibling pairs also showed wide variation in mental status. In addition, in one reported family [20],

115

the proband could not say any meaningful words, whereas her sister could speak sentences of two or three words. Although the speech ability varied between siblings and between families, all patients showed moderate to severe mental retardation. The convulsion state was consistent in all of seven sibling pairs, whereas two of seven sibling pairs differed in EEG findings. While one member of two sibling pairs had paroxysmal EEG discharges, their siblings showed no abnormality. Convulsion state was found in about half of the patients in the present study, as had been found in previous studies [1,12]. The familial FCMD patients showed relatively more severe motor disability than that in the sporadic FCMD patients, while in mental and convulsion states no significant difference was found between the two groups.

The wide variation in the life spans of FCMD patients which has also been reported by others [23] also suggests the broad clinical spectrum of FCMD. Among congenital anomalies other than those of muscle, eye and brain in patients with FCMD, cleft lip/palate, cryptorchidism, renal dysplasia and imperforate anus were also found in WWS [3]. This also suggests the close relationship between FCMD and WWS.

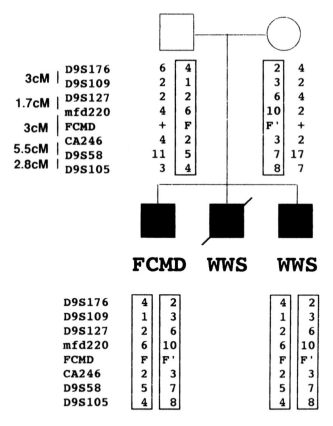

Fig. 9. Genotypes of the pedigree (Family #7) at polymorphic microsatellite loci flanking the FCMD locus. Each allele is indicated by numerals. 'F, F' and '+' denote FCMD alleles each with a mutation and a normal allele, respectively. The haplotype carrying the FCMD allele is boxed. The FCMD gene is presumed to lie within a region between D9S127 and CA246; mfd220 is the closest marker with no recombinants. Patient 1, with FCMD, and patient 3, with WWS, present the same genotype at marker loci surrounding the FCMD locus. (Reproduced from Toda et al. [15] with permission).

It is interesting that hydrocephalus was found in only one member of a sibling pair (Family #7) [16]. In this family, the proband showed typical CT findings of FCMD, whereas his brother showed marked dilatation of lateral ventricles and occipital encephalocele at birth. In fact, there have been several case reports of sporadic FCMD in which hydrocephalus or encephalocele was described [9,10,24,25]. As for the ophthalmological findings, in one sibling pair (#7) retinal detachment had developed in the proband at 3 years, whereas it had been present in his brother at birth. There are a few reports of retinal detachment in sporadic patients with FCMD [26,27].

Based on these observations, we conclude that the clinical spectrum of FCMD is much broader than we previously considered. These patients range from ambulatory to bedridden, and some are able to form sentences while others utter no meaningful words. Convulsions are found in about half of the patients. Hydrocephalus, encephalocele and retinal detachment are rare but pertinent findings in FCMD. The broad spectrum of FCMD seems to merge with that of 'mild' WWS or MEBD. There are arguments in favor of the concept of a continuum of diseases with the same etiology encompassing both typical FCMD and other types of CMD with ocular and central nervous system involvement (WWS and MEBD). Dobyns et al. [28] suggested that the unusual demography of these disorders may be caused by different alleles of the same developmental gene and by a founder effect in a relatively inbred population

Recently, Toda et al. [5] described mapping of the FCMD locus to distal 9q, using linkage analysis with microsatellite polymorphisms. Subsequently we used additional markers in this region to define the FCMD locus within a much smaller segment and also found evidence for strong linkage disequilibrium between FCMD and a polymorphic microsatellite marker, mfd220 [19]. In the present study, we showed that both patients with FCMD and with WWS, in Family #7 shared the identical combination of 9q31–33 chromosomal regions using these markers.

Since patients with FCMD and with WWS carry the identical combination of mutations on either allele of FCMD locus, these clinical conditions are caused by mutations in the same gene. The difference in clinical manifestations between FCMD and WWS may reflect the pleiotropy or variation of expressivity of the putative FCMD gene.

Acknowledgments

This work was supported, in part, by the Research Grant (8A-3) for Nervous and Mental Disorders, from the Ministry of Health and Welfare, Japan.

References

1. Fukuyama Y, Osawa M, Suzuki H. Congenital progressive muscular dystrophy of the Fukuyama type – clinical, genetic and pathological considerations. Brain Dev (Tokyo) 1981; 3: 1–29.
2. Santavuori P, Somer H, Sainio K, et al. Muscle-eye-brain disease (MEB). Brain Dev (Tokyo) 1989; 11: 147–153.
3. Dobyns WB, Pagon RA, Armstrong D, et al. Diagnostic criteria for Walker-Warburg syndrome. Am J Med Genet 1989; 32: 195–210.
4. Yoshioka M, Kuroki S. The clinical spectrum and genetic studies of Fukuyama congenital muscular dystrophy. Am J Med Genet 1994; 53: 245–250.

5. Toda T, Segawa M, Nomura Y, et al. Localization of a gene responsible for Fukuyama type congenital muscular dystrophy (FCMD) to chromosome 9q31-33 by linkage analysis. Nat Genet 1993, 5: 283–286.

6. Nihei K, Naitou H, Koizumi N, et al. Three cases of congenital muscular dystrophy with cardiac malformations. Brain Dev (Tokyo) 1989; 3: 241.

7. Ogihara Y, Yagi Y, Sawai N, et al. A case of Fukuyama congenital muscular dystrophy associated with imperforate anus (in Japanese). No To Hattatsu (Tokyo) 1989; 21: 392–393.

8. Kamoshita S, Konishi Y, Segawa M, Fukuyama Y. Congenital muscular dystrophy as a disease of the central nervous system. Arch Neurol 1975; 33: 513–516.

9. Kasubuchi Y, Haba S, Wakaizumi S, Shimada M. An autopsy case of congenital muscular dystrophy accompanying hydrocephalus (in Japanese). No To Hattatsu (Tokyo) 1974; 6: 36–41.

10. Miyake N, Goto A, Tsuchida M, Misugi N, Komiya K. An autopsy case of congenital muscular dystrophy associated with hydrocephalus and occipital dermal sinus (in Japanese). No To Hattatsu (Tokyo) 1977; 9: 212–219.

11. Ueda K, Ito T, Matsumoto K, et al. Hypotonic infant (in Japanese). Nihon Rinsho (Tokyo) 1968; 26: 143–168.

12. Yoshioka M, Okuno T, Nakano Y, Honda Y. Central nervous system involvement in progressive muscular dystrophy. Arch Dis Child 1980; 55: 589–594.

13. Yoshioka M, Saiwai S. Congenital muscular dystrophy (Fukuyama type): changes in the white matter low density on CT. Brain Dev (Tokyo) 1988; 10: 41–44.

14. Yoshioka M, Saiwai S, Kuroki S, Nigami H. MR imaging of the brain in Fukuyama-type congenital muscular dystrophy. Am J Neuroradiol 1991; 12: 63–65.

15. Toda T, Yoshioka M, Nakahori Y, Kanazawa I, Nakamura Y, Nakagome Y. Genetic identity of Fukuyama type congenital muscular dystrophy and Walker–Warburg syndrome. Ann Neurol 1995; 37: 99–101.

16. Yoshioka M, Kuroki S, Nigami H, Kawai T, Nakamura H. Clinical variation within sibships in Fukuyama-type congenital muscular dystrophy. Brain Dev (Tokyo) 1992; 14: 334–337.

17. Takada K, Nakamura H, Tanaka J. Cortical dysplasia in congenital muscular dystrophy with central nervous system involvement (Fukuyama type). J Neuropathol Exp Neurol 1984; 43: 395–407.

18. Svedberg B. Retrolental fibroplasia or congenital encephalo-ophthalmic dysplasia. Acta Pediatr Scand 1975; 64: 891–894.

19. Toda T, Ikegawa S, Okui K, et al. Refined mapping of a gene responsible for Fukuyama type congenital muscular dystrophy: evidence for strong linkage disequilibrium. Am J Hum Genet 1994; 55: 946–950.

20. Kuwajima K, Misugi N, Komiya K. A hydrocephalic girl with progressive muscular dystrophy: a case report (in Japanese). No To Hattatsu (Tokyo) 1974, 6: 29–35.

21. Itagaki Y, Sakamoto Y, Nishitani Y. Peculiar type of congenital muscular dystrophy (Fukuyama type) (in Japanese). Rinsho Shinkeigaku (Tokyo) 1980; 20: 897–903.

22. Riku S, Konagaya M, Ibi T, Sobue I. Unusual sibling cases of Fukuyama type congenital muscular dystrophy (in Japanese). Rinsho Shinkeigaku (Tokyo) 1982; 22: 216–222.

23. Mukoyama M, Hizawa K, Kagawa N, Takahashi K. The life spans, cause of death and pathological findings of Fukuyama type congenital muscular dystrophy – analysis of 24 autopsy cases (in Japanese). Rinsho Shinkeigaku (Tokyo) 1993; 33: 1154–1156.

24. Yamada H, Oi S. Follow-up of the hydrocephalic state in a case of congenital muscular dystrophy (Fukuyama type) – discussion of the change in white matter and functional prognosis after shunt procedure (in Japanese). CT Kenkyu (Tokyo) 1984; 7: 88–93.

25. Okudaira Y, Bandoh K, Wachi A, Sato K, Osawa M. A case of congenital muscular dystrophy associated with hydrocephalus – CSF dynamics and surgical treatment (in Japanese). No To Hattatsu (Tokyo) 1994; 26: 57–62.

26. Chijiiwa T, Nishimura M, Ushijima H, Yamana Y, Inomata H. Ocular manifestations of congenital muscular dystrophy (Fukuyama type) in two cases (in Japanese). Rinsho Ganka (Tokyo) 1982; 36: 21–25.

27. Hirata H, Mishima H, Shimizu S et al. Unusual fundus manifestations in a case with congenital muscular dystrophy (in Japanese). Rinsho Ganka (Tokyo) 1984; 38: 1241–1244.

28. Dobyns WB. Classification of the cerebro-oculo-muscular syndrome(s) – commentary to Kimura's paper. Brain Dev (Tokyo) 1993; 15: 242–244.

Y. Fukuyama, M. Osawa and K. Saito (Eds.), *Congenital Muscular Dystrophies*

CHAPTER 9

Characteristics of muscle involvement evaluated by computerized tomography scanning in early stages of progressive muscular dystrophy: comparison between Duchenne and Fukuyama types

YUMI ARAI, MAKIKO OSAWA and YUKIO FUKUYAMA

Department of Pediatrics, Tokyo Women's Medical College, Tokyo, Japan

Introduction

Computerized tomography (CT) of skeletal muscles has been widely applied to various neuromuscular disorders since 1977, when O'Doherty and colleagues first reported CT changes in patients with pseudohypertrophic muscular dystrophy [1], and the application of this technique has been established as a non-invasive means of in situ evaluation of muscle involvement. In Duchenne muscular dystrophy (DMD), a characteristic CT pattern of muscle involvement has been confirmed [1–11]. In addition, the distributions of affected muscles associated with other muscular diseases are also being elucidated [12–16].

Fukuyama type congenital muscular dystrophy (FCMD) is an autosomal recessive genetic disease which is characterized by an association of primary muscular dystrophy with central nervous system malformation [17,18]. In Japan, DMD is the most frequent type of muscular dystrophy in childhood, and FCMD has the second highest incidence [19]. However, few reports on the CT evaluation of the muscles in FCMD patients have been published [3,9,20]. In the present study, we examined skeletal muscle CT scans in cases of DMD and FCMD, two representative types of muscular dystrophy in childhood, to clarify the processes of muscular degeneration in early stages of these disorders. Furthermore, the anatomical distribution of affected muscles was compared between the two disorders.

Subjects and methods

The study subjects were 21 patients with DMD (between 6 months and 12 years of age, 26 examinations in total) and 18 patients with FCMD (between 5 months and 12 years of age, 22 examinations in total) who were managed as outpatients at the pediatric clinic of Tokyo Women's Medical College Hospital and whose parents/care givers gave informed consent for participation in this study. In both groups, 4 subjects underwent examination two or more times. Table 1 shows the frequency of examination for each age group. Each subject was followed for at least 2 years after the CT examination. Eighty percent of examinations were done before age 7 years. In other words, most examinations were carried out at such a stage of disease where a new motor function is still developing or the motor function is

Table 1

Frequency of examination for each age group

Age (years)	DMD	FCMD
0–<1	4	5
1–2	2	0
2–3	2	4
3–4	7	2
4–5	2	0
5–6	2	3
6–7	3	3
7–8	1	2
8–9	1	1
9–10	0	1
10–13	2	1
Total examinations	26	22

maintained at the maximum level, with the exception of 4 DMD and 3 FCMD cases which were in the declining stage at the time of CT examination (Fig. 1). Skeletal muscle CT scans of a 5-year-old child with mental retardation, who was brought to our clinic for evaluation of delayed motor development, but whose muscle biopsy ruled out muscular disease, served as the control.

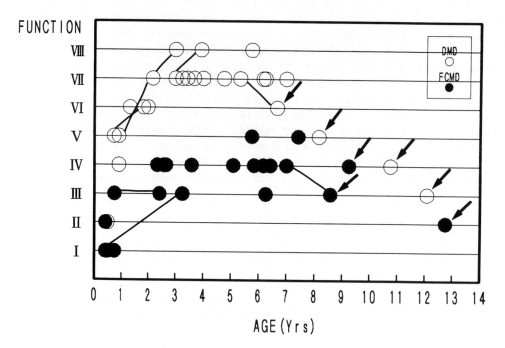

Fig. 1. Motor ability and age at CT examination. Subjects undergoing two or more examinations are denoted by the markers connected with a line. Cases showing clinical signs of motor deterioration are denoted by arrows. I, no head control; II, lifts head; III, remains sitting; IV, sliding on the buttocks while sitting; V, crawls on all fours; VI, ambulant; VII, climbs stairs with the aid of a railing; VIII, climbs stairs without assistance.

CT scans were carried out using Hitachi CT 600 apparatus operating at 120 kV and 300 mA, with a slice width of 10 mm and a scanning time of 4.5 s; slices were obtained transaxially at the levels of the 3rd lumbar vertebra (L3), the mid-position of the thigh, and the maximum circumference of the calf. Muscle images obtained at each slice level were assessed by visual inspection. During this evaluation, the extent of low density (LD) areas in muscle images as well as the severity of muscle atrophy (visible as enlargement of intermuscular spaces or a decrease in the cross-sectional area of muscle) was assessed.

Furthermore, using the image analysis program incorporated in the CT apparatus, the periphery of the each muscle or muscle group indicated in Fig. 2 was demarcated with the trackball of the monitor, and then the average CT numbers of the respective images were

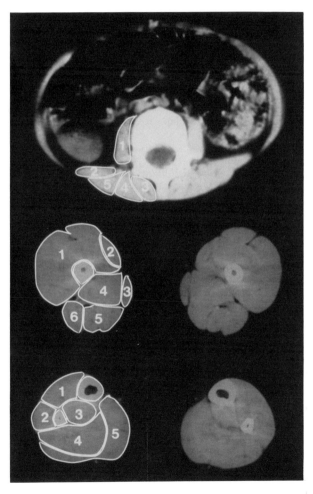

Fig. 2. Muscles evaluated at each slice level and showing normal CT appearance. Upper: L3 level: 1, M psoas major; 2, M quadratus lumborum; 3, Mm multifidi; 4, M longissimus thoracis; 5, M iliocostalis lumborum. Middle: thigh level: 1, M quadriceps; 2, M sartorius; 3, M gracilis; 4, M adductor magnus; 5, Mm semimembranosus et semitendinosus; 6, M biceps femoris. Bottom: calf muscle: 1, M tibialis anterior; 2, M peroneus; 3, M tibialis posterior; 4, M soleus; 5, M gastrocnemius.

calculated. As a rule, the calculation of CT number was based on the images obtained from muscles on the right side. The relationship between the average CT number of each muscle and age was analyzed statistically. The statistical significance of correlations between the two was then examined, at a 5% significance level, by means of Student's t-test. A regression line was obtained for muscles showing a significant correlation between CT number and age. Moreover, to explore inter-muscle differences in the rate of CT number decrease, we compared the slopes and Y intercepts of the age-CT number regression line between different muscles at the same slice level.

These parameters, for each muscle, were then compared between the DMD and FCMD groups. The significance of differences in these parameters was examined using the F distribution with a significance level of 5%.

Results

Macroscopical changes in muscle CT images

Fig. 2 shows a control CT image. In normal muscle images, contiguous muscles could not be distinguished and the intramuscular density appeared to be uniform. Figs. 3–5 show typical CT images of DMD and FCMD muscles.

L3 level

Fig. 3a shows a DMD case at the age of 6 months, and Fig. 3b, a FCMD case at the age of 5 months. In both infants, slightly widened spaces were visible between paravertebral muscles, but the density was essentially uniform within each muscle.

In a 3-year-old patient with DMD, the iliocostalis lumborum which is laterally situated within the paravertebral muscles, showed patchy low density (LD) areas of moth-eaten distribution (Fig 3c). A 3-year-old patient with FCMD (Fig. 3d) showed diffuse LD throughout the paravertebral muscles as well as patchy LD in the psoas major.

In a 6-year-old patient with DMD, patchy LD areas were also disseminated in the longissimus thoracis of the paravertebral muscles, although only mild LD was noted in other muscles (Fig. 3e). In the FCMD case shown in Fig. 3f, LD areas in the paravertebral muscles were extremely widespread, except in the multifidi, which showed a slight residual muscle shadow. Moreover, LD changes were also observed in the psoas major.

Thigh level

In the 6-month-old DMD patient shown in Fig. 4a, muscular density is well preserved, and the muscles appear to be normal. In a 5-month-old patient with FCMD, inter-muscular spaces suggesting atrophy are already apparent (Fig. 4b).

In a 3-year-old patient with DMD, a moth-eaten distribution of LD lesions was seen in each muscle, accompanied by mild atrophic changes (Fig. 4c). Another patient with FCMD also exhibited these changes in each muscle examined, but the changes were particularly pronounced in the adductor magnus (Fig. 4d).

Comparing with the findings in a 3-year-old DMD patient, a 6-year-old DMD patient showed more advanced LDs in all thigh muscles. Changes in the adductor magnus were especially marked (Fig. 4e). In a patient with FCMD, LD changes of the muscles were more extensive than those in DMD.

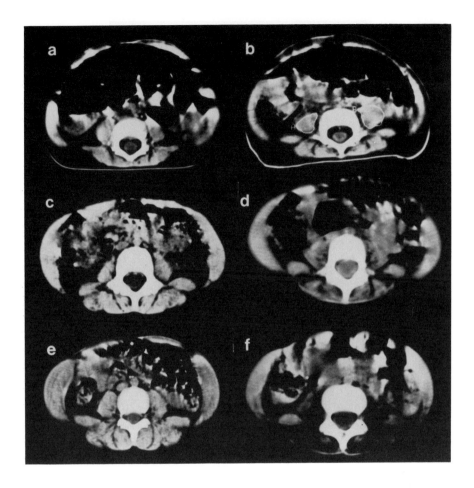

Fig. 3. Muscle CT scans at the level of the third lumbar vertebra. Left, DMD (a,c,e); right, FCMD (b,d,f). From the top: 6-month (a), 5-month (b), 3-year (c,d), and 6-year-old patients (e,f).

The changes were observed throughout the adductor magnus and hamstring muscles, although the sartorius and gracilis were relatively well preserved (Fig. 4f).

Calf level
A 6-month-old patient with DMD (Fig. 5a) and a 5-month-old patient with FCMD (Fig. 5b) show well-preserved intramuscular density, comparable to that of normal images.

In a 3-year-old patient (Fig. 5c) and a 6-year-old one with DMD (Fig. 5e), the gastrocnemius and soleus both show mildly moth-eaten LD and very slight muscle atrophy. Changes at the calf level were less severe than those at the thigh level in these cases.

In the FCMD group, the gastrocnemius and soleus were already occupied almost completely by LD at age 3 years (Fig. 5d). The anterior tibialis, peroneus and posterior tibialis were well preserved at age 3 years, but LDs were detected in these muscles at age 6 years (Fig. 5f).

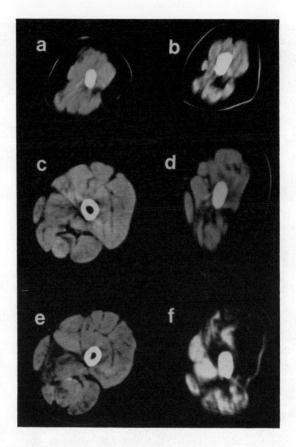

Fig. 4. Muscle CT scans at thigh level. Left, DMD (a,c,e); right, FCMD (b,d,f).

At each level, the changes were more marked in FCMD than in DMD cases. In the DMD group, the progression of changes was most conspicuous at the thigh level, while in the FCMD group, calf level changes were marked.

Relationship between average CT numbers of muscles and age

Figs. 6–8 show the relationship between the average CT number of a muscle and age at each level. Regression lines are also shown in those instances in which the correlation between the average CT number and age was statistically significant. Statistical analysis of the relationship between these two parameters is presented in Table 2.

L3 level (Fig. 6)
A significant negative correlation between the average CT number and age was recognized in all DMD muscles and in all but the quadratus lumborum in FCMD. The CT number clearly decreased with age.
    Comparison of the slopes of the regression lines in the DMD group revealed significant

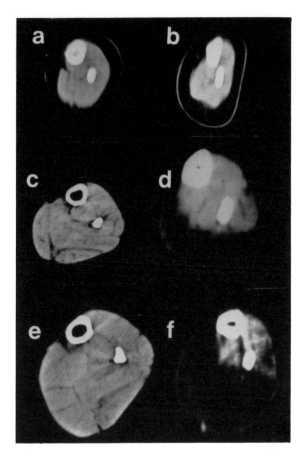

Fig. 5. Muscle CT scans at calf level. Left, DMD (a,c,e); right, FCMD (b,d,f).

differences between the multifidi, anatomically the most medially situated of the paraverte-bral muscles, and both the longissimus thoracis and the iliocostalis lumborum, 2 muscles which are situated laterally with respect to the multifidi (Table 3). Thus, rapid changes in the paravertebral group commence in the lateral muscles. A similar analysis in the FCMD group revealed that the age-related decreases in CT numbers were slower in the psoas major than in the paravertebral muscles.

Table 4 compares the regression lines in the DMD and FCMD groups for each muscle. The average rate of age-related decrease in the psoas major CT number was significantly more rapid in the DMD than in the FCMD group, while the rate in the multifidi was slower in the DMD than in the FCMD group. In examining the slopes of the regression lines of the longissimus thoracis and iliocostalis lumborum, no significant difference was detected be-tween the DMD and FCMD groups. However, the Y intercepts of the lines for these muscles were significantly different. Hence, for these muscles, corresponding lines in the DMD and FCMD groups were theoretically parallel, indicating that although the muscles of the DMD patients retained comparatively high CT numbers, their densities decreased at the same rates as those in the FCMD group.

126

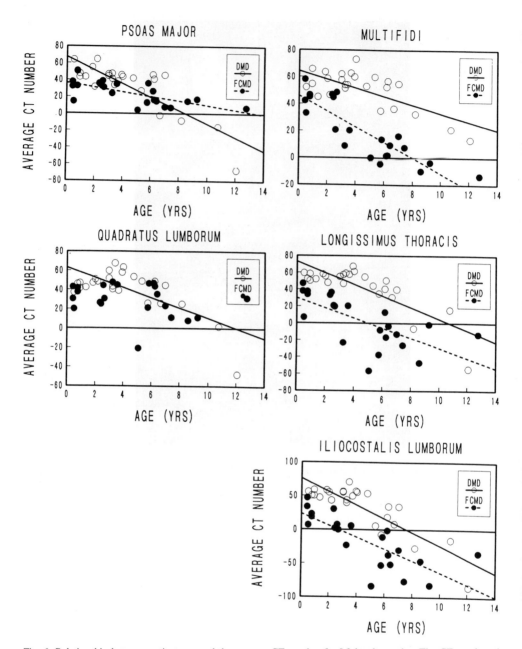

Fig. 6. Relationship between patient age and the average CT number for L3 level muscles. The CT numbers in DMD are denoted by open circles and those in FCMD by filled circles. Regression lines are shown for the muscles, between which statistically significant differences were observed (solid line, DMD; dashed line, FCMD).

Thigh level (Fig. 7)

Negative correlations between the average CT number and age were evident for all muscles except the gracilis in FCMD patients.

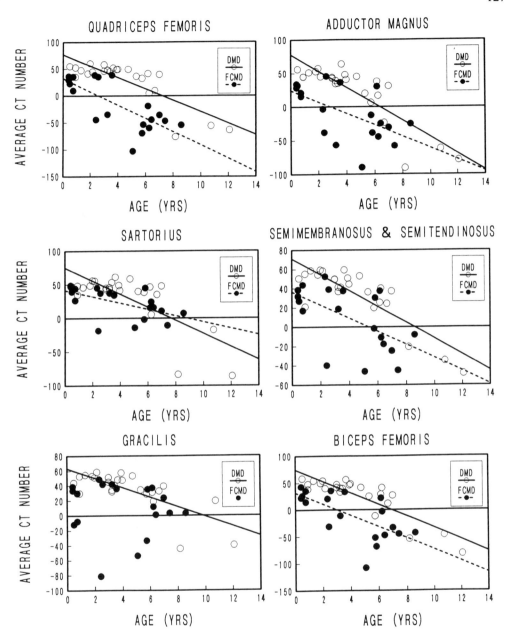

Fig. 7. Relationship between patient age and the average CT number for thigh level muscles.

In the DMD group, comparison of the slopes of the regression lines (Table 5) revealed a significant difference between the adductor magnus and gracilis. This observation indicates that the rate of CT number decrease was more rapid in the adductor magnus than in the gracilis, both of which belong to the adductor muscle group. Significant differences in this respect were also noticed between the adductor magnus and both the semimembranosus and semitendinosus. For the gracilis, the slope of the regression line differed significantly from

128

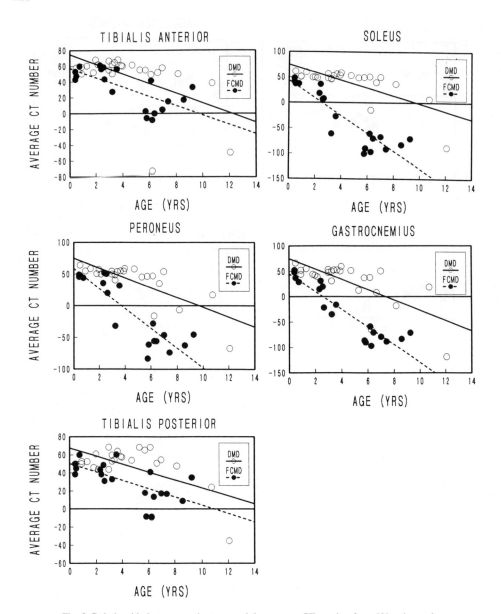

Fig. 8. Relationship between patient age and the average CT number for calf level muscles.

that for the quadriceps and biceps femoris; that is, the gracilis was relatively well preserved among the femoral muscles. There were no significant differences in the rates of CT number decreases among the extensors, such as the quadriceps and sartorius. Neither were any differences in rates observed among the flexors, i.e. the semimembranosus, semitendinosus and biceps femoris.

In the FCMD group, comparison of the slopes of the regression lines revealed a significant difference between the quadriceps and the sartorius, with the age-related decrease in

Table 2

Statistical correlation between patient age and the average CT number for each muscle

	Muscle	Regression line		P-value	
		DMD	FCMD	DMD	FCMD
L3	Psoas major	$y = 67.319 - 7.984x$	$y = 36.287 - 2.662x$	<0.01	<0.01
	Quadratus lumborum	$y = 63.101 - 5.252x$	NS	<0.01	NS
	Multifidi	$y = 64.231 - 3.135x$	$y = 45.857 - 5.748x$	<0.01	<0.01
	Longissimus thoracis	$y = 73.157 - 6.837x$	$y = 29.880 - 5.960x$	<0.01	<0.01
	Iliocostalis lumborum	$y = 75.971 - 10.027x$	$y = 23.536 - 8.738x$	<0.01	<0.01
Thigh	Quadriceps	$y = 76.776 - 10.646x$	$y = 32.263 - 12.389x$	<0.01	<0.01
	Sartorius	$y = 75.005 - 9.758x$	$y = 41.417 - 4.700x$	<0.01	<0.01
	Gracilis	$y = 63.141 - 6.413x$	NS	<0.01	NS
	Adductor magnus	$y = 77.956 - 12.238x$	$y = 24.371 - 8.512x$	<0.01	<0.01
	Semimembranosus et semitendinosus	$y = 70.931 - 8.257x$	$y = 36.484 - 6.811x$	<0.01	<0.02
	Biceps femoris	$y = 74.367 - 10.766x$	$y = 31.671 - 10.536x$	<0.01	<0.01
Calf	Tibialis anterior	$y = 74.680 - 6.097x$	$y = 57.305 - 5.902x$	<0.01	<0.01
	Peroneus	$y = 74.848 - 7.726x$	$y = 58.642 - 15.701x$	<0.01	<0.01
	Tibialis posterior	$y = 67.509 - 4.400x$	$y = 50.370 - 4.607x$	<0.01	<0.01
	Soleus	$y = 74.780 - 7.706x$	$y = 43.675 - 17.416x$	<0.01	<0.01
	Gastrocnemius	$y = 74.747 - 10.143x$	$y = 44.970 - 17.442x$	<0.01	<0.01

NS, not significant.

CT number in the quadriceps being more rapid than that in the sartorius. However, no significant differences were noted between any two of the other muscles.

Comparison of the slopes of the regression lines for each muscle between the DMD and the FCMD groups (Table 4) revealed no significant inter-group differences. The Y intercepts for all but the sartorius differed significantly between the 2 groups, indicating that the regression lines for all muscles, except the sartorius, showed a statistically significant parallel

Table 3

Statistical comparison of the regression slopes for CT numbers by age, for muscles at the L3 level in DMD and FCMD patients

	Psoas major (PM)	Quadratus lumborum (QL)	Multifidi (M)	Longissimus thoracis (LT)
Quadratus lumborum (QL)	NS (DMD)			
	– (FCMD)			
Multifidi (M)	M < PM***	NS		
	M > PM***	–		
Longissimus thoracis (LT)	NS	NS	LT > M***	
	LT > PM*	–	NS	
Iliocostalis lumborum (IL)	NS	IL > QL**	IL > M***	NS
	IL > PM***	NS	NS	NS

Top rows, DMD; bottom rows, FCMD. *$P < 0.05$; **$P < 0.01$; ***$P < 0.005$; NS, not significant. a > b indicates that the rate of CT number decrease for muscle "a" is theoretically more rapid than that for muscle "b".

Table 4

Statistical correlation between the regression lines for CT numbers by age in DMD and those in FCMD

	Muscle	Regression slopes	Y intercepts	Rates of CT number decrease
L3	Psoas major	$F < 0.005$	–	DMD > FCMD
	Multifidi	$F < 0.025$	–	FCMD > DMD
	Longissimus thoracis	NS	$F < 0.005$	DMD // FCMD
	Iliocostalis lumborum	NS	$F < 0.005$	DMD // FCMD
Thigh	Quadriceps	NS	$F < 0.005$	DMD // FCMD
	Sartorius	NS	NS	DMD = FCMD
	Adductor magnus	NS	$F < 0.005$	DMD // FCMD
	Semimembranosus et semitendinosus	NS	$F < 0.005$	DMD // FCMD
	Biceps femoris	NS	$F < 0.005$	DMD // FCMD
Calf	Tibialis anterior	NS	$F < 0.005$	DMD // FCMD
	Peroneus	$F < 0.005$	–	FCMD > DMD
	Tibialis posterior	NS	$F < 0.005$	DMD // FCMD
	Soleus	$F < 0.005$	–	FCMD > DMD
	Gastrocnemius	$F < 0.005$	–	FCMD > DMD

FCMD > DMD, the rate of CT number decrease in FCMD is more rapid than that in DMD; DMD // FCMD, regression lines in DMD and FCMD are theoretically parallel despite the retention of higher CT numbers in DMD as compared with the corresponding values in FCMD.

between the 2 groups and that the regression line for the sartorius was statistically identical in the 2 groups.

Calf level (Fig. 8)
Negative correlations between the CT number and age were recognized for all muscles in both groups of patients.

Comparison of the slopes of the regression lines (Table 6) revealed a significant difference between the posterior tibialis and the gastrocnemius in the DMD group, the rate of age-related CT number decrease being slower in the posterior tibialis. On the other hand, in the

Table 5

Statistical comparison of the regression slopes for CT numbers by age for thigh muscles in DMD and FCMD.

	Quadriceps (Q)	Sartorius (S)	Gracilis (G)	Adductor magnus (AM)	Semimembranosus, semitendinosus (SS)
Sartorius (S)	NS				
	S < Q**				
Gracilis (G)	G < Q*	NS			
	–	–			
Adductor magnus (AM)	NS	NS	AM > G***		
	NS	NS	–		
Semimembranosus et	NS	NS	NS	SS < AM*	
semitendinosus (SS)	NS	NS	–	NS	
Biceps femoris (BF)	NS	NS	BF >G**	NS	NS
	NS	NS	–	NS	NS

*P < 0.05; **P < 0.025; ***P < 0.01; NS, not significant.

Table 6

Statistical comparison of the regression slopes for CT numbers by age for calf muscles in DMD and FCMD.

	Tibialis anterior (TA)	Peroneus (P)	Tibialis posterior (TP)	Soleus (S)
Peroneus (P)	NS			
	P > TA****			
Tibialis posterior (TP)	NS	NS		
	NS	TP < P****		
Soleus (S)	NS	NS	NS	
	S > TA****	NS	S > TP****	
Gastrocnemius (G)	NS	NS	G > TP*	NS
	G > TA****	NS	G > TP****	NS

*$P < 0.05$; ****$P < 0.005$; NS, not significant.

FCMD group, significant differences in this respect were noted between the anterior tibialis and all calf muscles other than the posterior tibialis. There were also significant differences between the posterior tibialis and the other calf muscles, with the exception of the anterior tibialis. These observations indicate that the rate of age-related changes in CT numbers of the anterior and posterior tibialis were comparatively slow in calf muscles in FCMD patients.

Comparison of the regression lines between the DMD and FCMD groups (Table 4) revealed significant inter-group differences in the slopes for the peroneus, soleus and gastrocnemius, indicating that the rates of age-related decreases in the CT numbers of these muscles were more rapid in the FCMD than in the DMD group. No significant inter-group differences in the slopes of the regression lines were recognized for the anterior and posterior tibialis, though the Y intercepts of the lines for these 2 muscles were statistically significant. Hence, the corresponding lines in the DMD and FCMD groups were theoretically parallel.

Discussion

Since CT scanning first began to be applied to the examination of skeletal muscles, this technique has most frequently been used for the assessment of muscular dystrophy. Recent advances in the molecular genetic study of DMD have unveiled the gene deletion responsible for this disease [21]; that is, the inability to synthesize dystrophin (a protein which maintains muscular cell frames) leads to muscular collapse. It has been reported that the degeneration of muscles in DMD is already present in the preclinical stages or in the intrauterine period [22–24]. On the other hand, although FCMD does not involve a dystrophic defect, pathological features of FCMD muscles appeared to be identical to those of DMD. Takada et al. [25] reported that the muscles of a 23-week fetus were normal; however, considering that the clinical symptoms of FCMD manifest very early in infancy, it seems likely that muscle changes would already be present before birth. Thus, although muscular degeneration occurs in an early period in both diseases, patients acquire locomotive functions and become ambulatory in DMD, while FCMD patients can learn to crawl but not stand or walk. To clarify the processes of muscle involvement in these diseases during the development of motor function, it is necessary to carry out a detailed study of children with these diseases at early ages. In the present study, 85% of the patients from both the DMD and FCMD groups underwent CT scanning before their motor functional levels began to decline.

Macroscopic findings

DMD

The muscle CT findings in DMD first reported by O'Doherty et al. [1] presented an advanced stage, and were described as being characterized by diffuse LD in the calf, with preservation of the posterior tibialis. Subsequently, Hawley et al. [6] studied CT images of the thigh and calf muscles of DMD patients with mild to total disability. They reported that only slightly moth-eaten LD lesions were noted in patients who were ambulatory, but that patients who required assistance in walking showed more extensive LD; moreover, the gracilis and sartorius were preserved, revealing differences in the rates of progression of changes in various muscles. Such selective involvement of muscles in the mid-stage of DMD was confirmed by the studies of Stern et al. [7], as well as Kawai et al. [8]. Their results indicated that the gracilis and sartorius in the thigh region, as well as the peroneus, and anterior and posterior tibialis in the calf tend to remain intact until the late stages of the disease. As regards the paravertebral muscles, Kawai et al. [8], as well as Hadar et al. [26], reported that changes in the laterally situated muscles are pronounced, while the multifidi tend to be well preserved.

In the present study, the adductor magnus showed relatively extensive LD but the other muscles of the thigh were well preserved. Selective muscular involvement showing the aforementioned pattern was not yet macroscopically evident in either the thigh or the calf. However, the tendency for muscular changes to commence in the thigh earlier than in the calf [8] was also noted in the present study. Regarding the paravertebral muscles, LD changes were more marked in laterally, than in medially situated muscles, and the characteristic changes reported to be seen in older children were also noted in younger children as well.

FCMD

Sumida et al. [20] macroscopically evaluated CT images obtained from 16 FCMD cases, including some very young patients. They reported that changes were initially apparent in the calf muscles, and were particularly marked in the triceps surae muscles (specifically, the soleus and gastrocnemius). These changes were also reported by Ohiwa et al. [3], as well as Nagao et al. [9]. These characteristics of muscle involvement were confirmed in a pathological study reported by Saida et al. [27], on the basis of quantitative analysis of histological findings in the rectus femoris and gastrocnemius, which revealed that fatty infiltration was more marked in the calf than in the thigh. Sumida et al. [20] further reported that the sartorius and gracilis in the thigh and the posterior tibialis in the calf were well preserved, as had already been demonstrated in late stage DMD cases.

At the trunk level, changes in the paravertebral muscles were pronounced in an early period, followed by those of the psoas major; and rapid changes in the paravertebral group commenced in the lateral muscles, as in DMD.

The present study revealed that, as in previous reports, changes were most conspicuous at the calf level. In particular, the triceps muscles of the calf showed diffuse LD at 3 years of age. This accounts, in part, for most FCMD patients never becoming ambulant even though they can crawl, stand on their knees or remain standing when assisted with appliances. On the other hand, the anterior and posterior tibialis and peroneus in the calf, as well as the soleus and gracilis in the thigh, were well preserved; the pattern of muscular involvement in FCMD cases was identical to that noted in previous reports on DMD cases. Moreover, the degree of involvement varied, even within the same effector muscle group, and the muscles which were well preserved in our FCMD cases were consistent with the characteristic findings in older DMD patients.

Average CT numbers of muscles

Histopathologically, the replacement of muscle by fatty tissue, which follows destruction of the muscle, lower the CT density. Termote et al. [28] were the first to attempt the assessment of muscular lesions by determining the densities of muscle CT images. The method which these authors used for calculating CT numbers involved the free shifting of a small frame over the monitor screen of the computer, the arbitrary selection of a region of interest, and automatic computation of the CT number in the selected region. Most of the subsequent studies on muscle CT numbers were based on the same method, i.e. the use of a sample size CT number [7,12,29].

In the present study, since the CT numbers were obtained by demarcation of the images of entire muscles, the data obtained exhibit greater reliability with respect to the assessment of intramuscular lesions. In fact, our results revealed a close correlation between age and average CT number for almost all muscles examined in both diseases. Accordingly, analysis of the slopes of the regression lines allowed an objective comparison of the rates of age-related decreases in CT numbers (i.e., the severity of muscular lesions) between different muscles.

Comparison of the severity of muscular lesions in the DMD group
Stern et al. [7] compared the CT numbers of the thigh and calf muscles on the basis of data yielded from CT scans performed twice at an interval of 6 months in DMD patients ranging from 4 to 12 years of age. In almost all muscles scanned, the CT numbers observed on the second examination were lower than the corresponding numbers recorded on the first examination. The differences in the adductor magnus, semimembranosus and semitendinosus were reported to be particularly pronounced. However, this study was also based upon sample size CT numbers as indices of the degrees of involvement of the respective muscles.

In the present study, the decrease in the adductor magnus CT number was significantly more rapid than that of any other muscle, reflecting the macroscopic findings and confirming the report of Stern et al. [7]. However, the rates of decrease in semimembranosus and semitendinosus CT numbers did not differ from those of other muscles. Comparing the rates of CT number decreases revealed that the decrease in the gracilis tended to be comparatively slow, although this was not evident macroscopically. Thus, the selective involvement of muscles characteristic of the symptomatic stage was already partially evident in the preclinical stage.

Selective involvement of muscles was also noted in the paravertebral muscles at the L3 level; that is, the multifidi, the most medially situated muscles, tended to remain intact. However, this had already been noted macroscopically.

Comparison of the severity of muscular lesions in the FCMD group
In FCMD, only the psoas has been assessed using muscle CT numbers [20].

In our study, comparison of the slopes of the regression lines revealed that the CT number decrease in the psoas major was statistically slower than those in the paravertebral muscles. This result agrees with the macroscopic evaluation of our subjects and also with the report of Sumida et al. [20]. Clinically, even patients whose necks are unstable can acquire the ability to change their posture from the supine to the lateral decubitus position or to crawl on their backs, and they can bend their hip joints against gravity. Such clinical observations are supported by the findings of this study that the psoas major, the major hip joint flexor, tends to be well preserved. However, our statistical analysis of the slopes of the regression lines did not confirm the macroscopic findings of Sumida et al. [20] that changes commenced in the lateral muscles of the paravertebral group.

At the thigh level, the gracilis appeared macroscopically to have been relatively preserved as compared to the other muscles of the thigh; however, since the CT number of this muscle did not correlate significantly with age, this muscle was not included in the statistical comparison of muscles. Among the flexors, the sartorius differed significantly from the quadriceps in terms of muscle lesion severity, with no other inter-muscle differences being observed. Thus, selective muscle involvement, as seen in DMD, was not observed in the FCMD thigh muscles.

At the calf level, the anterior and posterior tibialis differed markedly from other muscles, indicating that the progression of muscle degeneration in the tibialis muscles was extremely mild, which reflected the macroscopic findings. This selective muscle involvement in the FCMD group was similar to that in the DMD group.

Comparison between DMD and FCMD

The present study demonstrated that CT numbers in FCMD were lower for all muscles, except the psoas major and sartorius, than the corresponding values in DMD patients. For the triceps muscles of the calf, as well as the multifidi of the paravertebral group, the rates of decrease in CT numbers were more rapid in FCMD than in DMD. For other muscles, the CT numbers in FCMD theoretically decreased in parallel with those in DMD, retaining comparatively low CT numbers; their densities decreased at the same rates as those in DMD during the same period.

Conclusion

The muscles which are well preserved in both DMD and FCMD are known to be preserved up to an advanced age in Becker type muscular dystrophy [12,28] and autosomal recessive distal muscular dystrophy [14]. For this reason, it has been speculated that selective involvement of muscles is not dependent solely on etiological factors. The present study verified this view that the decreases in muscle CT numbers were in parallel in the DMD and FCMD groups. Our results also suggest that selective involvement of muscles is also related to acquired factors such as anti-gravitation exercise.

Analyzing muscle CT numbers allowed an objective, detailed evaluation of changes which are not macroscopically visible in the early stages of muscular dystrophy.

Acknowledgments

We are grateful to assistant Professor Atsushi Kohno, Department of Roentogenology, Tokyo Women's Medical College, Tokyo, for his co-operation in the examination of skeletal muscle CT scanning. This study was supported by scientific research grants from the Ministry of Education (A No. 2857137, A No. 02404046), and research grants from the third research group on muscular dystrophy, sponsored by the Ministry of Health and Welfare of Japan.

References

1. O'Doherty DS, Schellinger D, Raptopoulos V. Computed tomographic patterns of pseudohypertrophic muscular dystrophy: preliminary results. J Comput Assist Tomogr 1977; 1: 482–648.
2. William C, Reno TNV. Computed tomography of muscle: a useful technique in the differential diagnosis and study of infantile hypotonia and a variety of neuromuscular disorders in children and adults (abstract). Ann Neurol 1980; 8: 233–234.
3. Ohiwa N, Kato T, Ando T, Mohri A, Yokoi K, Matsumoto H. CT findings of skeletal muscles in children with progressive muscular dystrophy (in Japanese). No To Hattatsu (Tokyo) 1981; 13: 156–159.
4. Tachino K, Nishimura A, Yamaguchi M. Computed tomographic patterns of progressive muscular dystrophy (in Japanese). Sogo Rehabilitation 1982; 10: 525–531.
5. Jones DA, Round JM, Edwards RHT, Grindwood SR, Tofts PS. Size and composition of the calf and quadriceps muscles in Duchenne muscular dystrophy. J Neurol Sci 1983; 60: 307–322.
6. Hawley RJ, Schellinger D, O'Doherty DS. Computed tomographic patterns of muscles in neuromuscular diseases. Arch Neurol 1984; 41: 383–387.
7. Stern LM, Caudrey DJ, Perrett LV, Boldt DW. Progression of muscular dystrophy assessed by computed tomography. Dev Med Child Neurol 1984; 26: 569–573.
8. Kawai M, Kunimoto M, Motoyoshi Y, Kuwata T, Nakano I. Computed tomography in Duchenne type muscular dystrophy – morphological stages based on the computed tomographical findings (in Japanese). Rinsho Shinkeigaku (Tokyo) 1985; 25: 578–590.
9. Nagao H, Takahashi M, Habara S, Nagai Y, Matsuda H. Computed tomography of skeletal muscles in neuromuscular diseases (in Japanese). Nippon Shonika Gakkai Zasshi (Tokyo) 1986; 90: 140–147.
10. Saitoh H. CT findings of muscular dystrophy: limb girdle type (LG), myotonic type (MYD) and Duchenne type (DMD) (in Japanese). Nippon Igaku Hoshasen Gakkai Zasshi (Tokyo) 1991; 51: 790–798.
11. Takahashi R, Matsui K, Fukushima N, Kurokawa T. Muscle CT in Duchenne muscle dystrophy in infants (in Japanese). No To Hattatsu (Tokyo) 1992; 24: 496–498.
12. Bulke JA, Crolla D, Termote JL, Baert A, Parmers Y, Bergh RVD. Computed tomography of muscle. Muscle Nerve 1981; 4: 67–72.
13. Mizusawa H, Inoue K, Toyokura Y, Nakanishi T. Distribution of skeletal muscle involvement in distal myopathy with rimmed vacuoles: a clinical and computed tomographic study (in Japanese). Rinsho Shinkeigaku (Tokyo) 1986; 26: 1174–1181.
14. Mizusawa H, Kobayashi F, Nakanishi T. Distribution of skeletal muscle involvement in autosomal recessive distal muscular dystrophy: a clinical and computed tomographic study (in Japanese). Rinsho Shinkeigaku (Tokyo) 1986; 26: 1174–1178.
15. Takahashi R, Imai T, Sadashima H, et al. Skeletal muscle CT of lower extremities in myotonic dystrophy (in Japanese). CT Kenkyu (Tokyo) 1988; 10: 73–79.
16. Takahashi R, Imai T, Sadashima H, et al. Computed tomographic findings of skeletal muscles in amyotrophic lateral sclerosis (in Japanese). CT Kenkyu (Tokyo) 1989; 11: 129–134.
17. Fukuyama Y, Kawazura M, Haruna H. A peculiar form of congenital progressive muscular dystrophy. Report of fifteen cases. Paediatr Univ Tokyo (Tokyo) 1960; 4: 5–8.
18. Fukuyama Y, Osawa M, Suzuki H. Congenital progressive muscular dystrophy of the Fukuyama type – clinical, genetic and pathological considerations. Brain Dev (Tokyo) 1981; 3: 1–29.
19. Osawa M. A genetic study of the Fukuyama type congenital muscular dystrophy (in Japanese). Tokyo Joshi Ikadaigaku Zasshi (Tokyo) 1978; 48: 204–241.

136

20. Sumida S, Osawa M, Okada N, et al. A study on the findings of muscle CT in patients with Fukuyama type congenital muscular dystrophy (FCMD) (in Japanese). Nippon Shonika Gakkai Zasshi (Tokyo) 1984; 88: 1763–1774.
21. Koenig M, Hoffmann EP, Bertelson CJ, Monaco AP, Feener C, Kunkel LM. Complete cloning of the Duchenne muscular dystrophy (DMD) cDNA and preliminary genomic organization of the DMD gene in normal and affected individuals. Cell 1987; 50: 509–517.
22. Pearson CM. Histopathological features of muscle in the preclinical stages of muscular dystrophy. Brain 1962; 85: 109–126.
23. Hudgson P, Pearce GW, Walton JN. Preclinical muscular dystrophy: Histopathological changes observed on muscle biopsy. Brain 1967; 90: 565–576.
24. Mahoney MJ, Haseltine FP, Hobbins JC, Banker BQ, Caskey CT, Golbus MS. Prenatal diagnosis of Duchenne's muscular dystrophy. N Engl J Med 1977; 287: 968–973.
25. Takada K, Nakamura H, Suzumori K, Ishikawa T, Sugiyama N. Cortical dysplasia in a 23-week fetus with Fukuyama congenital muscular dystrophy (FCMD). Acta Neuropathol (Berlin) 1987; 74: 300–306.
26. Hadar H, Gadoth N, Heifetz M. Fatty replacement of lower paraspinal muscles: normal and neuromuscular disorders. Am J Roentgenol 1983; 141: 895–898.
27. Saida K, Kyogoku M, Hojo H, Hirotani H, Nishitani H. Congenital muscular dystrophy (Fukuyama type). Quantitative histological study of distribution of affected muscles (in Japanese). Rinsho Shinkeigaku (Tokyo) 1973; 13: 587–596.
28. Termote JL, Baert A, Crolla D, Palmers Y, Bulcke JA. Computed tomography of the normal and pathological muscular system. 1980; 137: 439–444.
29. Nordal HJ, Dietrichson P, Eldevic P, Grønseth K. Fat infiltration, atrophy and hypertrophy of skeletal muscles demonstrated by X-ray computed tomography in neurological patients. Acta Neurol Scand 1988; 77: 115–122.

Y. Fukuyama, M. Osawa and K. Saito (Eds.), *Congenital Muscular Dystrophies*
© 1997 Elsevier Science B.V. All rights reserved

Longitudinal evaluation of leukoencephalopathy in congenital muscular dystrophy: data on a heterogeneous series of Western cases

CARLO P. TREVISAN[1], FRANCESCO MARTINELLO[1], MARINA FANIN[1],
CARLA CAROLLO[1], PAOLA PERINI[1], CORRADO ANGELINI[1],
PAOLA DRIGO[2], ANNA MARIA LAVERDA[2],
MARIA LUISA MOSTACCIUOLO[3], A. PATRIZIA TORMENE[4],
MICHEL FARDEAU[5] and FERNANDO M.S. TOMÉ[5]

[1]*Neurological Institute, University of Padua, Italy*
[2]*Department of Paediatrics, University of Padua, Italy*
[3]*Department of Biology, University of Padua, Italy*
[4]*Institute of Ophthalmology, University of Padua, Italy*
[5]*INSERM U.153 and CNRS ERS 064, Paris, France*

Introduction

The varied clinical appearance of congenital muscular dystrophy (CMD) has led to the distinction into subtypes of this heterogeneous disease [1–4]. Presently [5], the following clinical phenotypes can be defined: the Fukuyama type, with severe and progressive muscle deficit and clear-cut brain involvement [6]; the muscle-eye-brain disease (MEBd) [7] and the Walker–Warburg syndrome (WWS) [8], in which there is also clinical evidence of ocular involvement; the classical CMD (Cl-CMD), essentially characterized by muscular symptoms. In Cl-CMD, however, as was found in our previous investigations [9,10], there is frequent CNS involvement of a subclinical significance, mainly represented by white matter changes. These alterations, as discussed by Fardeau et al. in this book, characterize the subtype of Cl-CMD with merosin deficiency, recently identified by Tomé et al. [11].

In this study, we report some data on varied and heterogeneous brain involvement in an unselected group of 29 Western patients, with different clinical expressions of CMD, and evaluation of the leukoencephalopathy, the main alteration found in these cases. In some of them, the correlation of the brain abnormalities with the muscle expression of laminin α-2 chain (merosin) was also evaluated.

Subjects and methods

From 1981 to 1993, at the Neuromuscular Center of the Neurological Institute of the University of Padua, 29 patients, 13 males and 16 females, have been diagnosed as being affected by CMD. According to the criteria adopted by the International Consortium on CMD [5], 22 were considered to suffer from Cl-CMD and 3 from WWs. Four cases were diagnosed as having Fukuyama-like CMD: we considered these 4 patients to be similar to the cases with Fukuyama form of CMD because they presented, without ocular involvement, different degrees of mental retardation (4/4) and epilepsy (2/4) with evidence of severe brain alterations in neuroimaging studies, such as hydrocephalus (4/4), leukoencephalopathy (3/4) and pachygyria (2/4). However, differently from what was reported for cases with Fukuyama type CMD [14], their moderate (1/4) to severe (3/4) muscle involvement showed no progression at the time of the last clinical evaluation, at the age of 12–13.

The mean age at the time of diagnosis and at the time of the last evaluation of their CNS conditions, as well as the sex distribution of these 3 groups of cases, are reported in Table 1.

CNS evaluation

At the time of diagnosis, all 29 cases had a complete neurological and psychiatric examination. Intellectual ability was evaluated by clinical observation and, when possible, by means of intelligence tests such as the Raven Progressive Matrices, Stanford Binet Intelligence Scale and Wechsler Intelligence Scale for Children. Subsequently, all patients underwent EEG and brain CT or MRI. The same cerebral parameters were reevaluated in 18 of these patients after a mean period of 7 years (range 2–18 years). The same reevaluation is continuing in the others.

Immunocytochemistry of merosin

Indirect immunofluorescence microscopy, using monoclonal antibodies (Chemicon) anti-laminin α-2 chain (merosin) and antibodies (Gibco BRL) anti-laminin α-1 (4C7), was performed on cryosections from skeletal muscle biopsy specimens of 14 of the 22 patients with Cl-CMD, of the 3 cases with WWs, and of the 4 patients with Fukuyama-like CMD. This immunocytochemical investigation was performed according to the methods described by Tomé et al. elsewhere [11].

Results

As shown in Table 2, investigation of the CNS conditions of the 3 cases with WWs showed severe mental retardation and epilepsy in all of them (3/3). CT scanning at the time of diagnosis, in the first months of life, provided evidence of severe and diffuse leukoencephalo-

Table 1

Clinical forms of CMD observed in our series of 29 cases

	Number of cases	Males versus females	Mean age at diagnosis (years)	Mean age at CNS reevaluation (years)
Classical	22	11/11	2 11 (1 month–10 years)	(1–23)
Fukuyama-like	4	0/4	2 12 (1 month–2 years)	(12–13)
Walker–Warburg	3	2/1	3 months (1–7 months)	4 (2–5)

Criteria for diagnosis are reported under "Subjects and methods".

Table 2

Brain abnormalities in our 29 cases with CMD on neuroimaging studies

	Cl-CMD 22 cases (%)	Fukuyama-like 4 cases	WWs 3 cases
Mental retardation	6/22 (27)	4/4	3/3
– Mild	4/6	1/4	0/3
– Moderate	2/6	1/4	0/3
– Severe	0/6	2/4	3/3
Epilepsy	1/22 (5)	2/4	3/3
CT/MRI alterations	13/22 (59)	4/4	3/3
(a) White matter abnormalities	9/22 (41)	3/4	3/3
– Mild	4/9	1/4	0/3
– Moderate	4/9	0/4	0/3
– Severe	1/9	2/4	3/3
(b) Cerebellar alterations	5/22 (23)	0/4	2/3
(c) Ventricular dilatation	4/22 (18)	4/4	3/3
(d) Cortical atrophy	2/22 (9)	1/4	3/3
(e) Gyral abnormalities	1/22 (5)[a]	2/4	2/2
(f) Corpus callosum agenesis	0/22 (0)	0/4	1/3

[a]Evident on postmortem neuropathological examination (see [10]).

pathy and hydrocephalus in all of them (3/3). Lissencephaly and dilation of the cisterna magna and incisura posterior cerebelli was apparent in 2. CT reappraisal of one of the subjects, after 5 years, showed that the central white matter alteration was improved, whereas the other brain abnormalities were unchanged. Postmortem neuropathological examination in another, who died at age 4 years, showed that the leukoencephalopathy and other CNS alterations were unchanged. Immunocytochemistry of muscle merosin was normal in all of them.

At the time of diagnosis, a study of CNS conditions in the 4 cases with Fukuyama-like CMD (Table 2) showed in all of them mild to severe mental retardation, associated with epilepsy in 2. CT scanning showed hydrocephalus with cortical atrophy in all of them, mild (1/4) to severe (2/4) leukoencephalopathy in 3 and pachygyria in 2. In 3 of them, were also found alterations of visual evoked responses. CT and MRI reappraisal of the brain conditions in these 4 subjects, after a mean period of 9 years, showed evident improvement of the leukoencephalopathy in one but no changes in the central white matter conditions in the others. In the same 4 patients there was no modification of the other abnormalities. The MRI findings in one of these cases are presented in Fig. 1. In this case, as reported elsewhere [12], muscle merosin was undetectable by immunocytochemistry, while it was normal in the other 3 cases.

The CNS conditions in the 22 cases with Cl-CMD are summarized in Table 2: intellectual ability was normal in the vast majority (16/22). In a few cases, mild (4/22) to moderate (2/22) mental retardation was found: of these 6 patients, 1 exhibited no abnormalities on brain CT scanning, whereas 5 showed mild abnormalities as leukoencephalopathy, slight enlargement of the lateral ventricles or moderate cerebellar hypoplasia. At 3 years of age, one patient suffered from myoclonic jerks for a few days, that promptly ceased after treat-

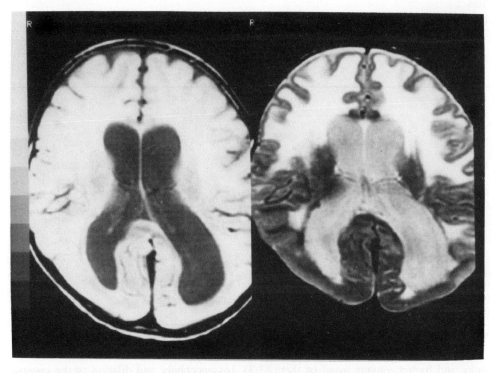

Fig. 1. Brain MRI of a merosin-negative case with Fukuyama-like CMD. This 9-year-old girl suffered from a severe congenital and non-progressive muscular deficit, mild mental retardation and epilepsy. Axial T2-weighted images (TR 2000; TE 30,90) show severe leukoencephalopathy, mainly in the anterior regions, associated with marked ventricular dilatation and pachygyria in the occipital cortex [12].

ment with valproate; her MRI was normal. Brain subclinical abnormalities were detected on CT or MRI in 9 of the 16 cases who had no symptoms or signs of CNS involvement. On the whole, in 13 of the 22 cases with Cl-CMD (59%) neuroimaging evaluation (CT or MRI) provided evidence of some abnormalities, mainly represented by white matter changes (41%) (Fig. 2), cerebellar hypoplasia (23%) or other minor alterations (Table 2). In 11 of them were detected abnormalities in visual evoked responses. Immunolabelling of muscle merosin was done only in 5 of the cases with white matter changes and showed an absence of the protein in all of them. Follow-up of the CNS conditions by CT or MRI, performed in 12 of the cases affected by Cl-CMD after a mean period of 8 years, showed that the central white matter conditions were mainly unchanged (9/12) like the other brain abnormalities, as reported elsewhere [15]. Leukoencephalopathy appeared to be improved in 2 cases and worse in another one, who at 6 years of age showed severe and slightly progressive muscle involvement without clinical symptoms of brain alterations. In the muscle of this patient with progressive leukoencephalopathy, there was no labelling with the antibody anti-laminin α-2 chain (merosin). The same immunocytochemical investigation showed partial merosin deficiency (Fig. 3) in another patient with Cl-CMD and improving and not severe leukoencephalopathy. On the contrary, muscle merosin was normal (Fig. 3) in her older sister, who presented improving but severe leukoencephalopathy associated with hydro-cephalus and pachygyria (Fukuyama-like). These two sisters have been extensively described elsewhere [13]. Two other patients with Cl-CMD and merosin deficiency presented static white matter changes. Nine patients with Cl-CMD showed a normal expression of muscle merosin; their MRI was either normal (6 cases) or mildly altered (3 cases). Table 3 presents the data on muscle and brain involvement in 7 of the 14 cases with Cl-CMD studied with antibodies anti-laminin subunits.

Discussion

Congenital muscular dystrophy (CMD) is a genetic heterogeneous disease [1–6] recently classified into 4 different forms according to the clinical manifestations accompanying the muscular deficit [5]. Severe CNS involvement characterizes the Fukuyama type of CMD with evidence on clinical grounds of moderate to profound mental retardation, frequently associated with epilepsy [6,14]. Clinical evidence of severe brain alterations is also a main feature of both WWs and MEBd, the muscular dystrophy types associated with clear-cut involvement of the ocular structures [1–5,7,8]. The similarity between WWs and Fukuyama CMD has often been stressed [5,6,8]. However, from our data it appears inconsistent since we found normal expression of merosin in muscles of the cases with WWs, in contrast to what was reported for cases with Fukuyama CMD in which muscle merosin is severely reduced [16].

In Western countries, classical CMD (Cl-CMD) shows usually clinical evidence of "pure" [5] muscular involvement, even if sporadic cases with mild to moderate mental re-

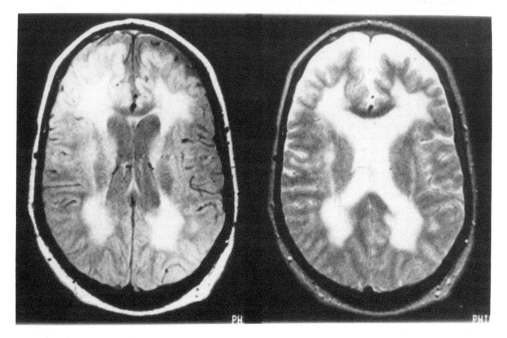

Fig. 2. Brain MRI of a merosin-negative classical CMD case. This 18-year-old non-ambulant young man suffered from severe congenital muscular deficit without clinical evidence of CNS involvement. Axial T2-weighted images (TR 2000; TE 30,90) provide evidence of moderate leukoencephalopathy in the periventricular regions, associated with mild ventricular enlargement and frontal cortical atrophy (from Trevisan et al., Brain Dev., submitted).

142

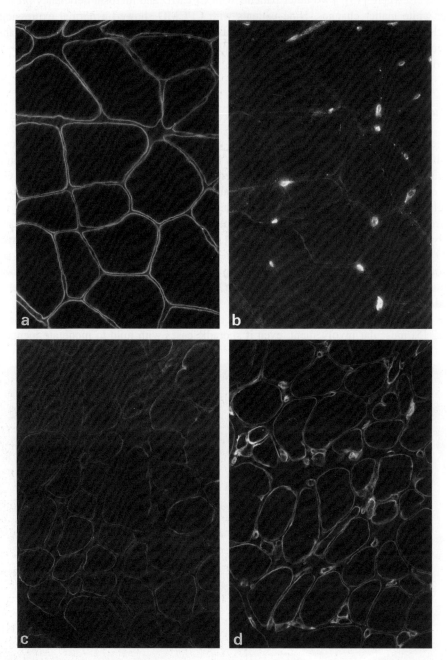

Fig. 3. Immunocytochemical analysis of merosin and laminin α-1 chain in muscle biopsy specimens from two sisters with CMD and different CNS involvement. In the older one, affected by a moderate muscle deficit and severe brain alterations (Fukuyama-like), there was normal staining with antibodies anti-merosin (a) and anti-laminin α-1 chain (b). In the younger one, affected by moderate muscle involvement associated with mild and subclinical brain alterations (Cl-CMD), merosin was evidently reduced (c) and laminin α-1 increased (d) (magnification ×375). These cases have been extensively described elsewhere [13].

Table 3

Correlation between clinical aspects and muscle content of merosin in 7 cases with Cl-CMD

	1	2	3	4	5	6	7
Sex	M	F	M	F	M	M	M
Age (years)	5	7	11	6	22	5	15
Age at biopsy (years)	4 months	6	3	2	10	1 month	14
Muscular weakness[a]	+	++	++	+	++	+++	++
Mental retardation	++	–	–	+	–	–	++
CT/MRI alterations[b]							
(a) Leukoencephalopathy	–	++	–	–	–	+++	–
(b) Ventricular dilatation	+	+	–	–	–	+	–
(c) Cortical atrophy	–	–	–	–	–	–	–
(d) Cerebellar alterations	–	–	–	–	–	–	+++
(e) Pachygyria	–	–	–	–	–	–	–
Muscle merosin[c]	N	–2	N	N	N	–3	N

[a]Muscle weakness is graded as mild (+), moderate (++) or severe (+++). Patients with severe weakness are not able to walk, patients with mild or moderate weakness can walk.
[b]The alterations are graded as absent (–), mild (+), moderate (++) or severe (+++).
[c]Immunostaining of muscle merosin is represented as normal (N), decreased (mildly: –1, moderately: –2) or absent (–3).

tardation have been described [1–5,17,19]. A systematic investigation of CNS conditions in an unselected group of Western cases of CMD reported some years ago [9,10] clearly indicated the high frequency of subclinical brain alterations in patients with Cl-CMD. As is also evident in subsequent reports [5,11], in this form of CMD, the most frequent CNS alteration found by MRI is represented by leukoencephalopathy that has no clinical expression. Tomé et al. [11] have recently identified a subtype of Cl-CMD with merosin deficiency: in the brain of all the patients affected by this form of the disease, white matter changes were characteristically found (see Fardeau et al., this volume), as was also evident in the merosin-deficient cases discussed here. Sometimes, Cl-CMD is differently classified depending on the presence or absence of CNS alterations: this distinction does not seem consistent considering the multiform CNS abnormalities found in Cl-CMD, irrespective of the merosin expression in muscle, as is evident in the cases reported here and in others described elsewhere [1–5,10,12,17–19]. Actually, there are cases with normal CT or MRI and mild mental retardation or epilepsy, as well as cases with no symptoms of CNS involvement and heterogeneous alterations on brain CT or MRI [15]. These include, other than various degrees of leukoencephalopathy that characterize CMD with merosin deficiency, mild cerebellar hypoplasia or cerebellar cysts, mild ventricular dilatation, mild cortical atrophy and focal pachygyria [9,10,15]. All these abnormalities may appear isolated or in various combinations.

In Western CMD, as evident in few of our series of patients as well as in others reported to date [1–5,15], brain involvement may not be mild and subclinical, but severe, with evidence of profound mental retardation and epilepsy on clinical grounds, and pachygyria, hydrocephalus, white matter changes and cortical atrophy at the neuroimaging level, as often described in cases with Fukuyama CMD [1–6,14]. We prefer to classify many of these cases as Fukuyama-like CMD, since they, like the 4 reported here, do not fully satisfy the criteria

144

adopted by the Japanese authors for the diagnosis of Fukuyama CMD [6,14]. Moreover, in contrast to typical cases of Fukuyama CMD, in which muscle merosin is dramatically reduced [16], our Fukuyama-like cases showed normal or absent expression of the same laminin subunit in muscle.

Central white matter changes, characteristic of Cl-CMD with merosin deficiency and very frequent in Fukuyama CMD, are also a common finding in patients with WWs [2–5]. In cases with MEBd the same alteration is less frequently reported [2–7].

Our follow-up data on the leukoencephalopathy in Western patients with different forms of CMD indicate that generally the white matter alteration does not progress. Actually, in our investigation, a non-progressive course of this abnormality after the first year of life was evident in the cases with WWs and in the patients with Fukuyama-like CMD, as reported for cases with Fukuyama CMD [14,21]. Also in Cl-CMD cases of our series, central white matter conditions showed a mainly stationary course. The predominantly non-progressive course of the leukoencephalopathy in CMD would indicate that it represents a secondary abnormality rather than a primary active degenerative process in the central myelin of these patients, as also suggested by Osawa et al. [14].

Acknowledgments

This work was supported by Grant n. 688 from Telethon-Italy.

References

1. Nonaka I, Chou SM. Congenital muscular dystrophy. In: Vinken PJ, Bruyn GW, eds. Handbook of clinical neurology, Vol 41. Amsterdam: North-Holland, 1979: 27–50.
2. Fardeau M. Congenital myopathies. In: Mastaglia FL, Walton J, eds. Skeletal muscle pathology. 2nd edn. Edinburgh: Churchill Livingstone, 1992: 237–281.
3. Gardner-Medwin D, Walton J. The muscular dystrophies. In: Walton J, Karpati G, Hilton-Jones D, eds. Disorders of voluntary muscle. 6th edn. Edinburgh: Churchill Livingstone, 1994: 553–594.
4. Fenichel GM. Clinical pediatric neurology. A signs and symptoms approach. Philadelphia, PA: Saunders, 1993.
5. Dubowitz V. 22nd ENMC sponsored workshop on congenital muscular dystrophy. Neuromusc Dis 1994; 4: 75–81.
6. Fukuyama Y, Osawa M, Suzuki H. Congenital progressive muscular dystrophy of the Fukuyama type. Clinical, genetic and pathological considerations. Brain Dev (Tokyo) 1981, 3: 1–29.
7. Santavuori P, Leisti J, Kruus J. Muscle, eye and brain disease. A new syndrome. Neuropaediatrie 1977; 8: 550–553.
8. Dobyns WB, Pagon RA, Armstrong J, et al. Diagnostic criteria for Walker–Warburg syndrome. Am J Med Genet 1989; 32: 195–210.
9. Trevisan CP, Segalla P, Drigo P, et al. Subclinical brain involvement in typical CMD. J Neurol Sci 1990; 98(Suppl.): 435.
10. Trevisan CP, Carollo C, Segalla P, Angelini C, Drigo P, Giordano R. Congenital muscular dystrophy: brain alterations in an unselected series of Western patients. J Neurol Neurosurg Psychiatry 1991; 54: 330–334.
11. Tomè FM, Evangelista T, Leclerc A, et al. Congenital muscular dystrophy with merosin deficiency. CR Acad Sci Paris 1994; 317: 351–357.
12. Trevisan CP, Martinello F, Fanin M, et al. Merosin expression in muscle of Western cases with Fukuyama-like congenital muscular dystrophy. Basic Appl Myol 1996; 6: 101–106.
13. Trevisan CP, Martinello F, Ferruzza E, Angelini C. Divergence of central nervous system involvement in two western sisters with congenital muscular dystrophy: a clinical and neuroradiological follow-up. Eur Neurol 1995; 35: 230–235.

14. Osawa M, Arai Y, Ikenaka H, et al. Fukuyama type congenital progressive muscular dystrophy. Acta Paediatr Jpn (Tokyo) 1991; 33: 261–269.
15. Trevisan CP, Martinello F, Ferruzza E, et al. Brain alterations in the classical form of congenital muscular dystrophy. Clinical and neuroimaging follow-up of 12 cases and correlation of merosin in muscle. Child Nerv Syst 1996; 12: 604–610.
16. Hayashi YK, Engvall E, Arikawa-Hirasawa E, et al. Abnormal localization of laminin subunits in muscular dystrophies. J Neurol Sci 1993; 119: 53–64.
17. Nogen AG. Congenital muscle disease and abnormal findings on computerized tomography. Dev Med Child Neurol 1980; 22: 658–663.
18. Egger J, Kendall BE, Erdohazi M, et al. Involvement of the central nervous system in congenital muscular dystrophies. Dev Med Child Neurol 1983; 25: 32–42.
19. Echenne B, Arthuis M, Billard C, et al. Congenital muscular dystrophy and cerebral CT scan anomalies. Results of a collaborative study of the Societè de Neurologie Infantile. J Neurol Sci 1986; 75: 7–22.
20. Topaloglu H, Yalaz K, Renda Y, et al. Occidental type cerebromuscular dystrophy: a report of eleven cases. J Neurol Neurosurg Psychiatry 1991; 54: 226–229.
21. Yoshioka M, Okuno T, Ito M, et al. Congenital muscular dystrophy (Fukuyama type). Repeated CT studies in 19 children. Comp Tomogr 1981; 5: 81–88.

Y. Fukuyama, M. Osawa and K. Saito (Eds.), *Congenital Muscular Dystrophies*
© 1997 Elsevier Science B.V. All rights reserved

CHAPTER 11

Congenital muscular dystrophy: clinical variability in Sicilian patients

ENRICO PARANO[1], LORENZO PAVONE[1], AGATA FIUMARA[1],
RAFFAELE FALSAPERLA[1] AND WILLIAM B. DOBYNS[2]

[1]*Pediatric Clinic, University of Catania, Catania, Italy*
[2]*Department of Neurology and Pediatrics, University of Minnesota, Minneapolis, MN, USA*

Introduction

Congenital muscular dystrophy (CMD) is a rare and unusual form of muscular dystrophy. It is characterized by generalized weakness, hypotonia and joint contractures from birth, and features of dystrophic changes on muscle biopsying. CMD is usually sporadic, although patients with autosomal recessive and rarely autosomal dominant inheritance have been reported. The disorder has a variable clinical course, but in most cases it is slow or slightly progressive. CK values may be elevated, slightly increased or within normal limits. EMG is usually myogenic and a muscle biopsy shows a typical dystrophic pattern with a normal dystrophin distribution [1–4]. Recently CMD patients with a deficiency of merosin, a specific basal lamina-associated protein, have been reported. These patients show severe hypotonia, weakness and often progressive contractures with normal mental development. CK is notably elevated, particularly in the early stages of the disease. CT-scanning and MRI show myelin changes in many areas of the white matter [5–7].

In this chapter we report 12 Sicilian patients affected by different types of CMD, showing the great clinical variability of this syndrome.

Case reports

Twelve patients (6 females and 6 males) affected by CMD were evaluated at the Pediatric Clinic, University of Catania, Italy. Their ages ranged from 1 to 13 years. Consanguinity was recorded in 5 cases. Hypotonia, weakness and joint contractures were present in most of the patients since birth and always within the first 2 years of life. Tendon reflexes were reduced or absent in all cases. Scoliosis was observed in 3 patients but none had calf hypertrophy. Mild cognitive impairment was present in 2 cases, while severe mental retardation was observed in 4 patients. Only 1 patient showed microcephaly and 2, macrocephaly. Seizures were present in 2 cases. CK was elevated in 5 cases, being slightly increased in 1 and normal in 4. Myopathic EMG and dystrophic changes in a muscle biopsy specimen with a normal dystrophin distribution (where performed) were observed in all cases. Retinal abnormality was present in 1 case, while 3 patients presented anterior chamber abnormalities and cataracts. Brain MRI disclosed the presence of a cobblestone cortex, white matter abnormality, hydrocephalus, a small brain stem and cerebellum, Dandy–Walker malformation and corpus callosum hypoplasia in 4 patients.

We briefly summarize the clinical histories of 2 patients who showed unreported clinical features associated with CMD.

Case 1. 13-year-old female

The parents are not consanguineous. The family history was unremarkable. The pregnancy was uneventful. The child was born at term by cesarean section. Fetal movements were absent. The birth weight was 2900 g. During the first month of life the patient showed muscle weakness, especially in the upper limbs. At the age of 6 months the diagnosis of homozygous beta-thalassemia was made, and so periodic blood transfusions were started. At the age of 18 months, hypotonia and muscle weakness were still present. Neurological examination at that time showed generalized hypotonia and muscle weakness also involving the facial muscles, in association with flexion contractures of the wrists, knees and elbows. Hyporeflexia was present. She could neither stand nor sit upright. Behavioral interaction was normal. Routine laboratory examinations showed a slight increase in the CK level (250 U/l; normal levels, <100). EMG revealed myogenic type findings. A nerve conduction study was normal. A muscle biopsy showed a dystrophic type pattern. Immunostaining of muscle for dystrophin, performed a few years later, was normal.

Case 2. 6-year-old male

The child was born at term after a normal pregnancy. The birth weight was 3500 g. The parents are not related. The family history was unremarkable. At birth, the infant was noted to be floppy, showing also torticollis and congenital hip subluxation. By age 6 months, the child had developed obvious skeletal deformities, generalized hypotonia and muscle weakness. At the age of 6 years, physical examination showed muscle wasting, hypotonia and facial muscle involvement. The tendon reflexes were poor. The child was unable to climb stairs or get up from the ground unassisted. Contractures of the elbows, shoulders, knees and wrists were present. CK and lactic acid were within normal limits. Skeletal X-rays showed severe scoliosis with metameric torsion along the axis in association with anterior deformation of the T5–T7 vertebral bodies. EMG was mixed, with neuropathic findings in the leg muscles and myopathic ones in the arms. A nerve conduction study was normal. A muscle biopsy revealed a dystrophic pattern. Immunostaining of muscle using antibodies to both the C- and N-terminals of dystrophin was normal. Brain MRI was normal but spinal cord MRI disclosed the presence of a smooth-walled thoracolumbar intramedullary cavity. The cavity appeared to be fluid-filled, consisting of a syringomyelic type of alteration.

Discussion

Three forms of CMD are actually distinguished, all characterized by a dystrophic pattern observed on muscle biopsy (Table 1). Type I or classical CMD includes patients with hypotonia and generalized muscle weakness present from birth or soon after, and multiple joint contractures. The clinical course is usually steady or only slowly progressive, and intelligence is normal or only moderately affected. There is no eye impairment, and CK is

Table 1

Classification of congenital muscular dystrophy: main manifestations

Type I: classical CMD
Clinical manifestations
– Onset at birth
– Hypotonia and generalized muscle weakness
– Multiple joint contractures
– Clinical course, not progressive or slowly progressive
– Normal or mildly impaired cognitive development
Muscle
– Dystrophic pattern
– Serum CK, normal or mildly increased
Brain
– Normal or white matter abnormalities only (delayed myelination)
Eyes
– Normal

Type II: Fukuyama congenital muscular dystrophy
Clinical manifestations
– Onset before 8 months
– IQ less than 50 or developmental delay if before 1 year old
– Seizures
– Delay of motor development
– Hypotonia and generalized muscle weakness
– Facial muscle involvement
– Tendon reflexes, decreased or absent
– Never able to walk
Muscle
– Dystrophic pattern
– Serum CK elevated
Brain
– white matter abnormalities; lissencephaly, polymicrogyria
Eyes
– myopia, optic atrophy, strabism, ptosis

Type III: Walker–Warburg syndrome and muscle-eye-brain disease
Clinical manifestations
– Onset at birth
– IQ less than 50 or developmental delay
– Hypotonia and generalized muscle weakness
– Seizures
Muscle
– Dystrophic pattern
– Serum CK elevated
Brain
– Lissencephaly, polymicrogyria, white matter abnormalities
– Dandy–Walker malformation, hydrocephalus, cerebellar involvement
Eyes
– Myopia
– Retinal abnormalities, anterior chamber malformations

normal or slightly increased. There are no anomalies on cerebral-MRI, with the exception of white matter abnormalities consisting of delayed myelination. This type of CMD would also include the recently reported form of CMD with a merosin deficiency[1–3,5–7]. Type II or Fukuyama congenital muscular dystrophy (FCMD) presents clinical manifestations usually not at birth but around or later than the first few months of life; CK is usually increased. MRI shows lissencephaly, polymicrogyria or both, and white matter abnormalities. Cerebellar_cortical dysplasia is usually observed on microscopic examination. Clinical manifestations include seizures, both partial and generalized, and muscle contractures, which may appear later. Occasionally, there are eye abnormalities consisting of mild myopia, optic atrophy, ptosis, strabism and weakness of the orbicularis oculi [1,8–10].

Type III is the most severe form of CMD, and includes patients reported as having Walker–Warburg syndrome (WWS), and muscle-eye-brain Santavuori (MEB) type [1,11, 12]. In this type of CMD the clinical symptoms are usually present from birth, with hypotonia and generalized weakness. CK is increased, and lissencephaly, polymicrogyria, white matter abnormalities and cerebellar involvement are evident on MRI. Eye abnormalities consist mainly of retinal abnormalities, mild myopia and anterior chamber malformations. Dysmorphic features such as cryptorchidism, and a cleft lip/palate may be present. Other severe anomalies of the brain are often also present: absence of the corpus callosum and septum pellucidum, Dandy–Walker malformation, hydrocephaly, and occipital cephaloceles. Patients often suffer from spasticity and seizures [1,11–13].

According to the present classification, 8 of our patients have classical CMD, including 2 cases with mildly impaired cognitive development. Merosin was not examined; however none of our patients had the combination of greatly elevated CK, normal mental development and white matter abnormalities, the main characteristics of classical CMD associated with a merosin deficiency. This specific form of CMD might be less common in Sicily than in France or England, where half of the classical CMD patients present a merosin deficiency [5–7]. The remaining 4 patients have CMD type III.

In the patients reported here, consanguineity was present in 5, including 2 sibs with classical CMD and 2 homozygous twins affected by WWS. Of particular interest were the patients, briefly summarized, in whom CMD was associated with unusual clinical manifestations never previously reported. The first patient, a 13-year-old girl, in addition to classical CMD, was also *homozygous* for beta-thalassemia. This association might be coincidental since beta-thalassemia is quite frequent in Sicily. However, the occurrence of these two diseases may be interesting for potential linkage studies. In the second patient, CMD was associated with kyphosis and skeletal anomalies; MRI of the spine showed a thoracic syringomyelia. This patient might have two separate diseases, but we think that the syringomyelia might be a consequence of central nervous system structural abnormalities that may occur as an expression of the basic defect that leads to CMD.

Many aspects of CMD remain unclear, but it is certain that, rather than a simple disease, CMD is a syndrome which includes several different entities.

References

1. Dubowitz V. Workshop Report: 22nd ENMC sponsored Workshop on Congenital Muscular Dystrophy, Baarn, The Netherlands, May 14–16 1993. Neuromusc Disord 1994; 4: 74–81.

2. Banker BQ. Congenital muscular dystrophy. In: Engel A , Banker BQ, eds. Myology. New York: McGraw-Hill, 1986: 1367–1382.

3. Lazaro RP, Fenichel GM, Kilroy AW. Congenital muscular dystrophy: case report and reappraisal. Muscle Nerve 1979; 2: 349–355.

4. Leyten QH, Gabreels FJM, Joosten EMG, et al. An autosomal dominant type of congenital muscular dystrophy. Brain Dev (Tokyo) 1986; 8: 533–537.

5. Arahata K, Hayashi YK, Koga R, et al. Laminin in animal models for muscular dystrophy: defect of laminin M in skeletal and cardiac muscle and peripheral nerve of the homozygous dystrophic dy/dy mice. Proc Jpn Acad (series B) 1993; 69: 259–264.

6. Tomé FMS, Evangelista T, Leclerc A, et al. Congenital muscular dystrophy with merosin deficiency. C R Acad Sci Paris/Life Sci 1994; 317: 351–357.

7. Dubowitz W, Fardeau M. Proceedings of the 27th ENMC sponsored Workshop on Congenital Muscular Dystrophy, 22–24 April 1994, The Netherlands (workshop report). Neuromusc Disord 1995; 5: 253–258.

8. Fukuyama Y, Osawa M, Suzuki H. Congenital progressive muscular dystrophy of the Fukuyama type – clinical, genetic and pathological consideration. Brain Dev (Tokyo) 1981; 3: 1–29.

9. Osawa M, Arai Y, Ikenaka H, et al. Fukuyama type congenital progressive muscular dystrophy. Acta Paediatr Jpn (Tokyo) 1991; 33: 261–269.

10. Toda T, Segawa M, Nomura Y, et al. Localization of a gene for Fukuyama type congenital muscular dystrophy to chromosome 9q31-33. Nature Genet 1993; 5: 283–286.

11. Dobyns WB, Pagon RA, Armstrong D, et al. Diagnostic criteria for Walker–Warburg syndrome. Am J Med Genet 1989; 32: 195–210.

12. Santavuori P, Somer H, Sainio K, et al. Muscle-eye-brain disease (MEB). Brain Dev (Tokyo) 1989; 11: 147–153.

13. Echenne B, Arthuis M, Billard C, et al. Congenital muscular dystrophy and cerebral CT scan anomalies: results of a collaborative study of the Societé de Neurologie Infantile. J Neurol Sci 1986, 7: 7–22.

Y. Fukuyama, M. Osawa and K. Saito (Eds.), *Congenital Muscular Dystrophies*

Merosin and clinical characteristics of congenital muscular dystrophy in an unselected group of Turkish patients

HALUK TOPALOĞLU[1], TERESINHA EVANGELISTA[2], SAFIYE GÖĞÜŞ[1], KALBIYE YALAZ[1] and FERNANDO M.S. TOMÉ[2]

[1]*Departments of Pediatrics, Neurology and Pathology, Hacettepe Children's Hospital, Ankara, Turkey*
[2]*INSERM U153 and CNRS ERS 064, Paris, France*

Introduction

Congenital muscular dystrophies (CMD) are heterogeneous, and characterized by an autosomal recessive inheritance, early onset hypotonia, multiple joint contractures, dystrophic changes in muscle, and a relatively non-progressive course. Several distinct clinical forms exist. One peculiar form, Fukuyama's CMD (FCMD) which is prevalent in Japan, invariably includes severe mental retardation and central nervous system (CNS) malformation. Recently, the gene for this form has been localized to chromosome 9q31-33 [1]. In "pure" classic type CMD there is always normal or sub-normal intelligence. There is also increasing evidence that CNS involvement in CMD may be more common than previously recognized [2–5]. An intermediate form with normal mental development and a leukodystrophic appearance on CT or MRI has been suggested, and named "occidental type cerebromuscular dystrophy" (OCMD), because this form appears to be prevalent in the West [6,7]. The immunostaining intensity and distribution of laminin subunits A, B1, B2, and M (merosin) have been studied in both FCMD and classical CMD. In both conditions, merosin has been found to be abnormal, being partially reduced in FCMD [8], and severely diminished or absent in many patients affected by the classical form [9]. In humans, the laminin M chain (merosin) gene has been linked to chromosome 6q22-23 [10]. Furthermore, a gene has been localized for merosin-negative CMD to chromosome 6q2 through both homozygosity mapping and linkage analysis [11]. In this report, we evaluate our clinical and neuroradiological findings in seven CMD cases whose merosin status in muscle was studied by means of immunocytochemistry.

Patients and methods

This study was carried out in 7 unselected families including cases with a clinicopathological diagnosis of CMD. They all fulfilled the criteria of the International Consortium on Congenital Muscular Dystrophy [12]. The clinical features are summarized in Table 1. All children presented hypotonia at birth and significant motor developmental delay afterwards. To assess mental development, the Bayley and Stanford–Binet tests were given to those under and above 3 years of age, respectively. WISC-R was used for those attending

154

Table 1

Clinical features of Turkish patients with congenital muscular dystrophy

	Merosin-positive			Merosin-negative			Merosin-reduced
Case:	1	2	3	4	5	6	7
Age at biopsy (years)	6	9	9	9 months	2	3	3
Sex	M	F	M	M	M	F	M
Onset	At birth	Early	At birth	At birth	At birth	At birth	At birth
JS	+	−	−	+	−	−	+
MMC	Walks w/o support	Walks w/o support	Walks w/o support	Poor head control	Sits w/o support	Walks w/o support	Stands w support
CK	230	117	139	3108	2779	630	387
DQ/IQ	N	N	N	N	N	N	N
CT/MRI	N	N	N	Abn.	Abn.	Abn.	Abn.

JS, joint stiffness; MMC, maximal motor capacity; w/o, without; w, with; N, normal; abn, abnormal

school. All patients had IQ or DQ scores of above 70 and thus were classified as normal. Cranial CT was performed using standard equipment with appropriate settings. Areas of white matter hypodensity, migration anomalies and ventricular dilatation with an Evans' index of more than 0.33 (normal 0.26–0.30) were the parameters sought. Cranial MRI was performed using a high field unit (0.5 T). Patients 1, 2 and 7 underwent CT, and the others MRI examinations (Fig. 1).

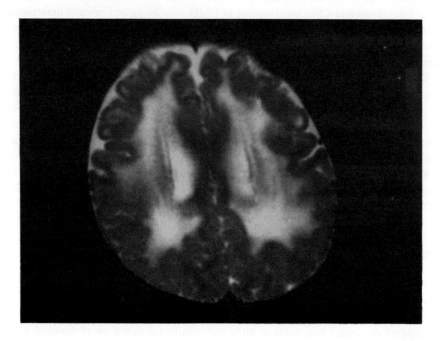

Fig. 1. Case 4. MRI scan obtained at age 18 months. T1 spin echo TR/TE = 500/20, T2-weighted images 3000/100. Evident signal abnormalities denote dysmyelination. Highly immature pattern for age.

Immunocytochemistry
Indirect immunofluorescence microscopy, using monoclonal antibodies, anti-dystrophin (DYS 2 and DYS 3; Novocastra), anti-merosin (laminin M-chain) (Chemicon), and anti-laminin A (4C7), B1 (4E10) and B2 (2E80) chains (Gibco BRL), was performed on cryosections from skeletal muscle biopsy specimens of the 7 patients as previously described [9]. For comparison, cryosections from normal controls were processed identically. The sections were examined under a Zeiss Axioplan fluorescence microscope. Photographs were taken under identical conditions with the same exposure time.

Results

In cases 1, 2 and 3, there was uniform labelling around each muscle fiber with the antibody against merosin (laminin M chain) (Fig. 2a). In these three cases, all the other antibodies used also showed labelling of the muscle tissue identical to that seen in normal controls. The anti-laminin A antibody strongly labelled the blood vessels, but the basement membrane of muscle fibers was very weakly stained or unstained (Fig. 2c). In cases 4, 5 and 6, there was no labelling with the anti-laminin M chain antibody (Fig. 2b) and an increased labelling around muscle fibers with the anti-laminin A chain antibody (Fig. 2d). In the latter 3 cases the anti-dystrophin antibodies showed normal labelling of the sarcolemma, and the anti-laminin B1 chain and B2 chain antibodies did not show significant changes. In case 7, merosin immunostaining was present, but was severely reduced, as judged on visual interpretation. In this specific case, laminin A chain staining was also upregulated.

The immunocytochemical studies allowed the identification of three "merosin-negative" cases of CMD. Thus, patients were grouped into "merosin-negative" and "merosin-positive" cases. The clinical features of our patients can be summarized as follows:

1. *Merosin-positive CMD group.* There were 3 patients in this group, aged 6–9 years at the time of muscle biopsy. One had joint contractures. All 3 were independently ambulant, beginning to walk between 18 months and 3 years and 6 months of age. Two had normal CK, and one had slightly elevated CK at 230 (normal 208 U/l). All had normal IQs and normal CT or MRI.

2. *Merosin-negative CMD group.* The 3 patients in this group were aged 9 months–3 years at the biopsy. All 3 showed definite motor retardation, however, 1 case was ambulant (she began to walk at 2 years and 9 months of age). All had significantly elevated CK levels ranging between 630 and 3108 U/l. The DQs were all normal. All 3 had abnormal MRI scans (Fig. 1).

3. *Merosin-diminished case.* The clinical features of this boy somewhat resembled those of group 2. His CK was mildly elevated (387 U/l). His DQ was normal, but he had abnormal CT with increased white matter hyperlucency resembling leukodystrophy.

Discussion

Tomé et al. reported 13 patients with the classical non-Japanese form of CMD along with 7 CMD cases which had normal merosin levels [9]. Thus, it is now possible to classify classical CMD into at least two separate groups, merosin-negative and merosin-positive CMD, on a clinico-pathological basis.

156

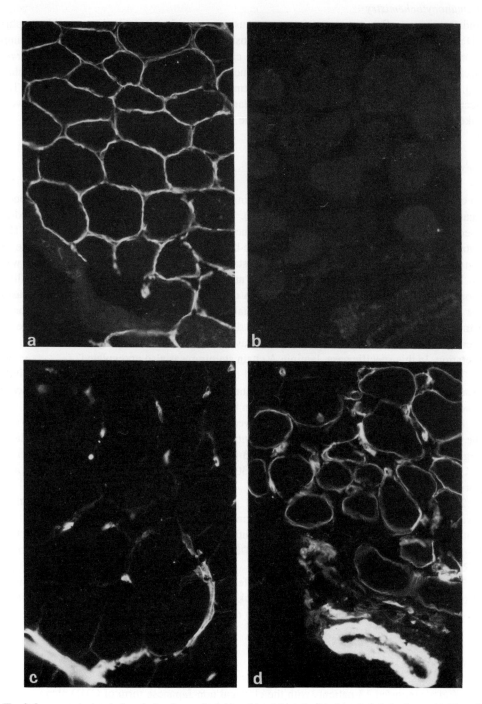

Fig. 2. Immunocytochemical analysis of merosin (a,b) and laminin A (c,d) in biopsied skeletal muscle. There is normal staining in (a) and (c) (case 3), and the absence of merosin and overexpression of laminin A around muscle fibers (case 6). Magnification ×375.

All our 3 merosin-negative cases and the merosin-diminished case had fairly homogeneous features; marked motor delay, significantly increased CK and associated white matter changes on MRI, but without clinical expression. These cases may be examples of the so-called occidental type cerebro-muscular dystrophy [6,7]. On the other hand, our merosin-positive group presented more "silent" features such as lower CK levels, becoming ambulant after age 3 years and 6 months (the latest), and normal CT or MRI scans. This latter group may be more heterogeneous both clinically and histopathologically. Similar observations have been documented by Tomé et al. [9], and Sewry et al. [13]. In Tomé et al.'s 7 published 7 and 18 unpublished cases without merosin deficiency, the clinical features were less severe and showed marked heterogeneity.

We are part of the group who reported the localization of merosin-negative CMD to chromosome 6q2 [11]. Merosin-negative cases 5 and 6 correspond to members of families 1663 and 1812, respectively, in that study, and they showed definite linkage, whereas merosin-positive case 3 is from family 1713, and did not show any linkage.

It has been shown that a laminin M (merosin) defect is primarily responsible for the pathogenesis of muscle fiber damage and dysmyelination in the dystrophic dy/dy mouse [14,15]. Expression of merosin is developmentally regulated, and it may play a crucial role in the differentiation and maturation of the neuromuscular system [16]. Thus, a selective merosin deficiency results in disruption of the linkage between the subsarcolemmal cytoskeleton and the extracellular matrix. The consequent sarcolemmal instability results in muscle cell necrosis.

The lack of merosin allows, therefore, the precise identification of a particular form of CMD, and suggests that defects of this protein may be the primary abnormalities leading to the lesions of the muscle tissue. It is possible that sub-clinical CNS involvement in CMD, i.e. the leukodystrophic abnormalities observed on CT/MRI, could be related to abnormal expression or localization of this protein.

In conclusion, Turkish merosin-negative CMD patients are clinically distinct from merosin-positive cases.

References

1. Toda T, Segawa M, Nomura Y, et al. Localization of a gene for Fukuyama type congenital muscular dystrophy to chromosome 9q 31-33. Nat Genet 1993; 5: 283–286.
2. Egger J, Kendall BE, Erdohazi M, Lake BD, Wilson J, Brett EM. Involvement of the central nervous system in congenital muscular dystrophies. Dev Med Child Neurol 1983; 25: 32–42.
3. Echenne B, Pages M, Marty-Double C. Congenital muscular dystrophy with white matter spongiosis. Brain Dev (Tokyo) 1984; 6: 491–495.
4. Leyten QH, Gabreels FJM, Reiner WO, ter Laak HJ, Sengers RCA, Mullaart RA. Congenital muscular dystrophy. J Pediatr 1989; 115: 214–221.
5. Trevisan C, Carollo CP, Segalla P, Angelini C, Drigo P, Giordiano R. Congenital muscular dystrophy: brain alterations in an unselected series of Western patients. J Neurol Neurosurg Psychiatry 1991; 54: 330–334.
6. Castro-Gago M, Diaz-Cardama I, Monasterio L, Fuster M, Perez-Becerra E, Pena J. Congenital muscular dystrophy with central nervous system involvement. An intermediate form? The Annals 1985; 7: 5–12.
7. Topaloglu H, Yalaz K, Renda Y, et al. Occidental type ccrebromuscular dystrophy. A report of eleven cases. J Neurol Neurosurg Psychiatry 1991; 54: 226–229.
8. Hayashi YK, Engwall E, Arikawa-Hirasawa E, et al. Abnormal localization of laminin subunits in muscular dystrophies. J Neurol Sci 1993; 119: 53–64.

158

9. Tomé FMS, Evangelista T, Leclerc A, et al. Congenital muscular dystrophy with merosin deficiency. CR Acad Sci Paris, Sci Vie/Life Sci 1994; 317: 351–357.

10. Vuolteenaho R, Nissien M, Sainio K, et al. Human laminin M chain (merosin): complete primary structure, chromosomal assignment, and expression of the M and A chain in human fetal tissues. J Cell Biol 1994; 124: 381–394.

11. Hillaire D, Leclerc A, Faure S, et al. Localization of merosin- negative congenital muscular dystrophy to chromosome 6q2 by homozygosity mapping. Hum Mol Genet 1994; 9: 1657–1661.

12. Dubowitz V. Workshop report, 22nd ENMC sponsored workshop on congenital muscular dystrophy held in Baarn, The Netherlands, 1993. Neuromusc Disord 1994; 4: 75–81.

13. Sewry CA, Philpot J, Mahony D, Wilson LA, Muntoni F, Dubowitz V. Expression of laminin subunits in congenital muscular dystrophy. Neuromusc Disord 1995; 5: 307–316.

14. Arahata K, Hayashi YK, Koga R, et al. Laminin in animal models for muscular dystrophy. Defect of laminin M in skeletal and cardiac muscles and peripheral nerve of the homozygous dystrophic dy/dy mice. Proc Jpn Acad 1993; 69: 259–264.

15. Sunada Y, Bernier SM, Kozak CA, Yamada Y, Campbell KP. Deficiency of merosin in dystrophic dy mice and genetic linkage of laminin M chain gene to dy locus. J Biol Chem 1994; 269: 13729–13732.

16. Edgar TS, Sunada Y, Lotz BP, Campbell KP, Rust RS. The role of the dystrophin-associated glycoprotein/laminin complex in congenital muscular dystrophies. Muscle Nerve 1994; Suppl: S180.

Y. Fukuyama, M. Osawa and K. Saito (Eds.), *Congenital Muscular Dystrophies*

159

CHAPTER 13

Rehabilitation of children with Fukuyama congenital muscular dystrophy

YAYOI OKAWA and SATOSHI UEDA

Department of Rehabilitation Medicine, Teikyo University Ichihara Hospital, Ichihara, Chiba, Japan

Introduction

The rehabilitation of children with Fukuyama congenital muscular dystrophy (FCMD) was started in 1965, just 5 years after the first report by Fukuyama [1]. After the accumulation of clinical experience, we constructed a classification scale for motor ability in FCMD based on the clinical records of 67 FCMD cases. It is a scale of 8 levels, from 0 to 8, and was revealed to be internally consistent and applicable to both the "upward" and "downward" phases of motor ability. Then the "natural history" of motor ability in FCMD was studied using this scale, 3 different groups being identified: (1) the "gait group"; (2) the "intermediate group"; and (3) the "poor motor development group". The most important finding in the natural history study was a marked sex difference in motor ability. It was found that female cases show a remarkably better motor ability course than males. Whereas many girls (39.5%) reached the walking levels of 6–8, often with adequate bracing, only one of 29 boys (3%) did so, and at that, only to the lowest level of 6.

The rehabilitation program for FCMD consists of prevention of contractures and enhancement of motor development along the general lines of the natural history, often with bracing. Psycho-social-educational rehabilitation is also very important. The latter consists of psychological support for the parents; stimulation of communication; socialization through attending nursery schools and/or kindergartens; education in regular or special schools along the general lines of normalization; social integration; and eventual working in sheltered workshops.

It was once considered that the disabilities, both motor and mental, in FCMD were too severe for rehabilitation to be of any value in improving the quality of life for children with this disease. However, our experience in rehabilitating them has proved that it is worthwhile in most cases.

Early clinical experience in rehabilitation of FCMD

One of the authors (SU) started seeing children with FCMD at the Central Rehabilitation Service of the University of Tokyo Hospital in 1965, just 5 years after the first report of 15 cases of "a peculiar form of congenital progressive muscular dystrophy" by Fukuyama et al. [1]. Dr. Fukuyama belonged to the Department of Pediatrics of the same hospital, and he and his associates referred many FCMD cases to us for rehabilitation. It was not an easy task, since the disease was entirely new, the natural history was not known, and a suitable rehabilitation program did not exist.

Fortunately, however, we had good enough experience of rehabilitation of Duchenne muscular dystrophy (DMD) cases based on studies of the classification of motor disability stages, first developed by Deaver et al. [2] and Swinyard et al. [3], and then adapted by Ueda [4] for the Japanese way of life, and on cases on DMD's natural history measured with respect to these stages [4,5]. The experiences of Nojima et al. [6,7], Ueda [5] and Ueda et al. [8], in rehabilitating children with DMD, had confirmed the effectiveness of bracing and the importance of locomotion by shuffling around on the (tatami) floor, in accordance with the Japanese way of life.

So it was natural for us to follow the same steps for FCMD. The first step was to try to get patients to stand with the aid of braces. It was relatively easy if the child had good sitting balance, and had not yet developed secondary hip and knee contractures. A FCMD boy could stand with so-called stabilizer-type standing braces, which consisted of bilateral long leg braces connected by a pelvic band and supported by two pillars attached to a board (Fig. 1). These standing braces, while they helped to increase the motivation of the parents by showing them that something can be done even for severe FCMD children, however, had no practical consequences. Children given this type of standing braces never become able to stand by themselves, let alone walk.

Then we experienced a slightly better case, who did not need the stabilizer-type standing braces, but could maintain a standing posture with the aid of bilateral long leg braces connected by a pelvic band. He needed a wooden frame, made by his father, for support (Fig. 2). This boy was unable to move around the floor by shuffling when he came to our rehabilitation clinic for the first time. However, he could already turn around on the same spot on the floor. So we tried to help, and motivate him, to shuffle by giving him a type of "sliding cart" consisting of 3 small casters attached to a triangular board with a handle-like hand support (Fig. 3). He liked it very much and used it to move around his home. His mother, taking the hint from this cart, bought him a light-weight tricycle. He liked this too and enjoyed moving around outside not using the pedals, but using his legs directly on the ground (Fig. 4). Eventually he became able to move around by shuffling without the sliding cart.

Then came a boy, the younger of siblings, who became able to maintain a standing posture with long leg braces connected by a pelvic band without any support (Fig. 5). However, he too showed no further development of motor ability.

His elder sister, however, was the first among our FCMD cases who walked. She walked with bilateral long leg braces with hand holding (Fig. 6). She needed to hold on with both hands most of the time, but sometimes she could walk holding on with only one hand, as shown in Fig. 6.

Then, finally, we found an even better case who could walk with long leg braces without any assistance for a long distance (Fig. 7). There were also a few exceptionally good cases who could walk without braces, and could even climb up and down stairs clutching handrails. But such cases invariably later developed an ankle equinovarus deformity due to shortening of the tibialis posterior muscle, which necessitated correction with short leg braces (Fig. 8). Fig. 9 shows the marked foot equinovarus deformity of the same girl after she had become unable to walk because the equinovarus deformity had become too severe to correct.

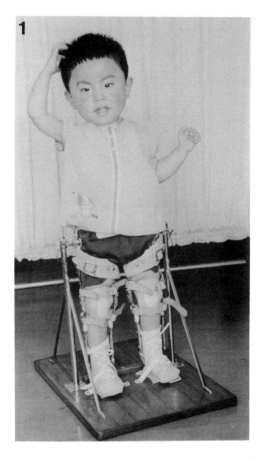

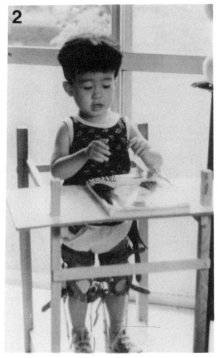

Fig. 1. A FCMD boy standing with stabilizer-type standing braces consisting of bilateral long leg braces connected by a pelvic band and supported by two pillars attached to a board.

Fig. 2. A FCMD boy who can maintain a standing posture with the aid of bilateral long leg braces connected by a pelvic band. He needs a wooden frame and table made by his father for support.

Classification of motor ability in FCMD

Based upon this clinical experience we tried to construct an accurate classification scale for motor ability in FCMD.

The clinical records of the 67 cases of FCMD who were seen at the outpatient rehabilitation clinics of the University of Tokyo Hospital and the Tokyo Metropolitan Rehabilitation Center during the period from 1966 to 1984, were analyzed to elucidate the underlying regularity, and the order of both the progression and regression of motor ability. As a result, a scale of 9 levels, from 0 to 9, was constructed that was confirmed to be internally consistent and applicable to both the "upward" and "downward" phases of this disease [9,10].

The levels are defined as in Table 1. It is very interesting that we could confirm later that the same classification scale, levels 0 to 8, can be fully applied to Werdnig–Hoffmann dis-

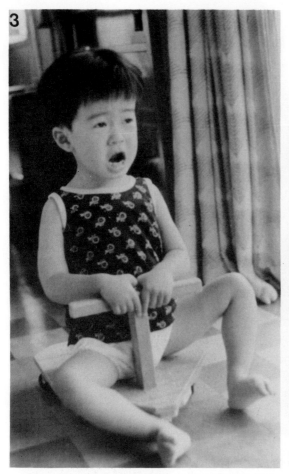
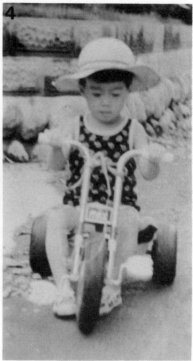

Fig. 3. The same FCMD boy as in Fig. 2 who can shuffle by means of a type of "sliding cart" consisting of three small casters attached to a triangular board with a handle-like support.

Fig. 4. The same FCMD boy as in Fig. 3, who enjoys moving around outside on a light-weight tricycle using his legs directly on the ground.

ease (the intermediate group), which is neurogenic but involves proximal muscles as in FCMD [11], and also to other congenital myopathies with proximal weakness [12].

Classification of "natural history"

We then tried to study the "natural history", or the course of motor ability in FCMD using this classification. It goes without saying that this is very important as the scientific basis for an effective rehabilitation program.

It was found that generally speaking there are 3 different groups as to the course of motor ability (Fig. 10).

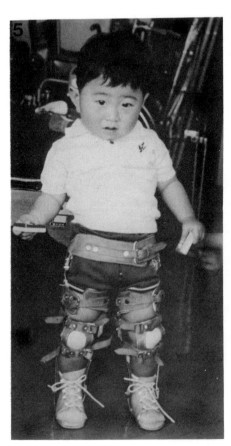
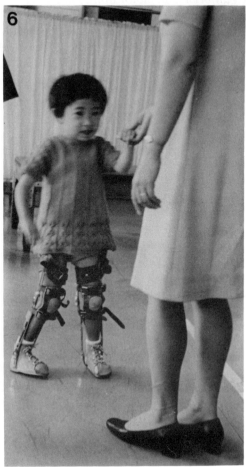

Fig. 5. A FCMD boy, the younger of siblings, who became able to maintain a standing posture with long leg braces connected by a pelvic band without any support.

Fig. 6. A FCMD girl, the elder sister of the boy in Fig. 5, who can walk with bilateral long leg braces with hand-holding. She needs to hold on with both hands most of the time, but sometimes she can walk holding on with only one hand, as shown.

Group 1 could be called the "gait group", showing two distinct "upward" and "downward" phases with slow, but steady initial motor progress, leading to some type of gait, then deteriorating in a down-hill fashion.

Group 2 could be called the "intermediate group", showing slower motor progress, reaching levels 3–5, staying generally longer at these levels than group 1, and then deteriorating slowly.

Group 3 could be called the "poor motor development group", showing very slow motor progress, and reaching only level 1 or 2.

Sex difference in motor ability in FCMD

It was found, very interestingly, that female cases show a remarkably better motor ability course than males. Whereas many girls reached the walking levels of 6–8, only one of 29 boys did so, and only to the lowest level of 6, at that. In other words, 39.5% of females reached levels 6–8, while only 3% of males did so (Table 2).

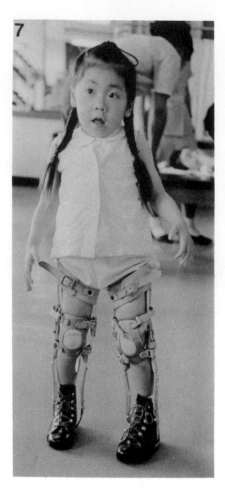 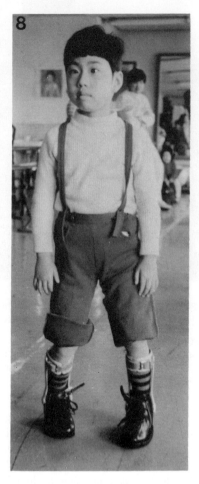

Fig. 7. A FCMD girl who can walk with long leg braces without any assistance for a long distance.

Fig. 8. An exceptionally good FCMD case, a girl who could walk and climb up and down stairs without braces, clutching handrails, but who later developed an ankle equinovarus deformity due to shortening of the tibialis posterior muscle, and thus she needed short leg braces.

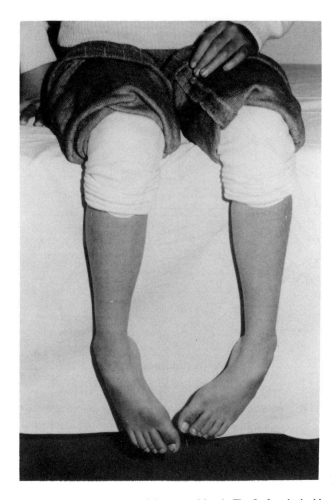

Fig. 9. The marked foot equinovarus deformity of the same girl as in Fig. 8 after she had become unable to walk because the deformity had become too severe to correct.

Table 1

Motor ability level scale for FCMD.

Level 8	Independent <u>stair climbing</u> with or without rails and/or braces (not applicable if hand-holding or trunk-support by another person is required)
Level 7	Independent <u>gait</u> on a level surface with or without braces
Level 6	<u>Gait</u> either by <u>clutching</u> to furniture or by <u>hand-holding</u>, with or without braces
Level 5	<u>Standing by clutching</u> to furniture, with or without short leg braces or high shoes, and/or crawling on <u>all-fours</u>
Level 4	Moving around the floor by <u>shuffling</u> in a squatting posture
Level 3	<u>Turning around</u> on the floor in a squatting posture
Level 2	<u>Unsupported squatting</u> on the floor
Level 1	<u>Neck control</u> in an upright held position (not necessarily in the supine or prone position)
Level 0	<u>No neck control</u> in an upright held position

166

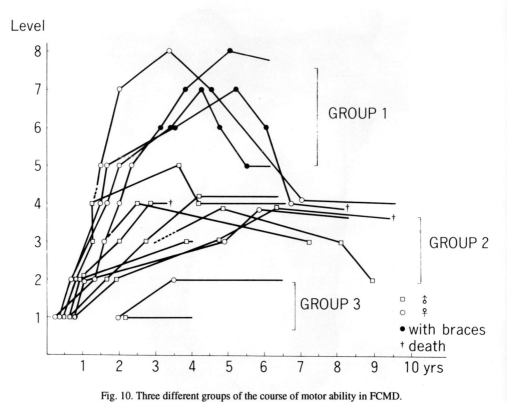

Fig. 10. Three different groups of the course of motor ability in FCMD.

Table 2

Sex difference in the highest motor ability level achieved in FCMD

Level	Male	Female	Total (%)
8	0	4	4 (6)
7	0	7	7 (10)
6	1	4	5 (8)
5	2	4	6 (9)
4	18	13	31 (47)
3	1	2	3 (5)
2	5	4	9 (12)
1	2	0	2 (3)
Total	29	38	67 (100)
Summary (%)			
6–8	1 (3)	15 (39.5)	16 (24)
1–5	28 (97)	23 (60.5)	51 (76)
Total	29 (100)	38 (100)	67 (100)

$P < 0.01$

The age of reaching the highest motor ability level

We then investigated the age at which FCMD children reached the highest motor ability level. It was found that the highest level of motor ability was reached in most males within 3 years of age, whereas in females it was reached even after 4 years in many cases. Also, in females, there was a tendency that the higher the highest level was, the later was the age when the highest level was reached with a Spearman's correlation coefficient of 0.60 (Table 3).

Rehabilitation program for FCMD children

The rehabilitation program for FCMD consists of many elements (Table 4).

Generally speaking, rehabilitation should be started as soon as the diagnosis is made. One of the most important points is prevention of secondary joint contractures. If started as early as possible, and targeted to the most frequent and most disabling location and type, i.e., hip and knee flexion contractures, ankle equinovarus contractures, elbow flexion and forearm pronation contractures, passive range-of-motion exercise, taught to and done by the parents at home, is quite effective for the prevention of contractures.

The enhancement of motor development proceeds along the general lines of motor development in FCMD, which was revealed by the "natural history" study. The training program along with the sequence of motor development in FCMD starts from neck control in the upright position, through maintenance of a squatting posture, proceeding to shuffling around on a tatami floor, standing, and then walking with braces, and finally, if possible, climbing up and down stairs.

Psycho-social-educational rehabilitation is also very important. It starts with psychological support for the parents, and goes through stimulation of communication, socialization through attending nursery schools, kindergartens, etc., education in regular or special schools along the general lines of normalization, social integration, and eventually working in sheltered workshops.

Table 3

Age at the highest level achieved in FCMD

Level	Male, age								Female, age							
	0	1	2	3	4	5	6	Total	0	1	2	3	4	5	6	Total
8												2	1	1		4
7										1	1		2	2		6
6				1				1					4			4
5				1				1			4					4
4		1	7	4	1		1	14		2	3	4		2		11
3				1				1				1			1	2
2		4	1					5	1	1	1					3
1		1	1					2								
Total		6	9	7	1		1	24	1	4	9	7	7	5	1	34

Table 4

Rehabilitation program for children with FCMD

Early stage
1. Should be started as soon as possible.
2. Prevention of joint contractures.
    (i)   Most important as early intervention.
    (ii) Should be targetted to the prevention of: hip and knee flexion contractures; ankle equino-varus contractures (shortening of tibialis posterior); and elbow flexion and forearm pronation contractures
    (iii) Should be taught to parents as home exercise.

Enhancement of motor development
1. Neck control in an upright held position.
2. Maintaining squatting posture without support.
3. Turning around in a squatting posture.
4. Moving (shuffling) on a (tatami) floor in a squatting posture; training with a "slider cart" or a light tricycle.
5. Standing with manual support, then holding onto firm objects (furniture) with braces.
6. Walking with long leg braces (LLB), short leg braces (SLB) or high shoes (HS), first with manual support, then without.
7. Climbing up and down stairs with or without rails.

Psycho-social-educational program
1. Psychological support of the parents.
2. Stimulation of verbal and non-verbal communication.
3. Socialization through attending nursery schools, kindergartens, etc.
4. Education in regular schools, special schools, and home schooling with occasions to study, and play together with regular children (normalization).
5. Social integration through social experiences, such as travel, going to zoos, aquariums, etc.
6. Working in sheltered workshops after graduation from special high schools.

Educational status in FCMD

In our survey in 1986 (Table 5), 3 of 18 cases of grade school age were attending regular schools. At junior high school age, only 1 in 7 were attending regular schools. At high school age, all cases were attending special schools.

Conclusion

Although the disabilities in FCMD were once considered too severe for rehabilitation to be of any value, our experience of many years in rehabilitating them has proved that it is worthwhile in most cases. Actually, many of them, mostly female cases, have become able to walk with braces. Even cases who cannot become ambulatory can also profit from early rehabilitation by gaining earlier the ability to move around by shuffling on the floor in a squatting posture and maintaining it longer than in cases who do not receive rehabilitation. In the traditional Japanese way of life, people are accustomed to squatting on a tatami mat, and thus children's moving around on a tatami-covered floor is not inappropriate. In such an environment, children with FCMD can enjoy greater freedom in moving around their homes.

Table 5

Educational status in FCMD

	8–7	6	5	4–3	2–1	Total
Grade school						
Level on admission	8–7	6	5	4–3	2–1	
Regular school	1		1	1		3
Regular-special school		1				1
Special school	1		2	3	4	10
Home schooling and regular school				1	3	4
Total	2	1	3	5	7	18
Junior high school						
Level on admission	8–7	6	5	4–3	2–1	
Regular school				1		1
Special school				2	2	4
Home schooling and regular school				1	1	2
Total				4	3	7
High school						
Level on admission	8–7	6	5	4–3	2–1	
Special school				1	2	3

In conclusion, we would like to state that comprehensive rehabilitation, including not only medical rehabilitation, but also educational, social, and even vocational rehabilitation, is as effective in achieving and maintaining a higher quality of life in children with FCMD as in those with any neuromuscular or musculoskeletal disabilities.

References

1. Fukuyama Y, Kawazura M, Haruna H. A peculiar form of congenital progressive muscular dystrophy. Report of fifteen cases. Paediatr Univ Tokyo (Tokyo) 1960; 4: 5–8.
2. Deaver GG, Greenspan L, Swinyard CA. Progressive muscular dystrophy, diagnosis and problems of rehabilitation. New York: Muscular Dystrophy Association of America, 1956.
3. Swinyard CA, Deaver GG, Greenspan L. Gradients of functional ability of importance in rehabilitation of patients with progressive muscular and neuromuscular diseases. Arch Phys Med 1957; 38: 574–579.
4. Ueda S. Rehabilitation in Duchenne progressive muscular dystrophy (in Japanese). Rigakuryohou to Sagyoryouhou (Tokyo) 1968; 2: 214–223.
5. Ueda S. Rehabilitation in Duchenne muscular dystrophy (in Japanese). Rehabilitation Igaku (Tokyo) 1972; 9: 286–291.
6. Nojima M, Shinno T, Ogimori K, et al. Rehabilitation in progressive muscular dystrophy (in Japanese). Rehabilitation Igaku (Tokyo) 1965; 2: 71–81.
7. Nojima M, Matsuka Y, Suto T, et al. Twenty-five years of rehabilitation in progressive muscular dystrophy (in Japanese). Rehabilitation Igaku (Tokyo) 1988; 25: 285–294.
8. Ueda S, Majima M, Okawa Y. Course and evaluation of motor disability of the lower extremities in Duchenne muscular dystrophy (in Japanese). Sogo Rehabilitation (Tokyo) 1983: 253–257.
9. Ueda S, Eto F, Kikuchi N. Rehabilitation in Fukuyama congenital muscular dystrophy. A clinical analysis of 50 cases (in Japanese). Sogo Rehabilitation (Tokyo) 1975; 3: 51–64.
10. Okawa Y, Ueda S, Eto F, Kikuchi N. Course of progression of motor disability in Fukuyama congenital muscular dystrophy (in Japanese). Rehabilitation Igaku (Tokyo) 1985; 22: 197–202.

11. Okawa Y, Eto F, Ueda S. Evaluation and course of progression of motor disability in Werdnig–Hoffmann disease (intermediate group) (in Japanese). Rehabilitation Igaku (Tokyo) 1986; 23: 115–120.
12. Kimura S, Okawa Y, Ueda S. Evaluation of motor ability in early infantile diseases characterized by proximal muscle weakness (in Japanese). Rehabilitation Igaku (Tokyo) 1992; 29: 231–233.

Y. Fukuyama, M. Osawa and K. Saito (Eds.), *Congenital Muscular Dystrophies*
1997 Elsevier Science B.V. All rights reserved

CHAPTER 14

Congenital muscular dystrophies: myo- and neuropathological studies

HANS H. GOEBEL[1], BERND REITTER[2], MICHAEL ALBANI[3],
ANTJE BORNEMANN[1], ROLF ROETTGER[4] and CHUNG W. CHOW[5]

[1]*Department of Neuropathology, University of Mainz Medical Center, Mainz, Germany*
[2]*Department of Paediatrics, University of Mainz Medical Center, Mainz, Germany*
[3]*Department of Paediatrics, Municipal Hospital, Wiesbaden, Germany*
[4]*Department of Pathology, Municipal Hospital Braunschweig, Germany*
[5]*Department of Anatomical Pathology, Royal Children's Hospital, Melbourne, Australia*

Introduction

Since the first report on an infantile muscular dystrophy which is credited to Frederick E. Batten [1] some 90 years ago, only later to be named congenital muscular dystrophy (CMD) [2], the spectrum has enormously expanded from an original single disease to several still ill-defined nosological entities. However, reports have drastically increased over the past 15 years [3], in certain years reaching more than 50 publications. Benign [4] and severe [5] forms attest to the variable clinical course and autosomal-recessive [6] and autosomal-dominant [7,8] types underscore the diversified nosography, as does the distinction into "CMD pure" and "CMD plus", the latter term not only invoking muscular and non-muscular symptoms but well-established extra-muscular pathology, largely of the brain and eyes, the group of cerebro-oculo-muscular dystrophies (COMD). Apart from the most recently observed abnormalities of merosin, the subunit M of laminin [9–11], the myopathology of CMD and COMD has been considered non-specific comprising variation in fiber diameters, necrosis, phagocytosis, regeneration of muscle fibers, and fibrosis, irrespective of the nosological form of CMD. To date, a large diagnostic armamentarium which includes clinical and genetic examinations, determination of creatine kinase (CK), electromyography, and muscle biopsy, but foremost a radiological study [12] of the nervous system, ophthalmological investigation, and even an occasional autopsy is necessary to confirm a patient's CMD or to exclude it because CMD has not only given the clinical impression of the floppy infant, but also of arthrogryposis multiplex congenita, the rigid-spine syndrome, early-onset dystrophinopathy [13,14] and even nemaline myopathy, conditions which may simulate CMD. Contrary to late-onset forms in congenital myopathies, which have contributed to the criticism concerning the concept of congenital myopathies, the CMD have one feature in common, i.e. the onset, at or even before birth, of clinical symptoms or the frank appearance of the CMD. The diagnosis of CMD may be based on the non-specific muscle pathology in conjunction with the age of the patient and the non-progressive character of the associated developmental defects of the central nervous system and the eye.

The non-specificity of mild pathological features may be augmented depending on when during the course of the disease and from where in the skeletal muscles a biopsy specimen has been taken (end-stage myopathy). One may encounter advanced replacement of muscle parenchyma by connective tissue and fat cells, or the changes may be mild without necrosis, phagocytosis and regeneration of myofibers.

The myopathology of CMD

Irrespective of the clinical form of CMD, the pathological spectrum in biopsied skeletal muscle is rather narrow and non-specific. It ranges from mild variation in fiber diameters to "dystrophic" changes, i.e. necrosis (Fig. 1), phagocytosis (Fig. 2), and regeneration (Fig. 3) of myofibers, occasionally comprising small groups of fibers (Fig. 3) to "end-stage" pathology with isolated fibers embedded in and surrounded by fibrous and fatty tissues (Fig. 4). The amount of endomysial connective tissue may vary, occasionally being rather mild, in other instances being rather pronounced. The wealth of fibroblast-like cells encountered among collagen fibrils, some of which were actually recorded within myofibroblast cytoplasm [15], in conjunction with accumulation of elastic fibrils within the endomysium sug-

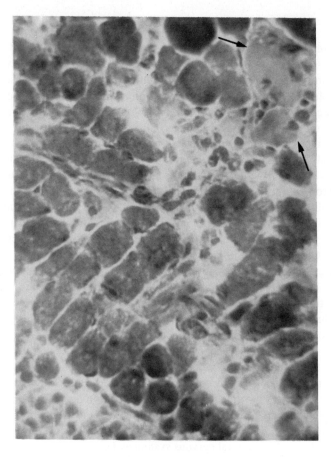

Fig. 1. Variation in fiber diameters and necrotic (arrows) fibers signify "dystrophic" changes, modified trichrome stain, ×410.

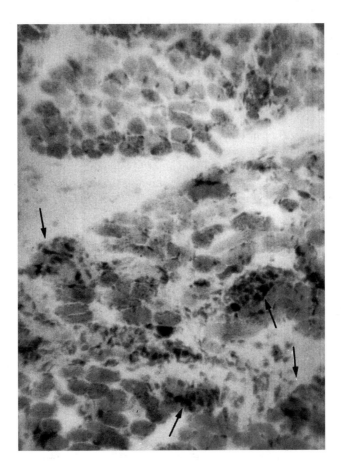

Fig. 2. Phagocytosis of muscle fibers is marked by dark acid phosphatase-positive macrophages within necrotic muscle fibers (arrows), ×168.

gested abnormal collagen synthesis. It has been thought that the merosin-deficient type of CMD appears particularly scarred. Unlike in congenital myopathies, among which CMD is occasionally classified [16], there have been no pathognomonic myopathological features in single or groups of CMD apart from the recently detected deficiency of subunit M, merosin, of the muscle fiber basal lamina laminin [11]. In spite of several such observations, it remains to be seen whether this complete absence of merosin in one group of CMD patients' muscle tissues is of similar nosological significance to that of the lack of dystrophin in Duchenne muscular dystrophy (DMD). Similarly, gaps in muscle fiber basal lamina have been observed at the ultrastructural level in Fukuyama type CMD (FCMD) [17]. Similarly, ultrastructural studies have not revealed any disease- or group-specific abnormalities, but only "streamed" Z-disks [18], loss of myofilaments, empty loops of muscle fiber basal lamina, and small round myofibers with few myofibrils as well as pairs of myofibers ensheathed by a common basal lamina [15] suggesting immaturity of muscle fibers. This latter aspect is also supported by the larger number of undifferentiated type-II C myofibers encountered in FCMD [19]. In FCMD, the authors [19] were not able to separate completely the myopathology of CMD from that of DMD [20]. The number of satellite cells has been found almost normal in FCMD [21]. Histochemical investigations have further shown type-I fiber predominance [18,22,23] with numerical decrease in type-II B fibers during progression of the disease [19]. Ringbinden have been a particular feature in benign CMD with autosomal-dominant heredity [8], but this pathological phenomenon, not emphasized in other reports and according to our own observations, may be more characteristic of these particular family members than of CMD in general or a specific nosological type. It is also interesting to note that in this report [8], nemaline bodies were encountered in several muscle fibers, although insufficient to justify the diagnosis of nemaline myopathy – and this is in accordance with our own observation, mentioned and illustrated below.

When antibodies against merosin, the subunit M of laminin, a component of the myofiber basal lamina became available, they accorded immunohistochemical parameters of greater specificity to the myopathological spectrum of CMD. One group of patients afflicted with "CMD pure" – although many of them also revealed delayed myelination of the cerebral white matter [24,25] – lacked merosin completely [26]. Thus, this new observation enabled the separation of "CMD pure" into merosin-deficient and merosin-positive forms, the deficiency of merosin in this group of CMD being almost complete, like that of dystrophin in DMD. Moreover, in FCMD the amount of merosin was found to be greatly reduced [9], but

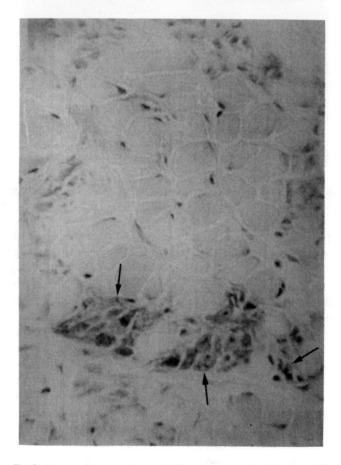

Fig. 3. A group of regenerating muscle fibers (arrows), Azur B-stain, ×450.

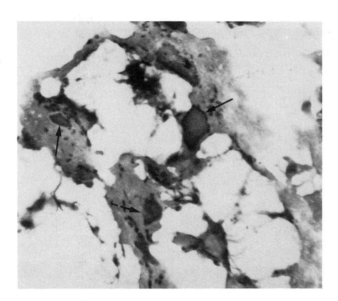

Fig. 4. "End stage" myopathology with replacement of muscle tissue by connective tissue and fat cells with a few myofibers (arrows) embedded in scarred fibrous tissue, modified trichrome stain, ×172.

this phenomenon was also observed when antibodies against dystrophin-associated proteins were applied [27] whereas dystrophin appeared normal [28]. Fetal myopathology in "CMD plus" does not yet seem to display any significant abnormalities [29].

Neuromuscular disorders simulating CMD

The non-specificity of myopathological features in the various forms of CMD may lead to the reclassification of a patient's congenital neuromuscular disorder if additional morphological studies were undertaken.

Several years ago [30], we observed four children from a large kinship, located in a German religious isolate, which we considered clinically and morphologically to suffer from CMD, subsequently registered as the Eichsfeld type of CMD, M 253850 in the McKusick catalogue [31]. However, more refined electron microscopic and immunohistochemical investigations later revealed the presence of desmin-related inclusions, called Mallory body-like inclusions [32], in each of the children's muscle. Moreover, in several children from other new families, the inclusions contained not only desmin, but also dystrophin [33]. Therefore, we now consider this former "Eichsfeld-type of CMD" one of the numerous congenital myopathies [34].

Similarly, the availability of antibodies against dystrophin led to the reclassification of a few patients' CMD when complete absence of dystrophin supported the diagnosis of a dystrophinopathy [13,35] as apparently early-infantile or even congenital variants within the clinical spectrum of DMD.

Conversely, the presence of dystrophin, demonstrated in muscle tissue originally thought to represent DMD in a young boy, also led to the transient reclassification of CMD. Despite a "dystrophic" myopathological pattern of an earlier biopsy specimen (Fig. 5a), a subse-

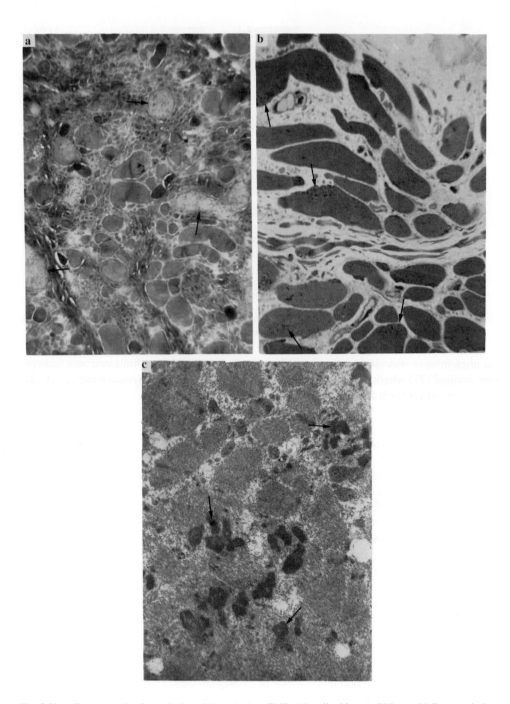

Fig. 5. Nemaline myopathy, formerly thought to represent CMD: (a) earlier biopsy of "dystrophic" myopathology with numerous necrotic muscle fibers (arrows), modified trichrome stain, ×550 (by courtesy of Professor Ketelsen, Freiburg/Germany); (b) in a second biopsy, 6 years later, several muscle fibers (arrows) display rods, 1-μm thick methylene-blue stained section, ×580; (c) several groups (arrows) of rods within the muscle fiber, depicted at the ultrastructural level, ×3040.

quent biopsy performed 6 years after the earlier one from the quadriceps muscle revealed unequivocal evidence of nemaline myopathy (Fig. 5b,c) emphasizing that within the spectrum of nemaline myopathy, an occasional patient may also exhibit clinical and morphological features of CMD.

"CMD plus"

Neuromuscular abnormalities are not infrequently components of multi-organ diseases. Among these, the single-organelle multi-organ diseases, i.e. mitochondrial encephalomyopathies and lysosomal disorders, foremost the type-II glycogenoses are such examples. Myotonic dystrophy is another multi-organ disease affecting the muscle, the brain, endocrine organs, and the eye, thus, a "muscle-eye-brain" disease (MEBD) in the broadest sense. Extramuscular symptoms have also been associated with other muscular dystrophies, e.g. DMD and the Bergia type of familial lethal cardiomyopathy and scapulo-peroneal muscular dystrophy [36]. The combination of mental retardation and X-linked lysosomal glycogen storage with normal acid maltase activity [37–39] and cardiomyopathy and myopathy with desmin accumulation [40] are further examples. Retinal abnormalities have been observed in myotonic dystrophy and facio-scapulo-humeral muscular dystrophy. Sensorineural hearing loss is a feature of childhood facio-scapulo-humeral muscular dystrophy [41]. In some such multi-organ disorders, common morphological features are encountered in different organs such as fibrillar glycogen in myofibers, hepatocytes and brain cells in type-IV glycogenosis and the polyglucosan body-related conditions or the lysosomal glycogen in the type-II glycogenoses which shows ubiquitous appearance.

Thus, it was a seminal observation [42] when the consistent association of CMD and CNS abnormalities was first reported. The linkage in clinical symptomatology and pathology of the CNS and the skeletal muscle subsequently accounted for additional syndromes, beside FCMD, the Walker–Warburg syndrome (WWS) [43], and the MEBD [44], predominantly seen in Finland [45,46]. In the latter two disorders, ocular abnormalities were consistently noted as part of the condition, cerebro-oculo-muscular dystrophies (COMD). The cerebral and ocular abnormalities usually overshadow the muscular symptoms evidenced by designation of the Walker–Warburg syndrome, named after a neurosurgeon (A. Earl Walker, USA) and an ophthalmologist (Mette Warburg, Denmark), whose descriptions first focused on the respective cerebral and ocular abnormalities which were only later found to be associated with muscle involvement. Occasionally, terms such as cerebro-oculo-muscular syndrome [47,48] or cerebro-ocular-dysplasia muscular dystrophy (COD-MD) syndrome [49] have been used to emphasize certain rather minor and thus morphologically possibly insignificant differences between the FCMD, WWS and MEBD groups.

Whether merosin-deficient CMD with increased white matter lucency is a "CMD pure" or a "CMD plus" remains to be seen by consecutive radiological studies, which seem to indicate reduction of the cerebral white matter lucency with the patient's age, and by neuropathological investigations to establish the anatomic basis of this cerebral white matter lucency. Thus, to speak of a "CMD with leukodystrophy" [50] currently appears unwarranted because of insufficient evidence that the radiological cerebral white matter lucency is evidence of a progressive demyelinating process, the definition of a leukodystrophy. Also it will have to be determined in individual patients whether associated mental retardation or seizures are coincidental (and based on morphological lesions) or form part of a more complex "CMD plus".

The neuropathology of "CMD plus"

Morphological lesions in the CNS have been repeatedly and amply described in "CMD plus" [51–55], including those in FCMD [56,57], the neuropathology of the various COMD forms has also been amply compared [50], and the neuropathological differences between FCMD and other forms of COMD have been emphasized [53,58]. The variability of the lesions, in particular the severity, have resulted in the large number of different terms applied [50]. The core neuropathology is type-II lissencephaly, a cerebro-cortical malformation, also recently termed "cobble-stone" cortex, and cerebellar malformations, Lissencephalic or agyric areas (Fig. 6a) may be complete or alternate with normal regions and pseudopolymicrogyric ones (Fig. 6b), termed type-II pachygyria and type-II polymicrogyria [51], based on lack of cortical lamination, fusion of gyri (Fig. 7), and extensive formation of glial and fibrous tissue which also extends into the subarachnoid space (Fig. 8a). Subarachnoid gliofibrous tissues may also be encountered subcortically (Fig. 8b). This outgrowth of fibroglial tissue into the subarachnoid space over the cerebral cortex and the brainstem may already be present prenatally (Fig. 9a,b) and serve as a marker for recognizing the WWS in an otherwise immature brain (Fig. 10).

Thus, our observations on fetal WWS neuropathology are in keeping with other reports [59] and are similar to the fetal pathology in FCMD [29]. This outgrowth of CNS parenchyma into the subarachnoid space is considered an essential process resulting in cortical dysplasia [29].

In the cerebellum, the cortex may also be malformed (Fig. 11), sometimes obvious at gross inspection, as well as in the prenatal stage [60].

Secondary to the severe dysplastic changes in the cerebral cortex, the corticofugal or efferent fibers forming the corticobulbar and corticospinal tracts are also affected by hypoplasia or possibly even aplasia accounting for the small basis of the pons, the flat ventral surface of the medulla and the bilateral grooves of the spinal cord at the level of the normal lateral corticospinal tracts (Fig. 12). However, no abnormalities of the motor neurons in the spinal anterior horns have been convincingly shown. Together with the myopathic or

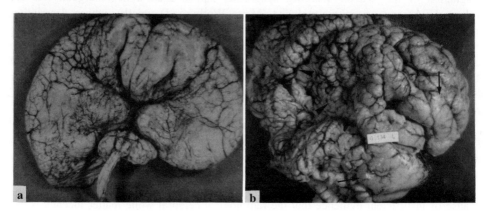

Fig. 6. Gross-surface pathology in the Walker–Warburg syndrome: (a) largely lissencephalic or agyric; (b) agyric (arrows) areas in addition to pseudopolymicrogyric (arrow heads) areas.

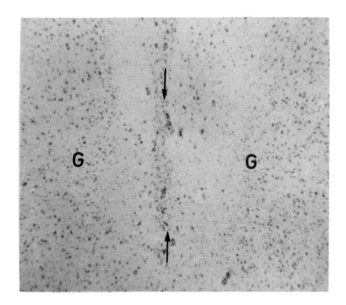

Fig. 7. Fusion (arrows) of two opposite cerebro–cortical gyri (G) in Walker-Warburg syndrome, Nissl stain, ×64.

"dystrophic" muscle pathology, reduction or absence of the pyramidal tracts has not been deemed responsible for the CMD pathology [20,61].

However, we recently observed [62] a patient who had agyria without gliofibrous out-growth into the subarachnoid space and without ocular pathology, thus different from the above-mentioned form of CNS pathology, but with aberrant pyramidal tracts and abnor-malities of spinal anterior-horn motor neurons. In conjunction with these findings a delay in maturation of muscle fiber types, i.e. a considerable number of type-II C myofibers, and

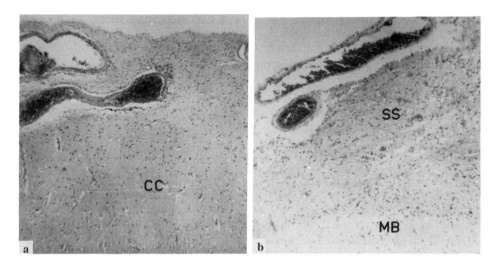

Fig. 8. Brain parenchyma in the subarachnoid space (SS), Walker–Warburg syndrome: (a) above the cerebral cortex (CC), hematoxylin-eosin stain, ×64; (b) above the mid-brain (MB), hematoxylin-eosin stain, × 80.

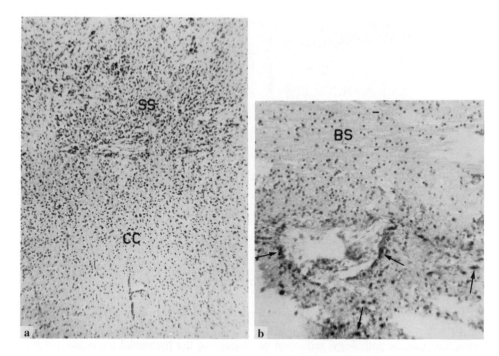

Fig. 9. Nineteen-week-old fetus with Walker–Warburg syndrome, outgrowth of cerebral tissue into the subarachnoid space (SS): (a) over cerebral cortex (CC), hematoxylin-eosin stain, ×80; (b) beneath brainstem (BS) with subarachnoid gliotic tissue (arrows), glial fibrillary acidic protein, peroxidase technique, ×172.

considerable variation in fiber diameters but no "dystrophic" changes, i.e. necrosis and regeneration of muscle fibers and endomysial fibrosis were noted. These myopathological findings indicated delay in maturation, but not necessarily in growth of muscle fibers in this 4-year-old boy which was present at autopsy in several muscles [62]. Lissencephaly type-I, likewise entailing dysplasia of the cerebral cortex, albeit of a different nosological connotation, was found associated with arthrogryposis multiplex congenita [63]. Thus, it cannot be completely ruled out that pyramidal tract abnormalities may somehow influence the development and/or subsequent pathology of respective muscles. Congenital absence of pyramids associated with non-lissencephalic microcephaly and an associated arthrogryposis has also been reported in two families [64].

Eye pathology
Pathological lesions in the eyes are plentiful and complex and they often differ among both eyes, most conspicuously in evidence as unilateral microphthalmia [43,49,51]. Almost every anatomic structure in the eye may be affected [65] entailing developmental defects of the cornea, the iris, the lens, and the retina. Apart from retinal non-attachment or detachment, retinal pathology encompasses either lack/loss of photoreceptors and retinal atrophy (Fig. 13a), even with proliferation and migration of retinal pigment epithelial cells (Fig. 13b), or severe reduction/absence of ganglion cells in the inner retina (Fig. 14a) with or without reduced retinal vasculature and dysplastic rosettes (Fig. 14b). Myopia, glaucoma, cataract, or optic hypotrophy/atrophy may be considered secondary to the widespread developmental

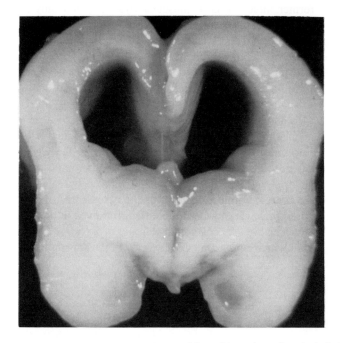

Fig. 10. Brain of a fetus with Walker–Warburg syndrome, sibling of the patient whose brain is depicted in Fig. 6b, at 19th week of gestation. Note large lateral ventricles.

abnormalities of the eyes. The complex pathologies of the CNS and the eye may also be separated into those representing primary and others representing secondary features, such as the absence of retinal ganglionic cells as a sequel of primary CNS maldevelopment similar to the abnormalities of the cerebral pyramidal system. Even lack or loss of outer retinal neurons may follow retrograde transneuronal degeneration in fetal life. Whether eye pathology in the WWS differs from that in FCMD only quantitatively, e.g. by frequency of appearance and by degree of severity, or also qualitatively is currently unknown as, to our knowledge, no post-mortem studies of the eyes have been reported from FCMD patients.

Conclusion

The term congenital muscular dystrophy (CMD), for decades considered a myological entity of early childhood, has now to be expanded to a variety of congenital muscular dystrophies. Even if only divided into "CMD pure" and "CMD plus" forms, the former still represents a heterogeneous group of conditions. Recent advances entail the subgroup of merosin-deficient CMD and another (or several?) group(s) of merosin-present CMD. The importance of this discovery is that nosologically different types of muscular dystrophies (DMD, BMD, SCARMD) seem to share the basic principle, a defective component of the dystrophin–sarcodystroglycan–merosin complex which extends across the sarcolemma of the myofiber. Structural defects outside the sarcolemmal region are not known in other nosological muscular dystrophies, e.g. oculo-pharyngeal muscular dystrophy (OPMD), Emery–Dreifuss muscular dystrophy (EDMD), limb-girdle muscular dystrophy (LGMD), and myotonic dystrophy (MtD). The former three forms of muscular dystrophy not only share a defective component of this trans-membraneous complex of proteins, but also the occurrence of spontaneously necrotic muscle fibers, a feature usually not seen in the latter muscular dystrophies. Thus, the structural defects in this trans-membraneous protein complex in CMD, DMD/BMD and SCARMD may possibly be related to the spontaneous necrosis of muscle fibers indicating that the absence of spontaneous necrosis may lead one to look for other than sarcolemmal defects in the above-mentioned non-necrotizing muscular dystrophies OPMD, EDMD, LGMD, and MtD.

Progress in the elucidation of CMD has also been made by unravelling the group of "CMD plus" as multi-organ diseases affecting skeletal muscle, the CNS, the eye and in some instances skeletal muscle and the skin [66,67]. Unlike other multi-organ diseases, such as lysosomal, mitochondrial and peroxisomal diseases, marked by defects in or of a single organelle, e.g. the lysosome, the mitochondrion, or the peroxisome, the common denominator in "CMD plus" has, however, not been identified. But even in the peroxisomal multi-organ disorder of Zellweger disease, developmental and progressive abnormalities, e.g. in the liver, can occur simultaneously, as in "CMD plus", because pathology of the CNS and

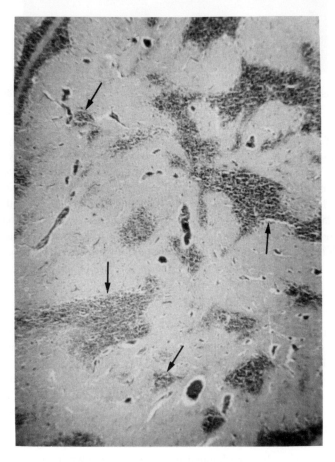

Fig. 11. Malformed cerebellar cortex in Walker–Warburg syndrome with numerous irregularly arranged islands of granule cells (arrows), hematoxylin–eosin, ×42.

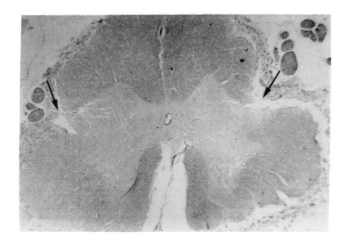

Fig. 12. Spinal cord in Walker–Warburg syndrome, note bilateral deep grooves (arrows) owing to a lack of lateral cortico-spinal tracts, Luxol-fast blue-PAS, ×13.5.

the eye in "CMD plus" largely consists of developmental abnormalities. The common pathogenetic principle in "CMD plus" is still unknown, but the formation of the different developmental defects in different parts of the CNS [47] suggests a common pathogenetic factor or principle that persists for a considerable prenatal period of time as would be expected from circulatory abnormalities such as the formation, spread and maturation of small vessels. Although a prenatal infectious process has been postulated [68], it now appears, based on the autosomal-recessive inheritance of "CMD plus", that genetic factors are the etiological basis of the "CMD plus". This growing awareness is also supported by the fact that the different clinical forms of "CMD plus", FCMD, WWS, and MEBD are similar in qualitative pathology, but different in quantitative pathology. However, so far, this seems to

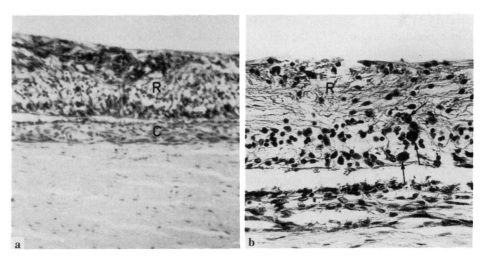

Fig. 13. Atrophic retina and loss of regular layers, Walker–Warburg syndrome: (a) severe (darkly stained) gliosis of the scarred retina (R), above the choroid (C), immunohistological preparation of glial fibrillary acidic protein, ×220; (b) severe loss of inner retinal (R) layer with displaced pigments (arrows), ×400.

184

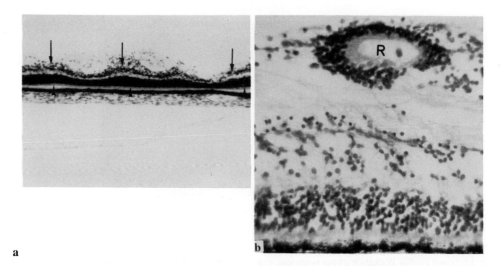

a   b

Fig. 14. Retina in Walker–Warburg syndrome: (a) wavy appearance of the bipolar layer (arrow) above the photo-receptor layer (arrowheads) without evidence of ganglion cell layer, hematoxylin–eosin stain, ×120; (b) a large rosette (R) at the internal surface of the retina, hematoxylin-eosin stain, ×400.

account rather for the pathology of the CNS than for that of the eye owing to a lack of ophthalmopathological reports, especially in FCMD for which ophthalmopathological data have not yet been published. Moreover, it seems that "CMD plus" share non-progression of CNS and eye lesions, but some progression of muscle abnormalities. Due to the incompleteness of pathological data in several forms of "CMD plus" in many patients, it may not be easy to distinguish variants from atypical groups or from atypical cases of "CMD plus".

The emergent nosological elucidation of CMD has also resulted in reclassification of certain CMD patients' neuromuscular conditions such as DMD, nemaline myopathy, EDMD, and certain patients afflicted with the rigid-spine syndrome may have a clinically particular CMD.

The experience that, in WWS, the cerebral and ocular abnormalities were discovered before skeletal muscle lesions were known or detected, emphasizes the need to study skeletal muscle in CNS diseases of even those conditions which do not primarily affect the spinal anterior horn cells.

Acknowledgments

These studies were financially supported by the "Deutsche Gesellschaft für Muskelkranke, Freiburg e.V." and the "Deutsche Forschungsgemeinschaft", Bonn (Go 185/14-1). Mr. W. Meffert provided photographs and Mrs. A. Wöber produced the manuscript. The financial generosity of the Tokyo Women's Medical College is also gratefully acknowledged.

References

1.   Batten FE. Three cases of myopathy, infantile type. Brain 1903; 26: 147–148.

2. Howard R. A case of congenital defect of the muscular system (dystrophia muscularis congenita) and its association with congenital talipes equino-varus. Proc R Soc Med 1908; 1 (Pathol Section): 157–166.
3. Fukuyama Y. Bibliography of congenital muscular dystrophies. Tokyo, 1994.
4. Zellweger H, Afifi A, McCormick WF, Mergner W. Benign congenital muscular dystrophy: a special form of congenital hypotonia. Clin Pediatr 1967; 6: 655–663.
5. Zellweger H. Afifi A, McCormick WF, Mergner W. Severe congenital muscular dystrophy. Am J Dis Child 1967; 114: 591–602.
6. Fukuyama Y, Osawa M. A genetic study of the Fukuyama type congenital muscular dystrophy. Brain Dev (Tokyo) 1984; 6: 373–390.
7. Leyten QH, Gabreëls FJM, Joosten EMG, et al. An autosomal dominant type of congenital muscular dystrophy. Brain Dev (Tokyo) 1986; 8: 533–537.
8. Schmalbruch H, Kamieniecka Z, Fuglsang-Frederiksen A, Trojaborg W. Benign congenital muscular dystrophy with autosomal dominant heredity: problems of classification. J Neurol 1987; 234: 146–151.
9. Arahata K, Hayashi YK, Mizuno Y, Yoshida M, Ozawa E. Dystrophin-associated glycoprotein and dystrophin co-localisation at sarcolemma in Fukuyama congenital muscular dystrophy. Lancet 1993; 342: 623–624.
10. Hayashi YK, Engvall E, Arikawa-Hirasawa E, et al. Abnormal localization of laminin subunits in muscular dystrophies. J Neurol Sci 1993; 119: 53–64.
11. Tomé FMS, Evangelista T, Leclerc A, et al. Congenital muscular dystrophy with merosin deficiency. CR Acad Sci Paris, Life Sci, Genet 1994; 317: 351–357.
12. Echenne B, Arthuis M, Billard C, et al. Congenital muscular dystrophy and cerebral CT scan anomalies. J Neurol Sci 1986; 75: 7–22.
13. Arikawa E, Arahata K, Sunohara N, Ishiura S, Nonaka I, Sugita H. Immunocytochemical analysis of dystrophin in muscular dystrophy. In: Kakulas BA, Howell JMcC, Roses AD, eds. Duchenne muscular dystrophy: animal models and genetic manipulation. New York: Raven Press, 1992: 81–87.
14. Beggs AH, Neumann PE, Arahata K. Possible influences on the expression of X chromosome-linked dystrophin abnormalities by heterozygosity for autosomal recessive Fukuyama congenital muscular dystrophy. Proc Natl Acad Sci USA 1992; 89: 623–627.
15. Fidzianska A, Goebel HH, Lenard HG, Heckmann C. Congenital muscular dystrophy (CMD) – a collagen formative disease? J Neurol Sci 1982; 55: 79–90.
16. Kaplan J-C, Fontaine B. Neuromuscular disorders: gene location (table). Neuromusc Disord 1994; 4: 393–395.
17. Wakayama Y, Shibuya S, Kumagai T, et al. Ultrastructural alterations of muscle plasma membranes in Fukuyama muscular dystrophy: comparative study with other types of muscular dystrophies (abstract). International Symposia of Child Neurologists, Tokyo, Japan, 1994.
18. Goebel HH, Fidzianska A, Lenard HG, Osse G, Hori A. A morphological study of non-Japanese congenital muscular dystrophy associated with cerebral lesions. Brain Dev (Tokyo) 1983; 5: 292–301.
19. Nonaka I, Sugita H, Takada K, Kumagai K. Muscle histochemistry in congenital muscular dystrophy with central nervous system involvement. Muscle Nerve 1982; 5: 102–106.
20. Fukuyama Y, Osawa M, Suzuki H. Congenital progressive muscular dystrophy of the Fukuyama type – clinical, genetic and pathological considerations. Brain Dev (Tokyo) 1981; 3: 1–29.
21. Terasawa K. Muscle regeneration and satellite cells in Fukuyama type congenital muscular dystrophy. Muscle Nerve 1986; 9: 465–470.
22. Kihira S, Nonaka I. Congenital muscular dystrophy. A histochemical study with morphometric analysis on biopsied muscle. J Neurol Sci 1985; 70: 139–149.
23. Heyer R, Ehrich J, Goebel HH, Christen H-J, Hanefeld F. Congenital muscular dystrophy with cerebral and ocular malformations (cerebro-oculo-muscular syndrome). Brain Dev (Tokyo) 1986; 8: 614–618.
24. Trevisan CP, Carollo C. Segalla P, Angelini C, Drigo P, Giordano R. Congenital muscular dystrophy: brain alterations in an unselected series of Western patients. J Neurol Neurosurg Psychiatry 1991; 54: 330–334.
25. Topaloglu H, Yalaz K, Renda Y, et al. Occidental type cerebromuscular dystrophy: a report of eleven cases. J Neurol Neurosurg Psychiatry 1991; 54: 226–229.
26. Fardeau M, Tomé FMS, Leclerc A, et al. Clinical and immunocytochemical evidence of heterogeneity in classical (occidental) congenital muscular dystrophies (abstract). International Symposia of Child Neurologists, Tokyo, Japan, 1994.
27. Matsumura K, Nonaka I, Campbell KP. Abnormal expression of dystrophin-associated proteins in Fukuyama-type congenital muscular dystrophy. Lancet 1993; 341: 521–522.

28. Leyten QH, ter Laak HJ, Gabreëls FJM, Renier WO, Renkawek K, Sengers RCA. Congenital muscular dystrophy. Acta Neuropathol (Berlin) 1993; 86: 386–392.

29. Takada K, Nakamura H, Suzumori K, Ishikawa T, Sugiyama N. Cortical dysplasia in a 23-week fetus with Fukuyama congenital muscular dystrophy (FCMD). Acta Neuropathol (Berlin) 1987; 74: 300–306.

30. Goebel HH, Lenard H-G, Langenbeck U, Mehl B. A form of congenital muscular dystrophy. Brain Dev (Tokyo) 1980; 2: 387–400.

31. McKusick VA. Mendelian inheritance in man. 10th edn, Vol 2. Baltimore, MD: Johns Hopkins University Press, 1992: 1567–1568.

32. Fidzianska A, Goebel HH, Osborn M, Lenard HG, Osse G, Langenbeck U. Mallory body-like inclusions in a hereditary congenital neuromuscular disease. Muscle Nerve 1983; 6: 195–200.

33. Fidzianska A, Ryniewicz B, Goebel HH. Familial desminopathy in children. (abstract). Muscle Nerve 1994; Suppl 1: S51.

34. Goebel HH, Lenard HG. Congenital myopathies. In: Rowland LP, DiMauro S, eds. Handbook of clinical neurology, Vol 18. Amsterdam: Elsevier, 1992: 331–367.

35. Kyriakides T. Gabriel G, Drousiotou A, Petrusa-Meznanic M, Middleton L. Dystrophinopathy presenting as congenital muscular dystrophy. Neuromusc Disord 1994; 4: 387–392.

36. Bergia B, Sybers HD, Butler IJ. Familial lethal cardiomyopathy with mental retardation and scapuloperoneal muscular dystrophy. J Neurol Neurosurg Psychiatry 1986; 49: 1423–1426.

37. Danon MJ, Oh SJ, DiMauro S, et al. Lysosomal glycogen storage disease with normal acid maltase. Neurology 1981; 31: 51–57.

38. Riggs JE, Schochet SS, Gutmann L, Shanske S, Neal WA, DiMauro S. Lysosomal glycogen storage disease without acid maltase deficiency. Neurology 1983; 33: 873-877.

39. Hart ZH, Servidei S, Peterson PL, Chang CH, DiMauro S. Cardiomyopathy, mental retardation and autophagic vacuolar myopathy. Neurology 1987; 37: 1065–1068.

40. Muntoni F, Catani G, Mateddu A, et al. Familial cardiomyopathy, mental retardation and myopathy associated with desmin-type intermediate filaments. Neuromusc Disord 1994; 4: 233–241.

41. Voit T, Lamprecht A, Lenard H-G, Goebel HH. Hearing loss in facioscapulohumeral dystrophy. Eur J Pediatr 1986; 145: 280–285.

42. Fukuyama Y, Kawazura M, Haruna H. A peculiar form of congenital progressive muscular dystrophy. Paediatria Universitatis Tokyo (Tokyo)1960; 4: 5–8.

43. Heggie P, Grossniklaus HE, Roessmann U, Chou SM, Cruse RP. Cerebro-ocular dysplasia-muscular dystrophy syndrome. Arch Ophthalmol 1987; 105: 520–524.

44. Korinthenberg R, Palm D, Schlake W, Klein J. Congenital muscular dystrophy, brain malformation and ocular problems (muscle, eye and brain disease) in two German families. Eur J Pediatr 1984; 142: 64–68.

45. Santavuori P, Leisti J, Kruus S, Raitta C. Muscle, eye and brain disease: a new syndrome. Docum Ophthal Proc Series 1978; 17: 393–396.

46. Santavuori P, Somer H, Sainio K, et al. Muscle-eye-brain disease (MEB). Brain Dev (Tokyo) 1989; 11: 147–153.

47. Dambska M, Wisniewski K, Sher J, Solish G. Cerebro-oculo-muscular syndrome: a variant of Fukuyama congenital cerebromuscular dystrophy. Clin Neuropathol 1982; 1: 93–98.

48. Sasaki M, Yoshioka K, Yanagisawa T, Nemoto A, Takasago Y, Nagano T. Lissencephaly with congenital muscular dystrophy and ocular abnormalities: cerebro-oculo-muscular syndrome. Childs Nerv Syst 1989; 5: 35–37.

49. Towfighi J, Sassani JW, Suzuki K, Ladda RL. Cerebro-ocular dysplasia-muscular dystrophy (COD-MD) syndrome. Acta Neuropathol (Berlin) 1984; 65: 110–123.

50. Dobyns WB, Pagon RA, Armstrong D, et al. Diagnostic criteria for Walker–Warburg syndrome. Am J Med Genet 1989; 32: 195–210.

51. Dobyns WB, Kirkpatrick JB, Hittner HM, Roberts RM, Kretzer FL. Syndromes with lissencephaly. II: Walker-Warburg and cerebro-oculo-muscular syndromes and a new syndrome with type II lissencephaly. Am J Med Genet 1985; 22: 157–195.

52. Federico A, Dotti MT, Malandrini A, Guazzi GC. Cerebro-ocular dysplasia and muscular dystrophy: report of two cases. Neuropediatrics 1988; 19: 109–112.

53. Leyten QH, Renkawek K, Renier WO, et al. Neuropathological findings in muscle-eye-brain disease (MEB-D). Neuropathological delineation of MEB-D from congenital muscular dystrophy of the Fukuyama type. Acta Neuropathol (Berlin) 1991; 83: 55–60.

54. Williams RS, Swisher CN, Jennings M, Ambler M, Caviness VS. Cerebro-ocular dysgenesis (Walker–Warburg syndrome): Neuropathologic and etiologic analysis. Neurology 1984; 34: 1531–1541.
55. Bordarier C, Aicardi J, Goutieres F. Congenital hydrocephalus and eye abnormalities with severe developmental brain defects: Warburg's syndrome. Ann Neurol 1984; 16: 60–66.
56. Takada K, Nakamura H, Tanaka J. Cortical dysplasia in congenital muscular dystrophy with central nervous system involvement (Fukuyama type). J Neuropathol Exp Neurol 1984; 43: 395–407.
57. Takada K, Nakamura H, Takashima S. Cortical dysplasia in Fukuyama congenital muscular dystrophy (FCMD): a Golgi and angioarchitectonic analysis. Acta Neuropathol (Berlin) 1988; 76: 170–178.
58. Osawa M, Arai Y, Ikenaka H, et al. Fukuyama type congenital progressive muscular dystrophy. Acta Paediatr Jpn (Tokyo) 1991; 33: 261–269.
59. Squier MV. Development of the cortical dysplasia of type II lissencephaly. Neuropathol Appl Neurobiol 1993; 19: 209–213.
60. Takada K, Nakamura H. Cerebellar micropolygyria in Fukuyama congenital muscular dystrophy: observations in fetal and pediatric cases. Brain Dev (Tokyo) 1990; 12: 774–778.
61. Nonaka I, Chou SM. Congenital muscular dystrophy. In: Vinken PJ, Bruyn GW, eds. Handbook of clinical neurology. Vol 41. Diseases of muscle, Part II. Amsterdam: North-Holland, 1979: 27–50.
62. Hori A, Bardosi A, Goebel HH, Roessmann U. Muscular alteration in agyria with pyramidal tract anomaly. Brain Dev (Tokyo) 1986; 8: 625–629.
63. Massa G, Casaer P, Ceulemans B. Van Eldere S. Arthrogryposis multiplex congenita associated with lissencephaly: a case report. Neuropediatrics 1988; 19: 24–26.
64. Chow CW, Halliday JL, Anderson RMcD, Danks DM, Fortune DW. Congenital absence of pyramids and its significance in genetic diseases. Acta Neuropathol (Berlin) 1985; 65: 313–317.
65. Warburg M. Ocular malformations and lissencephaly. Eur J Pediatr 1987; 146: 450–452.
66. Kletter G, Evans OB, Lee JA, Melvin B, Yates AB, Bock H-GO. Congenital muscular dystrophy and epidermolysis bullosa simplex. J Pediatr 1989; 114: 104–107.
67. Doriguzzi C, Palmucci L, Mongini T, et al. Congenital muscular dystrophy associated with familial junctional epidermolysis bullosa letalis. Eur Neurol 1993; 33: 454–460.
68. Saito K, Fukuyama Y, Ogata T, Oya A. Experimental intrauterine infection of Akabane virus. Brain Dev (Tokyo) 1981; 3: 65–80.

Y. Fukuyama, M. Osawa and K. Saito (Eds.), *Congenital Muscular Dystrophies*
© 1997 Elsevier Science B.V. All rights reserved

Brain pathology in Fukuyama type congenital muscular dystrophy with special reference to the cortical dysplasia and the occurrence of neurofibrillary tangles

JUNICHI TANAKA[1], MOTOYUKI MINAMITANI[1] and KUNIYASU TAKADA[2]

[1]*Division of Neuropathology, Institute of Neuroscience, The Jikei University School of Medicine, Tokyo, Japan*
[2]*Department of Clinical Neuropathology, Tokyo Metropolitan Institute for Neuroscience, Fuchu, Japan*

Introduction

Fukuyama type congenital muscular dystrophy (FCMD) with an autosomal recessive inheritance is now well known to involve not only the skeletal muscle but also the central nervous system [1,2]. Recently, Toda et al. [3] reported gene analysis in FCMD families and the mapping of the FCMD locus to the distal long arm of chromosome No 9 (9q31-33) with microsatellite polymorphism. The muscle pathology is similar to that in the Duchenne type [4], and the brain pathology comprises mainly cerebral and cerebellar cortical dysplasia [5] and the occurrence of Alzheimer's neurofibrillary tangles in young adults [6]. Hydrocephalus, focal interhemispheric fusion and hypoplasia of the corticospinal tracts are other reported abnormalities [7,8]. There has been comparative discussion on the neuropathological similarities between FCMD and other known disorders such as Walker–Warburg syndrome [9] and Santavuori disease [10].

Eleven brains from autopsy cases of FCMD ranging in age from 1 year 11 months to 34 years (Table 1), and one from a fetal case, a sibling with FCMD, at the gestational age of 23 weeks, were subjected to this investigation. Individual brain weights were within normal limits for each age group. Paraffin sections of the formalin-fixed brains were subjected to hematoxylin and eosin (H and E) staining, Klüver-Barrera staining, Gallyas' silver impregnation, and immunohistochemistry for glial fibrillary acidic protein (GFAP), neurofilaments and tau protein.

Cortical dysplasia

Cortical dysplasia was found in both the cerebrum and cerebellum to a greater or lesser extent in all the cases. The cerebral cortical dysplasia grossly varied from a lissencephalic appearance in extreme cases, to a polymicrogyric pattern which was commonly present in our series. Extensive areas with a lissencephalic appearance were observed over the surface of the cerebral hemispheres in the infant cases under the age of 10 years, with a preference for the temporal and parieto-occipital lobes (Fig. 1a). In other areas, the polymicrogyric pattern was frequently noted over the cortical surface, and was occasionally associated with a granular appearance, like brain warts. The primary sulci, such as the central, lateral and cal-

Table 1
Occurrence of Alzheimer's neurofibrillary tangles in FCMD

Age/sex	CC	PHC	HC	NBM	BST
1.9 F	−	−	−	−	−
2 F	−	−	−	−	−
6 F	−	−	−	−	−
10 F	−	−	−	−	−
11 F	−	−	−	−	−
17 M	−	−	−	−	−
22 M	−	−	−	+	−
23 M	−	+	−	+	−
26 F	−	+	−	+	++
29 M	+	++	−	++	++
34 F	+	++	−	++	+

CC, cerebral cortex; PHC: parahippocampal cortex; HC, hippocampus; NBM, nucleus basalis of Meynert; BST, brain stem tegmentum; (−), no tangles found; (+), a few tangles found; (++), several tangles found.

carine ones, were well delineated. In the juvenile and adult cases, the agyric areas were more focal and restricted to the occipital lobes. Cut sections through the lissencephalic areas revealed thickening of the cortical ribbons with shallowing of the sulci, suggesting pachygyria (Fig. 1b). The lateral and third ventricles were slightly dilated. Otherwise, the basal ganglia, thalamic nuclei, hippocampal formations and white matter appeared grossly normal.

Histologically the dysplastic changes in the cerebral cortex varied from site to site, even in the same brain. Polymicrogyric areas consisted of an acellular molecular layer and a single, thick, cellular layer with irregular folds, where a cortical structure was unlayered (Fig. 2). A peculiar dysplastic pattern was found which was characterized by the presence of a cellular nodule in the superficial layer, which was designated as verrucous dysplasia. Beneath the verrucous nodule, a normal 6-layered structure was evident. Another dysplastic pattern was a pachygyric formation consisting of 4 distinct layers: the outermost layer was a superficial thin myelinated layer; the second, a thick cellular layer; the third, a densely myelinated layer; and the deepest, an irregularly-arranged cellular layer. This cortical architecture showed some similarities to that of type 2 lissencephaly in Walker–Warburg syndrome [9,11].

This cortical dysplasia in the cerebrum was categorized into mainly 3 patterns, referred to as types 1, 2 and 3 [5]. Type 1 dysplasia comprises a verrucous nodule in the superficial cortical layer, chiefly on the medial aspect of the occipital lobes and on the lateral surface of the temporal lobes, type 2 a polymicrogyric pattern predominantly present in the frontal and parietal lobes, and type 3 a pachygyric one with a predilection for the occipital and temporal lobes. Even in a fetal case of 23 weeks gestational age, the conspicuous cortical dysplasia was manifest [12]. Nerve cells in the polymicrogyric area were small in size and primitive. The arachnoid membrane was markedly thickened due to proliferation of glial and fibrovascular components associated with verrucous protrusion of cortical neurons into the subarachnoid space. GFAP immunostaining demonstrated extensive proliferation of glial tissue in the subarachnoid space, where the external glial limitans in the pia mater was defective (Fig. 3). It is assumed that abnormal glio-mesenchymal interactions can contribute to the disorder of neuronal migration and finally result in the cortical dysplasia. The hypothesis is proposed that, if the external glial limitans happens to become defective in early embryonal life for whatever reason, either infection or vascular damage, migrating neurons could protrude or overrun into the subarachnoid space through the defective site and give rise to verrucous dysplasia, with disarrangement of the cortical lamination.

In the cerebellum, a smooth-surfaced cortical area was consistently found on the dorsal aspect of the hemispheres, most frequently in the superior semilunar lobules (Fig. 4a). In cut sections, the smooth-surfaced cortex was observed to consist of a conglomeration of irregular and tiny gyrations (Fig. 4b). The cerebellar polymicrogyria was microscopically characterized by numerous small zones of the molecular and granular layers, which were

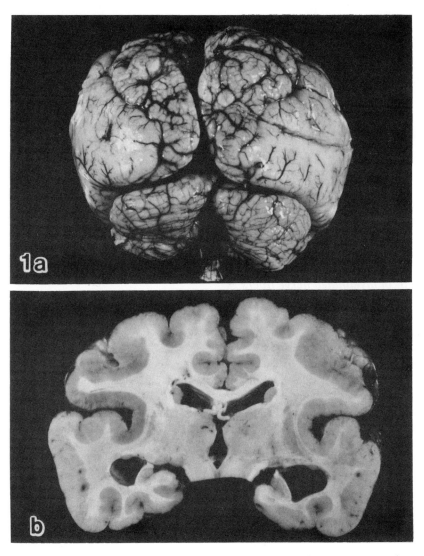

Fig. 1. Gross abnormalities of the cerebrum. (a) In a dorsal view, the cortical surface appears to be agyric and polymicrogyric over the temporo-occipital and parieto-occipital areas, respectively. (b) A coronal section reveals thickening of the cortical ribbons like pachygyria in the frontal and temporal lobes.

192

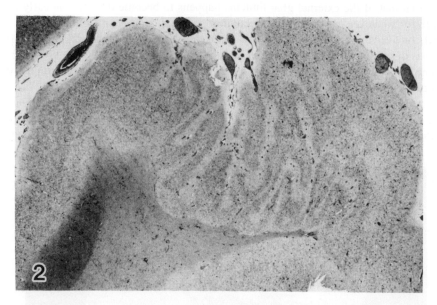

Fig. 2. Polymicrogyric formations in the cerebral cortex are composed of acellular and cellular layers associated with obliteration of the sulci. H and E stain, ×60.

irregularly intermingled with each other (Fig. 5). Purkinje cells were preferentially scattered at the border between these 2 layers. These dysplastic changes were more obvious in the fetal cerebellum.

Aberrancy of myelinated nerve fibers

In the subarachnoid space of the cerebellum, aberrant fascicles running along with small blood vessels were grossly found [5]. The aberrant fascicles were histologically composed of bundles of myelinated nerve fibers surrounded by a thick band of glial tissue, in which reactive astrocytes were verified by immunostaining for GFAP (Fig. 6). The origin of the aberrant fibers was pursued in serial histologic sections as far as possible and it was found that some of them arose from the pontine tegmentum near the root of the trochlear nerve and terminated in the polymicrogyric cortex in the superior semilunar lobule. Others originated from the white matter in the proximal lobules of the same hemisphere and also terminated in the polymicrogyric cortex. The presence of GFAP-immunoreactive astrocytes in these fascicles suggests that they are of central nervous system origin. No nerve cells were included in these fascicles. They were usually separated from the cerebellar parenchyma, and occasionally adhered to the subjacent polymicrogyric cortex. Although it remains unclear how such fascicles develop, it is implied that heterotopic white matter may extrude into the subarachnoid space through a defective site in the glial limitans in the pia mater. The formation of aberrant fascicles presumably follows the development of cerebellar folia by the twentieth week of gestation because the fascicles often override many normal folia. This may roughly coincide with the timing of cerebellar polymicrogyric formation in the late stage of the second trimester [13].

Alzheimer's neurofibrillary tangles

One more interesting finding was the early occurrence of Alzheimer's neurofibrillary tangles (NFTs) in adult cases [14]. The tangles within the nerve cells were stained slightly basophilic on H and E staining and more clearly demonstrated by Gallyas' silver impregnation (Fig. 7a). Immunohistochemically, they were reactive for neurofilaments (Fig. 7b) and tau protein. Senile plaques, as seen in aged brains, however, were not found in any cases of FCMD, nor Hirano bodies or granulovacuolar degeneration. NFTs in FCMD are distributed predictably in the nucleus basalis of Meynert, parahippocampal cortex, brain stem tegmentum including the locus ceruleus and substantia nigra, occasionally the cerebral neocortex and exceptionally the hippocampus. Electron microscopically NFT consisted of paired helical filaments with a maximal width of about 25 nm and regular constrictions at approximately 80 nm intervals. Their ultrastructure was almost identical to that in senile dementia of the Alzheimer type (SDAT), Down's syndrome [15], Hallervorden-Spatz disease [l6], infantile neuroaxonal dystrophy [17], Cockayne syndrome [18], and other neurological disorders, such as Parkinsonism-dementia complex of Guam, progressive supranuclear palsy,

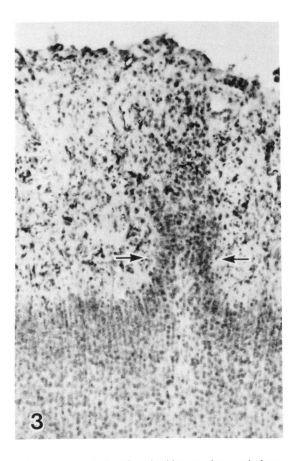

Fig. 3. Proliferation of astrocytes can be seen in the subarachnoid space where cortical neurons protrude through a defective site (between the two arrows) in the external glial linlitans. GFAP immunostain, ×150.

194

and subacute sclerosing panencephalitis (SSPE) [19]. As shown in Table 1, NFTs occurred earliest at the age of 22 years in our series, as well as in the previously reported case [20]. It is suggested that the precocious or accelerated aging process may be linked to the primary gene defect in some hereditary diseases, although the mental retardation was relatively mild in our studied cases. Moreover, the site predilection for NFTs in FCMD was quite different from that in SDAT [15]. The early occurrence of neurofibrillary tangles indicates that a peculiar neurodegenerative process may exist in FCMD.

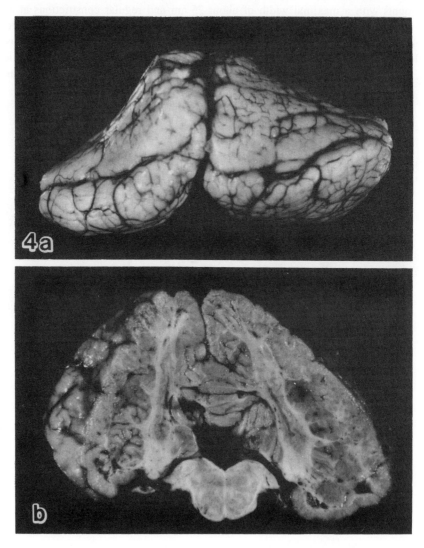

Fig. 4. Macroscopic appearance of the cerebellum. (a) The cortical surface is partly smooth on the dorsal aspect of the hemispheres. (b) On the cut surface, the cortex is thickened by irregular gyrations.

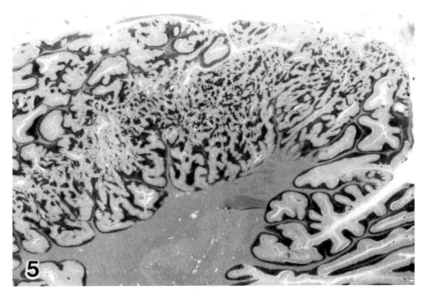

Fig. 5. Polymicrogyria in the cerebellum. Small gyrations are irregularly intermixed with each other. H and E stain, ×60.

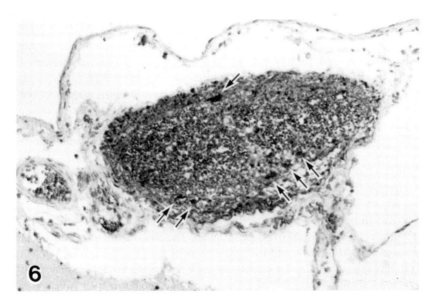

Fig. 6. In the cerebellar subarachnoid space, an aberrant fascicle of myelinated nerve fibers can be found to be surrounded by a band of glial tissue including astrocytes (arrows). Immunostain for GFAP, ×150.

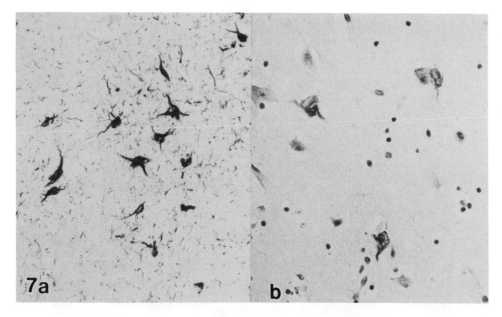

Fig. 7. Neurofibrillary tangles in the parahippocampal cortex. (a) The tangles are clearly demonstrated by silver impregnation. Gallyas' stain, ×150. (b) Neurofibrils are included in the neuronal cytoplasm. Immunostain for neurofilaments, ×150.

Conclusion

Twelve cases of FCMD ranging in age from 23 weeks gestation to 34 years have been studied neuropathologically. The brain pathology observed in this study can be summarized as follows: (1) various types of cortical dysplasia in the cerebrum, such as verrucous nodules, polymicrogyria and pachygyria; (2) polymicrogyria in the cerebellum; (3) gliomesenchymal proliferation in the subarachnoid space; (4) aberrant fascicles of myelinated fibers; and (5) the early occurrence of Alzheimer's neurofibrillary tangles in the nucleus basalis of Meynert, parahippocampal cortex and brain stem tegmentum. Although the pathogenesis of FCMD remains unresolved, it seems reasonable to postulate that a single pleiotrophic gene may account for both the muscular dystrophy and the brain lesions.

Acknowledgments

This study was in part supported by a Research Grant for Nervous and Mental Disorders from the Ministry of Health and Welfare of Japan. The authors are grateful to Profs. Yukio Fukuyama and Makiko Osawa, and to the members of the Organizing Committee for inviting them to this symposium, and are indebted to Dr. Nobutaka Arai, Department of Clinical Neuropathology, Tokyo Metropolitan Institute for Neuroscience, for taking the histologic pictures. This paper should have been read by Dr. Kuniyasu Takada, if he were alive. He was our best collaborator and had a special interest in the neuropathology of FCMD. We express our profound sorrow over his sudden death.

References

1. Fukuyama Y, Osawa M, Suzuki H. Congenital progressive muscular dystrophy of the Fukuyama type – clinical, genetic and pathological consideration. Brain Dev (Tokyo) 1981; 3: 1–29.

2. Osawa M, Arai M, Ikenaka H, et al. Fukuyama type congenital progressive muscular dystrophy. Acta Paediatr Jpn (Tokyo) 1991; 33: 261–269.

3. Toda T, Segawa M, Nomura Y, et al. Localization of a gene for Fukuyama type congenital muscular dystrophy to chromosome 9q31-33. Nat Genet 1993; 5: 283–286.

4. Nonaka I, Sugita H, Takada K, Kumagai K. Muscle histochemistry in congenital muscular dystrophy with central nervous system involvement. Muscle Nerve 1982; 5: 102–106.

5. Takada K, Nakamura H, Tanaka J. Cortical dysplasia in congenital muscular dystrophy with central nervous system involvement (Fukuyama type). J Neuropathol Exp Neurol 1984; 43: 395–407.

6. Takada K, Rin YS, Kasagi S, Sato K, Nakamura H, Tanaka J. Long survival in Fukuyama congenital muscular dystrophy: occurrence of neurofibrillary tangles in the nucleus basalis of Meynert and locus ceruleus. Acta Neuropathol 1986; 71: 228–232.

7. Kamoshita S, Konishi Y, Segawa M, Fukuyama Y. Congenital muscular dystrophy as a disease of the central nervous system. Arch Neurol 1976; 33: 513–516.

8. Ogasawara Y, Ito K, Murofushi K. Neuropathological studies on two cases of congenital muscular dystrophy, with special reference to morphological characteristics of micropolygyria found in the cerebral and cerebellar cortex (in Japanese). No To Shinkei (Tokyo) 1976; 28: 451–457.

9. Dobyns WB, Pagon RA, Armstrong D, et al. Diagnostic criteria for Walker–Warburg syndrome. Am J Med Genet 1989; 32: 195–210.

10. Santavuori P, Somer H, Sainio K, et al. Muscle-eye-brain disease (MEB). Brain Dev (Tokyo) 1989; 11: 147–153.

11. Takada K, Takashima S, Tanaka J. Is Walker–Walburg syndrome a severe type of Fukuyama type congenital muscular dystrophy (FCMD)? (in Japanese). No To Hattatsu (Tokyo) 1985; 17: 269–271.

12. Takada K, Nakamura H. Cerebellar micropolygyria in Fukuyama congenital muscular dystrophy: observations in fetal and pediatric cases. Brain Dev (Tokyo) 1990; 12: 774–778.

13. de Leon GA, Grover WD, Mestre GM. Cerebellar micropolygyria. Acta Neuropathol (Berlin) 1976; 35: 81–85.

14. Takada K. Early occurrence of Alzheimer's neurofibrillary tangles (NFT) in developmental brain damage and chronic brain diseases with early childhood onset. Neuropathology (Tokyo) 1993; 13: 333–335.

15. Wisniewski KE, Dalton AJ, McLachlan DRC, Wen GY, Wisniewski HM. Alzheimer's disease in Down's syndrome: clinicopathological study. Neurology 1985; 35: 957–961.

16. Eidelberg D, Sotrel A, Joachim C, et al. Adult onset Hallervorden-Spatz disease with neurofibrillary pathology. a discrete clinicopathological entity. Brain 1987; 110: 993–1013.

17. Hayashi S, Akasaki Y, Morimura Y, Takeuchi S, Sato M, Miyoshi K. An autopsy case of late infantile and juvenile neuroaxonal dystrophy with diffuse Lewy bodies and neurofibrillary tangles. Clin Neuropathol 1992; 11: 1–5.

18. Takada K, Becker LE. Cockayne's syndrome: two autopsy case report associated with neurofibrillary changes. Clin Neuropathol 1986; 5: 64–68.

19. Wisniewski K, Jervis GA, Moretz RC, Wisniewski HM. Alzheimer neurofibrillary tangles in disease other than senile and presenile dementia. Ann Neurol 1979; 5: 288–294.

20. Murakami T, Konishi Y, Takamiya M, Tsukagoshi H. Congenital muscular dystrophy associated with micropolygyria. Report of two cases. Acta Pathol Jpn (Tokyo) 1975; 25: 599–612.

Y. Fukuyama, M. Osawa and K. Saito (Eds.), *Congenital Muscular Dystrophies*

199

CHAPTER 16

Cytoarchitectonic alterations of the cerebral cortex in Fukuyama-type congenital muscular dystrophy and other cortical dysplasia syndrome

SACHIO TAKASHIMA and MASASHI MIZUGUCHI

Department of Mental Retardation and Birth Defect Research, National Institute of Neuroscience,
National Center of Neurology and Psychiatry, Koraira, Tokyo, Japan

Introduction

Fukuyama-type congenital muscular dystrophy (FCMD) [1] is associated with localized polymicrogyria of the cerebral and cerebellar hemispheres with the loss of a normal cytoarchitecture. Walker–Warburg syndrome (WWS) [2] exhibits a smooth cortical surface, diffuse polymicrogyria of the cerebrum and cerebellum, ocular dysplasia, and occasional findings such as hydrocephalus, arachnoid cysts of the posterior fossa or cerebellar hypoplasia. Classical lissencephaly is characterized by the absence of cerebral convolutions, which, with rare exceptions, is associated with extensive subcortical, inferior olivary and dentate neuronal heterotopias [3]. This report describes the cytoarchitecture of the cerebral cortex in FCMD, in comparison with with that in other cortical dysplasia syndromes, and discusses their pathogenetic relationships.

Materials and methods

Five children and a fetus with FCMD, and one case each of WWS and classical lissencephaly were neuropathologically examined. Representative samples were taken from the cerebral cortex, basal ganglia, thalamus, brainstem and spinal cord. The tissues were embedded in paraffin, cut at 7μm thickness, and then stained with hematoxylin and eosin, luxol fast blue and Mallory phosphotungstic acid. Blocks adjacent to those prepared for Golgi impregnation were cut at 4μm thickness and then stained with cresyl violet, and by immunohistochemical methods for glial fibrillary acidic protein (GFAP), myelin basic protein (MBP), neurofilament (NF) and synaptophysin.

At autopsy, 5 mm-thick sections of the right visual cortex containing the calcarine sulcus and a similar section taken from the frontal cortex were immediately immersed in Golgi fixative. The tissue were further processed using the rapid Golgi impregnation method [4]. The morphology of the neurons was observed and camera lucida drawings of the composite cortex were prepared, using methods similar to those we previously described [4].

Cerebral cytoarchitecture in FCMD

In the visual and frontal cortices of FCMD patients, the molecular layer was thin and contained occasional pyramidal neurons, while the second layer, consisting of pyramidal neurons, was tortuous and suggestive of polymicrogyria. Some parts of the molecular layer were buried in the intermediate zone of the superficial cellular layer. The irregular neuronal arrangement was marked in the superficial layer. In the deep cortex, there was a radial neuronal arrangement in some areas and markedly irregular arrangements of neurons in others, particularly in the occipital lobes (Fig. 1) [5].

In some cortical areas, 4 layers were recognized between the molecular layer and white matter. The border between the cortex and white matter was blurred, and myelinated fibers irregularly invaded the deepest cortical layer. There were nests of heterotopic neurons along the border between the cortex and white matter, especially in the most disorganized areas. Takada [6] classified these findings in FCMD into 3 types; superficial, upper-half and diffuse cortical dysplasias.

MBP-immunohistochemistry demonstrated a marked and irregular increase of positive myelin fibers in the superficial layer to the deep cellular cortex. The increase of MBP-immunoreactivity was more marked in the areas of severe cortical dysplasia than in those with a normal architecture. Synaptophysin immunohistochemistry revealed a multifocal and

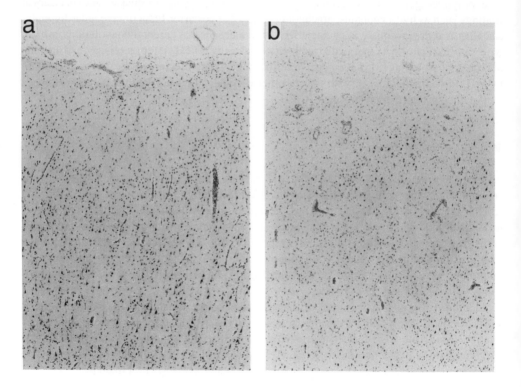

Fig. 1. Cortical dysplasia in a FCMD brain. (a) There are focal leptomeningeal glioneuronal heterotopias and irregular cellularity in the superficial cerebral cortex. (b) The cortex shows markedly irregular cell arrangement, which is predominant in the superficial layer. Nissl stain, ×60.

irregular increase of positive reactivity along the surface in the superficial layer, which suggested the disappearance or displacement of the molecular layer with abnormal migration.

On Golgi staining, pyramidal neurons were observed to be arranged either radially, obliquely or horizontally, and some adjacent neurons lay in opposite directions in parts of the areas of polymicrogyria. Irregular arrangement of neurons was predominant in the superficial cortex. The soma were variable in size but generally small. The basal dendrites were short in most of the pyramidal neurons. However, a few larger neurons had large soma and varicose apical or basal dendrites. Stellate neurons were small with irregularly shaped and short dendrites. Spines were few on the dendrites of small neurons and more numerous on large ones.; they were mushroom-shaped and very small. There were varicosities on some of the dendrites (Fig. 2) [5,6].

Cortical architecture in Walker–Warburg syndrome

In most areas of WWS, the cortical neurons were arranged in irregular cellular groups separated by less cellular areas or, occasionally, in radial columns. There were many astrocytes and pyramidal neurons in the subpial layer. The irregular cytoarchitecture was less marked in the frontal cortex than in the visual cortex. The neurons along the vertical myelin fibers were oriented either radially or obliquely.

Subcortical neuronal heterotopias at the border between the cortex and white matter contained small neurons and exhibited no characteristic arrangement of cells. On Golgi staining, the arrangement of neurons was observed as irregular and the individual neurons often showed an abnormal orientation in the entire cortex. Neuronal arrangements were related to neuronal groupings or the myelin fibers projecting into the cortex. Near the myelinated fibers, the neurons were arranged radially and apical dendrites projected toward the pial surface. In the groups next to the columns of myelin sheaths, neurons were arranged obliquely or inverted, with apical dendrites projecting toward the white matter. The soma were relatively small and the basal dendrites were short. The apical dendrites were somewhat tortuous. A few huge neurons were identified. Some pyramidal neurons showed abnormal branching of the basal dendrites with retraction to one side of the soma. In the subcortical nodules, pyramidal and stellate neurons had small soma and short basal dendrites. The pyramidal neurons formed an arc along the margins of the nodules. In the visual cortex, the neurons were smaller and shorter and their arrangement was more markedly irregular than in the frontal cortex. There were some immature and bipolar neurons [5].

Cortical architecture in classical lissencephaly

The visual cortex in classical lissencephaly had 4 layers: molecular, superficial cellular, sparsely cellular and deep cellular ones. A wide outer field of pyramidal cells and a narrow inner band of polymorphic cells were present in the superficial cellular layer. The deep cellular layer contained small, round cells and pyramidal neurons. Most of the neurons were radially aligned in columns. Some neurons were noted in subcortical or periventricular heterotopias, indicating premature arrest of their migration.

In an immunohistochemical study, the cortex with a smooth surface demonstrated characteristic patterns in the molecular, superficial cellular, sparse cellular and deep cellular

202

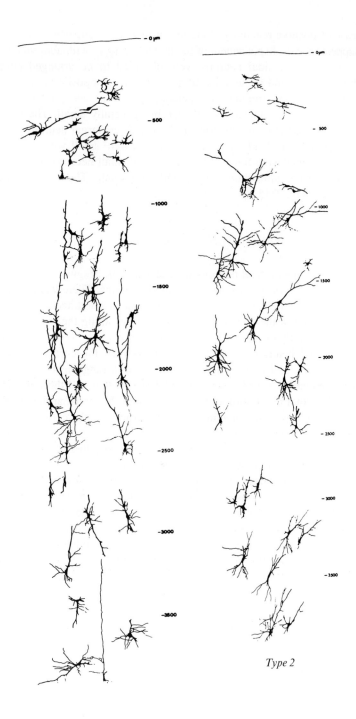

Type 1 dysplasia.

Fig. 2. Cytoarchitecture of cortical dysplasias, types 1 and 2 (Takada), in a FCMD brain Golgi stain and camera-lucida drawing.

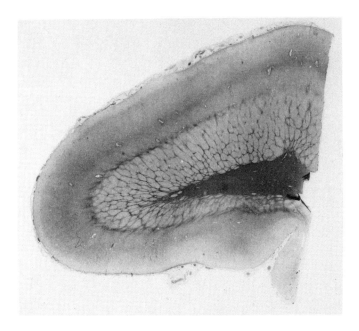

Fig. 3. In a classical lissencephaly brain, there are myelin basic protein positive bundles distributed regularly in the deep cellular layer of the cerebral cortex. Immunohistochemical (PAP) staining.

layers. The molecular layer showed abnormal positivity with synaptophysin. The superficial cellular layer was diffusely stained for synaptophysin. The molecular layer of these lissencephalic brains may contain many synapses on the terminals of the apical dendrites, which indicates abnormal neuronal development [7].

The sparse cellular layer exhibited less staining for synaptophysin, but was perivascularly positive for GFAP, and the linear myelination was stained positively for MBP. This reduced staining for synaptophysin indicates that this layer is similar to the molecular layer and white matter, although the perivascular astrocytosis may be consistent with the consequences of a laminar layer of necrotic tissue in early fetal life.

In the deep cellular layer, synaptophysin staining demonstrated multiple islets or a polylobular pattern, and MBP staining revealed a reticular pattern around neuronal columns separated by myelin sheaths. Below the cortex, there were areas of heterotopic cortical tissue of various sizes in the cerebral white matter (Fig. 3).

On Golgi staining most neurons were observed to be arranged radially, but some were aligned obliquely or inverted to the pial surface of the cortex. In the molecular layer, there were several pyramidal neurons with small soma and short, obliquely arranged dendrites. Spines were reduced in number on both the apical and basal dendrites, some of which had varicosities. In the heterotopic areas, there were pyramidal neurons with thick apical and short basal dendrites. Thus, the cortical neuronal arrangement in classical lissencephaly is quite different from that in FCMD or WWS (Fig. 4) [5].

Fetal cortical cytoarchitecture in FCMD

In a FCMD fetus of 23 weeks gestation, numerous bundles of neural tissues protruded to-

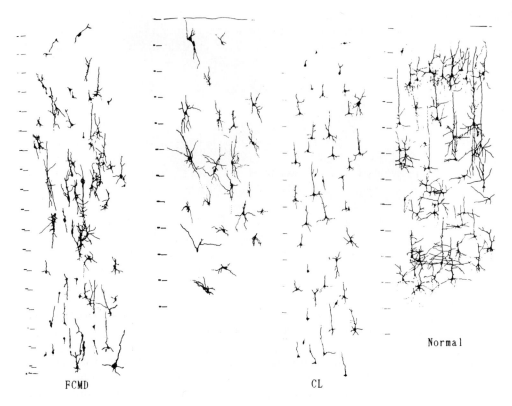

Fig. 4. Cytoarchitecture of the cerebral cortex in FCMD, Walker–Warburg syndrome and classical lissencephaly Golgi stain and camera-lucida drawing.

ward the leptoneninges through the original cortical surface and formed the superficial cellular layer, which showed an irregular cellular arrangement.

In the fetus, cortical dysplasia of various extents was distributed in the cortex, as Takada [8] illustrated 3 patterns of aberrant neuronal migration. This different expression of dysplasia among cortical regions may result from the varying maturity of the cortices at the beginning of the pathogenetic process.

GFAP-immunohistochemistry showed that positive glial cells were increased in number and irregularly scattered in the superficial cellular layer, while they were normally present in the remaining cortex and white matter. The increase of GFAP-positive glia may have induced or guided the formation of the superficial cellular layer, or it could be a secondary event with cell proliferation.

Neuronal migration is normally arrested by the integrity of the pial-glial barrier [9]. Damage to some components of this barrier, such as the glial end-feet, basement membrane or extracellular material, may allow the migration to continue into the subarachnoid space [10].

In fetal brains with type II lissencephaly, neurons formed an incomplete lamina beneath a horizontal vascular band, suggesting that early migration had been normal and a sort of primitive cortical plate had developed. As development continues, cells appear to burst through defects of the pial/glial barrier causing widespread neuronal and glial ectopias in the leptomeninges [11]. Experimental work has shown that selective damage to meningeal cells results in the loss of pial basal lamina and neuronal ectopias [12]. The association of FCMD, WWL and muscle-eye-brain disease with cerebral cortical dysplasia suggests a more generalized defect in some components of mesenchymal tissues [11].

Cortical angioarchitecture in FCMD

There is a close relationship between the cytoarchitecture and the angioarchitecture in the cerebral cortex. In the normal brain, the cortical perforating arteries consist of cortical, sub-cortical and medullary ones, which branch from the leptomeningeal arteries and supply the cerebral cortex, subcortical and deep white matter, respectively. The cortical arteries are the most abundant.

Takada and his colleagues [13] studied the angioarchitecture of cortical dysplasia of FCMD brains using the silver staining method of Hasegawa and Ravens. In type 1 dyspla-sia, perforating arteries consisting of many cortical and some subcortical vessels were mostly normal with irregular small vascular networks in superficial areas. In type 2 dyspla-sia, the cortical and subcortical vessels were distorted, particularly in the upper cortical layer. A normal perpendicular pattern was seen only in the deeper cortical layer. In type 3 dysplasia, vessels of relatively large caliber, which looked like leptomeningeal vessels, ran either vertically, obliquely or horizontally, branching laterally or radially into small and short vessels, which were interpreted as being cortical vessels (Fig. 5). Such an angioarchi-tecture of FCMD brains suggests overlying microgyri.

Conclusion

The cortical architecture of FCMD brains is characterized by bundles of cortical cells ir-regularly protruding into the superficial cellular layer, which form dysplasias of various

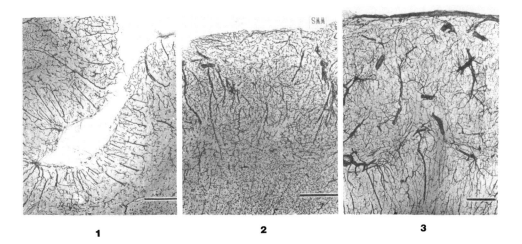

Fig. 5. Angioarchitecture in the cerebral cortex (types 1, 2 and 3) of FCMD [13].

degrees in different cortical regions, are associated with an increase of CFAP-positive glia in the superficial cellular layer, and result in the irregular neuronal arrangement and formation of microgyri. Therefore, the cortical dysplasias in FCMD, as well as WWS, may be due to an irregular overgrowth of cortical elements into the superficial cortical layer, while those in classical lissencephaly may involve regular neuronal heterotopias in the deep cellular layer. We need further studies to clarify the mechanism of cortical overgrowth in FCMD.

References

1. Fukuyama Y, Kawazura M, Haruna H. A peculiar form of congenital progressive muscular dystrophy. Report of fifteen cases. Paediatr Univ Tokyo (Tokyo) 1960; 4: 5–8.
2. Walker AE. Lissencephaly. Arch Neurol Psychiatry 1942; 48: 13–29.
3. Stewart RM, Richman DP, Caviness VS Jr. Lissencephaly and pachygyria an architectonic and topographical analysis. Acta Neuropathol (Berlin) 1975; 31: 1–12.
4. Takashima S, Chan F, Becker LE, Armstrong DL. Morphology of the developing visual cortex of the human infant. A quantitative and qualitative Golgi study. J Neuropathol Exp Neurol 1980; 39: 487–501.
5. Takashima S, Becker LE, Chan F, Takada K. A Golgi study of the cerebral cortex in Fukuyama-type congenital muscular dystrophy, Walker-type lissencephaly and classical lissencephaly. Brain Dev (Tokyo) 1987; 9: 621–626.
6. Takada K. Fukuyama congenital muscular dystrophy as a unique disorder of neuronal migration a neuropathological review and hypothesis. Yonago Acta Medica (Yonago) 1988; 31: 1–16.
7. Houdou S, Kuruta H, Konomi H, Takashima S. Structure in lissencephaly determined by immunohistochemical staining. Pediatr Neurol 1990; 6: 402–406.
8. Takada K, Nakamura H, Suzumori K, Ishikawa T, Sugiyaoa N. Cortical dysplasia in a 23-week fetus with Fukuyama congenital muscular dystrophy: a case analysis. Acta Neuropathol (Berlin) 1987; 74: 300–306.
9. Larroche JC, Razavi-Encha F. Cytoarchitectonic abnormalities. In: NC Myrianthospoulos, ed. Handbook of clinical neurology, Vol 6 (50). Malformations. Amsterdam: North-Holland 1987; 245–266.
10. Choi BH, Matthias SC. Cortical dysplasia associated with massive ectopia of neurons and glial cells within the subarachnoid space. Acta Neuropathol (Berlin) 1987; 73: 105–109.
11. Squier HV. Development of the cortical dysplasia of type II lissencephaly. Neuropathol Appl Neurobiol 1993; 19: 209–213.
12. Hartman D, Sievers J, Pehlemann FW, Berry H. Destruction of meningeal cells over the medial cerebral hemisphere of newborn hamsters prevents the formation of the infrapyramidal blade of the dentate gyrus. J Comp Neurol 1992; 320: 33–61.
13. Takada K, Nakamura H, Takashima S. Cortical dysplasia in Fukuyama congenital muscular dystrophy (FCMD) a Golgi and angioarchitectonic analysis. Acta Neuropathol (Berlin) 1988; 76: 170–178.

Y. Fukuyama, M. Osawa and K. Saito (Eds.), *Congenital Muscular Dystrophies*

207

CHAPTER 17

Neuronal and vascular involvement in Fukuyama type congenital muscular dystrophy

TERUHISA MIIKE[1], JUNICHIRO OHTA[1], SHIGETO SUGINO[1], JI-EN ZHAO[1] and TATSURO MUTOH[2]

[1]*Department of Child Development, University School of Medicine, Kumamoto, Japan*
[2]*Second Internal Medicine, Fukui Medical School, Fukui, Japan*

Introduction

It is known that muscle biopsy specimens from Fukuyama type congenital muscular dystrophy (FCMD) cases commonly show grouping of regenerating muscle fibers. These regenerating muscle fibers are at about the same stage, suggesting that grouping of necrotic fibers occurs prior to regeneration [1,2]. This grouping of necrotic and regenerating fibers is adequately explained by the vascular theory. Thus, we previously studied the behavior of blood vessels in biopsied FCMD muscles using electronmicroscopy and morphometric analysis, and reported capillary injury such as blister-like swelling of endothelial cells, and the extremely greater capillary, endothelial and pericyte areas in FCMD, respectively [3]. Subsequently, we immunohistochemically studied the behavior of the low affinity nerve growth factor receptor (LNGFR), which influences sympathetic neurons, and found a strong LNGFR reaction on the tunica adventitia of blood vessels [4]. The findings suggest a sympathetic nervous system process involving blood vessels in FCMD. LNGFR belongs to the nerve growth factor (NGF) family.

It is known that NGF is essential in the development and differentiation of not only neural tissues but also non-neural tissues [5]. To determine how neuronal factors, such as members of the NGF family, are involved in muscle degeneration and regeneration in FCMD, we studied biopsied muscle specimens with antibodies to NGF, LNGFR, high affinity NGFR with tyrosine kinase (p140[trk]), neurotrophin-3 (NT-3), and the tumor necrotic factor (TNF), immunohistochemically and immunoelectrophoretically.

Materials and methods

Muscle biopsy specimens from 6 FCMD patients were examined immunohistochemically using antibodies to the NGF family and TNF. Non-diagnostic (ND) age-matched muscle biopsy specimens and legally aborted fetus materials were observed as controls (Table 1). We used the following antibodies: (1) anti-nerve growth factor (NGF) antibody: rabbit polyclonal (provided by Professor Hayashi, Gifu Pharmaceutical University); (2) anti-low affinity NGF receptor (LNGFR) antibody ME 82–11 (provided by Dr. Soldano Ferrone); mouse monoclonal (AUSTRAL Biological); (3) anti-high affinity NGF receptor antibody

Table 1

Immunohistochemical reactivity of NGF family in FCMD and fetus

	NGF	LNGFR	p140^{trk}	NT3	TNFα	TNFβ	p60	p80
FCMD								
1. 2 m M	+	+++	R++	−	R++	−	R+~++	−
2. 7 m F	+	++	R+	−	R+	−	R+	−
3. 11 m F	+	++	R+	−	R+	−	R±	−
4. 11 m F	+	++	R+	−	R+	−	R±	−
5. 11 m F	+	++	R+	−	R+	−	R±	−
6. 19 m F	+	++	R+	−	R±	−	−	−
FETUS								
1. 12 w	+	+++	++	−	++	−	−	−
2. 14 w	++	++	+	−	+	−	−	−
3. 16 w	++	+	+	−	+	−	−	−
4. 17 w	++	+	±	−	±	−	−	−
5. 19 w	+	±	−	−	−	−	−	−
6. 36 w	+	−	−	−	−	−	−	−
7. 39 w	+	−	−	−	−	−	−	−

NGF, nerve growth factor; LNGFR, low affinity nerve growth factor receptor; p140^{trk}, high affinity NGF receptor; NT-3, neurotrophin-3; TNF, tumor necrotic factor; R, regenerating fibers; m, months; w, weeks.

(p140^{trk})(provided by Dr. Mutoh, Fukui University); (4) NT-3, mouse monoclonal (AUSTRAL Biological); (5) TNF-α and TNF-β, rabbit polyclonal (Genzyme); and (6) TNF receptor (60), mouse monoclonal (Genzyme), and TNF receptor (80), rat monoclonal (Genzyme).

For immunoassaying of the NGF family, using antibodies to NGF, LNGFR and p140^{trk}, the materials were homogenized in 15 μl of a proteolytic solution (1% SDS, 5% β-mercaptoethanol, 4 mM EDTA, 40 mM Tris, 0.1 M phenylmethylsulfonylfluoride (PMSF), 0.24 M glycine, 40% glycerine and 0.03% bromophenyl blue, pH 8.5), and then the supernatants (7–10 μl; 100 μg) were loaded onto 10-well SDS-polyacrylamide gels (1 mm × 10 × 9 cm), with the use of a 3% stacking gel and a 128 resolving gel. The fractionated proteins were transferred to nitrocellulose membranes and then incubated with the NGF family antibodies. Immune complexes were detected with affinity-purified rabbit anti-mouse IgG conjugated to avidine-DE biotinylated horseradish peroxidase (ABC method).

Results

Immunohistochemistry

Although NGF immunoreactivity was commonly observed on the muscle fiber membrane in both ND control and FCMD, younger fetuses showed strong activity around muscle fibers. As a common finding, LNGFR activity was seen on the perineurium of peripheral nerve bundles, peripheral nerve endings and some of the nerve fibers in all the specimens. Strong LNGFR immunoreactivity was seen on the tunica adventitia of blood vessels in FCMD. Positive LNGFR reactivity on the tunica adventitia of blood vessels was also seen in fetus muscles during fetal life, but disappeared after birth (data not shown). In addition to these findings, LNGFR activity on the membrane and p140^{trk} (Fig. 1a) in cytosomes of regener-

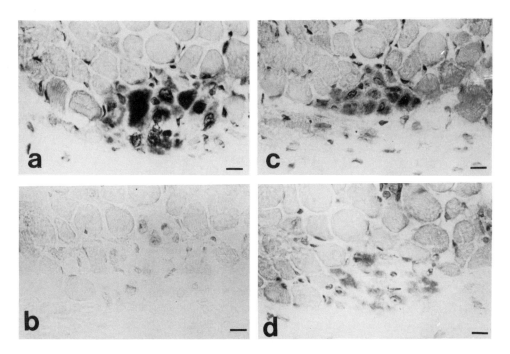

Fig. 1. Immunohistochemical study of regenerating muscle fibers in FCMD. Note the positive immunoreactivities of p140^{trk} (a) and TNF-α (c) on the regenerating muscle fibers (arrows) in FCMD. In contrast, p140^{trk} treated with p140^{trk}-antigen (b) and non-immune serum (d) showed negative reaction. Bar, 10 μm.

ating muscle fibers were seen in FCMD, and fetus muscles, especially before 17-weeks gestational age. In contrast, p140^{trk} treated with p140^{trk}-antigen and non-immune serum staining showed negative reaction on the regenerating muscle fibers (Fig. 1b,d). In controls, LNGFR and p104^{trk} activities were almost negative. Regenerating fibers in FCMD also showed positive TNF-α (Fig. 1c) and its receptor (p60) immunoreactivity, and fetal muscle before 17-weeks of age showed positive TNF-α immunoreactivity. NT-3, and TNF-β and its receptor (p80) showed no immunoreactivity at all, in any specimens.

Immunoelectrophoretical study

The immunoassaying of the NGF family using antibodies to NGF, LNGFR and p140^{trk} revealed a common band at 220 kDa (Fig. 2), which was considered to represent a heterodimer of these three components.

Discussion

In this study we observed positive NGF family immunoreactivity, especially in regenerating muscle fibers and fetus muscle fibers. It has been considered that only a heterodimer of three components (NGF, LNGF and p140^{trk}) exhibits the biological activity of NGF. On immunoassaying, we observed a positive band at 220 kDa, which is considered to represent a heterodimer of these three components, because all the three antibodies showed the same

210

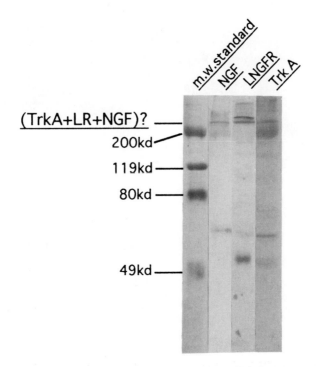

Fig. 2. Immunoblot analysis of NGF family. Note the common band at 220 kDa. NGF, nerve growth factor; LNGFR, low affinity nerve growth factor receptor; Trk A, high affinity NGF receptor (p140^{trk}).

band at 220 kDa. These findings suggested that the NGF family plays an important role in muscle development and/or differentiation in FCMD and fetuses. In addition, TNF-α and its receptor (p60) also showed a positive reaction in regenerating muscle fibers in FCMD. Although p60 was negative in fetus muscle, these results suggested that TNF-α, including p60, is also a kind of growth factor for muscle development and differentiation.

On the other hand, we previously observed vascular changes in FCMD, such as replication of the basement membrane, blister-like swelling of endothelial cells, and platelet adhesion and aggregation in small blood vessels [3]. Morphometric analysis of capillaries in biopsied muscles showed the extremely greater capillary, endothelial and pericyte areas in the FCMD patients than in controls [3]. Subsequently, we immunohistochemically studied the behavior of the LNGFR, which influences sympathetic neurons, and found a strong LNGFR reaction on the tunica adventitia of blood vessels, as previously found [4]. These findings suggest a sympathetic nervous system process involving blood vessels in FCMD, such as sensory and sympathetic nerve ganglia [6], and/or hypothalamus dysfunction, for example.

These results suggest two possibilities, either the vascular alterations comprise a primary lesion in FCMD or a secondary phenomenon after muscle degradation. We tried to observe blood vessels morphologically using an electron microscope after experimentally induced muscle degradation with marcaine, but failed to find any morphological changes in blood vessels [7]. It is well known that FCMD shows various clinical symptoms including central nervous system involvement. Recently, merosin negative congenital muscular dystrophy was reported. Both merosin [8] and dystrophin [9] are localized on the muscle fiber membrane. One may consider that both proteins also localize on the nervous system and smooth muscle cells [8,10,11]. If one tries to explain some of the symptoms in FCMD on the basis of only a defect of the muscle fiber membrane, it is not easy to explain other symptoms such as central nervous system involvement. We would like to emphasize that much more attention should be paid to the vascular hypothesis and/or sympathetic neurovascular hypothesis, because blood vessels are one of the most important tissues which exist in the entire body and it is much easier to explain various symptoms in various organs. Even if the vascular changes in FCMD are secondary phenomena, it is likely that the changes have an important influence on muscle regeneration and/or development.

References

1. Miike T, Tamari H, Ohtani Y, Nakamura H, Matsuda I, Miyoshino S. A fluorescent microscopy study of biopsied muscles from infantile neuromuscular disorders. Acta Neuropathol (Berlin) 1983; 59: 48–52.
2. Miike T. Maturational defect of regenerating muscle fibers in cases with Duchenne and congenital muscular dystrophies. Muscle Nerve 1983; 6: 545–552.
3. Sugino S, Miyatake M, Ohtani Y, Yoshioka K, Miike T, Uchino M. Vascular alterations in Fukuyama type congenital muscular dystrophy. Brain Dev (Tokyo) 1991; 13: 77–81.
4. Zhao J, Yoshioka K, Miike T, Kageshita T, Arao T. Nerve growth factor receptor immunoreactivity on the tunica adventitia of intramuscular blood vessels in childhood muscular dystrophies. Neuromusc Disord 1991; 1: 135–141.
5. Ernfors P, Wetmore C, Eriksdotter-Nilsson M, et al. The nerve growth factor receptor gene is expressed in both neuronal and non-neuronal tissues in the human fetus. Int J Dev Neurosci 1991; 9: 57–66.
6. Sobue G, Yasuda T, Mitsuma T, Pleasure D. Nerve growth factor receptor immunoreactivity in the neuronal perikarya of human sensory and sympathetic nerve ganglia. Neurology 1989; 39: 937–941.
7. Miike T, Nonaka I, Ohtani Y, Tamari H, Ishitsu T. Behavior of sarcotubular system formation in experimentally induced regeneration of muscle fibers. J Neurol Sci 1984; 65: 193–200.
8. Vuolteenaho R, Nissinen M, Saino K, et al. Human laminin M chain (merosin): complete primary structure, chromosomal assignment, and expression of the M and A chain in human fetal tissues. J Cell Biol 1994; 124: 381–394.
9. Hoffman EP, Brown RH Jr, Kunkel LM. Dystrophin: the protein product of the Duchenne muscular dystrophy locus. Cell 1987; 51: 919–928.
10. Byers TJ, Lidov HGW, Kunkel LM. An alternative dystrophin transcript specific to peripheral nerve. Nat Genet 1993; 4: 7781.
11. Miyatake M, Miike T, Zhao J, Yoshioka K, Uchino M, Usuku G. Possible systemic smooth muscle layer dysfunction due to a deficiency of dystrophin in Duchenne muscular dystrophy. J Neurol Sci 1989; 93: 11–17.

Y. Fukuyama, M. Osawa and K. Saito (Eds.), *Congenital Muscular Dystrophies*
213

Ultrastructural alterations of the muscle plasma membrane and related structures in Fukuyama muscular dystrophy: comparative study with other types of muscular dystrophies

Y. WAKAYAMA[1], S. SHIBUYA[1], T. KUMAGAI[2], T. KOBAYASHI[3],
S. YAMASHITA[4], N. MISUGI[5], S. MIYAKE[4], M. MURAHASHI[1],
T. JIMI[1] and H. ONIKI[6]

[1]*Division of Neurology, Department of Medicine, Showa University, Fujigaoka Hospital, Yokohama, Japan*
[2]*Division of Pediatric Neurology, Central Hospital, Aichi Prefectural Colony, Kasugai, Japan*
[3]*Department of Pediatrics, Yokohama City University, School of Medicine, Yokohama, Japan*
[4]*Department of Neurology, Kanagawa, Children's Medical Center, Yokohama, Japan*
[5]*Department of Orthopedics, Kanagawa, Children's Medical Center, Yokohama, Japan*
[6]*Electron Microscopic Laboratory, Showa University Fujigaoka Hospital, Yokohama, Japan*

Introduction

The pathophysiology of Fukuyama type congenital muscular dystrophy (FCMD) [1,2] is unknown, and it is possible that the myofiber surface membrane plays important roles in the pathogenesis of FCMD. An electron microscopic study of biopsied FCMD muscles was first reported by Misugi et al. [3]. However, the conventional electron microscopic findings for the FCMD muscle plasma membrane and related structures, such as the plasmalemmal undercoat and basal lamina, have not, so far, been described in detail. The purpose of this study is to investigate the ultrastructure of the myofiber plasma membrane and related structures in FCMD. We previously investigated the molecular architecture of the FCMD muscle plasma membrane by freeze fracture electron microscopy [4–6]. We compared the results of this study and those described previously [4–6] with those for other types of muscular dystrophies previously reported in the literature [7–13].

Materials and methods

For conventional electron microscopy, quadriceps femoris muscle biopsy specimens were obtained from 5 children with FCMD. The diagnosis of FCMD was made according to the criteria described previously [14,15]. Three histochemically normal quadriceps femoris muscle specimens were taken from children undergoing orthopedic operations. The muscle samples were fixed in a U-shaped muscle clamp at resting length with a chilled 2.5% glutaraldehyde solution for 1 h, washed three times, and then post fixed in chilled 1% osmium tetroxide for 1 h. These chemically fixed muscle specimens were dehydrated and then embedded in Epon. Ultrathin sections were stained doubly with uranyl and lead, and then examined under an electron microscope. The results were compared with the published data (7–9).

Freeze fracture studies were conducted by the methods described previously [4–6].

Results

The low power electron microscopic findings for the biopsied muscle specimens were the presence of small, variable sized myofibers with or without central nuclei, degenerating and regenerating myofibers, dense endomysial connective tissue, intramuscular nerve fibers, neuromuscular junctions and so on. Amongst these features, this study focused on the alterations of the muscle plasma membrane and related structures in FCMD. Fig. 1A shows the presence of a δ lesion of a FCMD myofiber, in which the rarefaction of myofibrils can be seen. Fig. 1B is a higher magnification electron micrograph of the indicated area (arrow) in Fig. 1A and shows the sarcolemma overlaying the δ lesion. The plasmalemma is disrupted and discontinuous (asterisk in Fig. 1B), whereas the basal lamina is preserved. The separation of the basal lamina from the plasma membrane can be seen and degenerating cell organelles are occasionally seen in the space between them (Fig. 1B). Figs. 2A and 3A show the plasma membrane and related structures overlaying a δ-lesion of FCMD myofibers, in which the plasmalemmal undercoat is rarefied when compared to that of the control myofibers (arrow in Fig. 2B). Interestingly, the basal lamina of FCMD myofibers is occasionally duplicated (asterisks in Fig. 3A). The muscle plasma membrane and its undercoat of a normal looking FCMD myofiber appear to be intact. On the other hand, the surface of regenerating FCMD myofibers contains cell organelles, such as many ribosomes, mitochondria and so on (asterisk in Fig. 3B). The plasma membranes of FCMD regenerating myofibers are continuous and the plasma membrane undercoats of these myofibers look dense (Fig. 3B and inset). The intramuscular myelinated (Fig. 4A) and unmyelinated (Fig. 4B) nerve fibers appeared to be intact. A neuromuscular junction was noted opportunistically in a FCMD muscle biopsy specimen and it also appeared to be normal, although the fiber type of an adjacent myofiber is unknown (Fig. 5A,B).

The freeze fracture technique enables us to observe the molecular architecture of the hydrophobic interior of the muscle plasma membrane of a FCMD myofiber. The split line of freeze fracture proceeds into the hydrophobic interior of the membrane and yields two leaflets, the protoplasmic (P) face and the extracellular (E) face. A low power electron micrograph of a fractured normal muscle plasma membrane showed the outline of a sarcomeric structure, and caveolae were universally distributed throughout the plasma membrane, being a little bit denser in the I band area (Fig. 6). Caveolae involve not only pinocytosis and exocytosis but also opening of the T-tubules. The results of statistical analysis of caveolar density between control and FCMD specimens was not significant (Table 1). A higher power magnification electron micrograph of a control membrane P face demonstrated a uniform distribution of individual intramembranous particles and orthogonal arrays composed of more than 4 subunit smaller particles (Fig. 7). A control membrane E face shows less numerous individual intramembranous particles and pits of orthogonal arrays (Fig. 8).

A higher magnification electron micrograph of a FCMD membrane P face revealed the marked depletion of orthogonal arrays, and decreases of intramembranous particles and orthogonal array subunit particles (Fig. 9). The decrease of intramembranous particles and depletion of pits of orthogonal arrays were also noted for a FCMD E face (Fig. 10). The

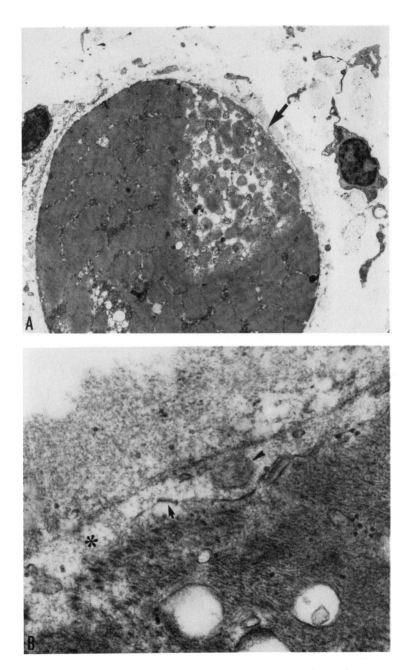

Fig. 1. (A) A low magnification electron micrograph shows the presence of a so-called δ lesion (arrow) in a Fu-kuyama congenital muscular dystrophy (FCMD) myofiber. The δ lesion contains rarefied myofilaments, mito-chondria and vesicular structures. (×6600). (B) A higher power view of the indicated (arrow) area in (A). The plasma membrane disclosed the presence of discontinuity (asterisk) and has a rarefied plasmalemmal undercoat (arrow). The separation of the muscle plasma membrane from the basal lamina can also be observed, and degener-ating cell debris (arrow head) can be seen in the space between them. (×82 500).

216

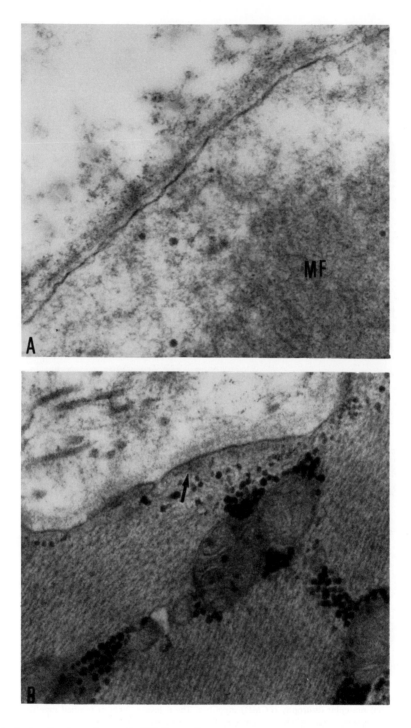

Fig. 2. Again the plasma membrane of a FCMD myofiber (A) contains a rarefied plasmalemmal undercoat; while a normal human myofiber (B) contains a dense plasmalemmal undercoat (arrow), and the plasma membrane and basal lamina are closely associated. (×82 500).

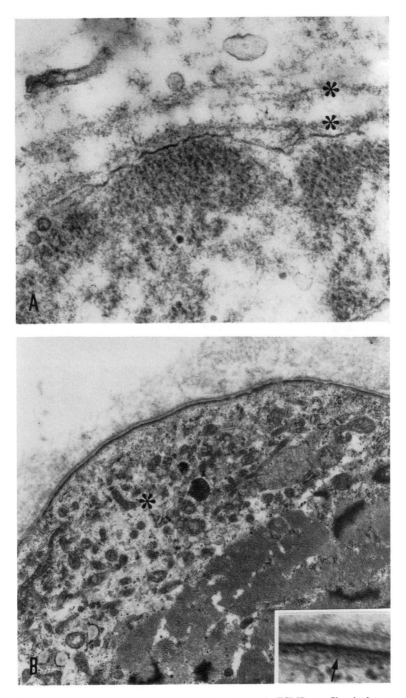

Fig. 3. (A) The situation of the plasma membrane and its undercoat in FCMD myofiber is the same as that in previous pictures, however, the basal lamina of this FCMD myofiber is duplicated (asterisks). (×82 500). (B) The plasma membrane of a regenerating FCMD myofiber covers the peripheral cytoplasm (asterisk) and contains a dense plasmalemmal undercoat, which is indicated by an arrow in the inset. (×16 500; inset ×82 500).

218

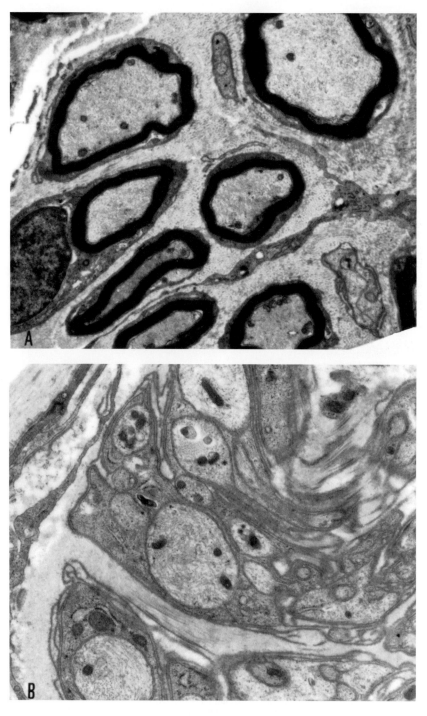

Fig. 4. Intramuscular myelinated (A) and unmyelinated (B) FCMD nerve fibers appear to be normal. ((A) ×8300; (B) ×16 500).

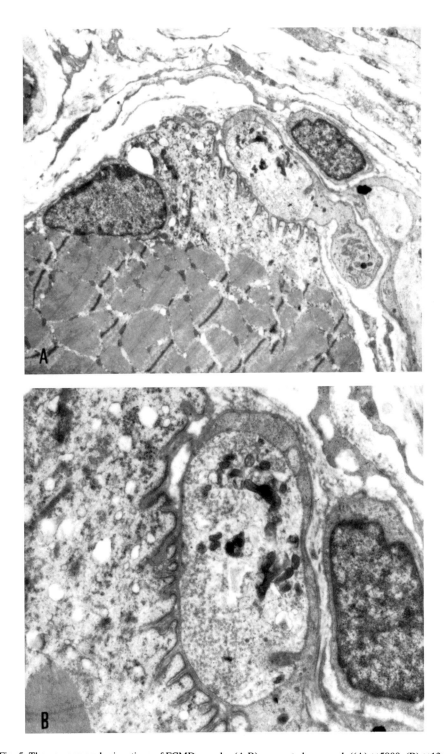

Fig. 5. The neuromuscular junctions of FCMD muscles (A,B) appear to be normal. ((A) ×5800; (B) ×13 200).

220

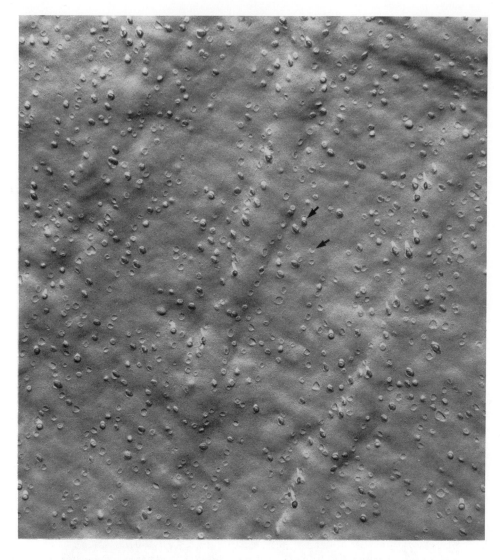

Fig. 6. A lower power electron micrograph of a freeze fractured normal human myofiber plasma membrane shows the sarcomere outline and the presence of numerous caveolae (arrows), which tend to exist more in the I band area. (×23 700).

results of statistical analysis are presented in Tables 2 and 3. In addition, the orthogonal array subunit particle density was 11.7 ± 0.7 (group mean $\pm$ SE) and 20.4 ± 0.3 in the FCMD and control groups, respectively. The decrease in the subunit number was significant ($P < 0.001$, two-tailed t-test).

Digitonin forms cholesterol-digitonin complexes inside the muscle plasma membrane and the cholesterol-digitonin complexes are observed as rod-like structure in higher magnification electron micrographs (Fig. 11). The percentage of plasma membrane area with the complexes expressed as the group mean percentage $\pm$ standard error of the mean was $52.1 \pm 4.7\%$ and $31.9 \pm 2.9\%$ in the FCMD and control groups, respectively, and a statisti-

Table 1

Caveolae density per μm^2 of normal and Fukuyama- type congenital muscular dystrophy (FCMD) muscle plasma membranes

Case[a]	Normal	FCMD
1	18.35 ± 5.19[b]	19.76 ± 6.23[b]
2	15.25 ± 3.23	16.42 ± 7.36
3	18.17 ± 3.74	19.77 ± 5.88
4	21.32 ± 2.91	15.55 ± 5.59
5	23.11 ± 7.48	23.44 ± 5.31
6	12.46 ± 1.67	20.54 ± 8.01
Mean	18.11 ± 1.59[c,d]	19.25 ± 1.18[c,d]

[a]Case no. of respective condition.
[b]Mean ± standard deviation for each case.
[c]Group mean ± standard error of the mean.
[d]$P > 0.5$ (two-tailed t-test).

cally significant increase of cholesterol in the FCMD myofiber plasma membrane was observed ($P < 0.01$, two-tailed t-test). The overall features on freeze fracture analyses in human muscular dystrophies are summarized in Table 4.

Discussion

The pattern of inheritance of FCMD is autosomal recessive and the gene for FCMD has recently been localized to 9q31-33 [16], but the gene product of FCMD remains unknown. The disease frequency is estimated to be 6.9–11.9:100 000 [14], which is about half that of X-linked recessive Duchenne muscular dystrophy (DMD), in which the defective gene product is a 427 kDa protein called "dystrophin" [17]. Dystrophin comprises the membrane cytoskeleton present just inside the muscle plasma membrane [18–39]. The δ lesion was first described in degenerating muscle fibers in boys with DMD by Mokri and Engel [7], who pointed out disruption of the muscle plasmalemma overlaying the δ lesions. Subsequently, but almost simultaneously, Schmalbruch [8] reported a similar finding in DMD muscles, and we even observed the finding in the myofiber plasma membranes of asymptomatic preclinical boys [9]. In these reports, electron micrographs, depicting the situation of muscle plasma membranes and related structures, revealed more or less the rarefied muscle plasmalemmal undercoat, although this finding was not pointed out by the authors. We reexamined ultrastructurally the muscle plasmalemmal undercoat of degenerating myofibers in DMD and found a rarefied plasmalemmal undercoat as well (Murahashi et al., manuscript in preparation). However, the plasmalemmal undercoats of normal looking DMD myofibers appeared to be intact, this situation being similar to that observed in FCMD in this study. Therefore, the rarefied muscle plasma membrane undercoat observed in FCMD myofibers is a non-specific and secondary phenomenon, although dystrophin in FCMD myofibers is expressed irregularly [40].

The dense plasma membrane undercoat seen in regenerating myofibers in FCMD may imply the enhanced synthesis of a membrane cytoskeleton composed of the plasmalemmal undercoat, and the increased content of utrophin [41,42] may contribute to this dense plasmalemmal undercoat in regenerating myofibers.

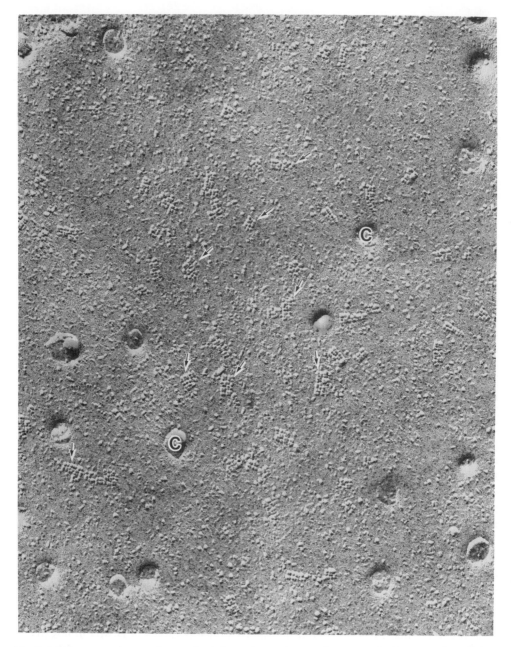

Fig. 7. A higher power electron micrograph of a freeze fractured normal human muscle plasma membrane P face reveals the presence of individual intramembranous particles, many orthogonal arrays (arrows), and caveolae (c). (×160 000).

Freeze fracture replica images of FCMD myofiber plasma membranes showed significant decreases of intramembranous particles and orthogonal arrays, and an increased content of membrane cholesterol. Of special interest is the remarkable decrease in orthogonal arrays

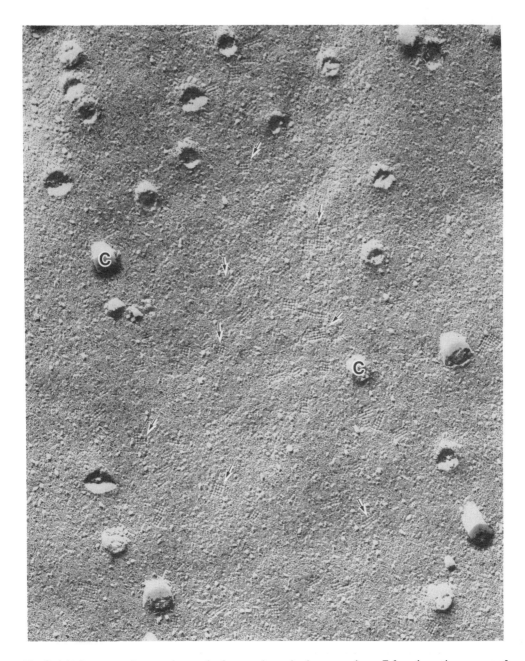

Fig. 8. A higher power electron micrograph of a normal muscle plasma membrane E face shows the presence of individual intramembranous particles, numerous pits of orthogonal arrays (arrows), and caveolae (c). (×160 000).

[4]. These findings were very similar to those in DMD membranes [10], except for the caveolae density. We examined the molecular architecture of the muscle plasma membrane in DMD [10,13], Becker muscular dystrophy (BMD) [43], FCMD [4–6], facioscapulo-

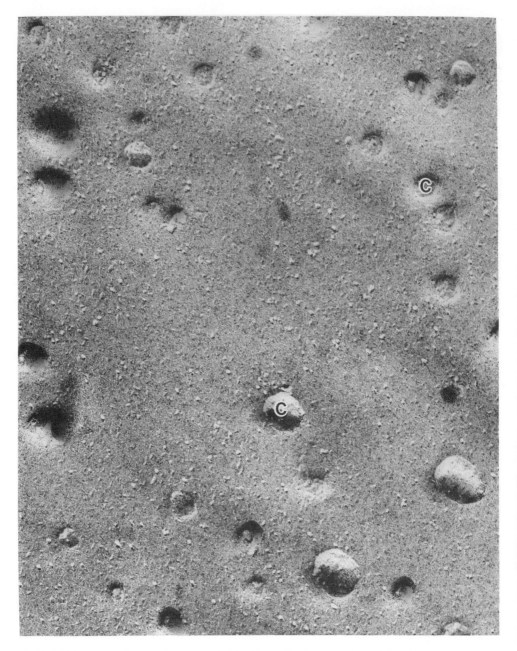

Fig. 9. A higher power electron micrograph of a FCMD muscle plasma membrane P face demonstrates the decreased number of individual intramembranous particles and the markedly decreased orthogonal arrays. In the field, no orthogonal arrays are evident. c, caveolae. (×160 000).

humeral muscular dystrophy (FSH) [10], and myotonic dystrophy [10]. The results are summarized in Table 4. In addition, in the MDX mouse, the animal model of dystrophin deficiency, the muscle plasma membrane exhibited similar findings to those in FCMD and

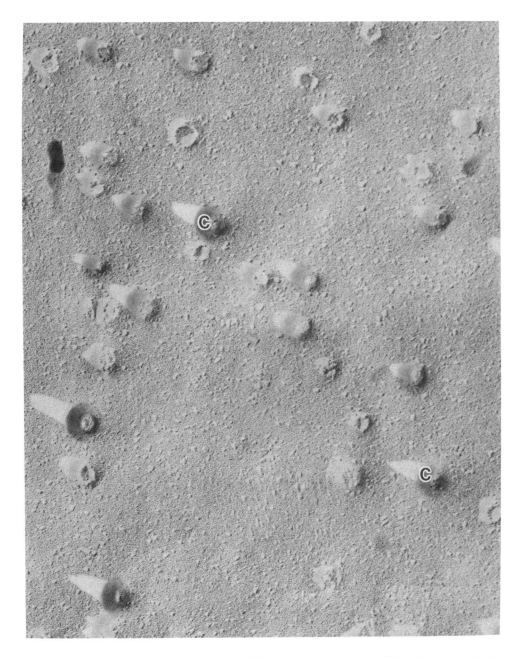

Fig. 10. A higher power electron micrograph of a FCMD muscle plasma membrane E face demonstrates the decrease of intramembranous particles, especially the pits of orthogonal arrays. In the field, no pits of orthogonal arrays are evident. c, caveolae. (×160 000).

DMD, although the depletion of intramembranous particles (IMP) and orthogonal arrays was not as severe as in FCMD and DMD [44,45].

Table 2

Particle density per μm^2 of normal and Fukuyama-type congenital muscular dystrophy (FCMD) muscle plasma membranes

Case	Normal			FCMD		
	P face[a]	P face[b]	E face	P face[a]	P face[b]	E face
1	2178 ± 285[c]	2826 ± 333[c]	798 ± 246[c]	1483 ± 363[c]	1534 ± 399[c]	950 ± 124[c]
2	1517 ± 336	2186 ± 212	834 ± 156	1238 ± 357	1271 ± 326	730 ± 169
3	2095 ± 123	2980 ± 488	1049 ± 222	1721 ± 381	1760 ± 394	726 ± 141
4	1916 + 359	2367 ± 492	881 ± 75	1342 ± 326	1360 ± 329	559 ± 176
5	1782 ± 354	2583 ± 651	945 ± 166	1270 ± 234	1270 ± 234	704 ± 164
6	1895 ± 415	2626 ± 308	800 ± 157	1465 ± 630	1490 ± 640	678 ± 156
Mean	1897 ± 96*,d	2595 ± 119**,d	885 ± 40***,d	1420 ± 73*,d	1448 ± 77**,d	725 ± 52***,d

[a]Excluding subunit particles of orthogonal arrays.
[b]Including subunit particles of orthogonal arrays.
[c]Mean ± standard deviation for each case.
[d]Group mean ± standard error of the mean.
*$P < 0.01$ (two-tailed t-test).
**$P < 0.001$ (two-tailed t-test).
***$P < 0.05$ (two-tailed t-test).

The intramuscular nerve fibers and neuromuscular junctions of FCMD muscles appeared to be normal, but this finding is not definite or final, because only small numbers of these structures were examined in this study. However, this does not necessarily rule out a functional defect of motor nerve fibers, although this finding is consistent with the results of a histochemical study of FCMD muscles [46]. But the neuromuscular junction structure differs in different fiber types, and the type 2 fiber junction has more complex secondary synaptic clefts [47], so more work is needed to draw a conclusion. Even if these structures are intact, we cannot exclude the defective functional influence of nerves on the myofiber macromolecular organization. In fact, denervated muscle plasma membranes exhibited similar freeze fracture findings to FCMD and DMD membranes [48].

Recently, dystrophin-associated glycoproteins (DAGs) were identified, and 156 and 43 kDa DAGs have been cloned and their sequences determined [49]. The proteins were derived from the same 97 kDa precursor protein, which yielded the two DAGs through posttranslational modifications. The 156 kDa DAG is an extracellular protein that binds to laminin [49], and the 43 kDa DAG has a transmembranous and cytoplasmic domain which links directly to dystrophin [50–53]. SCARMD is the severe autosomal recessive muscular

Table 3

Orthogonal array density per square micron of normal and Fukuyama- type congenital muscular dystrophy (FCMD) muscle plasma membranes

	Median	Midrange (25–75%)
Normal (6)	13.52*	6.46–19.83
FCMD (6)	0.54*	0–1.10

*$P < 0.001$ (Wilcoxon rank sum test). The numbers in parentheses represent the number of cases in each group.

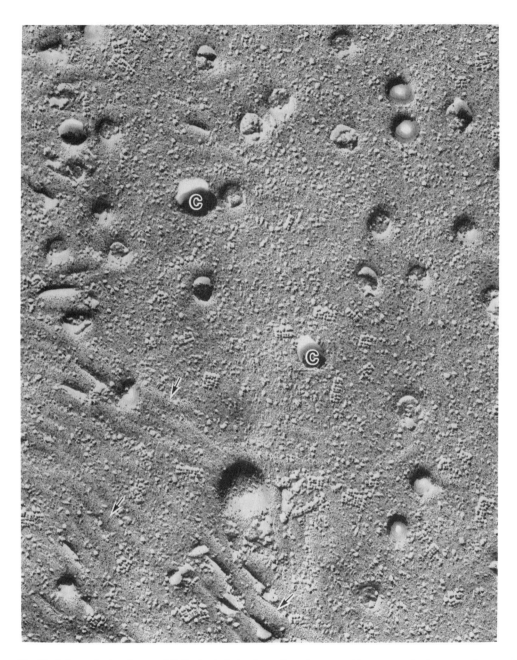

Fig. 11. A freeze fracture image of digitonin-cholesterol complexes in a normal human muscle plasma membrane. The complexes can be seen as rod like structures (arrows). c, caveolae. (×160 000).

dystrophy prevalent in Africa, in which the 50 kDa DAG is reported to be deficient [54]. Merosin has been very recently found to be deficient in another animal model, *dy/dy* mouse [55,56], and found to be abnormal in congenital muscular dystrophy [57]. Therefore, whatever point(s) in these molecular complexes from cytoplasmic dystrophin through muscle

228

Table 4
Summary of freeze fracture analyses of muscle plasma membranes in human muscular dystrophies

	Caveolae	IMP–OASP	IMP+OASP	OA	OASP	Cholesterol
Fukuyama dystrophy	→	↓	↓↓	↓↓↓	↓	↑
Duchenne dystrophy	↑	↓	↓↓	↓↓↓	↓	↑
Becker dystrophy	↑	→	→	↓↓	↓	
FSH dystrophy	→	→	→	↓		
Myotonic dystrophy	→	→	→	→		

IMP, intramembranous particles; OA, orthogonal arrays; OASP, orthogonal array subunit particles; FSH dystrophy, facioscapulohumeral dystrophy.

plasmalemma to extracellular laminin are defective, the dystrophic muscle feature and dystrophic phenotype will appear. Therefore, it is possible that the FCMD gene products are included in these macromolecular complexes present in and around the muscle plasma membrane.

Acknowledgments

The authors wish to thank Mrs. U. Suzuki for her skillful technical assistance and Mrs. T. Mitani for typing the manuscript.

References

1. Fukuyama Y, Kawazura M, Haruna H. A peculiar form of congenital progressive muscular dystrophy. Report of fifteen cases. Paediatria Universitatis Tokyo (Tokyo) 1960; 4: 5–8.
2. Fukuyama Y, Osawa M, Suzuki H. Congenital muscular dystrophy of the Fukuyama type – clinical, genetic and pathological considerations. Brain Dev (Tokyo) 1981; 3: 1–29.
3. Misugi N. Light and electron microscopic studies of congenital muscular dystrophy. Brain Dev (Tokyo) 1980; 2: 191–199.
4. Wakayama Y, Kumagai T, Shibuya S. Freeze fracture studies of muscle plasma membrane in Fukuyama type congenital muscular dystrophy. Neurology 1985; 35: 1587–1593.
5. Wakayama Y, Kumagai T, Jimi T. Small size of orthogonal array in muscle plasma membrane of Fukuyama type congenital muscular dystrophy. Acta Neuropathol 1986; 72: 130–133.
6. Wakayama Y, Kumagai T, Jimi T, Shibuya S. Freeze fracture analysis of cholesterol in muscle plasma membrane of Fukuyama type congenital muscular dystrophy. Acta Neuropathol 1987; 75: 46–50.
7. Mokri B, Engel AG. Duchenne dystrophy: electron microscopic findings pointing to a basic or early abnormality in the plasma membrane of the muscle fiber. Neurology 1975; 25: 1111–1120.
8. Schmalbruch H. Segmental fibre breakdown and defects of the plasma-lemma in diseased human muscles. Acta Neuropathol 1975; 33: 129–141.
9. Wakayama Y, Bonilla E, Schotland DL. Muscle plasma membrane abnormalities in the early stages of Duchenne muscular dystrophy. Neurology 1983; 33: 1368–1370.
10. Schotland DL, Bonilla E, Wakayama Y. Freeze fracture studies of muscle plasma membrane in human muscular dystrophy. Acta Neuropathol 1981; 54: 189–197.
11. Bonilla E, Fischbeck K, Schotland DL. Freeze-fracture studies of muscle caveolae in human muscular dystrophy. Am J Pathol 1981; 104: 167–173.
12. Fischbeck KH, Bonilla E, Schotland DL. Freeze-fracture analysis of plasma membrane cholesterol in Duchenne muscle. Ann Neurol 1983; 13: 532–535.

13. Wakayama Y, Okayasu H, Shibuya S, Kumagai T. Duchenne dystrophy: reduced density of orthogonal array subunit particles in the muscle plasma membrane. Neurology 1984; 34: 1313–1317.

14. Osawa M. A genetical and epidemiological study on congenital progressive muscular dystrophy (Fukuyama type) (in Japanese). Tokyo Joshi Ikadaigaku Zasshi (Tokyo) 1978; 48: 112–149.

15. Nonaka I, Chou SM. Congenital muscular dystrophy. In: Vinken PJ, Bruyn GW, eds. Handbook of clinical neurology, Vol 41. Diseases of muscle. Amsterdam: North-Holland, 1979: 27–50.

16. Toda T, Segawa M, Nomura Y, et al. Localization of a gene for Fukuyama type congenital muscular dystrophy to chromosome 9q31-33. Nat Genet 1993; 5: 283–286.

17. Hoffman EP, Brown RH Jr, Kunkel LM. Dystrophin: the protein product of the Duchenne muscular dystrophy locus. Cell 1987; 51: 919–928.

18. Arahata K, Ishiura S, Ishiguro T, et al. Immunostaining of skeletal and cardiac muscle surface membrane with antibody against Duchenne muscular dystrophy peptide. Nature 1988; 333: 861–863.

19. Bonilla E, Samitt CE, Miranda AF, et al. Duchenne muscular dystrophy: deficiency of dystrophin at the muscle cell surface. Cell 1988; 54: 447–452.

20. Koenig M, Monaco AP, Kunkel LM. The complete sequence of dystrophin predicts a rod-shaped cytoskeletal protein. Cell 1988; 53: 219–228.

21. Miranda AF, Bonilla E, Martucci G, Moraes CT, Hays AP, DiMauro S. Immunocytochemical study of dystrophin in muscle cultures from patients with Duchenne muscular dystrophy and unaffected control patients. Am J Pathol 1988; 132: 410–416.

22. Zubrzycka-Gaarn EE, Bulman DE, Karpati G, et al. The Duchenne muscular dystrophy gene product is localized in sarcolemma of human skeletal muscle. Nature 1988; 333: 466–469.

23. Watkins SC, Hoffman EP, Slayter HS, Kunkel LM. Immunoelectron microscopic localization of dystrophin in myofibres. Nature 1988; 333: 863–866.

24. Shimizu T, Matsumura K, Hashimoto K, et al. A monoclonal antibody against a synthetic polypeptide fragment of dystrophin (amino acid sequence from position 215 to 264). Proc Jpn Acad (Tokyo) 1988; 64B: 205–208.

25. Hoffman EP, Kunkel LM. Dystrophin abnormalities in Duchenne/Becker muscular dystrophy. Neuron 1989; 2: 1019–1029.

26. Miike T, Miyatake M, Zhao J, Yoshioka K, Uchino M. Immunohisto-chemical dystrophin reaction in synaptic regions. Brain Dev (Tokyo) 1989; 11: 344–346.

27. Cullen MJ, Walsh J, Nicholson LVB, Harris JB. Ultrastructural localization of dystrophin in human muscle by using gold immunolabelling. Proc R Soc London (Biol) 1990; 240: 197–210.

28. Uchino M, Araki S, Miike T, Teramoto H, Nakamura T, Yasutake T. Localization and characterization of dystrophin in muscle biopsy specimens from Duchenne muscular dystrophy and various neuromuscular disorders. Muscle Nerve 1989; 12: 1009–1016.

29. Wakayama Y, Jimi T, Misugi N, et al. Dystrophin immunostaining and freeze-fracture studies of muscles of patients with early stage amyotrophic lateral sclerosis and Duchenne muscular dystrophy. J Neurol Sci 1989; 91: 191–205.

30. Wakayama Y, Jimi T, Takeda A, et al. Immunoreactivity of antibodies raised against synthetic peptide fragments predicted from mid portions of dystrophin cDNA. J Neurol Sci 1990; 97: 241–250.

31. Samitt CE, Bonilla E. Immunocytochemical study of dystrophin at the myotendinous junction. Muscle Nerve 1990; 13: 493–500.

32. Wakayama Y, Shibuya S. Observations on the muscle plasma membrane-associated cytoskeletons of mdx mice by quick-freeze, deep-etch, rotary-shadow replica method. Acta Neuropathol 1990; 80: 618–623.

33. Byers TJ, Kunkel LM, Watkins SC. The subcellular distribution of dystrophin in mouse skeletal, cardiac, and smooth muscle. J Cell Biol 1991; 115: 411–421.

34. Wakayama Y, Shibuya S. Antibody-decorated dystrophin molecule of murine skeletal myofiber as seen by freeze-etching electron microscopy. J Electron Microsc 1991; 40: 143–145.

35. Wakayama Y, Shibuya S. Gold-labelled dystrophin molecule in muscle plasmalemma of mdx control mice as seen by electron microscopy of deep etching replica. Acta Neuropathol 1991; 82: 178–184.

36. Masuda, T, Fujimaki N, Ozawa E, Ishikawa H. Confocal laser microscopy of dystrophin localization in guinea pig skeletal muscle fibers. J Cell Biol 1992; 119: 543–548.

37. Minetti C, Beltrame F, Marcenaro G, Bonilla E. Dystrophin at the plasma membrane of human muscle fibers shows a costameric localization. Neuromusc Disord 1992; 2: 99–109.

38. Porter GA, Dmytrenko GM, Winkelmann JC, Bloch RJ. Dystrophin colocalizes with δ spectrin in distinct subsarcolemmal domains in mammalian skeletal muscle. J Cell Biol 1992; 117: 997–1005.

39. Straub V, Bittner RE, Leger JJ, Voit T. Direct visualization of dystrophin network on skeletal muscle fiber membrane. J Cell Biol 1992; 119: 1183–1191.

40. Arikawa E, Ishihara T, Nonaka I, Sugita H, Arahata K. Immunocytochemical analysis of dystrophin in congenital muscular dystrophy. J Neurol Sci 1991; 105: 79–87.

41. Karpati G, Carpenter S, Morris GE, Davies KE, Guerin C, Holland P. Localization and quantitation of the chromosome 6-encoded dystrophin-related protein in normal and pathological human muscle. J Neuropathol Exp Neurol 1993; 52: 119–128.

42. Mizuno Y, Nonaka I, Hirai S, Ozawa E. Reciprocal expression of dystrophin and utrophin in muscles of Duchenne muscular dystrophy patients, female DMD-carriers and control subjects. J Neurol Sci 1993; 119: 43–52.

43. Shibuya S, Wakayama Y, Jimi T, et al. Freeze fracture analysis of muscle plasma membrane in Becker's muscular dystrophy. Neuropathol Appl Neurobiol 1994; 20: 487–494.

44. Shibuya S, Wakayama Y. Freeze-fracture studies of myofiber plasma membrane in X chromosome-linked muscular dystrophy (mdx) mice. Acta Neuropathol 1988; 76: 179–184.

45. Shibuya S, Wakayama Y. Changes in muscle plasma membranes in young mice with X chromosome-linked muscular dystrophy: a freeze-fracture study. Neuropathol Appl Neurobiol 1991; 17: 335–344.

46. Nonaka I, Sugita H, Tanaka K, Kumagai K. Muscle histochemistry in congenital muscular dystrophy with central nervous system involvement. Muscle Nerve 1982; 5: 102–106.

47. Santa T, Engel AG. Histometric analysis of neuromuscular junction ultrastructure in rat red, white and intermediate muscle fibers. In: Desmedt JE, ed. New developments of electromyography and clinical neurophysiology, Vol 1. Basel: Karger, 1973: 41–54.

48. Jimi T, Wakayama Y. Effect of denervation on regenerating muscle plasma membrane integrity: freeze fracture and dystrophin immuno-staining analysis. Acta Neuropathol 1990; 80: 401–405.

49. Ibraghimov-Beskrovnaya O, Ervasti JM, Leveille CJ, Slaughter CA, Sernett SW, Campbell KP. Primary structure of dystrophin-associated glycoproteins linking dystrophin to the extracellular matrix. Nature 1992; 355: 696–702.

50. Suzuki A, Yoshida M, Yamamoto H, Ozawa E. Glycoprotein-binding site of dystrophin is confined to the cysteine-rich domain and the first half of the carboxy-terminal domain. FEBS Lett 1992; 308: 154–160.

51. Suzuki A, Yoshida M, Hayashi K, Mizuno Y, Hagiwara Y, Ozawa E. Molecular organization at the glycoprotein-complex-binding site of dystrophin. Three dystrophin-associated proteins bind directly to the carboxy-terminal portion of dystrophin. Eur J Biochem 1994; 220: 283–292.

52. Wakayama Y, Jimi T, Takeda A, Shibuya S, Nakamura Y, Oniki H. Immunoelectron microscopic localization of C-terminus of 43 kDa dystrophin associated glycoprotein in normal human skeletal myofibers. J Electron Microsc, in press.

53. Wakayama Y, Shibuya S, Takeda A, Jimi T, Nakamura Y, Oniki H. Ultrastructural localization of C-terminus of 43 kDa dystrophin associated glycoprotein, and its relation to dystrophin in normal murine skeletal myofiber. Am J Pathol, in press.

54. Matsumura K, Tomé FMS, Collin H, et al. Deficiency of the 50 k dystrophin-associated glycoprotein in severe childhood autosomal recessive muscular dystrophy. Nature 1992; 359: 320–322.

55. Arahata K, Hayashi YK, Koga R, et al. Laminin in animal models for muscular dystrophy defect of laminin M in skeletal and cardiac muscles and peripheral nerve of the homozygous dystrophic dy/dy mice. Proc Jpn Acad (Tokyo) 1993; 69B: 259–264.

56. Sunada Y, Bernier SM, Koazak CA, Yamada Y, Campbell KP. Deficiency of merosin in dystrophic dy mice and genetic linkage of laminin M chain gene to dy locus. J Biol Chem 1994; 269: 13729–13732.

57. Hayashi YK, Engvall E, Arikawa-Hirasawa E, et al. Abnormal localization of laminin subunits in muscular dystrophies. J Neurol Sci 1993; 119: 53–64.

Y. Fukuyama, M. Osawa and K. Saito (Eds.), *Congenital Muscular Dystrophies*

Walker–Warburg syndrome in Japan: a comparative study with Fukuyama type congenital muscular dystrophy

SEIJI KIMURA[1], YOSHIROU SASAKI[2], SHOTA MIYAKE[3],
NOBUKO MISUGI[2], TAKUYA KOBAYASHI[1,2],
ETSUKO YAMAGUCHI[4] and TAKASHI HAYASHI[4]

[1]*Department of Pediatrics, Urafune Hospital of Yokohama City University, Yokohama, Japan*
[2]*Division of Pathology, Kanagawa Children's Medical Center, Yokohama, Japan*
[3]*Division of Neurology, Kanagawa Children's Medical Center, Yokohama, Japan*
[4]*Department of Pediatrics, Yamaguchi University, Ube, Yamaguchi, Japan*

Introduction

Walker–Warburg syndrome (WWS), a syndrome of type II lissencephaly with hydrocephalus, cerebellar hypoplasia and eye abnormalities, is synonymous with Walker's lissencephaly [1] or Warburg's syndrome [2], in which muscular lesions have recently been recognized [3]. Other terms, such as cerebro-oculo-muscular syndrome [4], cerebro-ocular dysplasia muscular dystrophy syndrome [5], and HARD±E [6] have also been used to describe the condition in patients having congenital muscular dystrophy (CMD) accompanied by central nervous system (CNS) and ocular dysplasias. However, we think these syndromes are forms of WWS, as mentioned previously [7].

Fukuyama type congenital muscular dystrophy (FCMD), first described by Fukuyama et al. in 1960 [8], is a definite disease entity of CMD accompanied by CNS involvement. FCMD is common in Japan, the relative prevalence ratio of FCMD to Duchenne muscular dystrophy being 1:2.1 [9]. Recently, the location of the gene for FCMD was discovered on chromosome 9q [10].

Despite the progress in the genetical analysis of CMD, the classification of CMD is not yet clear, and it is still a matter of discussion whether WWS and FCMD belong to the same category or not. The main reason for this is thought to be that comparative studies have been very few [11,12] because WWS is very rare in Japan and FCMD is extremely rare outside Japan. In Japan, only 6 patients with WWS have been reported [13–18] until now. In this study, we analyze the clinical and neuropathological findings in the 6 Japanese WWS patients in comparison with those in FCMD patients.

Materials and methods

Six previously reported Japanese patients with WWS [13–18], 3 of whom were our own cases and the other 3 from the literature, were analyzed. The CNS of all 6 patients showed lissencephaly, congenital hydrocephalus and severe cerebellar dysplasia, with severe eye lesions. The muscle pathology in all patients was consistent with muscular dystrophy. The results for these 6 patients were compared with those for our 11 FCMD patients, who had been examined either on autopsy or by MRI.

Clinical findings

The clinical outline is summarized in Table 1. The male/female ratio was 3:3. All were full term infants. One of the 6 was of low birth weight, and 1 was relatively large for age. Each patient had a large head, severe muscle weakness and eye lesions that were recognized just at or soon after birth. The large head was due to obstructive hydrocephalus, and 3 of the 6 patients had undergone ventriculo-peritoneal shunt. The other 3 patients did not have the shunt operation because of their poor general condition. The muscle weakness was very severe. All patients had difficulty in swallowing and 4 of the 6 showed respiratory distress in the neonatal period. The eye lesions were variable. All had cataracts but no information on the optic fundus in 2 of the patients was available. Microphthalmia and buphthalmos were seen in 2 and 1 patient(s), respectively. Retinal dysplasia or detachment was seen in 3. The other abnormalities were chorioretinitis, an albino-like pale retina, a persistent pupillary membrane artery and glaucoma. Multiple joint contractures were seen in 4. Five out of 5 had minor anomalies, such as a high-arched palate, low set ears, a small jaw, retentio testes, a small penis and an abnormal palpable fissure. Convulsions were also seen in these 5. All had severely abnormal electroencephalograms (EEG) showing markedly slow dysryhthmic basic activity with multifocal spikes. The age at death ranged from 25 days to 9 months. One patient was still alive at 23 months. The CK levels were more than 10 times higher than the upper normal limit (Table 1). All exhibited abnormal electromyography with a myogenic pattern.

On the contrary, the clinical findings in FCMD (Table 2) were much milder than those in WWS. The age at death of the youngest patient, having a large porencephalic cyst in the right hemisphere, was 2 years, at which time he had disseminated intravascular coagulation followed by intracranial hemorrhage. The maximal motor development varied from no head fixation to walking alone. Maximum speech ability also varied, from no meaningful words to simple conversations.

Muscle pathology

Muscle tissue specimens obtained from multiple sites in each patient at biopsy and/or autopsy showed similar findings consistent with muscular dystrophy. A biopsied specimen from the femoral muscle (Patient 2, Fig. 1a), showed fiber size variation, opaque fibers, central nuclei, and an increase in connective tissue. Focal perivascular lymphocyte infiltrations was sporadically seen in this patient (Fig. 1b). This patient had a high serum IgM value at birth. The muscle pathology at autopsy of Patient 3 showed more prominent fiber size variation and further increased connective tissue (Fig. 1c). These findings were similar to those in FCMD.

Magnetic resonance imaging (MRI) of the brain

Brain MRI is very useful for diagnosing WWS. Only one patient (Patient 6) diagnosed by means of MRI had been reported in Japan. This 12-day-old male patient showed typical findings of WWS (Fig. 2); diffuse agyria, hydrocephalus with agenesis of the septum pellu-

Table 1

Clinical summary of 6 Japanese patients with Walker–Warburg syndrome

	Patient [Ref.]					
	(1) [13]	(2) [14]	(3) [17]	(4) [15]	(5) [16]	(6) [18]
Sex	Male	Female	Male	Female	Male	Male
Gest./BW[a]	40 weeks / 3280 g	42 weeks / 2490 g	40 weeks / 2500 g	40 weeks / 2900 g	Full / 4004 g	Full / 3500 g
Perinatal	Respiratory distress (patients (1)–(4))					
	Poor sucking in all 6 patients					
Onset/muscle power	Severe muscle weakness appeared just/soon after birth in all 6 patients					
Head	Large head due to obstructive hydrocephalus (patients (2)–(6))					
Eye lesions	Cataracts[b]	Cataracts	Cataracts	Cataracts[b]	Cataracts	Cataracts
		Chorioretinitis	Albino-like retina	Microphthalmia	Buphthalmos	Microphthalmia
		Retinal detachment	Optic nerve atrophy	Retinal dysplasia	Retinal dysplasia	
		Glaucoma		Retinal detachment	Retinal detachment	
		Optic nerve atrophy			Optic nerve atrophy	
Joint contracture	Multiple	Multiple	Multiple	?	Multiple	No
Minor anomaly	High-arched palate	Double uteri	Small jaws	?	Palpable fissure ab.	Small penis
	Retentio testes	Small jaw	Low set ears			Retentio testes
		High-arched palate	High-arched palate			
		Low set ears				
Convulsion	Present	Present	Present	Present	?	Present
Age at death	9 months	3 months	25 days	Alive (23 months)	?	5 months
Serum CK	248 IU	300 mg/dl (<4)	1785 IU/l	3000 U/l	2645 IU/l (<170)	5484 U (<260)

[a]Gest., gestational period; BW, body weight.
[b]Optic fundus was not examined. All patients have no family history.

Table 2

Clinical summary of our 11 patients with Fukuyama type congenital muscular dystrophy

	Patients										
	(1)[a]	(2)	(3)	(4)	(5)	(6)	(7)	(8)	(9)	(10)	(11)
Sex	Male	Male	Male	Male	Female	Female	Male	Female	Male	Female	Male
Age at death	2 years	8 years	14 years	15 years	21 years	27 years	Alive 2 years	Alive 2 years	Alive 3 years	Alive 4 years	Alive 12 years
Cause of death	DIC, ICH	Pulmonary hemorrhage	Chronic respiratory failure (patients (3)–(6))			CCF					
Family history	No	No	No	Sister[b]	Brother[b]	Sister[b]	No	No	No	No	No
Perinatal accident	No	No	No	Asphyxia	No	No	Asphyxia	Asphyxia	No	No	No
Max motor milestone	No head fix	Sit	Sit	Sit	Sit	Walk	No head fix (patients (7)–(10))				Sit
Meaningful words	None	Few	Few	Few	Many[c]	Many	No	No	No	No	Many[c]
Hydrocephalus	No	No	No	No	No	No	No	No	No	No	No
Eye lesion	No	No	No	No	No	Myopia	No	No	No	No	No

CCF, chronic cardiac failure; DIC, disseminated intravascular coagulation; ICH, intracranial hemorrhage.

[a]Patient 1 had porencephaly.

[b]Sister/brother of each patient was affected by Fukuyama type congenital muscular dystrophy (these patients were not included in this table).

[c]Can communicate verbally, though naively.

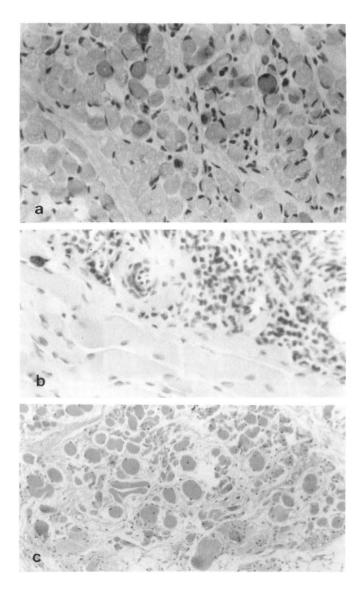

Fig. 1. Muscle pathology of WWS. A biopsied muscle specimen from Patient 2 shows fiber size variation, opaque fibers, central nuclei, and mild connective tissue increase ((a) ×640, frozen section, HE stain). Perivascular chronic inflammatory cell infiltrations can be sporadically seen ((b) Patient 2, ×1200, HE stain). Muscles at autopsy shows a marked increase in connective tissue ((c) Patient 3, ×640, paraffin embedded HE stain). Fig. 1b reproduced with permission from [12].

cidum and hypoplasia of the corpus callosum, a small dysplastic cerebellum and brain stem, and eye lesions. His left eyeball was small and its intraocular density was abnormal. These findings fulfill the diagnostic criteria of WWS. Band heterotopias and a large cystic lesion were also observed in this patient.

On the contrary, the general configuration of the FCMD brain was well preserved (Fig. 3), but the severity differed. In the most severely affected patient, there was mild ventricular dila-

236

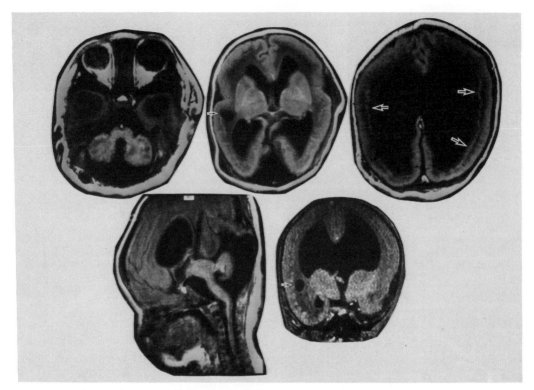

Fig. 2. MRI of WWS (Patient 6) shows diffuse agyria, hydrocephalus with agenesis of the septum pellcidum and hypoplasia of the corpus callosum, a small dysplastic cerebellum and brain stem, and eye lesions. The left eyeball is small and its intraocular density is abnormal. Band heterotopias (large arrows) and a large cystic lesion (small arrow) can also be observed in this patient. Reproduced with permission from [18].

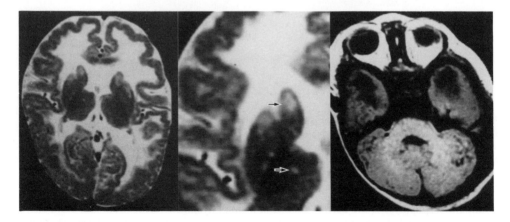

Fig. 3. MRI of FCMD. T2-weighted MRI of Patient 10 (8 months old) shows diffuse dysmyelination and abnormal cortical structures. Spotty lesions in the basal ganglia isointense to the white matter signal (arrows), which are thought to be aberrant cortico-spinal pathways, can be observed. Abnormal irregular intensities of the cortex indicates the structural abnormality. The cerebellum (T1-weighted image) exhibits multiple abnormal intensed lesions (focal polymicrogyria).

tation due to the hypoplastic brain. However, even in this patient, the cerebellum was not hypoplastic, and the corpus callosum and septum pellucidum looked normal. The most characteristic features were dysmyelination and abnormal cortical structures (Fig. 3). Pachygyric lesions were usually observed on computed tomographic or T1-weighted MR scanning, but actually the pachygyric lesions were proved to comprise micropolygyria on T2-weighted imaging. Abnormal small spotty lesions in the basal ganglia isointense to white matter, which were thought to be aberrant cortico-spinal pathways, were observed. The cortex in FCMD exhibited irregular nodular and/or linear abnormal intensities, which indicated an abnormal cortical structure. Irregular small nodular protrusions from the cortical surface were also present. The myelination observed on MRI was usually completed at around 3–4 years, although the process was irregular. The general configuration of the cerebellum in FCMD was normal, but there were focal nodular hetrotopic lesions. The brain MRI findings were quite different between WWS and FCMD.

Neuropathology

An autopsy was performed in 3 of the 6 patients with WWS. Two were our patients and the other was reported by Kasubuchi et al. [13]. Each showed quite similar pathology. In this paper, we describe the neuropathology of our 2 patients (Patients 2 and 3) with WWS and our 6 autopsied patients with FCMD (Table 2).

The leptomeninges of the WWS brain were thick and looked turbid. With regard to gross appearance, the WWS cerebrum had a diffuse smooth surface, although there were very small and shallow gyrations. The olfactory bulbs could not be identified in Patient 3. The cerebellum of each patient was severely dysplastic and had a coarse irregular nodular surface. The vermis was partially absent (Fig. 4). The Sylvian fissures were identified, but were shallow. A cut section showed hydrocephalus, the absence of a septum pellucidum, and marked hypoplasia of the corpus callosum. The basal ganglia were also hypoplastic (Fig. 5).

On the other hand, the general configuration of the FCMD brain was well preserved in all autopsied patients (Fig. 6), but exhibited diffuse or focal polymicrogyria, which was of somewhat different severity in each patient. Some had pachygyric lesions. The cerebellum was not hypoplastic. There was no evidence of obstructive hydrocephalus, septum pellucidum agenesis or corpus callosum hypogenesis.

The cut surface of the WWS brain showed a diffuse smooth surface with abnormal features of the temporal lobe. The cortico-medullary junction was very irregular. Many heterotopic nodules were present. In Patient 3, multicystic lesions were observed (Fig. 7a). On the other hand, some parts of the cortical surface of FCMD were very smooth, but the pachygyric lesions actually consisted of many fused microgyri (Fig. 7b). Thus, true pachygyria is thought to be rare in the FCMD brain.

On histological examination, the WWS brain was found to be covered with thickened leptomeninges, which was most extreme over the mesencephalon. The cytoarchitecture of the cerebral cortex was extremely disorganized in all areas. It showed no laminar neuronal differentiation, and individual neurons were oriented in abnormal directions, i.e. horizontally or invertedly. Frequently, the cortex was separated into irregular lobules by narrow strands of glial and connective tissue (Fig. 8). The white matter exhibited no myelination and the stroma was very loose (Fig. 9a). Numerous heterotopic neurons were seen in the white matter (Fig. 9b). The cortical histology of the FCMD brain was basically similar to that in WWS, however, the severity varied in each patient and in each cortical region. The arrangement of cortical cells was distorted. Myelinated fibers were occasionally seen on the cortical surface (Fig. 10a). Ir-

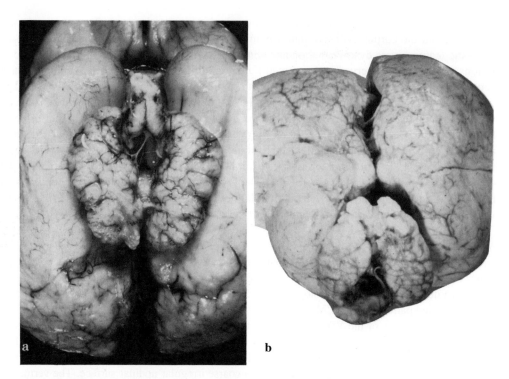

Fig. 4. WWS (Patients 2 and 3; right and left, respectively). The leptomeninges are very thick and turbid. In gross appearance, the surface is smooth all over the cerebrum, but there are very small and shallow gyrations. The olfactory bulb cannot be identified in Patient 3. The cerebellum of each patient is severely dysplastic and has a coarse irregular nodular surface. The vermis is partially absent. Fig. 4a reproduced with permission from [12] and Fig. 4b reproduced with permission from [17].

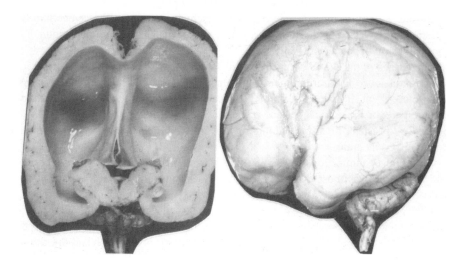

Fig. 5. WWS (Patient 3). The surface is smooth. The Sylvian fissure can be identified, but is very shallow. The cut section shows hydrocephalus, the absence of a septum pellucidum, and marked hypoplasia of the corpus callosum. The basal ganglia are also hypoplastic. Reproduced with permission from [12].

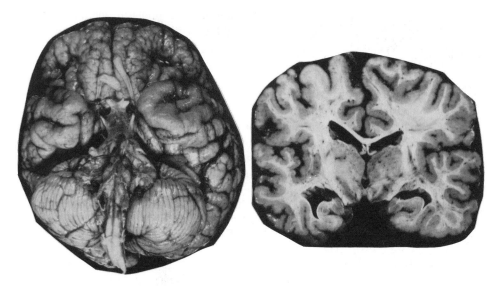

Fig. 6. The FCMD brain (left, Patient 3; right, Patient 4) shows a diffuse migration abnormality. Polymicrogyria is dominant in the frontal portion, and the temporal and occipital lobes look pachygyric. The cerebellum is not hypoplastic. The cut section shows a normal configuration with diffuse polymicrogyria. Reproduced with permission from [12].

regular masses of fused microgyri were frequently observed (Fig. 10b), which also proved that true pachygyria was rare in FCMD. In contrast to WWS, subcortical heterotopia was rarely seen.

The cerebellar cortex was diffusely disorganized in WWS. On the other hand, the FCMD cerebellum was well organized, but had some focal micropolygyria (Fig. 11). The cerebellar white matter in WWS was rather well organized compared to the cortex, however, the dentate nuclei were small and exhibited gliosis. The white matter of FCMD cerebellum showed no abnormality.

The mid brain, pons, medulla oblongata, and spinal cord in WWS were dysplastic. Meningeal gliomesenchymal overgrowth was marked. The pyramidal tract could not be identified in our 2 patients (Fig. 12). Diffuse gliosis was present. In FCMD, the general configurations of the brain stem and spinal cord were well preserved, and the pyramidal tracts could easily be identified. However, their pathways were usually aberrant and asymmetric (Fig. 13). Subependymal gliomesenchymal proliferations were also present, but were much less severe than those in WWS.

Peripheral nerve pathology
The peripheral nerves were examined in 1 patient with WWS, and 3 patients with FCMD. In FCMD, there was no remarkable finding. On the other hand, the peripheral nerves at multiple sites including intramuscular nerve fibers in the patient with WWS (Patient 3) were severely abnormal, although the nerve conduction velocity was normal. On light microscopy, bizarre myelin balls, sheaths consisting of loops and folds of compact myelin, and big naked axons were frequently observed. In some nerve fibers sectioned longitudinally, the segmental absence of myelination around thick axons was observed. Isolated loops or ovoids of myelin within the axoplasm of a nerve fiber were frequently seen (Fig. 14). On electron

240

microscopy, large naked axons, surrounded by Schwann cell cytoplasm, and tortuously proliferated myelin sheaths, which indented the axoplasm or protruded into the Schwann cell cytoplasm, were observed in every section. Coexistence of naked and myelinated axons in a single nerve fiber was also observed (Fig. 15). In one lesion, a Schwann cell had many myelin sheaths having no neurofilaments or microtubules inside, and in contrast, absence of myelination around normal axons were also observed (Fig. 16). The paranodal lesions and ones at the node of Ranvier were predominant (Fig. 17). Some myelin loops were evaginated and terminated abruptly within the Schwann cell cytoplasm, and did not surround axons. Some of them were seen as isolated ovoids of myelin in the Schwann cell cytoplasm. In longitudinal sections, the segmental absence of myelin was frequently observed. Neither myelinoclastic lesions nor onion bulb formation was observed in this patient.

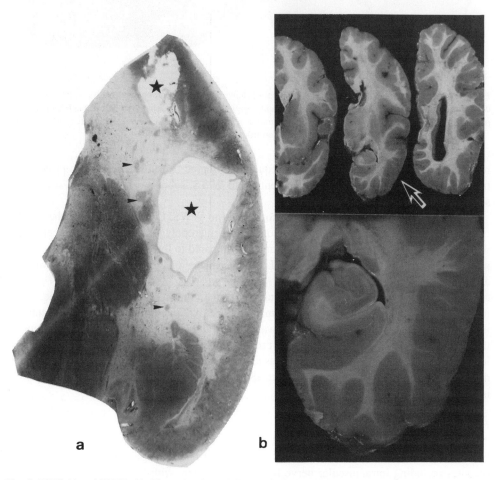

a   b

Fig. 7. WWS (a) and FCMD (b). The cut surface of the WWS (Patient 3) brain shows a diffuse smooth surface with abnormal infolding of the temporal lobe. The density of the cortex and the cortico-medullary junction are very irregular. Many heterotopic nodules (arrowheads) are present. In this patient, multicystic lesions (*) can be observed. On the other hand, some parts of the cortical surface in FCMD are very smooth (arrow), but this pachygyric lesion actually consists of many fused microgyri (right lower). Thus, true pachygyria is thought to be rare in the FCMD brain. Fig. 7a reproduced with permission from [12].

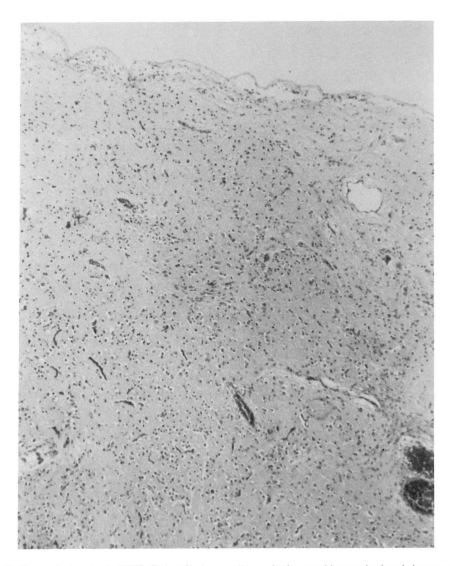

Fig. 8. The cerebral cortex in WWS (Patient 3) shows a disorganized cytoarchitecture in the whole cortex; no laminar neuronal differentiation, and individual neurons are oriented in abnormal directions, and are separated into irregular lobules by narrow strands of glial and connective tissue (×121, HE stain). Reproduced with permission from [12].

Discussion

The clinical characteristics of the 6 Japanese patients with WWS were: (1) neonatal onset; (2) congenital obstructive hydrocephalus; (3) severe muscle weakness, with respiratory distress and/or swallowing difficulty; and (4) severe eye lesions. In addition, most patients had multiple minor anomalies and seizures. Only one patient was still alive at the age of

242

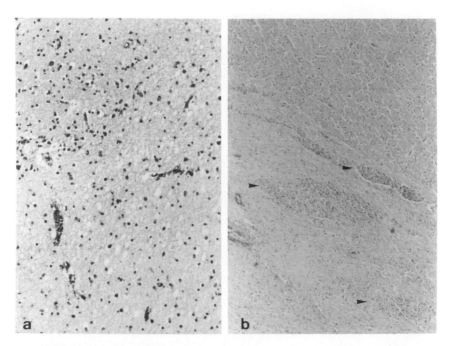

Fig. 9. The white matter (WWS, Patient 2) exhibits no myelination and the stroma is very loose ((a) ×300, LFB stain). Numerous heterotopic neurons (arrowheads) can be seen in the white matter ((b) ×121, LFB stain).

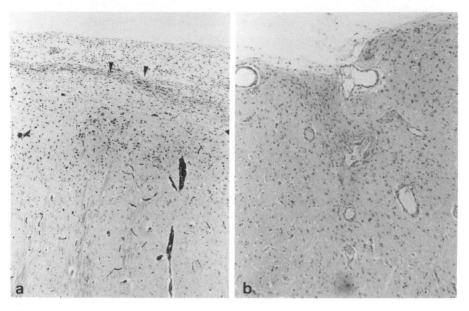

Fig. 10. The cortical histology of FCMD (right, Patient 5; left, Patient 1) is basically similar to that of WWS, however, the severity varies in each cortical region. The arrangement of cortical cells is distorted. Myelinated fibers can be seen on the cortical surface (arrowheads). Irregular masses of fused microgyri can be frequently observed, which also proves that true pachygyria is rare in FCMD. Subcortical heterotopias are rare. Fig. 10a reproduced with permission from [12].

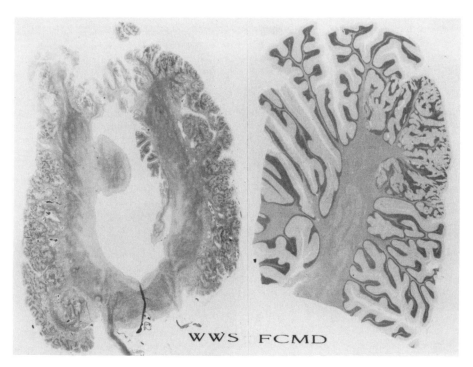

Fig. 11. The cerebellar cortex is diffusely disorganized in WWS (Patient 2), and that in FCMD (Patient 6) is well organized but exhibits polymicrogyria. The subcortex in WWS is rather well organized compared to the cortex, however, the dentate nuclei are small and exhibit gliosis. The white matter in FCMD shows no abnormality.

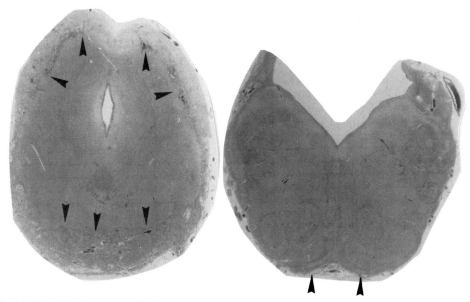

Fig. 12. The mid brain, pons, and medulla oblongata in WWS (Patient 3) are dysplastic. The meningeal gliomesenchymal proliferation is marked (left; arrowheads). The pyramidal tract cannot be identified (right; arrowheads) under the olivery nuclei.

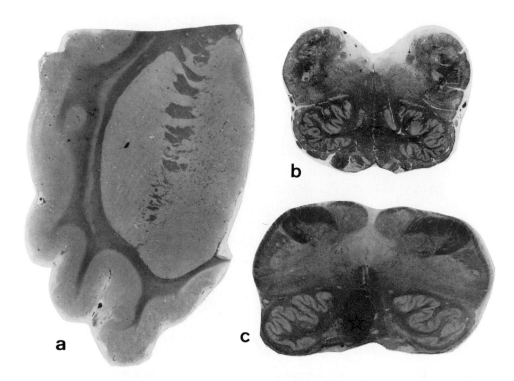

Fig. 13. In FCMD, the general configuration in all patients was well preserved, and the pyramidal tracts can be easily identified. However, their pathways were usually aberrant; mild in Patient 6 (b), and only one large pyramidal tract in Patient 1 (c). A lot of nerve fibers, probably cortico-spinal tracts, can be seen in the basal ganglia in Patient 4 (a). Fig. 13c reproduced with permission from [12].

23 months; the other patients died between 25 days and 9 months. These clinical symptoms were much severer than those of FCMD.

On MRI and neuropathology, WWS showed diffuse agyria (lissencephaly), obstructive hydrocephalus with dysgenesis of the corpus callosum and septum pellucidum, and diffuse dysplasia of the cerebellum. Dysplasia of the brain stem and the spinal cord was also present. These MRI and neuropathological findings in WWS are quite characteristic.

On the other hand, a diffuse cortical migration anomaly of the cerebrum, focal polymicrogyria of the cerebellum, and aberrant pathways of the pyramidal tracts comprise the basic neuropathology in FCMD. In the most severe case, moderate dilatation of the ventricles due to hypoplasia of the brain was observed, but even in such a case, there was no obstructive hydrocephalus, agenesis of the septum pellucidum or dysgenesis of the cerebellum.

The cortical dysplasia in WWS was severe, and diffuse and monotonous, but in FCMD the severity varied in each cortex and in each patient. The cortical dysplasia in WWS was similar to the severest pattern of the cortical dysplasia seen in FCMD, however, the mildest pattern in FCMD was not found in patients with WWS, as mentioned previously [11,19]. The white matter pathology in FCMD and WWS was different; the former showed no specific abnormality, and the latter showed no myelination, loose edematous white matter, and the presence of prominent heterotopias. However, these changes cannot be used for differential diagnosis, because the ages at autopsy were quite different.

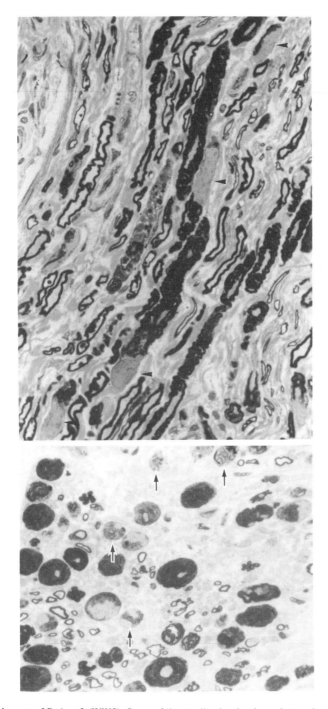

Fig. 14. Femoral nerve of Patient 3 (WWS). Some of the myelin sheaths show abnormal and tortuous proliferation, giving a rosary-like appearance. The absence of myelin segmentally around large axons can frequently be seen (arrowheads). Isolated loops or ovoids of myelin within the axoplasm of a nerve fiber can frequently be seen (arrows). Epon-embedded toluidine blue stain, upper, ×800; lower, ×1000.

246

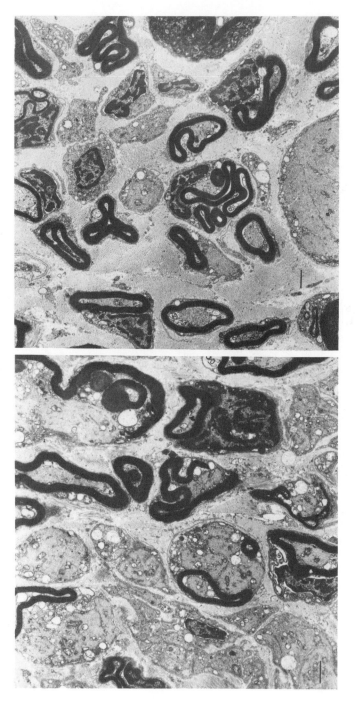

Fig. 15. Large naked axons surrounded by Schwann cell cytoplasm, and tortuously proliferated myelin sheaths, that indented the axoplasm or protruded into the Schwann cell cytoplasm, can be observed in every section. The coexistence of naked and myelinated axons in a single nerve fiber can also be observed. The myelin sheaths of some nerve fibers are located on only one side. Bar, 1 μm.

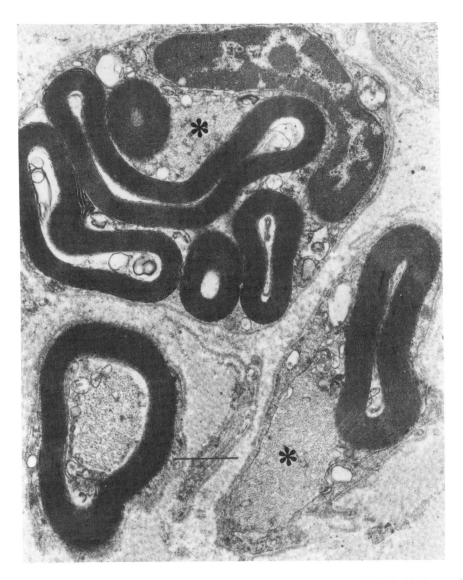

Fig. 16. One Schwann cell has five myelin sheaths with no neurofilaments or microtubules inside them, and in contrast, the absence of myelination around normal-looking axons (*) can also be observed. Bar, 1 μm. Reproduced with permission from [17].

We had examined the peripheral nerve pathology in only 1 patient with WWS. The findings were very characteristic: (1) myelin sheaths were markedly and tortuously proliferated, and showed variable contours consisting of loops and folds of compact myelin, which indented the axoplasm or protruded into the Schwann cell cytoplasm; depending on the plane of the section, they were seen as isolated ovoids of myelin within the axoplasm or Schwann cell cytoplasm; (2) the absence of myelin was seen segmentally around large axons; (3) in one section plural myelinated and/or unmyelinated axons were observed in one nerve fiber; (4) some Schwann

248

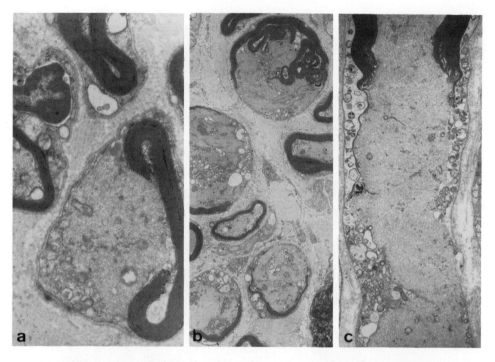

Fig. 17. Paranodal lesions and ones at the node of Ranvier are predominant. Some myelin loops are evaginated and terminate abruptly within the Schwann cell cytoplasm, and have no connection to other myelin sheaths (a). Some can be seen as isolated ovoids of myelin in the Schwann cell cytoplasm (b). In a longitudinal section, the segmental loss of myelination can be observed (c). Bar, 1 μm. Fig. 17a reproduced with permission from [17].

cells had many myelin sheaths which had no neurofilaments inside them; and (5) in some Schwann cells, the coexistence of the absence of myelin around normal looking axons and of abnormally proliferated myelin sheaths having no axonal elements inside them was seen. Although these findings were reported in the previous papers on experimental demyelination [21] or experimental allergic neuritis [22] in animals, the absence of myelinoclastic lesions or onion bulb formation might indicate that the lesion did not comprise degeneration in this patient but a congenital abnormality of myelination or Schwann-axon connection. If these findings are common in WWS, WWS is a completely different disease from FCMD. Thus, peripheral nerves should be more examined at autopsy of patients with these conditions.

The clinical and neuropathological findings in WWS and FCMD are quite different. The neuropathology of WWS can be summarized as diffuse dysplasia or disorganization of the CNS with or without peripheral nerve involvement, and that of FCMD as a diffuse or focal migration disorder, mainly of the brain cortex.

Recently, the gene for FCMD was localized to 9q31-33 [10], thus FCMD was proved to be a genetic disorder. The location of the gene has not been determined in WWS. However, we think that WWS and FCMD are different diseases because: (1) the clinical and neuropathological findings are quite different; and (2) no familial occurrence of WWS and FCMD has been reported (a familial occurrence was reported by Yoshioka et al. [20]; however, the WWS case in their report does not seem to be a true WWS case, but FCMD with an encephalocele, because the patient did not show pellucidum agenesis or cerebellar dysplasia). If FCMD and

WWS are the same genetic disorder, WWS should be more common in Japan, compared to the number of FCMD patients, because there are so many FCMD patients in Japan. We summarize the clinical and pathological differences between WWS and FCMD in Table 3.

We think that WWS is a genetically determined disorder different from FCMD, because the clinico-pathological appearance of WWS involving the CNS, eyes and muscle is monotonous and the familial incidence is very high [7]. However, the possibility of intrauterine infection cannot be ruled out completely. The presence of sclerosing meningoencephalitis-like lesions and cystic lesions, and a high frequency of an elevated serum IgM titer at birth (2 of 6 Japanese WWS patients) may suggest the presence of intrauterine infection. In addition, one of our WWS patients had focal chronic inflammatory cell infiltrations in the muscle, which has also been reported in the literature on WWS [7,23]. The proportion having a high serum IgM value at birth and chronic inflammatory cell infiltrations in the muscle in WWS is high compared to in FCMD.

Recently, the diagnostic criteria for WWS were widened compared to those of previously reported by Dobyns et al. [24], muscle-eye-brain disease (MEB) [25] being included in WWS. The reason is that MEB exhibited brain anomalies similar to WWS, as follows: (1) progressive hydrocephalus; (2) the absence of a septum pellucidum; and (3) cerebellar hypoplasia. Although we do not have a patient with MEB, we have some questions regarding this conclusion. According to Santavuori et al. [25], the main clinical and pathological manifestations of MEB are: (1) severe mental retardation and motor development delay; (2) deterioration beginning around age 5 years, including spasticity and contractures; (3) a constant (100%) finding of progressive myopia; (4) high amplitude visual evoked potentials and abnormal electroretinography develop gradually and parallel the retinal change; (5) dilatation of the ventricles and low white matter density; and (6) death usually occurs at 6–16 years of age. This clinical severity is very different from in WWS, and the clinico-pathological features of the CNS and eye lesions

Table 3

Clinical and pathological comparison between Walker–Warburg syndrome (WWS) and Fukuyama type congenital muscular dystrophy (FCMD)

	WWS	FCMD
Clinical manifestation		
Age at onset	Just/soon after birth	Usually manifest with delayed development
Respiratory distress	Present in all	Appears at later stage
Max. motor milestone	No head fixation	Variable (no head fixation – walking)
Meaningful word	No	Variable (no – practically communicable)
Muscle	Dystrophic	Dystrophic
Neuropathology		
Cerebrum	Diffuse agyria, obstructive hydrocephalus, aplasia of septum pellucidum, dysplasia of corpus callosum	Polymicrogyria
Cerebellum	Diffuse and severe dysplasia, partial agenesis of vermis	Focal polymicrogyria
Brain stem and spinal cord	Diffuse and severe dysplasia, absence of pyramidal tract	Aberrant pathway of the pyramidal tract
Peripheral nerve	Severe dysplasia	Not remarkable
Comment	Diffuse dysplasia of CNS with or without peripheral nerve involvement	Diffuse or focal migration anomaly located in CNS cortex

250

are progressive. These findings may indicate a degenerative disorder of unknown etiology. In addition, the muscle pathology of MEB looks much milder than those of FCMD and our patients with WWS. The age at death of typical WWS and MEB patients are quite different, and transitional cases have rarely been reported. If WWS and MEB are the same genetical disorder, how can we explain the difference in clinical severity between them. We think that the clinical severity should be included in the criteria for the diseases in addition to the pathological findings. As the genetical abnormality and a detailed CNS pathology of MEB remain obscure, discussion on their precise differences should continue.

References

1. Walker AE. Lissencephaly. Arch Neurol Psychiatry 1942; 48: 13–29.
2. Warburg M. Hydrocephaly, congenital retinal non-attachment and congenital falciform fold. Am J Ophthalmol 1978; 85: 88–94.
3. Krijgsman JB, Barth PG, Stam FC, Slooff JL, Jaspar HHJ. Congenital muscular dystrophy and cerebral dysgenesis in a Dutch family. Neuropaediatrics 1980; 11: 108–120.
4. Dambska M, Wisniewski K, Sher J, Solish G. Cerebro-oculo-muscular syndrome: a variant of Fukuyama congenital muscular dystrophy. Clin Neuropathol 1982; 1: 93–98.
5. Towfighi J, Sasanni JM, Suzuki K, Ladda BL. Cerebro-ocular dysplasia muscular dystrophy (COD-MD) syndrome. Acta Neuropathol 1984; 65: 110–123.
6. Pagon RA, Chandler JW, Collie WR, et al. Hydrocephalus, agyria, retinal dysplasia, encephalocele (HARD±E) syndrome: an autosomal recessive condition. Birth Defects 1978; 14: 233–241.
7. Dobyns WB, Kirkpatrick JB, Hittner HM, et al. Syndrome with lissencephaly. II. Walker–Warburg and cerebro-oculo-muscular syndromes and a new syndrome with type II lissencephaly. Am J Med Genet 1985; 22: 157–195.
8. Fukuyama Y, Kawazura M, Haruna A. A peculiar form of congenital progressive muscular dystrophy. Report of fifteen cases. Paediatr Univ Tokyo (Tokyo) 1960; 4: 5–8.
9. Fukuyama Y, Osawa M, Suzuki H. Congenital progressive muscular dystrophy of Fukuyama type: clinical, genetic and pathological considerations. Brain Dev (Tokyo) 1981; 3: 1–29.
10. Toda T, Segawa M, Nomura Y, et al. Localization of a gene for Fukuyama type congenital muscular dystrophy to chromosome 9q31-33. Nat Genet 1993; 5: 283–286.
11. Takada K, Becker LE, Takashima S. Walker–Warburg syndrome with skeletal muscle involvement: a report of three patients. Pediatr Neurosci 1987; 13: 202–209.
12. Kimura S, Sasaki Y, Kobayashi T, et al. Fukuyama-type congenital muscular dystrophy and the Walker–Warburg syndrome. Brain Dev 1993; 15: 182–191.
13. Kasubuchi Y, Hara S, Wakaizumi S, et al. An autopsy case of congenital muscular dystrophy accompanying hydrocephalus (in Japanese). No to Hattatsu (Tokyo) 1974; 6: 36–41.
14. Miyake S, Goto A, Tsuchida M, et al. An autopsy case of congenital muscular dystrophy associated with hydrocephalus and occipital dermal sinus (in Japanese). No to Hattatsu (Tokyo) 1977; 9: 212–219.
15. Tachi N, Tachi M, Sasaki K, Tanabe C, Minagawa K. Walker–Warburg syndrome in a Japanese patient. Pediatr Neurol 1988; 4: 236–240.
16. Sasaki M, Yoshioka K, Yanagisawa T, Nemoto A, Takasago W, Nagano T. Lissencephaly with congenital muscular dystrophy and ocular abnormalities: cerebro-oculo-muscular syndrome. Child Nerv Syst 1989; 5: 35–37.
17. Kimura S, Kobayashi T, Sasaki Y, et al. Congenital polyneuropathy in Walker–Warburg syndrome. Neuropediatrics 1992; 23: 14–17.
18. Yamaguchi E, Hayashi T, Kondoh H, et al. A case of Walker–Warburg syndrome with uncommon findings. Double cortical layer, temporal cyst and increased serum IgM. Brain Dev 1993; 15: 61–66.
19. Takada K, Nakamura H, Tanaka J. Cortical dysplasia in congenital muscular dystrophy with central nervous system involvement (Fukuyama type). J Neuropathol Exp Neurol 1984; 43: 395–407.
20. Yoshioka M, Kuroki S, Nigami H, Kawai T, Nakamura H. Clinical variation within sibships in Fukuyama-type congenital muscular dystrophy. Brain Dev (Tokyo) 1992; 14: 334–337.

21. Webster HdeF, Spiro D. Phase and electron microscopic studies of experimental demyelination. I. Variations in myelin sheath contour in normal guinea pig sciatic nerve. J Neuropathol Exp Neurol 1960; 19: 42–69.

22. King RHM, Thomas PK. Aberrant remyelination in chronic relapsing experimental allergic neuritis. Neuropathol Appl Neurobiol 1975; 1: 367–378.

23. Shevell MI, Rosenblatt B, Silver K. Inflammatory myositis and Walker–Warburg syndrome; etiologic implications. Can J Neurol Sci 1993; 20: 227–229.

24. Dobyns WB, Pagon RA, Armstrong D, et al. Diagnostic criteria for Walker–Warburg syndrome. Am J Med Genet 1989; 32: 195–210.

25. Santavuori P, Somer H, Sainio K, et al. Muscle-eye-brain disease (MEB). Brain Dev (Tokyo) 1989; 11: 147–153.

Y. Fukuyama, M. Osawa and K. Saito (Eds.), *Congenital Muscular Dystrophies*
253

CHAPTER 20

Membrane abnormality in Fukuyama congenital muscular dystrophy

ERI ARIKAWA-HIRASAWA[1,2], YUKIKO K. HAYASHI[1,2],
YOSHIKUNI MIZUNO[1,2], IKUYA NONAKA[1]
and KIICHI ARAHATA[1]

[1]*Department of Neuromuscular Research, National Institute of Neuroscience, NCNP, Tokyo, Japan*
[2]*Department of Neurology, Juntendo University School of Medicine, Tokyo, Japan*

Introduction

Congenital muscular dystrophy (CMD) is the name given to a heterogeneous group of disorders characterized by severe muscle wasting from birth or early infancy.

CMD has been classified into several types according to clinical histological differences: Fukuyama type CMD (FCMD), Walker–Warburg syndrome (WWS), Santavuori's muscle eye and brain disease (MEB), and the classical form of CMD. In FCMD, WWS and MEB, there are structural brain abnormalities (brain malformations and/or hydrocephalus) and associated intellectual retardation.

FCMD is endemic to Japan but is rarely observed in other countries [1–3], and the incidence of FCMD in Japan is approximately half that of Duchenne muscular dystrophy [4]. FCMD is an autosomal recessive disorder and the chromosome localization for the disease has been assigned to 9q31-33 [5]. Although the chromosome localization for FCMD is different from that for DMD, the histopathological changes of the skeletal muscle in FCMD patients are grossly similar to those seen in DMD or even more severe compared with age-matched patient muscles [1,2,6–8], and muscle biopsy specimens show dystrophic features with necrotic and regenerating fibers, increased fibrous and fatty tissues, and progressive loss of muscle fibers. In both CMD and DMD, cytochemical and immunocytochemical studies of skeletal muscle have shown increased calcium overloaded fibers, which suggest a membrane abnormality of the fibers [9].

Dystrophin is the DMD gene product [10,11], and is normally localized to the inner surface of the muscle fiber plasma membrane. Dystrophin has not been detected in DMD [12–17]. In this study, we compared the immunocytochemical pattern of the dystrophin protein on the surface membrane of skeletal muscle from 49 patients with CMD (FCMD and non-FCMD), 5 with DMD and 17 with SMA.

Materials and methods

Clinical materials

Skeletal muscle specimens (mostly biceps brachii, and in some younger patients rectus femoris) from 49 patients with CMD (34 FCMD; 15 non-FCMD), 17 with SMA and 5 with DMD were examined for diagnostic purposes, with informed consent. All clinical diagnoses were based on conventional criteria. Each CMD case demonstrated progressive muscle weakness and hypotonia, with or without joint contractures, from birth or early infancy. All exhibited a dystrophic muscle histopathology and myopathic electromyographic findings. Forty-seven of the 49 CMD patients exhibited elevated creatine kinase (CK) activity. All the FCMD patients showed intellectual impairment, abnormal CT findings in the brain (16 of 18 cases examined), and epileptic convulsions (3 cases).

Immunocytochemistry

Dystrophin immunostaining was performed with a monoclonal 4C5 anti-dystrophin anti-body, which was raised against a synthetic peptide corresponding to amino acids 3495–3544 of the carboxy terminus of human fetal skeletal muscle dystrophin [14]. In some cases, ad-ditional region specific antibodies were used. The immunostaining patterns found with 4C5 were not significantly different than those found with other domain specific anti-dystrophin antibodies [13,14].

Indirect immunoperoxidase methods used were as described previously [13,14]. Each coverslip carried 4–6 frozen sections from different biopsy specimens, and included sections from normal muscle and a known DMD patient, as controls.

Qualitative and quantitative analysis of immunostaining

Quantitative analysis of the immunostaining signals for dystrophin and spectrin was accom-plished by assigning one of 5 patterns to each biopsy specimen: negative, fluffy (fluffy staining of the plasma membrane, with or without diffuse and faint cytoplasmic staining), normal, partially deficient, and intense (Fig. 1). Serial cryostat sections were examined for acridine orange-RNA fluorescence (AO), desmin and C9, together with a battery of

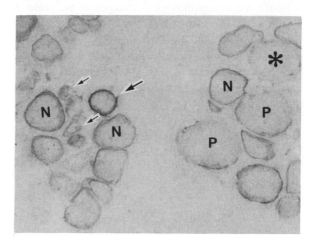

Fig. 1. Qualitative assignment of the immunoperoxidase staining pattern for dystrophin was accomplished by classifying each immunoreactive fiber into five groups with; negative (asterisk), fluffy (small arrows), normal (N), intense (large arrow), and partially deficient (P) immunostaining (FCMD, ×420). (Reproduced with permission from [18]).

histochemical stains, which included acid and alkaline preincubated ATPase for characterization of the abnormally reacting muscle fibers to dystrophin and spectrin (data not shown) [18].

For quantitative analysis, a total of 395–650 muscle fibers from each specimen was analyzed at random, and the number of immunoreacting fibers was determined according to the 5 different patterns described above. Five age-matched patients were selected from each patient group.

Immunocytochemistry of dystrophin and spectrin

In control SMA patients, the dystrophin immunoreaction was detected as a continuous ring around the periphery of all muscle fibers (Fig. 2h). Dystrophin was not detected in the muscle from patients with DMD (Fig. 2f). Non FCMD patients showed almost the normal immunostaining pattern for dystrophin (Fig. 2d). The muscle from 34 FCMD patients generally exhibited positive immunostaining for dystrophin, however a subset of fibers in all 34 specimens showed an abnormal dystrophin pattern (Figs. 1, 2b). The abnormal pattern included: (1) negatively stained necrotic, degenerating or immature fibers; (2) fluffy staining in some small basophilic type 2C fibers which also reacted strongly with AO, and were classified as early regenerating fibers; (3) partially deficient thus degenerating fibers; and (4) intense staining in some hypercontracted opaque fibers. However, not every dystrophin negative fiber was necrotic, not every fluffy fiber was positive for AO, and not every partially defective fiber was degenerating [18].

Spectrin immunostaining in the FCMD muscle fibers was identical to that of dystrophin when consecutive cryostat sections were examined. Similar results were obtained for spectrin and dystrophin in other CMD muscles (Fig. 3). The spectrin immunoreaction was well preserved in the dystrophin-deficient DMD muscle (Fig. 3).

Quantitative analysis of the immunocytochemical dystrophin and spectrin staining patterns

FCMD muscle showed a significantly higher number of abnormally immunoreactive fibers for both dystrophin (17.4–43.5%; mean, 28.0) and spectrin (18.0–33.9%; mean, 24.5) (Fig. 3). In contrast, other CMD muscle showed only a few abnormally immunoreactive fibers for dystrophin (1.2–7.8%; mean, 4.0) and spectrin (1.0–6.9%; mean, 3.8) (Fig. 3). DMD muscle also showed a significantly smaller percentage of abnormally immunoreactive fibers for spectrin (3.9–16.6%; mean, 9.0).

Discussion

Plasma membrane breakdown has been suggested as an early event in muscle fiber damage in both CMD and DMD [1,19]. To further investigate the possible membrane abnormality in skeletal muscle from patients with CMD and DMD, we examined two components of the membrane-associated cytoskeleton, dystrophin and spectrin, immunocytochemically.

A high percentage (28.0%) of abnormally immunoreactive muscle fibers to dystrophin, was found in the FCMD patients, while other types of CMD patients (non-FCMD) had only 4.0%. Similar results were obtained on the spectrin immunostaining.

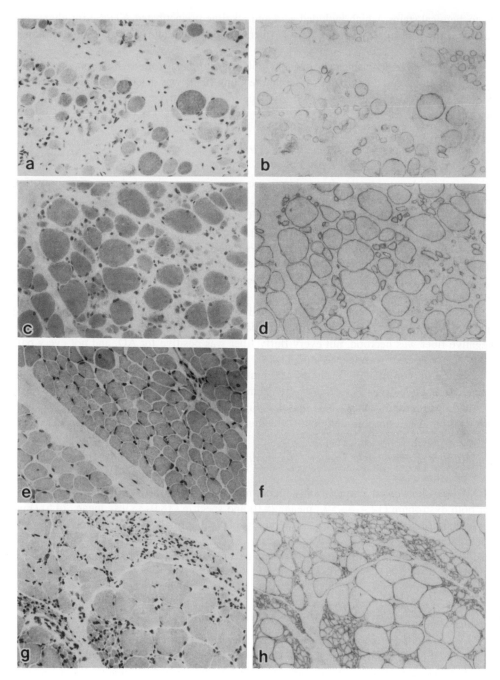

Fig. 2. Consecutive frozen sections of biopsied skeletal muscle specimens from FCMD (a,b), non-FCMD (c,d), DMD (e,f), and SMA (g,h) patients stained with hematoxylin and eosin (a,c,e,g) or immunoreacted for dystrophin (b,d,f,h). Note the heterogeneous immunostaining pattern in FCMD muscle, i.e negative, fluffy, normal, intense and partially deficient fibers in one section. In contrast, normal immunostaining of the surface membrane was observed in most of the non-FCMD and SMA muscle fibers. Dystrophin was not detected in DMD (×370). (Reproduced with permission from [18]).

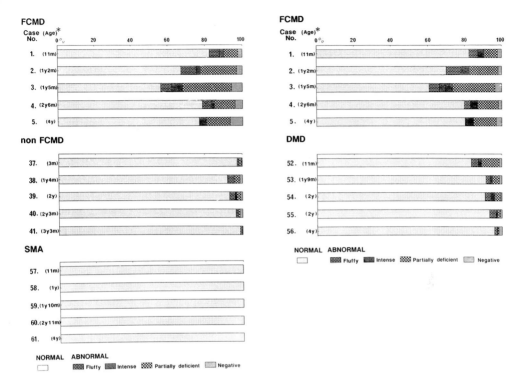

Fig. 3. Quantitative comparison of dystrophin (a) and spectrin (b) immunostaining patterns of muscles between each of 5 age-matched patients with FCMD, non-FCMD (other CMD), SMA, and DMD. Each bar represents the percentage of a different pattern of dystrophin or spectrin immunostaining. In FCMD muscle, immunostaining pattern of dystrophin (a) is considered to be similar to that of spectrin (b). Note the higher percentage of abnormally reacted fibers for both dystrophin and spectrin in the FCMD muscle. (Reproduced with permission from [18]).

Most of the abnormally immunoreactive fibers to dystrophin and spectrin, were acridine orange-positive early regenerating fibers or C9-positive necrotic fibers. However, there were occasional normal-looking non-necrotic fibers that showed no C9 immunostaining.

In conclusion, the present study demonstrated the following. First, CMD patients other than FCMD showed normal dystrophin and spectrin expression patterns on the surface membrane of skeletal muscle. On the other hand, the FCMD patients exhibited a high percentage of abnormally immunoreactive muscle fibers to both dystrophin and spectrin. Muscles from patients with DMD showed a lower percentage (9%) of abnormally immunoreactive fibers to spectrin compared to that in FCMD (25%). These observations strongly suggest the presence of intrinsic factor(s) that produce an abnormality of the plasma membrane of FCMD muscle. The immunocytochemical abnormality in FCMD muscle could reflect a primary abnormality of the muscle fiber surface membrane or could be a secondary consequence of generalized fiber damage.

We have recently reported a marked reduction of laminin subunits (particularly laminin $\alpha2$ or M chain) in most muscle fibers of FCMD patients [20]. These results again suggest the presence of intrinsic factors that produce a primary abnormality of the plasma membrane and/or basal lamina of FCMD muscle, although the $\alpha2$ chain abnormality in FCMD is considered to be a secondary phenomenon to muscle fiber damage, since the chromosome localization for FCMD has been assigned to 9q31-33, while the gene for the $\alpha2$ chain has been localized to chromosome 6q22-23 [21].

References

1. Fukuyama Y, Kawazura M, Haruna H. A peculiar form of congenital progressive muscular dystrophy. Paediatr Univ Tokyo (Tokyo) 1960; 4: 5–8.
2. Nonaka I, Chou SM. Congenital muscular dystrophy. In: Vinken PJ, Bruyn GW, eds. Handbook of clinical neurology, Vol 41. Amsterdam: North Holland 1979: 27–50.
3. Dubowitz V. Congenital muscular dystrophy. In: Dubowitz V, ed. Muscle disorders in childhood. Chicago, IL: Year Book Med Publ 1989: 52–65.
4. Fukuyama Y, Osawa M, Suzuki H. Congenital progressive muscular dystrophy of the Fukuyama type: clinical, genetic and pathologic considerations. Brain Dev (Tokyo) 1981; 13: 1–29.
5. Toda T, Segawa M, Nomura Y, et al. Localization of a gene for Fukuyama type congenital muscular dystrophy to chromosome 9q31-33. Nat Genet 1993; 5: 283–286.
6. Segawa M. Histological, histochemical and electron microscopical studies of biopsied muscle of congenital muscular dystrophy with mental retardation and facial muscle involvement (in Japanese). No To Hattatsu (Tokyo) 1971; 3: 21–36.
7. Nonaka I, Miyoshino S, Miike T, et al. An electron microscopical study of the muscle in congenital muscular dystrophy. Kumamoto Med J (Kumamoto) 1972; 25: 68–75.
8. Saida K, Kyogoku M, Hojo H, Hiroya H, Nishitani H. Congenital muscular dystrophy (Fukuyama type). Quantitative histological study of distribution of affected muscles (in Japanese). Rinsho Shinkeigaku (Tokyo) 1973; 13: 587–596.
9. Cornelio F, Dones I. Muscle fiber degeneration and necrosis in muscular dystrophy and other muscle diseases: cytochemical and immunocytochemical data. Ann Neurol 1984; 16: 694–701.
10. Hoffman EP, Knudson CM, Campbell KP, Kunkel LM. Subcellular fractionation of dystrophin to the triads of skeletal muscle. Nature 1987; 330: 754–758.
11. Hoffman EP, Brown RH Jr, Kunkel LM. Dystrophin: the protein product of Duchenne muscular dystrophy locus. Cell 1987; 51: 919–928.
12. Arahata K, Ishiura S, Ishiguro T, et al. Immunostaining of skeletal and cardiac muscle surface membrane with antibody against Duchenne muscular dystrophy peptide. Nature 1988; 333: 466–469.
13. Arahata K, Hoffman EP, Kunkel LM, et al. Dystrophin diagnosis: comparison of dystrophin abnormalities by immunofluorescent and immunoblot analyses. Proc Natl Acad Sci USA 1989; 86: 7154–7158.
14. Arahata K, Beggs AH, Honda H, et al. Preservation of the C-terminus of dystrophin molecule in the skeletal muscle from Becker muscular dystrophy. J Neurol Sci 1991; 101: 148–156.
15. Bonilla E, Samitt CE, Miranda AP, et al. Duchenne muscular dystrophy: deficiency of dystrophin at the muscle cell surface. Cell 1988; 54: 447–452.
16. Sugita H, Arahata K, Ishiguro T, et al. Negative immunostaining of Duchenne muscular dystrophy (DMD) and *mdx* mouse muscle surface membrane with antibody against synthetic peptide fragment predicted from DMD cDNA. Proc Jpn Acad 1988; 64: 210–212.
17. Watkins SC, Hoffman EP, Slayter HS, Kunkel LM. Immunoelectron microscopic localization of dystrophin in myofibers. Nature 1988; 333: 863–866.
18. Arikawa E, Ishihara T, Nonaka I, Sugita H, Arallata K. Immunocytochemical analysis of dystrophin in congenital muscular dystrophy. J Neurol Sci 1991; 105: 79–87.
19. Morandi LM, Mora M, Gussoni E, Tedeschi S, Cornelio F. Dystrophin analysis in Duchenne and Becker muscular dystrophy carries: correlation with intracellular calcium and albumin. Ann Neurol 1990; 28: 674–679.
20. Hayashi YK, Engvall E, Arikawa-Hirasawa E, et al. Abnormal localization of laminin subunits in muscular dystrophies. J Neurol Sci 1993; 119: 53–64.
21. Vuolteenaho R, Nissinen M, Sainio K, et al. Human laminin M chain (merosin): complete primary structure, chromosomal assignment, and expression of the M and A chain in human fetal tissues. J Cell Biol 1994; 124: 381–394.

Y. Fukuyama, M. Osawa and K. Saito (Eds.), *Congenital Muscular Dystrophies*
© 1997 Elsevier Science B.V. All rights reserved

259

CHAPTER 21

Laminin α2 (or M) chain abnormality in congenital muscular dystrophy

YUKIKO K. HAYASHI, IKUYA NONAKA and KIICHI ARAHATA

National Institute of Neuroscience, NCNP, Tokyo, Japan

Introduction

The muscle basal lamina is a specialized extracellular matrix ensheathing each muscle fiber, and it is thought to contribute more than the mechanical properties of muscle. Laminin is one of the major components of the basal lamina, together with type IV collagen, heparan-sulfate proteoglycan and entactin/nidgen. The large laminin (~800 kDa) comprises a heterotrimer arranged in the shape of a cross. "Classical" laminin (or laminin-1) has one long chain, $\alpha 1$ (or A, 300–400 kDa), and two short chains (180–200 kDa) $\beta 1$ (or B1) and $\gamma 1$ (or B2), but in mature skeletal muscle basal lamina, laminin has an $\alpha 2$ (or M) long chain instead of an $\alpha 1$ one [1], and comprises an $\alpha 2$-$\beta 1$-$\gamma 1$ heterotrimer named laminin-2. The $\alpha 2$ chain is thought to interact with receptor proteins on the plasma membrane of muscle fiber, such as α-dystroglycan (156 kDa dystrophin-associated glycoprotein; 156DAG) [2].

We previously showed that skeletal muscle in Fukuyama type congenital muscular dystrophy (FCMD) patients exhibited a higher percentage of fibers that were immunostained abnormally for both dystrophin and spectrin [3], and for β-dystroglycan (43DAG) [4]. These results suggested the presence of instability of the membrane cytoskeleton in FCMD.

We have examined each laminin subunit ($\alpha 1$, $\alpha 2$, $\beta 1$ and $\gamma 1$) and type IV collagen, together with dystrophin and spectrin, in muscles from various neuromuscular diseases.

Materials and methods

A total of 64 limb-muscle specimens (mostly biceps brachii, and in some cases rectus femoris) were examined for diagnostic purposes, with informed consent. The subjects included: 17 patients with FCMD, 13 with other congenital muscular dystrophy unrelated to FCMD (other CMD), 16 with Duchenne muscular dystrophy (DMD), and 18 with other neuromuscular diseases (OND) as controls. OND included spinal-muscular atrophy, nemaline myopathy, myotubular myopathy, mitochondrial myopathy, inflammatory myopathies, and patients with non-specific muscle weakness. Table 1 lists the clinical profiles of the patients. For quantitative analysis, each of 5 age-matched patients with FCMD, other CMD, DMD and OND were selected (mean age, 2 years 1 month to 3 years 1 month).

The antibodies used in this study were as follows: monoclonal antibodies for each laminin subunit, $\alpha 1$, $\alpha 2$, $\beta 1$ and $\gamma 1$ chains (kindly provided by E. Engvall, La Jolla Cancer Research Foundation) [5]; monoclonal antibody for dystrophin, 4C5 [6,7]; rabbit antiserum

Table 1

Clinical profiles of the patients

Clinical diagnosis	Number of patients	Sex		Age[a]		CK(U/l)	
		M	F	Range	Mean	Range	Mean
FCMD	17	12	5	4 m–6 y	1 y 9 m	763–10130	3618
Other CMD	13	6	7	5 m–12 y	2 y 1 m	176–3786	1271
DMD	16	16	0	1 y–12 y	4 y	6480–64855	10508
OND	18	8	10	5 m–39 y	8 y 9 m	18–05980	3064

FCMD, Fukuyama congenital muscular dystrophy; other CMD, Congenital muscular dystrophy unrelated to FCMD; DMD, Duchenne muscular dystrophy; OND, other neuromuscular diseases include nemaline myopathy (3), myotubular myopathy (1), mitochondrial myopathy (3), motor neuron disease (1), polymyositis (1), dermato-myositis (1), McArdle disease (1), congenital fiber type disproportion (1), neuropathic changes (3) and non-specific myopathy (3); CK, creatine kinase (normal range: 12–75U/l). (Reproduced with permission from [8].)
[a]m, months; y, years.

for human type IV collagen (Advance Inc., Tokyo); and human erythrocyte spectrin (Transformation Res. Inc., MA).

Affinity-purified fluorescein isothiocyanate (FITC)-labeled goat F(ab')2 anti-mouse and anti-rabbit IgG (Tago Inc., CA) were used as the second layer antibodies.

Immunocytochemistry was performed as previously described [8].

Quantitative densitometric analysis of the immunostaining intensity was performed as follows: the immunolabeling intensity of the fluorescence of the sarcolemma was calculated with an IBAS Rel. 2.0 automatic image analyzer (Carl Zeiss Vision Co. Ltd.) with appropriate control. A total of 3264 pixels of a randomly chosen rectangular region ($56006.25 \mu m^2$) in each muscle specimen was examined. Positive immunostaining for the vascular basal lamina was erased from the screen before the analysis, and the mean cytoplasmic gray level was subtracted before the calculation. The total plasma membrane length of a given region was determined to express the immunolabeling intensity per unit plasma membrane length.

Results

In control OND and other CMD muscles, laminin $\alpha2$, $\beta1$ and $\gamma1$ clearly showed a delineated ring around each muscle fiber. Laminin $\alpha1$ was not detected around muscle fibers except for a few regenerating fibers exhibiting faint immunoreaction (Fig. 1A(a–d, i–l)). The endoneurial basement membrane of intramuscular nerves and intrafusal spindle fibers was also stained for laminin $\alpha2$, $\beta1$ and $\gamma1$, whereas the perineurial basement membrane was stained for all antibodies (Fig. 2). Intramuscular small blood vessels showed no immunoreaction at all for laminin $\alpha2$, but were reactive for laminin $\alpha1$, $\beta1$ and $\gamma1$.

Dystrophin-deficient, DAGs-reduced DMD muscle showed similar immunostaining patterns for laminin $\alpha2$, $\beta1$ and $\gamma1$ to those observed in controls. In addition, DMD muscle showed faint but definite immunoreactivity for laminin $\alpha1$ in over 90% of the muscle fibers (Fig. 1A(m–p)). Occasional degenerating fibers showed abnormal immunostaining for spectrin, but laminin $\alpha2$, $\beta1$ and $\gamma1$ were preserved in these fibers.

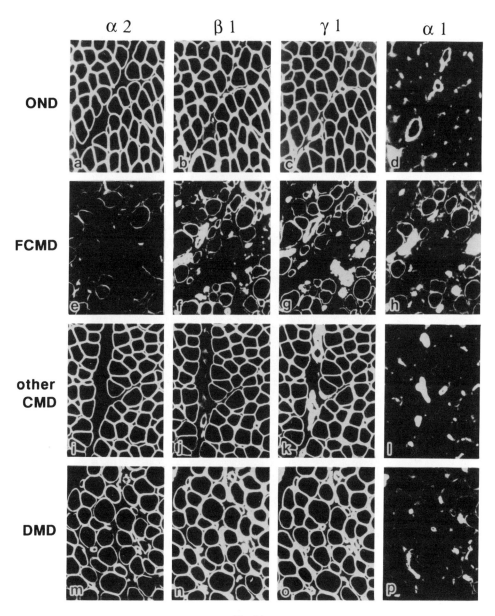

Fig. 1A.

In FCMD muscle, a dramatic reduction of the immunostaining intensity for laminin $\alpha 2$ was observed, only approximately 26% of the levels seen in controls, on quantitative analysis. Similar but much milder changes were seen for laminin $\beta 1$ and $\gamma 1$ immunoreaction, while blood vessel staining for laminin $\alpha 1, \beta 1$ and $\gamma 1$ appeared normal. In addition, laminin $\alpha 1$ was detected around most (~90%) muscle fibers (Fig. 1A(e–h)). Interestingly, the immunoreaction for laminin $\alpha 2, \beta 1$ and $\gamma 1$ of intrafusal spindle fibers and peripheral nerves was well preserved (Fig. 2).

262

B

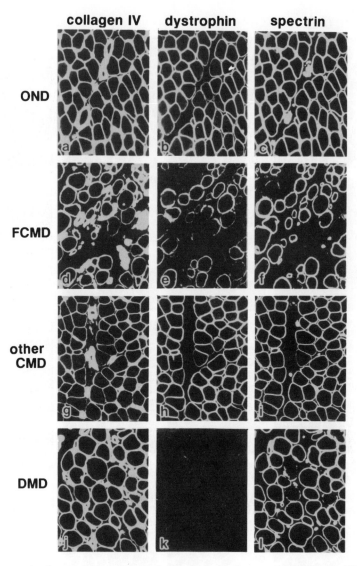

Fig. 1. (A) Consecutive frozen sections of biopsied skeletal muscles from control OND (a–d), FCMD (e–h), other CMD (i–l), and DMD (m–p) patients immunoreacted for laminin $\alpha 2$ (a,e,i,m), $\beta 1$ (b,f,j,n), $\gamma 1$ (c,g,k,o), and laminin $\alpha 1$(d,h,l,p). Note the faint and deranged pattern of immunostaining for laminin $\alpha 2$ on the muscle fiber basal lamina in FCMD. Laminin $\beta 1$ also show abnormal immunostaining patterns in FCMD muscle, but the reduction of the immunoreactivity is less marked compared to laminin $\alpha 2$. In contrast, strong and clear immunostaining of the basal lamina for laminin $\alpha 2$, $\beta 1$ and $\gamma 1$ is equally observed in the other diseases examined including DMD. Laminin $\alpha 1$ is not detected around muscle fibers in OND or other CMD muscles, but is found in FCMD and DMD. Intramuscular blood vessels are not reactive for laminin $\alpha 2$, whereas they are immunostained for laminin $\alpha 1$, $\beta 1$ and $\gamma 1$ in all diseases examined, with variable staining for $\beta 1$ (×300). (B) Consecutive frozen sections of the specimen as in A. Sections from control OND (a–c), FCMD (d–f), other CMD (g–i), and DMD (j–l) patients are immunostained for type IV collagen (a,d,g,j), dystrophin (b,e,h,k), and spectrin (c,f,i,l). In FCMD muscle, abnormally immunoreacted fibers for each of the antibodies is occasionally observed. The vascular basal lamina is equally immunostained for type IV collagen in these diseases (×300). (Reproduced with permission from [8].)

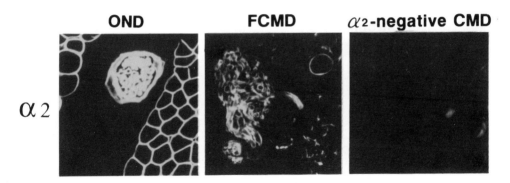

Fig. 2. Indirect immunofluorescence staining of frozen sections of control OND, FCMD and laminin $\alpha2$ chain-negative CMD muscle. In FCMD muscle fibers, immunostaining for laminin $\alpha2$ is apparently fainter than in control OND. The endoneurial basal lamina of intramuscular nerves of OND and FCMD patients is intensely stained for laminin $\alpha2$, $\beta1$ (not shown), and $\gamma1$ (not shown). Laminin $\alpha2$ chain-negative CMD muscle exhibits no laminin $\alpha2$ staining for the basal lamina of either muscle fibers or peripheral nerves ($\times300$). (Reproduced with permission from [8].)

Type IV collagen, like laminin $\gamma1$, was clearly preserved on the basal lamina of muscle fibers and blood vessels in control OND, other CMD and DMD muscles (Fig. 1B(a,g,j)). In FCMD muscle, although the staining intensity for type IV collagen was not significantly different from those in other diseases, most muscle fibers (~83%) showed an abnormal immunostaining pattern (Fig. 1B(d)).

We also examined muscles of 18-week DMD and 23-week FCMD fetal cases. At 18-weeks, DMD fetal muscle showed laminin $\alpha2$ immunoreaction clearly around each muscle fiber. However, FCMD fetal muscle at 23-weeks showed extremely faint immunoreaction for laminin $\alpha2$ (Fig. 3).

During our examination, we found two CMD patients who exhibited no immunoreaction for the laminin $\alpha2$ chain in muscle, intrafusal spindle fibers or intramuscular peripheral nerves (Fig. 2). The immunostaining intensity for laminin $\beta1$ and $\gamma1$ were reduced. The patients were clinically diagnosed as having "atypical FCMD", because mental involvement was not observed at the time of muscle biopsy.

Discussion

We found that in FCMD muscle, the immunostaining intensity for the laminin $\alpha2$ chain on the muscle fiber basal lamina was significantly reduced compared to that in normal control muscle fibers and other diseased controls, including dystrophin-deficient DMD. The changes for laminin $\beta1$ and $\gamma1$ were less marked compared to those for the $\alpha2$ chain. Furthermore, the reduction of laminin $\alpha2$ in muscle was apparent even in a 23-week FCMD fetus, while an 18-week DMD fetus showed clearly visible immunostaining for laminin $\alpha2$. Thus, among the basal lamina components examined, the laminin $\alpha2$ chain showed the most striking and consistent change, suggesting an early role for laminin $\alpha2$ in the muscle fiber breakdown in FCMD.

Two patients with CMD who exhibited no immunostaining for laminin $\alpha2$ were of note. The absence of immunostaining for the $\alpha2$ chain in skeletal muscle and peripheral nerves

264

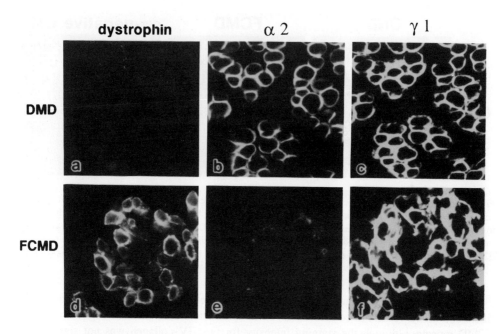

dystrophin $\alpha\,2$ $\gamma\,1$

DMD

FCMD

Fig. 3. Indirect immunofluorescence staining of consecutive frozen sections of DMD (a–c) and FCMD (d–f) fetal*
(18 and 23 weeks, respectively) muscle. In DMD, although dystrophin is not detected (a), laminin $\alpha2$ (b) is easily
observed. In contrast, although the FCMD muscle exhibits clear dystrophin staining (d), the laminin $\alpha2$ is dramatically reduced (e). Laminin $\beta1$ (not shown) and $\gamma1$ (c,f) are equally immunostained in both diseases (×400).
(Reproduced with permission from [8].) *Details of the FCMD fetus have been reported previously [10].

was similar to that previously reported in 13 French patients with $\alpha2$ chain negative CMD
[9], although in the French patients, the laminin $\beta1$ and $\gamma1$ chains were immunostained normally, while in our patients, the immunostaining for $\beta1$ and $\gamma1$ chains appeared to be decreased.

It will be quite important to compare $\alpha2$ chain-negative CMD and $\alpha2$ chain-positive but
reduced FCMD. The two diseases show several clinical and immunocytochemical similarities. Clinically, these are severe forms of CMD; patients show a floppy tendency at birth,
their motor milestones are delayed, serum CK activity is moderately to markedly elevated,
and the patients usually are not able to walk. CT/MRI scan abnormalities of diffuse low
density areas in the brain appear frequently in both diseases, although the $\alpha2$ chain-negative
CMD patients show no intellectual retardation. Severe intellectual retardation is considered
a characteristic clinical feature of FCMD. The chromosomal localization of the responsible
genes in each disease is different. In laminin $\alpha2$ chain-negative CMD, the chromosome localization has been assigned to 6q, where the gene for the laminin $\alpha2$ chain is located, and
mutation(s) of the $\alpha2$ chain gene may exist. In FCMD, the $\alpha2$ chain abnormality is a phenomenon secondary to an unknown course, because the gene is localized at chromosome 9q.
Nonetheless, the immunocytochemical similarities of these diseases lead us to speculate that
there is a similar underlying mechanism responsible for the muscle fiber breakdown.

References

1. Leivo I, Engvall E. Merosin, a protein specific for basement membrane of Schwann cells, striated muscle, and trophoblast, is expressed late in nerve and muscle development. Proc Natl Acad Sci USA 1988; 85: 1544–1548.

2. Ibraghimov-Beskrovnaya O, Ervasti JM, Leveille CJ, Slaughter CA, Sernett SW, Campbell KP. Primary structure of dystrophin-associated glycoproteins linking dystrophin to the extracellular matrix. Nature 1992; 355: 696–702.

3. Arikawa E, Ishihara T, Nonaka I, Sugita H, Arahata K. Immunocytochemical analysis of dystrophin in congenital muscular dystrophy. J Neurol Sci 1991; 105: 79–87.

4. Arahata K, Hayashi YK, Ozawa E. Dystrophin-associated glycoprotein and dystrophin co-localisation at sarcolemma in Fukuyama congenital muscular dystrophy. Lancet 1993; 342: 623–624.

5. Sanes JR, Engvall E, Butkowski R, Hunter DD. Molecular heterogeneity of basal lamina: isoforms of laminin and collagen IV at the neuromuscular junction and elsewhere. J Cell Biol 1990; 111: 1685–1699.

6. Arahata K, Hoffman EP, Kunkel LM, et al. Dystrophin diagnosis: comparison of dystrophin abnormalities by immunofluorescence and immunoblot analyses. Proc Natl Acad Sci USA 1989; 86: 7154–7158.

7. Arahata K, Beggs AH, Honda H, et al. Preservation of the C-terminus of dystrophin molecule in the skeletal muscle from Becker muscular dystrophy. J Neurol Sci 1991; 101: 148–156.

8. Hayashi YK, Engvall E, Arikawa-Hirasawa E, et al. Abnormal localization of laminin subunits in muscular dystrophies. J Neurol Sci 1993; 119: 53–64.

9. Tomé FMS, Evangelista T, Leclerc A, et al. Congenital muscular dystrophy with merosin deficiency. CR Acad Sci III, Sciences de la vie/Life Sci 1994; 317: 351–357.

10. Takada K, Nakamura H, Suzumori K, Sugiyama N. Cortical dysplasia in a 23-week fetus with Fukuyama congenital dystrophy (FCMD). Acta Neuropathol 1987; 74: 300–306.

Y. Fukuyama, M. Osawa and K. Saito (Eds.), *Congenital Muscular Dystrophies*

267

Peripheral nerve dystroglycan: its function and potential role in the molecular pathogenesis of neuromuscular diseases

KIICHIRO MATSUMURA[1], HIROKI YAMADA[1], SACHIKO FUJITA[1],
HIROKO FUKUTA-OHI[1], TAKESHI TANAKA[2], KEVIN P. CAMPBELL[3]
and TERUO SHIMIZU[1]

[1]*Department of Neurology and Neuroscience, Teikyo University School of Medicine, Tokyo, Japan*
[2]*Saitama Red Cross Blood Center, Yono, Japan*
[3]*Howard Hughes Medical Institute and Department of Physiology & Biophysics, University of Iowa College of Medicine, Iowa City, USA*

Introduction

Dystrophin is a large cytoskeletal protein encoded by the Duchenne muscular dystrophy (DMD) gene [1,2]. In skeletal muscle, dystrophin exists in a large oligomeric complex tightly associated with several novel sarcolemmal proteins, including an extracellular glycoprotein of 156 kDa (α-dystroglycan) and a transmembrane glycoprotein of 50 kDa (adhalin) [3–8]. The 156 kDa α-dystroglycan binds laminin, a major component of the basement membrane [7,9,10]. It is heavily glycosylated, two-thirds of its molecular mass being accounted for by sugar residues [7,9,10]. The glycoprotein-binding site exists in the cysteine-rich/C-terminal domains of dystrophin [11,12]. Dystrophin also interacts with F-actin through the actin binding site(s) in the N-terminal domain [10,13–15]. These findings indicate that the dystrophin-glycoprotein complex spans the sarcolemma to link the subsarcolemmal actin-cytoskeleton with laminin meshwork in the basement membrane in skeletal muscle [6,7,10,16].

Utrophin, an autosomal homologue of dystrophin, is localized exclusively to the neuromuscular junction in adult skeletal muscle [17–19]. Utrophin, which has the cysteine-rich/C-terminal domains highly homologous to those of dystrophin [17], is associated with sarcolemmal proteins identical, or immunologically homologous to the dystrophin-associated proteins in the neuromuscular junction [19]. The recent demonstration that α-dystroglycan binds the basement membrane component agrin, which mediates the clustering of acetylcholine receptor in the neuromuscular junction, suggests that the utrophin-glycoprotein complex may play a role in peripheral synaptogenesis [20–23].

Distal transcripts of the DMD gene have been identified and their protein products have been shown to be expressed differently from the full-size 400 kDa dystrophin [24,28]. A protein of 71 kDa called Dp71 (also called apo-dystrophin-1) is expressed in non-muscle tissues, such as brain and liver [24–27]. A protein of 116 kDa called Dp116 (also called apo-dystrophin-2) is expressed in Schwann cells of peripheral nerve [28]. While physiological functions of these proteins remain unknown, the fact that both Dp71 and Dp116 share the cysteine-rich/C-terminal domains of dystrophin, which are involved in the interaction with the glycoprotein complex, suggests that Dp71 and Dp116 may exist in a similar complex as the dystrophin-glycoprotein complex of skeletal muscle.

Results

Here we report on (1) the status of expression of α-dystroglycan, adhalin, dystrophin and utrophin, and (2) the biochemical characterization of α-dystroglycan, in peripheral nerve [29, 30]. Immunohistochemical analysis demonstrated intense staining of peripheral nerve by antibodies against the C-terminal domains of dystrophin or utrophin [29]. Staining was positive surrounding myelin sheath of nerve fibers [29]. A similar staining pattern was obtained with antibody against α-dystroglycan [29]. In sharp contrast, antibody against the N-terminal domain of dystrophin and antibody against adhalin did not stain peripheral nerve [29].

On immunoblot analysis of SDS-extracts of peripheral nerve, antibodies against the C-terminal domains of dystrophin stained a band with a molecular mass of 110–120 kDa, but full-size 400 kDa dystrophin was not detected [29]. This 110–120 kDa band was not stained by antibody against the N-terminal domain of dystrophin [29]. These findings, together with the immunohistochemical data described above, indicate that this 110–120 kDa band is Dp116. Antibody against the C-terminus of utrophin, on the other hand, stained full-size

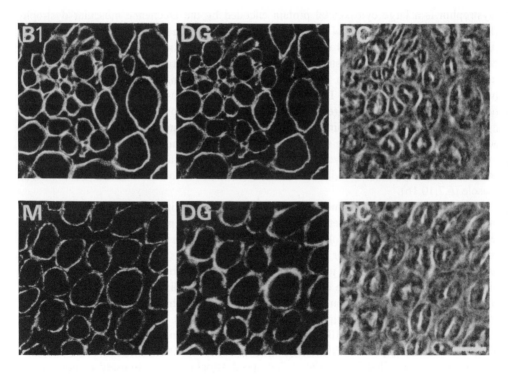

Fig. 1. Co-localization of dystroglycan and merosin in peripheral nerves. Shown are the double-immunostaining analyses of dystroglycan/merosin B1 chain and dystroglycan/merosin M chain. Confocal laser scanning microscopy fluorescent and phase-contrast (PC) images are shown. DG, B1 and M indicate dystroglycan, the M and B1 chains, respectively. Dystroglycan and merosin were co-localized surrounding myelin sheath of peripheral nerve fibers. Bar, 10 μm.

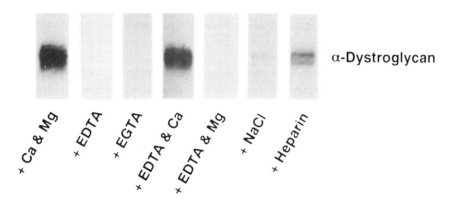

Fig. 2. Laminin-binding properties of peripheral nerve dystroglycan.. Nitrocellulose transfers of the digitonin extracts of peripheral nerve membranes were incubated, in the presence of 1 mM $CaCl_2$ and 1 mM $MgCl_2$, with mouse EHS laminin (+Ca and Mg). The binding of laminin to the 120 kDa peripheral nerve α-dystroglycan was inhibited by the inclusion of 10 mM EDTA (+EDTA) or EGTA (+EGTA) in the overlay medium. Addition of 20 mM $CaCl_2$ (+EDTA and Ca), but not 20 mM $MgCl_2$ (+EDTA and Mg), in the overlay medium containing 10 mM EDTA restored laminin binding. The binding of laminin was significantly reduced by the presence of 0.5 M NaCl (+NaCl) or 1 000-fold excess (wt/wt) of heparin (+Heparin) in the overlay medium.

400 kDa utrophin in peripheral nerve [29]. Antibody against α-dystroglycan stained a band of 120 kDa in peripheral nerve, while it stained a band of 156 kDa in skeletal muscle [29]. Antibody against adhalin did not stain a band in peripheral nerve while it stained a band of 50 kDa in skeletal muscle [29].

Taken together, these findings demonstrate the expression of Dp116, utrophin and α-dystroglycan surrounding myelin sheath of peripheral nerve fibers [29]. However, full-size dystrophin and adhalin are undetectable in peripheral nerve, suggesting that the putative complex which could involve Dp116, utrophin and α-dystroglycan may lack adhalin in peripheral nerve [29].

In the next step towards the elucidation of the cellular functions of this putative complex, we investigated the biochemical activities of the 120 kDa peripheral nerve α-dystroglycan. Immunocytochemical analysis demonstrated the co-localization of α-dystroglycan and merosin, a laminin heterotrimer comprised of the M, B1 and B2 chains [31–36], surrounding myelin sheath of peripheral nerve fibers (Fig. 1) [30]. Immunocytochemical analysis of teased peripheral nerve fibers demonstrated homogeneous staining for α-dystroglycan on the surface of myelin sheath but not in the node of Ranvier, suggesting the localization of α-dystroglycan in the outer membrane of myelin sheath [30].

Immunoblot analysis demonstrated that the 120 kDa α-dystroglycan was enriched in peripheral nerve membranes and was extracted by non-ionic detergent such as digitonin [30]. The 120 kDa α-dystroglycan was quantitatively absorbed by WGA-Sepharose, indicating that it is a membrane-associated glycoprotein with N-acetyineuraminic acid/N-acetylglucosamine residues [30]. In the presence of 1 mM $CaCl_2$ and 1 mM $MgCl_2$, laminin- and merosin-Sepharose removed the 120 kDa α-dystroglycan from the digitonin extracts of peripheral nerve membranes [30]. α-Dystroglycan was eluted by 10 mM EDTA [30]. When overlaid with laminin or merosin on the nitrocellulose transfers, the eluted α-dystroglycan bound both these proteins [30]. In order to confirm laminin and merosin binding of peripheral nerve α-dystroglycan, the nitrocellulose transfers of the digitonin extracts of peripheral nerve membranes were overlaid with laminin or merosin. The 120 kDa α-dystroglycan bound laminin and merosin in the presence of 1 mM $CaCl_2$ and 1 mM $MgCl_2$ (Fig. 2) [30]. The binding of laminin and merosin was inhibited by the inclusion of 10 mM EDTA or EGTA in the overlay medium (Fig. 2) [30]. Addition of 20 mM $CaCl_2$, but not 20 mM $MgCl_2$, in the overlay medium containing 10 mM EDTA restored binding of laminin and merosin (Fig. 2) [30]. These results demonstrate Ca^{2+}-dependency of binding of laminin and merosin. The binding of laminin and merosin was inhibited by the presence of 0.5 M NaCl or 1000-fold excess (wt/wt) of heparin in the overlay medium (Fig. 2) [30].

Discussion

Together, our results indicate that α-dystroglycan is a novel merosin-binding protein in peripheral nerve, most likely in the myelin sheath membrane. The size of α-dystroglycan varies among different tissues [7,9,10]. The molecular mass of peripheral nerve α-dystroglycan is comparable to that of brain form (120 kDa), and is smaller, by about 40 kDa, than that of striated muscle or lung form (156 kDa) [7,9,10,37]. This is presumed to be due to differences in the posttranslational modification, such as glycosylation, of α-dystroglycan [7,9,10,29,30]. However, the binding activities of laminin and merosin to the 120 kDa α-dystroglycan are similar to the laminin-binding activities of the 156 kDa α-dystroglycan [10,30].

Recently, the specific reduction of merosin M chain was demonstrated in skeletal muscle of patents with Fukuyama-type congenital muscular dystophy (FCMD), a disease characterized by brain anomaly and muscular dystophy [38]. The abnormality in the expression of α-dystroglycan in the sarcolemma of FCMD patients implicates the disturbance of the interaction between α-dystroglycan and merosin in the molecular pathogenesis of FCMD [39]. The M chain is also deficient in skeletal muscle and peripheral nerve of dy mice [40–42], which have muscular dystophy and peripheral nerve dysmyelination [40–42]. Intriguingly, laminin is known to promote Schwann cell myelination [43,44]. Furthermore, the expression of merosin is upregulated during development of peripheral nerve [31], and merosin is expressed in differentiated Schwann cell neoplasms, with the exception of 6 detectable in undifferentiated malignant Schwannomas [45]. These findings indicate that the expression of laminin/merosin in the basement membrane is associated with Schwann cell differentiation and myelination. Taken together, our results raise intriguing possibilities that α-dystroglycan may be involved in the regulation of Schwann cell myelination and that the disturbance of the interaction between α-dystroglycan and merosin may play a role in the pathogenesis of peripheral neuropathy in dy mice. At present it is unknown if α-dystroglycan exists in a complex associated with Dp116, utrophin or other dystrophin-associated proteins, or if this putative complex is involved in signal transduction. Further research is currently underway in our laboratory to address these important questions.

Finally, adhalin is deficient in the sarcolemma of patients with severe childhood autosomal recessive muscular dystrophy with DMD-like phenotype (SCARMD) [46–51], and all the dystrophin-associated proteins, including adhalin, are greatly reduced in the sarcolemma of DMD patients [12,52]. These findings suggest that the deficiency of adhalin may be the common denominator leading to muscle cell necrosis in these diseases [16,46]. Interestingly, SCARMD patients never present with nervous system dysfunction which is found in a substantial percentage of DMD patients. Taking our results into consideration, one hypothesis to explain this phenotypic difference could be that adhalin is not expressed in the nervous system [8,29,53,54], and thus, its specific deficiency causes only muscular dysfunction.

Acknowledgments

Kevin P. Campbell is an Investigator of the Howard Hughes Medical Institute. This work was supported by the Muscular Dystrophy Association, grants from Ichiro Kanahara Foundation, Nakatomi Foundation and Japan Foundation for Neuroscience and Mental Health, Research Grant (5A-2) for Nervous and Mental Disorders from the Ministry of Health and Welfare, and Grants-in-Aid for Scientific Research on Priority Areas, for Scientific Research (05454262, 06454280, 06670670 and 06770463) and for Scientific Research on developmental areas (05557037) from the Ministry of Education, Science and Culture.

References

1. Hoffman EP, Brown RH, Kunkel LM. Dystrophin: the protein product of the Duchenne muscular dystrophy locus. Cell 1987; 51: 919–928.
2. Koenig M, Monaco AP, Kunkel LM. The complete sequence of dystrophin predicts a rod-shaped cytoskeletal protein. Cell 1988; 53: 219–228.
3. Campbell KP, Kahl SD. Association of dystrophin with an integral membrane glycoprotein. Nature 1989; 338: 259–262.
4. Ervasti JM, Ohlendieck K, Kahl SD, Gaver MG, Campbell KP. Deficiency of glycoprotein component of the dystrophin complex in dystrophic muscle. Nature 1990; 345: 315–319.
5. Yoshida M, Ozawa E. Glycoprotein complex anchoring dystrophin to sarcolemma. J Biochem 1990; 108: 748–752.
6. Ervasti JM, Campbell KP. Membrane organization of the dystrophin-glycoprotein complex. Cell 1991; 66: 1121–1131.
7. Ibraghimov-Beskrovnaya O, Ervasti JM, Leveille CJ, Slaughter CA, Sernett SW, Campbell KP. Primary structure of dystrophin-associated glycoproteins linking dystrophin to the extracellular matrix. Nature 1992; 355: 696–702.
8. Roberds SL, Anderson RD, Ibraghimov-Beskrovnaya O, Campbell KP. Primary structure and muscle-specific expression of the 50 kDa dystrophin-associated glycoprotein (adhalin). J Biol Chem 1993; 268: 23739–23742.
9. Ibraghimov-Beskrovnaya O, Milatovich A, Ozcelik T, Yang B, Francke U, Campbell KP. Human dystroglycan: skeletal muscle cDNA, genomic structure, origin of tissue specific isoforms and chromosomal localization. Hum Mol Genet 1993; 2: 1651–1657.
10. Ervasti JM, Campbell KP. A role for the dystrophin-glycoprotein complex as a transmembrane linker between laminin and actin. J Cell Biol 1993; 122: 809–823.
11. Suzuki A, Yoshida M, Hayashi K, Mizuno Y, Hagiwara Y, Ozawa E. Molecular organization at the glycoprotein-complex-binding site of dystrophin: three dystrophin-associated proteins bind directly to the carboxy-terminal portion of dystrophin. Eur J Biochem 1994; 220: 283–292.
12. Matsumura K, Tome FMS, Ionasescu VV, et al. Deficiency of dystrophin-associated proteins in Duchenne muscular dystrophy patients lacking C-terminal domains of dystrophin. J Clin Invest 1993; 92: 866–871.
13. Levine BA, Moir AJD, Patchell VB, Perry SV. Binding-sites involved in the interaction of actin with the N-terminal region of dystrophin. FEBS Lett 1992; 298: 44–48.
14. Way M, Pope B, Cross RA, Kendrick-Jones J, Weeds AG. Expression of the N-terminal domain of dystrophin in *E. coli* and demonstration of binding to F-actin. FEBS Lett 1992; 301: 243–245.
15. Hemmings L, Kuhimann PA, Critchley DR. Analysis of actin-binding domain of α-actinin by mutagenesis and demonstration that dystrophin contains a functionally homologous domain. J Cell Biol 1992; 116: 1369–1380.

272

16. Matsumura K, Campbell KP. Dystrophin-glycoprotein complex: its potential role in the molecular pathogenesis of muscular dystrophies. Muscle Nerve 1994; 17: 2–15.

17. Tinsley JM, Blake DJ, Roche A, et al. Primary structure of dystrophin-related protein. Nature 1992; 360: 591–593.

18. Ohlendieck K, Ervasti JM, Matsumura K, Kahl SD, Leveille CJ, Campbell KP. Dystrophin-related protein is localized exclusively to neuromuscular junctions of adult skeletal muscle. Neuron 1991; 7: 499–508.

19. Matsumura K, Ervasti JM, Ohlendieck K, Kahl SD, Campbell KP. Association of dystrophin-related protein with dystrophin-associated proteins in mdx mouse muscle. Nature 1992; 360: 588–591.

20. Bowe MA, Deyst KA, Leszyk JD, Fallon JR. Identification and purification of an agrin receptor from torpedo postsynaptic membranes: a heteromeric complex related to the dystroglycans. Neuron 1994; 12: 1173–1180.

21. Campanelli JT, Roberds SL, Campbell KP, Scheller RH. A role for dystrophin-associated glycoproteins and utrophin in agrin-induced AChR clustering. Cell 1994; 77: 663–674.

22. Gee SH, Montanaro F, Lindenbaum MH, Carbonetto S. Dystroglycan-α, a dystrophin-associated glycoprotein, is a functional agrin receptor. Cell 1994; 77: 675–686.

23. Sugiyama J, Bowen DC, Hall ZW. Dystroglycan binds nerve and muscle agrin. Neuron 1994; 13: 103–115.

24. Blake DJ, Love DR, Tinsley J, et al. Characterization of a 4.8 kb transcript from the Duchenne muscular dystrophy locus expressed in Schwannoma cells. Hum Mol Genet 1992; 1: 103–3519.

25. Lederfein D, Levy Z, Augier N, et al. A 71 kd protein is a major product of the Duchenne muscular dystrophy gene in brain and other non-muscle tissues. Proc Natl Acad Sci USA 1992; 89: 5346–3350.

26. Hugnot JP, Gilgenkrantz H, Vincent N, et al. Distal transcript of the dystrophin gene initiated from an alternative first exon and encoding a 75 kDa protein widely distributed in nonmuscle tissues. Proc Natl Acad Sci USA 1992; 89: 7506–7510.

27. Fabbrizio E, Nudei U, Hugon G, Robert A, Pons F, Mornet D. Characterization and localization of a 77 kDa protein related to the dystrophin gene family. Biochem J 1994; 299: 359–365.

28. Byers TJ, Lidov HGW, Kunkel LM. An alternative dystrophin transcript specific to peripheral nerve. Nature Genet 1993; 4: 77–81.

29. Matsumura K, Yamada H, Shimizu T, Campbell KP. Differential expression of dystrophin, utrophin and dystrophin-associated proteins in peripheral nerve. FEBS Lett 1993; 334: 281–285.

30. Yamada H, Shimizu T, Tanaka T, Campbell KP, Matsumura K. Dystroglycan is a binding protein of laminin and merosin in peripheral nerve. FEBS Lett 1994; 352: 49–53.

31. Leivo I, Engvall E. Merosin, a protein specific for basement membranes of Schwann cells, striated muscle, and trophoblast, is expressed late in nerve and muscle development. Proc Natl Acad Sci USA 1988; 85: 1544–1548.

32. Ehrig K, Leivo I, Argraves WS, Rouslahti E, Engvall E. Merosin, a tissue-specific basement membrane protein, is a laminin-like protein. Proc Natl Acad Sci USA 1990; 87: 3264–3268.

33. Vuolteenaho R, Nissinen M, Sainio K, et al. Human laminin M chain (merosin): complete primary structure, chromosomal assignment, and expression of the M and A chain in fetal tissues. J Cell Biol 1994; 124: 381–394.

34. Sanes JR, Engvall E, Butkowski R, Hunter DD. Molecular heterogeneity of basal laminae: isoforms of laminin and collagen IV at the neuromuscular junction and elsewhere. J Cell Biol 1990; 111: 1685–1699.

35. Engvall E, Earwicker D, Haaparanta T, Ruoslahti E, Sanes JR. Distribution and isolation of four laminin variants; tissue restricted distribution of heterotrimers assembled from five different subunits. Cell Regul 1990; 1: 731–740.

36. Jaakkola S, Savunen O, Halme T, Uitto J, Peltonen J. Basement membranes during development of human nerve: Schwann cells and perineurial cells display marked changes in their expression profiles for laminin subunits and β1 and β4 integrins. J Neurocytol 1993; 22: 215–230.

37. Gee SH, Blacher RW, Douville PJ, Provost PR, Yurchenco PD, Carbonetto S. Laminin-binding protein 120 from brain is closely related to the dystrophin-associated glycoprotein, dystroglycan, and binds with high affinity to the major heparin binding domain of laminin. J Biol Chem 1993; 268: 14972–14980.

38. Hayashi YK, Engvall E, Arikawa-Hirasawa E, et al. Abnormal localization of laminin subunits in muscular dystrophies. J Neurol Sci 1993; 119: 53–64.

39. Matsumura K, Nonaka I, Campbell KP. Abnormal expression of dystrophin-associated proteins in Fukuyama-type congenital muscular dystrophy. Lancet 1993; 341: 521–522.

40. Arahata K, Hayashi YK, Koga R, et al. Laminin in animal models for muscular dystrophy: defect of laminin M in skeletal and cardiac muscles and peripheral nerve of the homozyous dystrophic *dy/dy* mice. Proc Jpn Acad B 1993; 69: 259–264.

41. Sunada Y, Bernier SM, Kozak CA, Yamada Y, Campbell KP. Deficiency of merosin in dystrophic *dy* mice and genetic linkage of laminin M chain gene to *dy* locus. J Biol Chem 1994; 269: 13729–13732.

42. Xu H, Christmas P, Wu X-R, Wewer UM, Engvall E. Defective muscle membrane and lack of M-laminin in the dystrophic *dy/dy* mouse. Proc Natl Acad Sci USA 1994; 91: 5572–5576.

43. Eldridge CF, Bunge MB, Bunge RP. Differentiation of axon-related Schwann cells *in vitro*. II. Control of myelin formation by basal lamina. J Neurosci 1989; 9: 625–628.

44. Reichardt LF, Tomaselli KJ. Extracellular matrix molecules and their receptors: functions in neural development. Ann Rev Neurosci 1991; 14: 531–570.

45. Leivo I, Engvall E, Laurila P, Miettinen M. Distribution of merosin, a laminin-related tissue-specific basement membrane protein, in human Schwann cell neoplasms. Lab Invest 1989; 61: 426–432.

46. Matsumura K, Tome FMS, Collin H, et al. Deficiency of the 50K dystrophin-associated glycoprotein in severe childhood autosomal recessive muscular dystrophy. Nature 1992; 359: 320–322.

47. Azibi K, Bachner L, Beckmann JS, et al. Severe childhood autosomal recessive muscular dystrophy with the deficiency of the 50 kDa dystrophin-associated glycoprotein maps to chromosome 13q12. Hum Mol Genet 1993; 2: 1423–1428.

48. Fardeau M, Matsumura K, Tome FMS, et al. Deficiency of the 50 kDa dystrophin associated glycoprotein (adhalin) in severe autosomal recessive muscular dystrophies in children native from European countries. CR Acad Sci Paris 1993; 316: 799–804.

49. Zatz M, Matsumura K, Vainzof M, et al. Assessment of the 50 kDa dystrophin-associated glycoprotein in Brazilian patients with severe childhood autosomal recessive muscular dystrophy. J Neurol Sci 1994; 123: 122–128.

50. Sewry CA, Sansome A, Matsumura K, Campbell KP, Dubowitz V. Deficiency of the 50 kDa dystrophin-associated glycoprotein and abnormal expression of utrophin in two south Asian cousins with variable expression of severe childhood autosomal recessive muscular dystrophy. Neuromusc Disord 1994; 4: 121–129.

51. Higuchi I, Yamada H, Fukunaga H, et al. Abnormal expression of laminin suggests disturbance of sarcolemma-extracellular matrix interaction in Japanese patients with autosomal recessive muscular dystrophy. J Clin Invest 1994; 94: 601–606.

52. Ohlendieck K, Matsumura K, Ionasescu VV, et al. Duchenne muscular dystrophy: deficiency of dystrophin-associated proteins in the sarcolemma. Neurology 1993; 43: 795–800.

53. Mizuno Y, Yoshida M, Yamamoto H, Hirai S, Ozawa E. Distribution of dystrophin isoforms and dystrophin-associated proteins 43DAG (A3a) and 50DAG (A2) in various monkey tissues. J Biochem 1993; 114: 936–941.

54. Yamamoto H, Mizuno Y, Hayashi K, Nonaka I, Yoshida M, Ozawa E. Expression of dystrophin-associated protein 35DAG (A4) and 50DAG (A2) is confined to striated muscles. J Biochem 1994; 115: 162–167.

Y. Fukuyama, M. Osawa and K. Saito (Eds.), *Congenital Muscular Dystrophies*
© 1997 Elsevier Science B.V. All rights reserved

Distribution and organization of utrophin and the laminin $\alpha 2$ chain in normal and dystrophic skeletal muscle fibers

VOLKER STRAUB[1], RALF HERRMANN[2], REGINALD BITTNER[3],
LOUISE ANDERSON[4], JEAN J. LÉGER[5] and THOMAS VOIT[2]

[1]*Department of Pediatrics, University of Düsseldorf, Moorenstrasse 5, D-40225 Düsseldorf, Germany*
[2]*Department of Paediatrics, University of Essen, Hufelandstr. 55, D-45122 Essen, Germany*
[3]*Institute of Anatomy, Department 3, University of Vienna, Waehringer Straße 13, A-1090 Vienna, Austria*
[4]*Muscular Dystrophy Group Research Laboratories, Regional Neurosciences Centre,
Newcastle General Hospital, Newcastle-upon-Tyne NE4 6BE, UK*
[5]*INSERM, Unité 300, Faculté de Pharmacie, Avenue Charles Flahaut, F-3400 Montpellier, France*

Introduction

Mutations of the X-chromosome encoded dystrophin gene may cause Duchenne muscular dystrophy (DMD) and the milder allelic Becker muscular dystrophy. Dystrophin, its 427 kD protein product, is a member of the spectrin-superfamily of large cytoskeletal proteins with significant sequence similarities between dystrophin, spectrins and α-actinins [1–3]. These proteins show conservation at their amino-terminal ends [4], where they are thought to bind to actin filaments, and across the central rod-domain. The sequence of the carboxyl-terminal end seemed to be unique to the protein until Love and colleagues screened a fetal muscle cDNA library with probes covering the carboxyl-terminal coding region of the dystrophin transcript [5]. They isolated a homologous cDNA which detected a 13 kb transcript in human fetal and adult muscle, and localized it to human chromosome band 6q24 and mouse chromosome 10 [5,6]. The protein product was first termed the DMD-like protein [7], dystrophin-related protein (DRP) [8–10], 6-dys [11], and recently, utrophin, due to its ubiquitous expression in human and mouse tissue [12]. Cloning and further sequence analysis revealed a high homology of utrophin over the N-terminal, rod, and C-terminal domains to dystrophin. Furthermore, studies of the neuromuscular junction (NMJ) region have demonstrated that utrophin may replace dystrophin as the cytoskeletal anchor of the dystrophin-glycoprotein complex (DGC). In the sarcolemmal DGC, dystrophin serves as the cytoskeletal linker between the actin-cytoskeleton and dystroglycan, a transmembrane component consisting of α- and β-subunits (156 and 43 kDa) [13]. Recently, direct interaction between dystrophin and β-dystroglycan has been demonstrated by in vitro binding studies and the interaction sites were narrowed down to the C-terminal 15 amino acids of β-dystroglycan and a large C-terminal region of dystrophin, encompassing the second half of hinge 4 and the cysteine-rich domain [14]. The heterotrimeric basement membrane protein laminin-2 is the extracellular ligand for α-dystroglycan at the sarcolemma [13]. Laminins are composed of three subunits: a 400 kDa heavy α chain and two distinct 200 kDa light chains designated as β and γ [15]. The laminins vary in their subunit structure and composition, and in their tissue distribution. Laminin-2 (merosin), which differs from laminin-1 in that the α1 chain is replaced by a partially homologous α2 chain, is predominantly expressed in skeletal muscle [15–17], and was shown to be deficient in congenital muscular dystrophy (CMD) of the classical or occidental type [18,19]. A subcomplex of four single transmembrane glycoproteins, called the sarcoglycan complex, is closely associated with the DGC. It consists of α-, β-, γ-, and δ-sarcoglycan components. Mutations in each of the four sarcoglycan genes have been shown to cause autosomal recessive limb-girdle muscular dystrophy [20–24].

In normal adult skeletal muscle, utrophin is expressed at low overall levels, being concentrated at NMJs and myotendinous junctions (MTJs). MTJs show similarities with synapses, where utrophin is colocalized with agrin-induced acetylcholine receptors [25]. Laser microscopical studies indicated that dystrophin and utrophin may exhibit slightly different distribution patterns at NMJs of normal muscle. In contrast to normal muscle, utrophin appears to spread out of the NMJ region, and is expressed throughout the sarcolemma in muscle fibers from DMD patients, *mdx* mice and dystrophin deficient fibers of female DMD-carriers. By means of immunofluorescence staining of single teased skeletal muscle fibers and semi-thin cryosections with specific antibodies against utrophin, we showed that utrophin is organized in a similar costameric network to that described for dystrophin in normal muscle, and seems to replace dystrophin in its spatial organization.

Because costameres form a structural linkage between contractile myofibrils and the extracellular environment, we also investigated the organization of laminin-2 in normal skeletal muscle, performing immunofluorescence staining of single teased muscle fibers with specific antibodies against the α2 chain of laminin-2.

Methods

Tissue sources

We examined human control subjects by observing muscle tissue obtained from orthopaedic surgery for non-muscle-related reasons. Muscle specimens from DMD patients and female DMD-carriers were obtained from diagnostic biopsies and had been shown to lack dystrophin completely, or to express the mosaic dystrophin staining pattern of female DMD-carriers on immunofluorescence staining [26,27]. We used diagnostic biopsy specimens from patients with a clinical picture of CMD, dysmyelination on brain magnetic resonance imaging, and histological evidence of muscular dystrophy as controls for laminin α2 chain staining of single teased fibers. Immunofluorescence analysis of skeletal muscle cryosections revealed complete lack of the laminin α2 chain in the CMD patients.

Western blotting

Western blotting was carried out as described [27,28]. Briefly, proteins from total muscle homogenates were resolved by sodium dodecyl sulfate-polyacrylamide gel electrophoresis on linear 4–20% gradient gels using a 3.5% stacking gel and then tank blotted onto nitrocellulose sheets as described. As a detection system after antibody incubation, we used peroxidase/diaminobenzidine. The amount of different proteins loaded per lane was controlled by laser densitometry (Ultro Scan X, Pharmacia LKB, Freiburg, Germany).

Single teased muscle fibers

Skeletal muscle specimens were carefully dissected immediately after removal and single muscle fibers were teased out in a phosphate-buffered saline (PBS) solution in the presence of protease inhibitors [24] before fixation in 0.3 M ethylacetimidate for 20 min (Sigma Chemical GmbH, Deisenhofen, Germany). After fixation, the fibers were placed on gelatin-coated glass slides and protein staining was performed with the primary antibodies in PBS for 2 h. Washing in PBS was followed by incubation with the biotinylated secondary antibodies for 1 h, and streptavidin Texas red (Amersham Buchler GmbH, Braunschweig, Germany) or streptavidin fluorescein isothiocyanate (FITC; Amersham Buchler GmbH, Braunschweig, Germany). Specimens stained for immunofluorescence were viewed and photographed under a Zeiss III RS photomicroscope equipped for epifluorescence.

Antibodies

For immunofluorescence and Western blotting, the following antibodies to dystrophin were used, as already described: dys1, dys2, and dys3 [30,31] (Novocastra Laboratories, Newcastle-upon-Tyne, UK). These monoclonal antibodies are specific for dystrophin and do not cross-react with utrophin expressed in the muscle of DMD patients who lack dystrophin. Monoclonal antibodies C.4G10 and H.5A3 raised against chicken dystrophin (rod domain and C-terminus, respectively) with known cross-reaction to utrophin were used for utrophin-detection by means of immunofluorescence in dystrophin-deficient muscle as described [32]. Furthermore, specific monoclonal antibodies were produced to selective fusion proteins expressing the C-terminal utrophin sequence in *E. coli* [33], and mAbs to utrophin (DRP1/12B6) were generated by immunizing CD1 mice with a synthetic peptide containing the C-terminal 11 amino acids of utrophin as described previously [34]. The primary antibodies were detected using biotinylated secondary antibodies and streptavidin Texas red or streptavidin FITC. For double staining, mouse monoclonal antibodies to utrophin were combined with rabbit polyclonal antibodies to α-actinin (ICN Biomedicals GmbH, Meckenheim, Germany). The specificity of anti-utrophin mAb DRP1/12B6, which exclusively labelled a 400 kDa band, was shown previously [35].

The monoclonal antibody, DRP1/12B6, also labelled blood vessels and intramuscular nerves in sections.

Monoclonal mouse anti-human merosin (M-chain) antibodies were commercially available (Chemicon International, Inc., Temecula, USA).

Double staining of dystrophin and utrophin in skeletal muscle from a female carrier of DMD was achieved by incubation with anti-utrophin mAb DRP1/12B6, followed by incubation with biotinylated anti-mouse IgG. A third incubation was carried out with a mixture of Texas red coupled to streptavidin, along with fluorescein conjugated anti-dystrophin purified mAbs [35].

Results

Staining of 5 μm cryosections of normal human skeletal muscle with monoclonal antibodies dys1, dys2, and dys3 revealed a homogenous dystrophin staining pattern around the entire muscle fibers (Fig. 1a). Using these antibodies to stain longitudinal semi-thin cryosections, dystrophin revealed the previously described periodic signal accumulation at the sar-

278

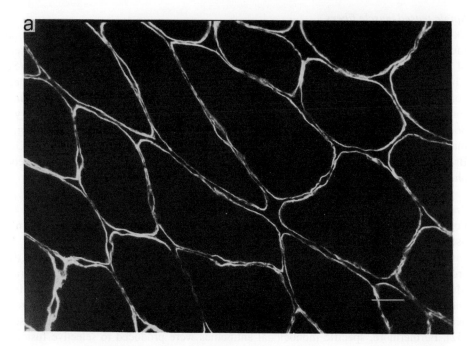

Fig. 1a.

Fig. 1b.

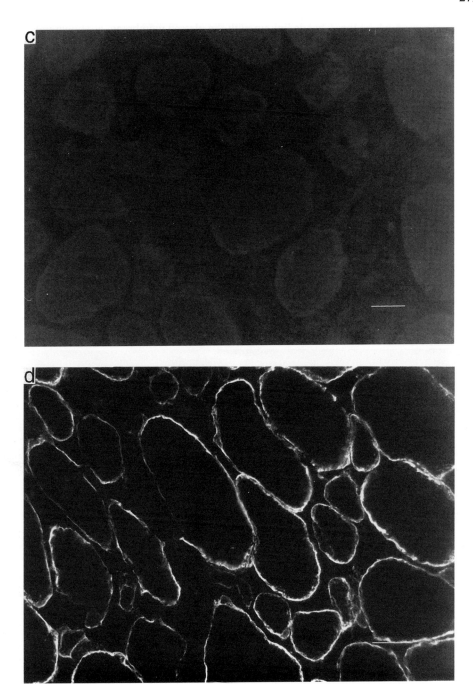

Fig. 1. Immunofluorescence labeling of 5 μm cryosections of normal muscle (a,b) and DMD muscle from a patient with dystrophin-deficiency (c,d) using antibodies to dystrophin and utrophin. (a,c) mAb dys 2 raised against the C-terminus of human dystrophin revealed homogenous expression of dystrophin around the sarcolemma of normal muscle fibers (a), but showed a complete lack of staining in DMD muscle (c). (b,d) mAb DRP1/12B6 raised against the C-terminus of utrophin demonstrated restriction of utrophin to the NMJs in normal muscle fibers (b), but showed utrophin expression around the entire sarcolemma of DMD muscle fibers (d). Bar, 10 μm.

280

colemma region where the Z-bands link up with the plasma membrane, as shown previously [29].

Staining of DMD muscle fibers showed no expression of dystrophin and served as a negative control for immunofluorescence (Fig. 1c).

Immunofluorescence staining of 5 μm cryosections showed that utrophin was localized almost exclusively to the NMJ region in normal human skeletal muscle, but was not detectable at the sarcolemma (Fig. 1b). The results of different groups suggested that utrophin represents a specialized form of dystrophin which is restricted to the membrane cytoskeleton underlying the NMJs [10,34].

In contrast to normal muscle, utrophin was homogenously expressed along the sarcolemma in cryosections of DMD muscle fibers (Fig. 1d). The reciprocal image on staining with anti-dystrophin and anti-utrophin antibodies, when muscle tissue of control subjects and DMD patients was compared, was in accordance with the results obtained by several groups [9,32,36,37].

It thus seemed that upregulation of utrophin occurred as a result of dystrophin deficiency. In order to further determine if this upregulation was a phenomenon occurring at the single skeletal fiber level, we investigated the expression of dystrophin and utrophin in skeletal muscle of female DMD carriers with known mosaicism of dystrophin expression, using double labeling (Fig. 2). In these biopsy specimens, the majority of fibers expressed dystro-

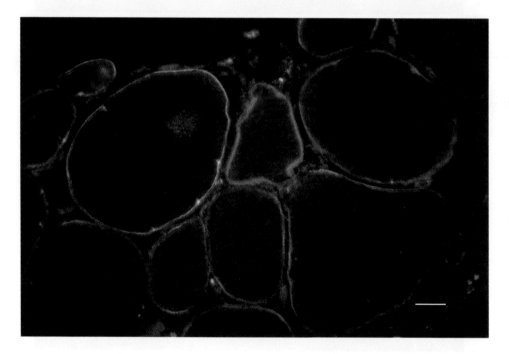

Fig. 2. Immunofluorescence double labeling of a 5 μm cryosection from a female carrier for DMD with monoclonal dys2 anti-dystrophin antibodies and monoclonal DRP1/12B6 anti-utrophin antibodies. Double exposure for dystrophin (FITC, green) and utrophin (Texas red) revealed combined expression of both proteins in an irregular fashion. Some fibers expressed dystrophin around their entire surface, while in others dystrophin was partly or not expressed at all around the fiber circumference. Reciprocal expression was seen for utrophin, with partial expression in partially dystrophin-deficient, and strong expression in completely dystrophin-deficient fibers. Bar, 10 μm.

phin with normal staining intensity, and these fibers characteristically lacked utrophin expression at the sarcolemma. In contrast, the majority of dystrophin-deficient fibers expressed utrophin on their fiber surface. Utrophin expression was strongest in dystrophin-negative fibers, which also expressed neonatal myosin (not shown) and were, therefore, thought to be regenerating fibers. In addition to these two fiber populations, some fibers showed reduced dystrophin expression as well as increased utrophin expression (Fig. 2). This coexpression of dystrophin and utrophin seemed to occur in reciprocal alternation over some areas of the sarcolemma but also as spatially inseparable coexpression, at the light microscopic level, in other areas. It thus seemed that utrophin upregulation in dystrophin-deficient muscle was indeed a phenomenon occurring at the single fiber level. We therefore attempted to determine the subcellular distribution of utrophin in these single fibers, in comparison to dystrophin.

By staining single teased muscle fibers, we had demonstrated that dystrophin forms a co-stameric network spanning the entire fiber. It consists of major transversal rings running perpendicular to the longitudinal axis of the muscle fiber and finer interspersed interconnections with transversal and longitudinal alignment relative to the long axis of the fiber (Fig. 3a) [29]. The protein scaffold of dystrophin was not evenly stained using immunofluorescence on single teased fibers, but was interrupted by round or oval-shaped dystrophin negative holes, which seemed to be surrounded by a dystrophin ring (Fig. 3a). These holes were shown to be occupied by peripheral myonuclei and therefore were called myonuclear lacunae [29].

Staining of single teased fibers of normal human skeletal muscle with specific antibodies against utrophin using immunofluorescence microscopy showed no detectable fiber surface staining in the absence of NMJs (Fig. 3b).

Because dystrophin is distributed in an uneven complex pattern around the muscle fiber surface [29,38,39], we were interested in the subcellular distribution of utrophin in dystrophin-deficient skeletal muscle. We obtained single teased muscle fiber preparations of DMD skeletal muscle and stained them for utrophin using specific, as well as cross-reacting, antibodies. The staining signals revealed an uneven distribution of utrophin on the muscle fiber surface similar to the distribution of dystrophin on normal skeletal muscle (Fig. 3c). The utrophin staining pattern displayed periodic organization in costameres running perpendicular to the long axis of the fibers and irregularly interspersed interconnections of lower intensity (Fig. 3c). As shown for the costameric dystrophin organization, the structure and orientation of these interconnections seemed to depend on the state of contraction of the fibers. The entire surface of DMD muscle fibers was covered by utrophin costameres except for areas where peripheral myonuclei were localized. Here the utrophin network was interrupted by utrophin-negative lacunae, which were surrounded by a utrophin ring and occupied by myonuclei (Fig. 3c).

To correlate the periodical staining pattern of utrophin costameres, with a distance of approximately 1.5–2.5 μm between the costameres, to the periodicity of the underlying contractile apparatus and the sarcomeres, we performed double labelling investigations [29]. Staining of longitudinal semi-thin cryosections of DMD skeletal muscle with antibodies against utrophin and α-actinin, a protein localized in the Z-disks of striated muscle, revealed focal concentration of utrophin at the region where the end of the Z-bands would link up with the plasma membrane (not shown). Double exposure for utrophin and α-actinin showed the one to one juxtapositioning of the predominant utrophin bands, seen as dots in the semi-thin cryosections, and the Z-bands. The fluorescent signals of lower intensity be-

282

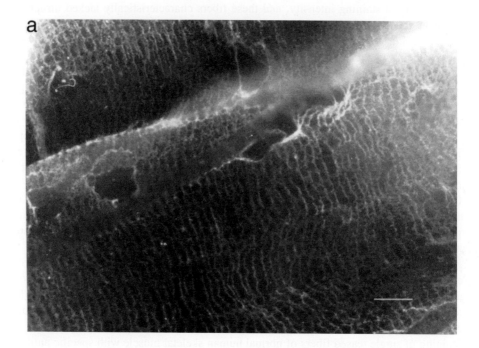

Fig. 3a.

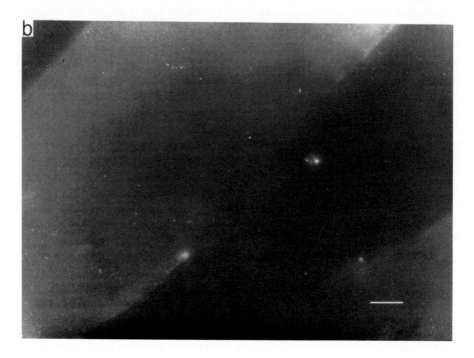

Fig. 3b.

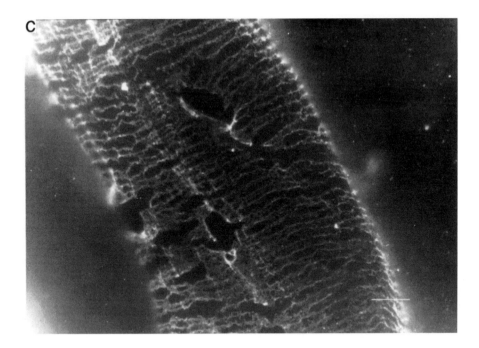

Fig. 3. Immunofluorescence labeling of single teased muscle fibers of normal muscle (a,b) and DMD muscle from a patient with dystrophin-deficiency (c) using monoclonal dys 2 anti-dystrophin antibodies and monoclonal DRP1/12B6 anti-utrophin antibodies. (a) The dystrophin staining pattern of normal muscle fibers (a) revealed a costameric network with major rings running transversal to the long axis of the fibers and myonuclear lacunae. (b,c) The utrophin staining pattern displayed reciprocal expression with a lack of staining in normal muscle fibers (b), but showed a costameric network with myonuclear lacunae on DMD muscle fibers (c). Bar, 10 μm.

tween the major utrophin accumulations probably corresponded to the fine interconnections of the costameric network seen in single teased muscle fibers. If areas of the sarcolemma were in the plane of the section, the costameric network of utrophin was detected on semi-thin cryosections as well. If it happened that a myonucleus was in the plane of the section, double staining of semi-thin cryosections confirmed that in the presence of peripheral myonuclei the assumed insertion of the Z-bands into the sarcolemma was prevented and the staining pattern of utrophin changed (not shown).

From these results, which showed reciprocal expression of dystrophin and utrophin on normal and dystrophin-deficient skeletal muscle, it seems that utrophin may partly compensate for the absence of dystrophin in DMD muscles in preventing dystrophic changes. The pathological dystrophic alterations in DMD muscle, however, were present in dystrophin-deficient fibers, although utrophin had developed the characteristic costameric organization, surrounding the entire fibers. In utrophin-positive single teased fibers of DMD muscle, we sometimes found structural disintegration of the utrophin network (Fig. 3c), depending on the pathological stage of muscle fiber degeneration in the dystrophic muscle. Some fibers just exhibited a dispersed, unsteady structure of the costameric scaffold, whereas others showed a stage of pathology with focal disintegration and partial loss of the costameres or longitudinal clefts emanating from the myonuclei and splitting the sarcolemma. On fibers in the final dystrophic stage, there was a complete loss of the periodical, regular costameric

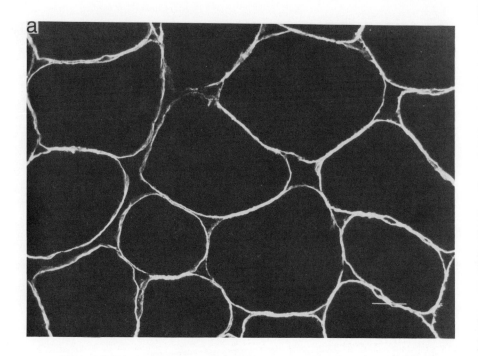

Fig. 4a.

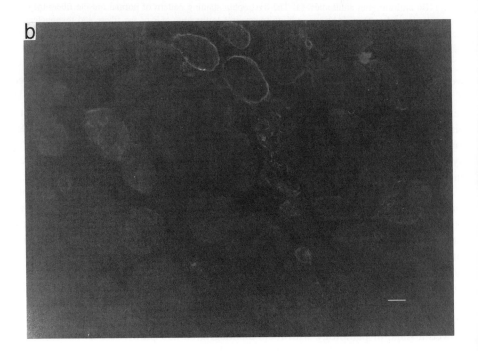

Fig. 4b.

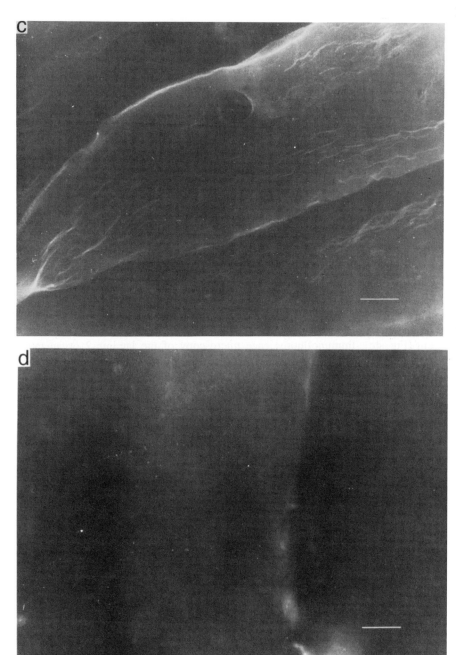

Fig. 4. Immunofluorescence labeling of normal skeletal muscle (a,c) and skeletal muscle from a patient with merosin-deficient CMD of the classical or occidental type (b,d) using monoclonal antibodies against merosin. (a,b) Immunofluorescence staining of 5 μm cryosections with monoclonal anti-merosin antibodies revealed homogenous expression of merosin around the sarcolemma of normal muscle fibers (a), but showed a complete lack of staining in CMD muscle except for some isolated fibers which were weakly positive for merosin (b). (c,d) Staining of single teased muscle fibers with anti-merosin antibodies demonstrated the homogenous expression of merosin (c), but showed a lack of merosin expression on the surface of CMD skeletal muscle fibers (d). Bar, 10 μm.

organization of utrophin. No comparable changes were found in single teased fibers of normal skeletal muscle and, therefore, these changes did not seem to be due to preparation artefacts.

Colocalization of membrane-associated proteins, such as dystrophin and vinculin, to costamere sites imply that costameres are composite structures, containing one set of proteins whose function is to anchor the Z-discs to the sarcolemma, and another set of proteins involved in mechanically coupling the Z-discs to the extracellular matrix (ECM) [40]. As laminin-2 forms the extracellular binding site of the DGC in normal skeletal muscle, we were interested in the subcellular distribution of laminin-2 on the fiber surface. Immunocytochemical investigations using specific anti-α2 chain antibodies showed uniform labelling around normal human skeletal muscle fibers in 5–7 μm cryosections (Fig. 4a), as well as labelling of intramuscular nerves. In contrast, there was no such labelling in a group of patients with CMD of the classical or occidental type (Fig. 4b).

Performing indirect immunofluorescence microscopy of single teased skeletal muscle fibers, we wanted to determine whether laminin-2 was organized in a costameric network as described for dystrophin in normal and utrophin in DMD-muscle, or whether this expression pattern was specifically restricted to components of the subsarcolemmal cytoskeleton. Immunocytochemical analysis of the α2 chain of laminin-2 on single teased fibers of normal human skeletal muscle revealed non-costameric, homogenous expression of this extracellular protein (Fig. 4c). Immunofluorescence microscopy of the laminin-2 organization did not show any structural alignment regarding the longitudinal or transversal axis of the muscle fibers. Laminin-2 coated the muscle fiber surface evenly and without interruption (Fig. 4c).

Control single teased fibers from α2 chain-deficient CMD patients did not reveal fiber surface staining with antibodies to the α2 chain (Fig. 4d), but the costameric expression of dystrophin was preserved (not shown).

Discussion

Costameres, submembranous transverse ribs, are composite structures made up of several different protein components, and were first described by Pardo and co-workers as vinculin-containing, electrodense plaques, located between the cell membrane and Z-discs in cardiac muscle and certain types of skeletal muscle [41]. The term "costamere" was used to characterize the rib-like distribution of vinculin when immunostained with an anti-vinculin antibodies. Recently, we were able to show a comparable costameric organization for dystrophin on normal human and mouse skeletal muscle [29], and similar results were obtained by other groups [38,39]. Dystrophin showed a sarcomeric distribution; that is, linear arrays of bands or rings, aligned perpendicularly to the longitudinal axis of the myofibrils, with a spacing of approximately 1.5–2.5 μm, the distance between adjacent Z-lines. Double staining for dystrophin and α-actinin, a major component of the Z-lines, in semi-thin cryosections revealed one to one juxtapositioning of the dystrophin costameres and the Z-lines of the subjacent myofibrils. It was speculated that in so far as costameres may be a link between the sarcolemma and the underlying contractile apparatus, and may thereby allow the lateral transmission of force along the myofibers, dystrophin might play an important role in sarcolemmal stabilization. Thus the absence of dystrophin results in sarcolemmal instability and eventually leads to muscle cell necrosis.

Utrophin and dystrophin exhibit great sequence homology and have similar molecular weights, however, they differ in both their tissue distribution and expression in DMD. While utrophin is ubiquitously expressed, it is localized exclusively to NMJs in normal adult skeletal muscle. In contrast to normal muscle, utrophin was homogeneously expressed along the sarcolemma in $5\,\mu$m cryosections of DMD muscle fibers. The reciprocal image on staining with anti-dystrophin and anti-utrophin antibodies, when muscles of control subjects and DMD patients were compared, was demonstrated by several groups [9,32,36,37]. This was further corroborated by our double staining results for dystrophin and utrophin on muscle fibers of female carriers for DMD, which showed that utrophin upregulation occurs in dystrophin-deficient fibers at the single fiber level.

Interestingly, our single fiber preparation results showed that utrophin was expressed throughout the sarcolemma in the form of a costameric network in muscle fibers from DMD patients. The costameric organization of utrophin seen on single teased muscle fibers of DMD patients was indistinguishable from that seen for dystrophin in normal skeletal muscle.

Double staining of semi-thin cryosections of DMD muscle fibers for utrophin and α-actinin confirmed the sarcomeric arrangement of utrophin and the one to one juxtaposition of the major transversal utrophin rings to the underlying adjacent Z-lines. The same subcellular localization of utrophin to the inner face of the plasma membrane of DMD muscle to that of dystrophin in normal muscle was previously demonstrated by immunoelectron microscopy [50].

The identification of utrophin, with its sequence homology to the carboxyl-terminal domain of dystrophin, has led to the investigation of the functional similarity of these related proteins. Kevin Campbell's group showed that dystrophin, isolated from skeletal muscle membranes using wheat germ agglutination chromatography, was found to exist in a large, tightly associated oligomeric complex of proteins and glycoproteins [42–44]. The carboxyl-terminal domain of dystrophin appears to be functionally critical in that its absence is associated with a severe clinical phenotype, and it is involved in the binding of dystrophin to the sarcolemma via the DGC [14]. The similar costameric network of utrophin in DMD muscle to that of dystrophin in normal skeletal muscle supports the idea that the two proteins could have the same binding epitope to bind to the sarcolemma. It was shown that the corresponding site of utrophin shares 80% of the amino acid-sequence of the DGC-anchoring site of dystrophin [45], and Matsumura and co-workers demonstrated the association of utrophin with a complex of glycoproteins which seemed to be the same or similar complex of glycoproteins to the one associated with dystrophin [46].

Bittner and co-workers reported two patients with large intragenic in frame deletions, who were still able to express grossly truncated, but stable dystrophin molecules with preserved C-terminal domains. These semi-functional proteins still bound through the DGC-binding sites to the sarcolemma and thus prevented sarcolemmal expression of utrophin, thereby supporting the idea that "available" DGC binding sites are necessary for sarcolemmal expression of utrophin [47].

Whereas the amount of the sarcoglycans is markedly reduced in DMD muscle [22,43,48–50], it was shown by Ozawa's group that β-dystroglycan was distinctly preserved [49]. It has also been demonstrated that β-dystroglycan binds directly to dystrophin [14,51,52]. Tinsley and colleagues have shown that the locus of utrophin corresponding to the anchoring site of dystrophin exhibits 80% amino acid homology [45] and combined with the costameric network of utrophin, it seems plausible that utrophin provides an anchoring site for β-dystroglycan in a manner similar to dystrophin anchoring. As costameres form a mechanical linkage between the contractile myofibrils and the ECM, these data suggest that the DGC may be involved in maintaining sarcolemmal stabilization and integrity, and destruction of the costameric organization would lead to damage of the plasma membrane, followed by dystrophic muscle changes. The group of Kay Davies has recently demonstrated that the expression of high levels of utrophin in *mdx* mice leads to the restoration of all of the DGC components [53]. Furthermore, they showed evidence that muscle pathology in *mdx* mice was corrected by utrophin overexpression. These results provide the first evidence that, at least in mice, utrophin can functionally replace dystrophin.

Interestingly, our results for laminin-2 expression around the muscle fiber surface demonstrated that the extracellular binding site of the DGC is not organized in the form of a costameric network. Until now it was not known whether the costameric organization of proteins is restricted to elements of the subsarcolemmal cytoskeleton or involves components of the ECM. It was supposed that absence of the laminin α2 chain could disrupt the linkage between the subsarcolemmal cytoskeleton and the ECM, according to a mechanism common to DMD and the sarcoglycan deficient limb-girdle muscular dystrophies.

However, the dystrophin scaffold remained intact in the laminin α2 chain-deficient CMD muscle fibers we looked at, indicating that a laminin α2 chain deficiency does not primarily cause disruption or disorganization of the costameric network. On the other hand, the even, non-costameric organization of the laminin α2 chain on the fiber surface also indicates important interaction with other proteins which are non-costameric in their distribution. While the existing evidence shows that alterations of the skeletal muscle sarcolemma due to extracellular (laminin-2), intramembrane (sarcoglycans) or intracellular (dystrophin) components can cause muscular dystrophy, modulating factors which would explain the differences in the clinical features of these forms of muscular dystrophy remain to be identified.

Acknowledgments

This study was supported by a grant from the Deutsche Forschungsgemeinschaft (Vo 392/2–3). We are grateful to Andrea Lauterbach for her excellent technical assistance.

References

1. Davison MD, Critchely DR. Alpha-actinins and the DMD protein contain spectrin-like repeats. Cell 1988; 52: 159–260.
2. Blanchard A, Ohanian V, Critchely D. The structure and function of α-actinin. J Muscle Res Cell Motil 1989; 10: 280–289.
3. Koenig M, Kunkel LM. Detailed analysis of the repeat domain of dystrophin reveals four potential hinge segments that may confer flexibility. J Biol Chem 1990; 265:4560–4566.
4. Byers TJ, Husain-Chishiti A, Dubreuil RR, Branton D, Goldstein LSB. Sequence similarity of the amino-terminal domain of *Drosophila* beta spectrin to alpha actinin and dystrophin. J Cell Biol 1989; 109: 1633–1641.
5. Love DR, Hill DF, Dickson G, et al. An autosomal transcript in skeletal muscle with homology to dystrophin. Nature 1989; 339: 55–58.
6. Buckle VJ, Guenet JL, Simon-Chazottes D, Love DR, Davies KE. Localization of a dystrophin-related autosomal gene to 6q24 in man and to mouse chromosome 10 in the region of the dystrophia muscularis (dy) locus. Hum Genet 1990; 85: 324–326.

7. Spence MA, Spurr NK, Field LL. Report of the committee on the genetic constitution of chromosome 6. Cytogenet Cell Genet 1989; 51: 149–165.

8. Khurana TS, Hoffman EP, Kunkel LM. Identification of a chromosome 6-encoded dystrophin-related protein. J Biol Chem 1990; 265: 16717–16720.

9. Khurana TS, Watkins SC, Chafey P, et al. Immunolocalization and developmental expression of dystrophin related protein in skeletal muscle. Neuromusc Disord 1991; 1: 185–194.

10. Ohlendieck K, Ervasti JM, Matsumura K, Kahl SD, Leveille CJ, Campbell KP. Dystrophin-related protein is localized to neuromuscular junctions of skeletal muscle. Neuron 1991; 7: 1–20.

11. Ishiura S, Arahata K, Tsukahara T, et al. Antibody against the C-terminal portion of dystrophin crossreacts with the 400 kDa protein in the pia mater of dystrophin-deficient *mdx* mouse brain. J Biochem 1990; 107: 510–513.

12. Blake DJ, Love DR, Tinsley J, et al. Characterization of a 4,8 kb transcript from the Duchenne muscular dystrophy locus expressed in Schwannoma cells. Hum Mol Genet 1992; 1: 103–109.

13. Henry MD, Campbell KP. Dystroglycan: an extracellular matrix receptor linked to the cytoskeleton. Curr Opin Cell Biol 1996; 8: 625–631.

14. Jung D, Yang B, Meyer J, Chamberlain JS, Campbell KP. Identification and characterization of the dystrophin anchoring site on β-dystroglycan. J Biol Chem 1995; 270: 27305–27310.

15. Engvall E. Laminin variants: why, where and when? Kidney Int 1993; 43: 2–4.

16. Engvall E, Earwicker D, Haaparanta T, Ruoslahti E, Sanes JR. Distribution and isolation of four laminin variants; tissue restricted distribution of heterodimers assembled from five subunits. Cell Regul 1990; 1: 731–740.

17. Sanes JR, Engvall E, Butkowski R, Hunter DD. Molecular heterogeneity of basal laminae: isoforms of laminin and collagen IV at the neuromuscular junction and elsewhere. J Cell Biol 1990; 11: 1685–1699.

18. Tomé FMS, Evangelista T, Leclerc A, et al. Congenital muscular dystrophy with merosin deficiency. C R Acad Sci 1994; 317: 351–357.

19. Helbling-Leclerc A, Zhang X, Topaloğlu H, et al. Mutations in the laminin α2-chain gene (LAMA2) cause merosin-deficient congenital muscular dystrophy. Nat Genet 1995; 11:216–218.

20. Roberds SL, Leturcq F, Allamand V, et al. Missense mutations in the adhalin gene linked to autosomal recessive muscular dystrophy. Cell 1994; 78: 625–633.

21. Bönnemann CG, Modi R, Noguchi S, et al. β-sarcoglycan (A3b) mutations cause autosomal recessive muscular dystrophy with loss of the sarcoglycan complex. Nat Genet 1995; 11: 266–272.

22. Lim LE, Duclos F, Broux O, et al. β-sarcoglycan: characterization and role in limb-girdle muscular dystrophy linked to 4q12. Nat Genet 1995; 11: 257–265.

23. Nigro V, de Sá Moreira E, Piluso G, et al. Autosomal recessive limb-girdle muscular dystrophy, LGMD2F, is caused by a mutation in the δ-sarcoglycan gene. Nat Genet 1996; 14: 195–198.

24. Noguchi S, McNally EM, Othmane KB, et al. Mutations in the dystrophin-associated protein γ-sarcoglycan in chromosome 13 muscular dystrophy. Science 1996; 270: 819–822.

25. Campanelli JT, Roberds SL, Campbell KP, Scheller RH. A role for dystrophin-associated glycoproteins and utrophin in agrin-induced AChR clustering. Cell 1994; 77: 663–674.

26. Koenig M, Monaco AP, Kunkel LM. The complete sequence of dystrophin predicts a rod-shaped cytoskeletal protein. Cell 1988; 53: 219–228.

27. Voit T, Stüttgen P, Cremer M, Goebel HH. Dystrophin as a diagnostic marker in Duchenne and Becker muscular dystrophy. Correlation of immunofluorescence and Western blot. Neuropediatrics 1991; 22: 152–162.

28. Voit T, Patel K, Dunn MJ, Dubowitz V, Strong PN: Distribution of dystrophin, nebulin and Ricinus communis I (RCA I)-binding glycoprotein in tissues of normal and *mdx* mice. J Neurol Sci 1989; 89: 199–211.

29. Straub V, Bittner RE, Léger JJ, Voit T. Direct visualization of the dystrophin network on skeletal muscle fiber membrane. J Cell Biol 1992; 119: 1183–1191.

30. Nicholson LVB, Davison K, Falkous G, et al. Dystrophin in skeletal muscle I. Western blot analysis using a monoclonal antibody. J Neurol Sci 1989; 94: 125–136.

31. Nicholson LVB, Johnson MA, Davison K, et al. Dystrophin or a "related protein" in Duchenne muscular dystrophy? Acta Neurol Scand 1992; 86: 8–14.

32. Voit T, Haas K, Leger JOC, Pons F, Léger JJ. Xp21 dystrophin and 6q dystrophin-related protein. Am J Pathol 1991; 139: 969–976.

33. Fabbrizio E, Leger J, Anoal M, Léger JJ, Mornet D. Monoclonal antibodies targeted against the C-terminal domain of dystrophin or utrophin. FEBS Lett 1993; 322: 10–14.

34. Pons F, Nicholson LVB, Robert A, Voit T, Léger JJ. Dystrophin and dystrophin-related protein (utrophin) distribution in normal and dystrophin-deficient skeletal muscles. Neuromusc Disord 1993; 3: 507–514.

35. Love DR, Morris GE, Ellis JM, et al. Tissue distribution of the dystrophin-related gene product and expression in the *mdx* and *dy* mouse. Proc Natl Acad Sci USA 1991; 88: 3243–3247.

36. Helliwell TR, Man NT, Morris GE, Davies KE. The dystrophin-related protein, utrophin, is expressed on the sarcolemma of regenerating human skeletal muscle fibres in dystrophies and inflammatory myopathies. Neuromusc Disord 1992; 3: 177–184.

37. Porter GA, Dymtrenko GM, Winkelmann JC, Bloch RJ. Dystrophin colocalizes with B-spectrin in distinct subsarcolemmal domains in mammalian skeletal muscle. J Cell Biol 1992; 117: 997–1005.

38. Bewick GS, Nicholson LVB, Young C, O'Donell E, Slater CR. Different distribution of dystrophin and related proteins at nerve-muscle junctions. NeuroReport 1992; 3: 857–860.

39. Minetti C, Beltrame F, Marcenaro G, Bonilla E. Dystrophin at the plasma membrane of human muscle fibers shows a costameric localization. Neuromusc Disord 1992; 2: 99–109.

40. Danowski BA, Imanaka-Yoshida K, Sanger JM, Sanger JW. Costameres are sites of force transmission to the substratum in adult rat cardiomyocytes. J Cell Biol 1992; 118: 1411–1420.

41. Pardo JV, Siciliano JD, Craig SW. A vinculin-containing cortical lattice in skeletal muscle: transverse lattice elements ("costameres") mark sites of attachment between myofibrils and sarcolemma. Proc Natl Acad Sci USA 1983; 80: 1008–1012.

42. Campbell KP, Kahl SD. Association of dystrophin and an integral membrane glycoprotein. Nature 1989; 338: 259–262.

43. Ervasti JM, Ohlendieck K, Kahl SD, Gaver MG, Campbell KP. Deficiency of a glycoprotein component of the dystrophin complex in dystrophic muscle. Nature 1990; 345: 315–319.

44. Ohlendieck K, Ervasti JM, Snook JB, Campbell KP. Dystrophin-glycoprotein complex is highly enriched in isolated skeletal muscle sarcolemma. J Cell Biol 1991; 112: 135–148.

45. Tinsley JM, Blake DJ, Roche A, et al. Primary structure of dystrophin-related protein. Nature 1992; 360: 591–593.

46. Matsumura K, Ervasti JM, Ohlendieck K, Kahl SD, Campbell KP. Association of dystrophin-related protein with dystrophin-associated proteins in mdx mouse muscle. Nature 1992; 360: 588–591.

47. Bittner RE, Shorny S, Ferlings R, et al. Sarcolemmal expression of dystrophin C-terminus but reduced expression of 6q-dystrophin-related protein in two DMD patients with large deletions of the dystrophin gene. Neuromusc Disord 1995; 5: 81–92.

48. Ibraghimov-Breskrovnaya O, Ervasti JM, Leveille CJ, Slaughter CA, Sernett SW, Campbell KP. Primary structure of dystrophin-associated glycoproteins linking dystrophin to the extracellular matrix. Nature 1992; 355: 696–702.

49. Mizuno Y, Yoshida M, Nonaka I, Hirai S, Ozawa E. Expression of utrophin (dystrophin-related protein) and dystrophin-associated glycoproteins in muscle from patients with Duchenne muscular dystrophy. Muscle Nerve 1994; 17: 206–216.

50. Jung D, Duclos F, Apostol B, et al. Characterization of δ-sarcoglycan, a novel component of the oligomeric sarcoglycan complex involved in limb-girdle muscular dystrophy. J Biol Chem 1996; 271: 32321–32329.

51. Yoshida M, Ozawa E. Glycoprotein complex anchoring dystrophin to sarcolemma. J Biochem 1990; 108: 748–752.

52. Suzuki A, Yoshida M, Hayashi K, Mizuno Y, Hagiwara Y, Ozawa E. Molecular organization at the glycoprotein-complex-binding site of dystrophin. Three dystrophin-associated proteins bind directly to the carboxy terminal binding site of dystrophin. Eur J Biochem 1994; 220: 283–292.

53. Tinsley JM, Potter AC, Phelps SR, Fisher R, Trickett JI, Davies KE. Amelioration of the dystrophic phenotype of *mdx* mice using a truncated utrophin transgene. Nature 1996; 384: 349–353.

Y. Fukuyama, M. Osawa and K. Saito (Eds.), *Congenital Muscular Dystrophies*
291

CHAPTER 24

Laminin in animal models for muscular dystrophy: deficiency of the laminin α2 chain in the homozygous dystrophic dy/dy mouse

KIICHI ARAHATA[1], YUKIKO K. HAYASHI[1], RITSUKO KOGA[1], HIROKO ISHII[2] and TETSUYA MATSUZAKI[1]

[1]*National Institute of Neuroscience, NCNP, Tokyo, Japan*
[2]*Tokyo Metropolitan Higashiyamato Medical Center for Disabilities, Tokyo, Japan*

Introduction

We have previously shown a significant reduction in the amount of the laminin α2 (or M) chain (a tissue-restricted basal lamina protein expressed in striated muscle, Schwann cells and placental trophoblasts) in the skeletal muscle in Fukuyama type congenital muscular dystrophy (FCMD) [1]. To examine the role of laminin α2 chain in the process of muscular dystrophies, we examined the changes of laminin α2 and other protein components of the basal lamina, together with the membrane-associated cytoskeletal proteins, dystrophin and utrophin, in the C57BL/6J-*dy/dy* mouse and other animal models of muscular dystrophy [2].

A progressive fatal murine muscular dystrophy was discovered to be due to a spontaneous mutation in the strain 129 mouse at the Jackson Laboratories in 1955, and was designated as dystrophia muscularis (*dy*) [3]. The disease is transmitted in an autosomal recessive manner and the gene responsible for *dy* has been assigned to mouse chromosome 10, where the gene for utrophin is located [4]. Utrophin, however, is present in the muscle membrane of the *dy/dy* mouse [5]. In a milder allelic dystrophic mouse (*dy²ᴶ*), a mutation in the α2 chain has been identified [6]. Dystrophin and/or dystrophin-associated glycoproteins (DAGs) have been well studied in muscular dystrophy models, e.g., the *mdx* mouse [7–9], BIO 14.6 hamster [10,11], line 413 chicken [12], and *dy/dy* mouse [5]. The homozygous affected *dy/dy* mouse shows morphological similarities to severe human muscular dystrophies such as Duchenne (DMD) and FCMD types, except dysmyelination in the proximal part of sciatic nerves and the ventral and dorsal spinal roots in the *dy/dy* mouse [13–15].

Materials and methods

Materials

Tissue specimens from dystrophic homozygous *dy/dy* mice (C57BL/6J-*dy/dy*) were obtained as described previously [2]. Tissues from dystrophic chicken (line 413), hamster (BIO 14.6), and mouse (*mdx*) were studied together. All samples were flash frozen in isopentane chilled with liquid nitrogen.

Antibodies

The rabbit anti-laminin $\alpha2$ chain antiserum was raised against the 14-mer peptide (CNNFGLDLKADDKI) deduced from the human $\alpha2$ chain cDNA sequence (2456–2468) with an extra Cys to the N-terminus. Antibodies against type IV collagen (Advance Inc., Tokyo) and dystrophin 6–10 were also used simultaneously. Affinity-purified fluorescent isothiocyanate (FITC)-labeled goat F(ab')^2 anti-mouse and anti-rabbit IgG were obtained from Tago Inc., and used as second layer antibodies. Preimmune rabbit serum and control mouse myeloma IgG served as controls.

Immunocytochemistry

Immunocytochemical analysis of each muscle sample was accomplished as described [1], using the antibodies.

Immunoblot analysis of the laminin $\alpha2$ chain

Immunoblot detection of the $\alpha2$ chain was performed as described previously [1]. In brief, skeletal muscle laminin $\alpha2$ chain was extracted with EDTA-containing buffers. Samples were transferred to nitrocellulose sheets and allowed to react with the anti-laminin $\alpha2$ antiserum overnight, and then visualized with an ABC kit (Vector Lab., USA).

Analysis of laminin $\alpha2$ chain mRNA

Total RNA was extracted from biopsied muscle samples by the acid guanidium thiocyanate-phenol-chloroform (AGPC) method. The reverse transcription polymerase chain reaction (RT-PCR) method was used to analyze expression of the $\alpha2$ chain in the skeletal muscle. We designed primer sets for the human $\alpha2$ chain mRNA. We also designed two primer sets, for beta-actin and muscle-specific creatine kinase (CK) cDNA, as internal standards. Two μg (5 μl) of total RNA was primed with 2 μl (1 OD/ml) of random hexamers at 70°C for 10 min, and then transcribed to cDNA copy, using 1 μl (200 U/μl) of M-MLV-Reverse Transcriptase (GIBCO/BRL), as recommended in the manufacturer's protocol, and then diluted to 100 μl with distilled water. A 5.0 μl aliquot of cDNA was then used as a template for each PCR amplification in a reaction mixture of 50 μl, using reagents from Takara Co. Ltd., with 100 ng of each primer, 2.5 units of rTaq polymerase and dNTPs. The amplification conditions were as follows: 94°C, 3 min for denaturation, followed by 30 cycles of 94°C, 1 min; 55°C, 1 min; 72°C, 1 min 30 sec (step cycle), with a final elongation cycle for 5 min. Reverse transcriptase was omitted to examine genomic DNA contamination. The reaction products (15 μl) were separated on 1.2% agarose gel and then visualized with ethidium bromide. The gels were subsequently subjected to Southern hybridization with cDNA probes for the human $\alpha2$ chain. The amplified DNA was transferred to Hybond N+ (Amersham), and hybridization was allowed to proceed overnight at 65°C. The membrane was then thoroughly washed in 1× SSC/0.1% SDS for 1 h at 60°C, followed by ECL direct nucleic acid labeling and detection system kit (Amersham) for 3 min as suggested by the manufacturer's protocol.

Electron microscopy

Two percent glutaraldehyde fixation was used to obtain optimal preservation of fine structures. Semithin 1 μm-thick resin sections were stained with methylene blue for observation, and gray-colored ultrathin sections were cut with diamond knives, stained with uranyl acetate and lead citrate, and then examined under a Hitachi H-7100 electron microscope.

Results

Immunofluorescence analysis of the laminin α2 chain (Figs. 1,5)

In the homozygous *dy/dy* mouse, no detectable immunostaining for the α2 chain was found in muscle. Spinal nerve roots, intramuscular peripheral nerves and intrafusal spindle fibers also exhibited no immunoreaction at all for the α2 chain. The laminin α1 chain, which was not detected around normal mature muscle fibers, was upregulated in the muscle fibers of the α2 chain-deficient *dy/dy* mouse. Dystrophin, utrophin and type IV collagen were normally immunostained in muscle in all animals examined, including the *dy/dy* mouse.

In contrast, in muscles from non affected heterozygous *Dy/dy* mice and the other dystrophic animal models examined, the laminin α2 chain, but not the α1 chain, was clearly immunostained as a sharply delineated ring around each muscle fiber. In these controls, intramuscular blood vessels showed no reaction for the α2 chain, but were normally immunoreactive for the α1 chain. The endoneurial basement membranes (BMs) of intramuscular nerves and intrafusal spindle muscles were also intensely stained for the α2 chain in the controls.

Immunoblot analysis of the laminin α2 chain (Fig. 2)

The homozygous *dy/dy* mice exhibited a barely detectable or extremely faint immunoreactive band for the anti-α2 chain antibody, while the control mice exhibited a clearly visible 300 kDa band.

Messenger RNA analysis of the laminin α2 chain (Fig. 3)

Laminin α2 chain mRNA is detected by RT-PCR amplification from day-12 embryos in both *dy/dy* mice and controls. In both the dystrophic *dy/dy* and control mice, the amount of α2 chain mRNA was not reduced throughout the examined coding sequence. Messenger RNA for beta-actin was simultaneously amplified in all samples examined. All of the amplified products of the α2 chain hybridized with the corresponding cDNA probes for the human α2 chain (data not shown).

Electron microscopic findings (Fig. 4)

In the control muscles, the BM was observed as a continuous, uniformly dense structure above the muscle fiber plasma membrane. In the α2 chain-deficient *dy/dy* mouse, in contrast, non-necrotic muscle fibers consistently showed a highly abnormal BM, with a thinner

294

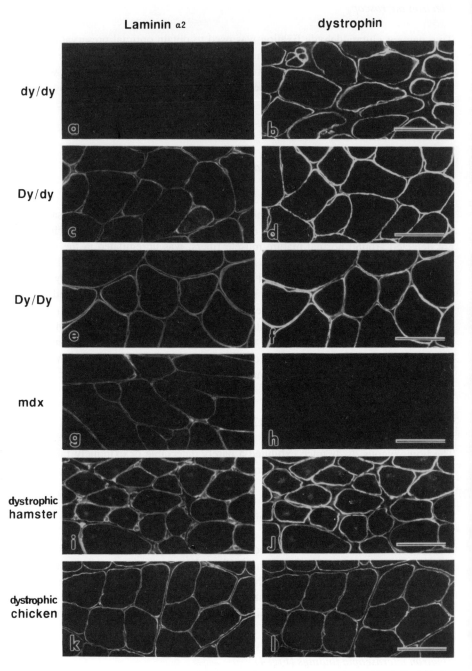

Fig. 1. Consecutive frozen sections of biopsied skeletal muscles from homozygous dystrophic *dy/dy* (a,b), heterozygous non-affected *Dy/dy* (c,d), control *Dy/Dy* (e,f), and *mdx* (g,h) mice, dystrophic BIO 14.6 hamsters (i,j) and line 413 chickens (k,l) immunoreacted for laminin α2 (a,c,e,g,i,k), and dystrophin (b,d,f,h,j,l). Note the defect of immunostaining for laminin α2 in the *dy/dy* mice (a), and for dystrophin in the *mdx* (h) mice. In contrast, clear immunostaining for laminin α2 and dystrophin can be similarly observed in the other specimens. Bar, 50 μm. (Reproduced with permission from [2]).

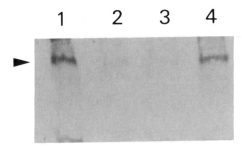

Fig. 2. Immunoblot analysis of the laminin α2 chain. An immunoreactive component of a molecular weight of 300 kDa laminin α2 chain (arrowhead) can be clearly observed in the control *Dy/Dy* (lanes 1, 4) mice, but is barely detectable in the muscles from *dy/dy* mice (lanes 2, 3).

and often disruptive appearance, without detectable defects of the underlying plasma membrane.

Discussion

In the α2 chain-deficient *dy/dy* mouse, structural abnormality of the BM has become evident as shown by EM studies. This observation suggests that, in the α2 chain-deficient *dy/dy* mouse, the muscle fiber BM becomes fragile, and this, in turn, possibly produces plasma membrane instability, and finally causes muscle fiber breakdown. The laminin α2 chain is observed predominantly in the BM of skeletal and cardiac muscles, Schwann cells and placental trophoblasts [16]. The BM is a specialized extracellular matrix composed mainly of laminins, type IV collagen, heparan sulfate proteoglycan and entactin/nidgen, and both agrin and laminin have been shown to bind to a putative cellular receptor, alpha-dystroglycan (156 kDa DAG) [17,18].

A primary abnormality of dystrophin is known to cause Duchenne/Becker muscular dys-

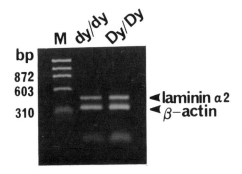

Fig. 3. Messenger RNA analysis of muscle tissues from *dy/dy* and control *Dy/Dy* mice. RT-PCR amplification products of part of the G domain of the laminin α2 chain and beta-actin are equally detectable in both the *dy/dy* and *DY/Dy* mice as the expected 468 bp and 344 bp bands, respectively.

296

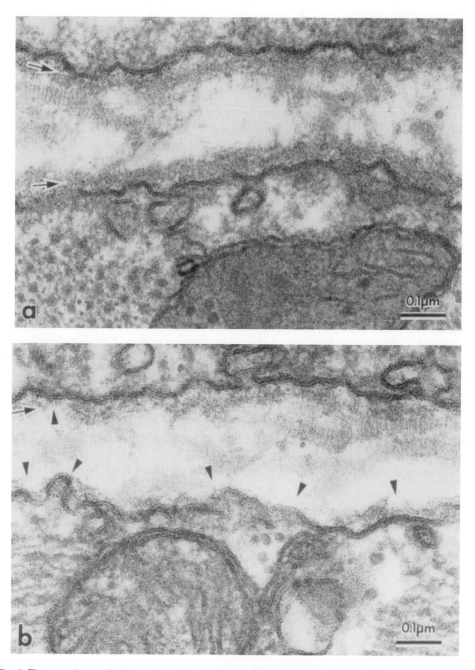

Fig. 4. Electron microscopic observation of the skeletal muscle of control *Dy/Dy* (a) and homozygous *dy/dy* (b) mice. In the control, the BM on the surface of a muscle fiber is intact (arrow). On the contrary, thinner and disrupted (arrowhead) BM is seen in the *dy/dy,* while the underlying plasma membrane is preserved. Bar, 0.1 μm. (Reproduced with permission from [2]).

dy/dy   Dy/Dy

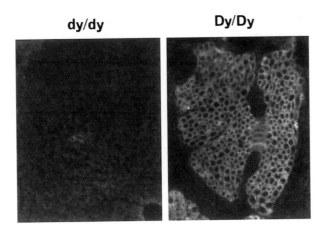

Fig. 5. Frozen sections of homozygous *dy/dy* and control *Dy/Dy* mouse muscle reacted with the anti-laminin $\alpha2$ antibody. In the control, a clearly detectable laminin $\alpha2$ immunoreaction is present in the spinal nerve root (lumbar), while in the dystrophic *dy/dy* mouse, no detectable immunostaining can be observed.

trophy (DMD/BMD) [7,19–20]. The 156 kDa DAG is an extracellular subunit of the dystrophin-associated membrane protein complex (DAPs) [21], and one of the DAPs (adhalin) is deficient in a form of muscular dystrophy called SCARMD (severe childhood autosomal recessive muscular dystrophy) [22]. Thus, it is conceivable that, in the muscle of $\alpha2$ chain-deficient *dy/dy* mouse, the DAPs may become deranged, although other still unidentified molecule(s) which are closely related with the $\alpha2$ chain could also be involved in the process of muscle fiber breakdown in the $\alpha2$ chain-deficient mouse.

Recently, other groups have detected the $\alpha2$ chain deficiency in the autosomal recessive dystrophic *dy/dy* mouse [23,24]. These results raised the question of whether $\alpha2$ chain-deficient human neuromuscular diseases exist or not. Therefore, we started to screen muscles from CMD patients unrelated to FCMD for the $\alpha2$ chain. During our search, a deficiency of the $\alpha2$ chain was found in patients with classical (occidental) CMD in Europe [25], and this disease entity is now known as merosinnegative (or $\alpha2$ chain-negative) CMD. Linkage studies involving homozygosity mapping and linkage analysis have revealed a possible linkage of the disease to chromosome 6q22–23 [26], where the $\alpha2$ chain gene has been mapped [27]. Thus, a subset of patients with classical CMD is considered to have merosinnegative CMD, although mutation(s) of the gene for the $\alpha2$ chain have not yet been identified. At the moment, however, analysis of the $\alpha2$ chain in CMD muscles seems to be essential for the accurate differential diagnosis of muscular dystrophies.

More recently, we have examined 40 Japanese patients with CMD to elucidate the frequency and molecular genetic abnormalities in merosin-negative CMD. Twelve overlapping primer sets for human $\alpha2$ chain mRNA which cover most (>99%) of the coding sequence were prepared [28]. One of the 40 patients had no detectable laminin $\alpha2$ chain by immunocytochemical, immunoblot and mRNA analysis. These findings suggest a crucial role of the $\alpha2$ chain in the process of muscle fiber breakdown. Finally, intramuscular peripheral nerves of our merosin-negative CMD patient also exhibited no immunoreaction for the $\alpha2$ chain. A similar result was found in the $\alpha2$ chain-defective *dy/dy* mouse, in which dysmyelination of the spinal nerve roots has been identified (Fig. 5). Indeed, we found another merosin-negative CMD patients who showed delayed MCV and SCV with minimum sensory disturbance (data not shown). This observation indicates that the $\alpha 2$ chain deficiency also could produce peripheral neuropathy.

Acknowledgments

We wish to thank Dr. Tastuji Nomura (Director of the Central Institute for Experimental Animals, Kawasaki, Japan) who contributed a great deal to the establishment of a system for supplying *dy* mouse in Japan, and Drs. Setsuro Ebashi (National Institute for Physiological Sciences, Okazaki, Japan) and Hideo Sugita (National Center of Neurology and Psychiatry, Tokyo, Japan) for their helpful discussion and advice. This research was supported by grants from the National Center of Neurology and Psychiatry of the Ministry of Health and Welfare, Japan, and the Ministry of Education, Science, Sports and Culture, Japan.

References

1. Hayashi YK, Engvall E, Arikawa-Hirasawa E, et al. Abnormal localization of laminin subunits in muscular dystrophies. J Neurol Sci 1993; 119: 53–64.
2. Arahata K, Hayashi YK, Koga R, et al. Laminin in animal models for muscular dystrophy: defect of laminin M in skeletal and cardiac muscles and peripheral nerve of the homozygous dystrophic *dy/dy* mice. Proc Jpn Acad 1993; 69(Ser B): 259–264.
3. Michelson AM, Russell ES, Harman PJ. Dystrophia muscularis: a hereditary primary myopathy in the house mouse. Proc Natl Acad Sci USA, 1955; 41: 1079–1084.
4. Buckle VJ, Guenet JL, Simon-Chazottes D, Love DR, Davies KE. Localization of a dystrophin-related autosomal gene to 6q24 in man, and to mouse chromosome 10 in the region of the dystrophia muscularis (*dy*) locus. Hum Genet 1990; 85: 324–326.
5. Ohlendieck K, Ervasti JM, Matsumura K, Kahl SD, Leveille CJ, Campbell KP. Dystrophin-related protein is localized to neuromuscular junctions of adult skeletal muscle. Neuron 1991; 7: 499–508.
6. Xu H, Wu X-R, Wewer UM, Engvall E. Murine muscular dystrophy caused by a mutation in the laminin $\alpha 2$ (Lama α) gene. Nat Genet 1994; 8: 297–302.
7. Arahata K, Ishiura S. Ishiguro T, et al. Immunostaining of skeletal and cardiac muscle surface membrane with antibody against Duchenne muscular dystrophy peptide. Nature 1988: 333: 861–863.
8. Hoffman EP, Hudecki MS, Rosenberg PA, Pollina CM, Kunkel LM. Cell and fiber-type distribution of dystrophin. Neuron 1988; 1: 411–420.
9. Ohlendieck K, Campbell KP. Dystrophin-associated proteins are greatly reduced in skeletal muscle from mdx mice. J Cell Biol 1991; 115: 1685–1694.
10. Homburger F. Myopathy of hamster dystrophy: history and morphologic aspects. Ann N Y Acad Sci 1979; 317: 2–17.
11. Roberds SL, Anderson RD, Ibraghimov-Beskrovnaya O, Campbell KP. Primary structure and muscle-specific expression of the 50 kDa dystrophin-associated glycoprotein (adhalin). J Biol Chem 1993; 268: 11496–11499.
12. Asmundson VS, Doerr L. Inherited muscle abnormality in the domestic fowl. J Hered 1956; 47: 248–252.
13. Woo M, Tanabe Y, Ishii H, Nonaka I, Yokoyama M, Esaki K. Muscle fiber growth and necrosis in dystrophic muscles: a comparative study between *dy* and *mdx* mice. J Neurol Sci 1987; 82: 111–122.
14. Bradley WG, Aguayo AJ. Quantitative ultrastructural studies of the axon-Schwann cell abnormality in nerve roots from dystrophic mice. J Neurol Sci 1973; 18: 227–247.
15. Bradley WG, Jaros E. Involvement of peripheral and central nerves in murine dystrophy. Ann N Y Acad Sci 1979; 317: 132–142.
16. Engvall E, Earwicker D, Day A, Muir D, Manthorpe M, Paulsson M. Merosin promotes cell attachment and neurite outgrowth and is a component of the neurite-promoting factor of RN22 Schwannoma cells. Exp Cell Res 1992; 198: 115–123.

17. Gee SH, Montanaro F, Lindenbaum MH, Carbonetto S. Dystroglycan-α, a dystrophin associated glycoprotein, is a functional agrin receptor. Cell 1994; 77: 675–686.

18. Campanelli JT, Roberds SL, Campbell KP, Scheller RH. A role for dystrophin-associated glycoprotein and utrophin in agrin-induced AchR clustering. Cell 1994; 77: 663–74.

19. Koenig M, Hoffman EP, Bertelson CJ, Monaco AP, Feener C, Kunkel LM. Complete cloning of the Duchenne muscular dystrophy (DMD) cDNA and preliminary genomic organization of the DMD gene in normal and affected individuals. Cell 1987; 50: 509–517.

20. Hoffman EP, Brown RH, Kunkel LM. Dystrophin: the protein product of the Duchenne muscular dystrophy locus. Cell 1987; 51: 919–928.

21. Ibraghimov-Beskrovnaya O, Ervasti JM, Leveille CJ, Slaughter CA, Sernett SW, Campbell KP. Primary structure of dystrophin-associated glycoproteins linking to the extracellular matrix. Nature 1992; 355: 696–702.

22. Roberds SL, Leturcq F, Allamand V, et al. Missense mutations in the adhalin gene linked to autosomal recessive muscular dystrophy. Cell 1994; 78: 625–633.

23. Sunada Y, Bernier SM, Kozak CA, Yamada Y, Campbell KP. Deficiency of merosin in dystrophic *dy* mice and genetic linkage of laminin M chain gene to *dy* locus. J Biol Chem 1994; 269: 13729–13732.

24. Xu H, Christmas P, Wu X-R, Wewer UM, Engvall E. Defective muscle basement membrane and lack of M-laminin in the dystrophic *dy/dy* mouse. Proc Natl Acad Sci USA 1994; 91: 5572–5576.

25. Tomé FMS, Evangelista T, Leclerc A, et al. Congenital muscular dystrophy with merosin deficiency. CR Acad Sci Paris, Sciences de la vie/Life Sci 1994; 317: 351–357.

26. Hillaire D, Leclerc A, Faure S, et al. Localization of merosin-negative congenital muscular dystrophy to chromosome 6q2 by homozygosity mapping. Hum Mol Genet 1994; 3: 1657–1661.

27. Vuolteenaho R, Nissinen M, Sainio K, et al. Human laminin M chain (merosin): complete primary structure, chromosomal assignment, and expression of the M and A chain in human fetal tissues. J Cell Biol 1994; 124: 381–394.

28. Hayashi YK, Koga R, Tsukahara T, et al. Deficiency of laminin α2 chain mRNA in muscle in a patient with merosin-negative congenital muscular dystrophy. Muscle Nerve 1996; 18: 1027–1030.

Y. Fukuyama, M. Osawa and K. Saito (Eds.), *Congenital Muscular Dystrophies*
© 1997 Elsevier Science B.V. All rights reserved

CHAPTER 25

Toward identification of the Fukuyama type congenital muscular dystrophy gene

TATSUSHI TODA[1], MASASHI MIYAKE[1], YUTAKA NAKAHORI[1],
MASAYA SEGAWA[2], YOSHIKO NOMURA[2], IKUYA NONAKA[3],
SHIRO IKEGAWA[4], ERI KONDO[5], KAYOKO SAITO[5], MAKIKO OSAWA[5],
YUKIO FUKUYAMA[5], MIEKO YOSHIOKA[6], TERUO SHIMIZU[7],
ICHIRO KANAZAWA[8], YUSUKE NAKAMURA[4] and YASUO NAKAGOME[1]

[1]*Department of Human Genetics, University of Tokyo, Tokyo, Japan*
[2]*Segawa Neurological Clinic for Children, Segawa, Japan*
[3]*National Institute of Neuroscience, NCNP, Japan*
[4]*Institute of Medical Science, University of Tokyo, Tokyo, Japan*
[5]*Department of Pediatrics, Tokyo Women's Medical College, Tokyo, Japan*
[6]*Department of Pediatrics, Kobe General Hospital, Kobe, Japan*
[7]*Department of Neurology, Teikyo University, Teikyo, Japan*
[8]*Department of Neurology, University of Tokyo, Tokyo, Japan*

Introduction

Since the discovery of the Duchenne muscular dystrophy (DMD) gene product, "dystrophin" [1], by the "positional cloning" approach, intensive investigations have been under way for resolution of the pathophysiology of muscular dystrophy and improvement of therapeutic approaches.

Another muscular dystrophy, Fukuyama type congenital muscular dystrophy (FCMD), is an autosomal recessive disorder characterized by severe congenital muscular dystrophy associated with central nervous system involvement. The syndrome was first described in 1960 [2]. The phenotype consists of muscular dystrophy combined with brain anomalies due to a defect in the migration of neurons [3]. It is the second most common form of childhood muscular dystrophy in Japan; the incidence is 7–12/100 000. One in a hundred persons is presumed to be a heterozygous carrier [3,4].

Patients with FCMD manifest weakness of facial and limb muscles, and general hypotonia before nine months of age. Functional disabilities are more serious in patients with FCMD than in DMD patients; usually the maximum motor function is shuffling, and most patients are never able to walk. Simultaneously, they exhibit severe mental retardation and they require careful nursing as there is no effective therapy. Patients usually become bedridden before 10 years of age because of generalized muscle atrophy and joint contractures, and most of them die by the age of 20 [3].

The cause of this pathology is unknown. No strong hypothesis has emerged with respect to the biochemical defect responsible for FCMD, and no cytogenetic defects are obvious. It is necessary for us to resolve the pathophysiology of this tragic disease as early as possible. It is unknown why two organs, the brain and skeletal muscle, are affected simultaneously,

302

but abnormalities in the skeletal muscle suggest developmental defects, as in the brain. So, the identification of the primary defect in FCMD should yield a better understanding of the pathophysiology of muscular dystrophy, and provide insights into normal development of the brain and skeletal muscle.

As a first step to elucidate the genetic defect of FCMD, we performed genetic linkage analysis of FCMD, using the homozygosity mapping method [5] mainly, which takes advantage of consanguineous marriages. Here we report initial mapping of the FCMD locus to chromosome 9q31–33 [6], and further describe refined mapping within a region of approximately 5 cM, and evidence for strong linkage disequilibrium between FCMD alleles and a polymorphic microsatellite marker, mfd220 [7].

Homozygosity mapping

When we examine autosomal recessive disorders such as FCMD by means of conventional linkage analysis, it is necessary to collect more than two hundred family members. We, therefore, adopted homozygosity mapping [5]. This method needs about 10 patients to obtain similar results. Fig. 1 shows the principle of homozygosity mapping. In an inbred family carrying a recessive disease gene, a patient inherits two identical copies of the disease allele (here denoted by "f") from a carrier ancestor. That is, the patient is "homozygous by descent". A flanking marker allele, here denoted by "1", is also likely to be "homozygous by descent". In other words, a marker, for which many inbred patients are homozygous, is suggested to be linked to the disease. Highly polymorphic markers such as microsatellite polymorphisms are necessary for this purpose, since at a marker exhibiting low heterozygosity many inbred patients will be homozygous, even if the marker is not linked to FCMD.

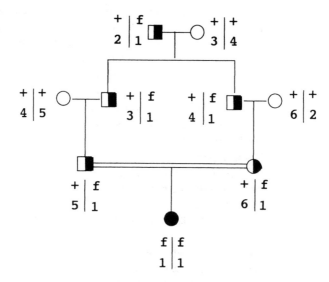

Fig. 1. Principle of homozygosity mapping. In an inbred family carrying a recessive disease gene, a patient inherits two identical copies of the disease allele (here denoted by "f") from a carrier ancestor. A flanking marker allele, here denoted by "1", is also likely to be "homozygous by descent". A marker, for which many inbred patients are homozygous, is suggested to be linked to the disease.

The human genome has many di- or tri-nucleotide repeat sequences, the number of each repeat being different in each individual. Microsatellite markers (di- or tri-nucleotide repeats) take advantage of this high polymorphism [8]. We can easily detect each allele of a given microsatellite marker by PCR. Nowadays, more than 2 000 microsatellite markers have been described and catalogued [9].

Linkage analysis

We collected affected patients from inbred families and affected siblings from non-consanguineous families, mainly. Of 35 families, 15 are consanguineous and include 17 inbred patients. DNA was extracted from whole blood, biopsied skeletal muscle, and formalin-fixed and paraffin-embedded autopsy specimens. Individuals were genotyped with polymorphic microsatellite markers, as described [6]. We performed genetic linkage analysis with the LINKAGE program, version 5.2 [10]. All complex matings were dealt with by breaking the loops and inserting a genetically identical person, i.e., double individual, into the pedigree. The gene frequency for the FCMD allele was assumed to be 0.0052, as reported [4]. We noticed that all patients from inbred families were homozygous at the D9S59 locus located on distal 9q. The frequency of homozygosity in non-consanguineous patients was similar to that in the general population. This suggests a possible linkage of this locus to FCMD.

Subsequently, linkage analysis of this marker, D9S59, in all FCMD families revealed a significant pairwise lod score of 4.33 [6]. We, furthermore, used additional markers in this region to define the FCMD locus. The order of these markers was estimated to be as follows: centromere–D9S176–3 cM–(D9S109, D9S127)–1.7 cM–mfd220 [11]–3 cM–CA246 (Toda et al., unpublished data)–5.5 cM–D9S58–2.8 cM–D9S105–4.9 cM–D9S59–telomere [12–15]. Significant lod scores as to the FCMD locus were also obtained at all adjacent markers examined (Table 1). Strikingly, two markers, D9S127 and mfd220, revealed maximum lod scores of 10.34 at 1% recombination frequency and 17.49 at 0%, respectively. In other words, linkage of this marker, mfd220, with FCMD is 10^{18} more likely than an accidental event. It was noteworthy that there were no obligate recombinants between FCMD and mfd220 [7].

These markers have been mapped to chromosome 9q31–33 by fluorescent in-situ hybridization (FISH; Fig. 2). The genetic distances between each marker are also shown in

Table 1

Pairwise lod scores of 9q31–33 markers with FCMD

Recombination fraction (θ)

Marker	0.00	0.01	0.05	0.10	0.15	0.20	0.30	0.40	Z_{max}	θ
D9S176	$-\infty$	6.00	6.95	6.32	5.31	4.22	2.26	0.84	6.95	0.05
D9S109	$-\infty$	9.47	8.61	7.07	5.57	4.20	2.02	0.63	9.47	0.01
D9S127	$-\infty$	10.34	9.65	8.27	6.84	5.46	3.04	1.20	10.34	0.01
mfd220	17.49	16.97	14.93	12.46	10.14	7.98	4.32	1.65	17.49	0.00
CA246	6.34	7.20	7.22	6.25	5.09	3.95	2.01	0.69	7.42	0.03
D9S58	$-\infty$	6.31	8.00	7.61	6.51	5.27	2.75	0.92	8.04	0.06
D9S105	$-\infty$	3.10	4.91	4.81	4.15	3.32	1.72	0.57	4.99	0.07

304

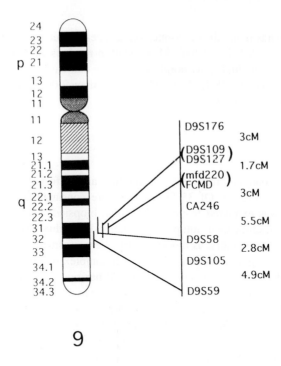

9

Fig. 2. Physical and genetic locations of chromosome 9q31–33 markers flanking FCMD [12–15].

Fig. 2. A marker, mfd220, showing a high lod score and no recombination is located on 9q31.

Recombination and homozygosity analysis

To further investigate the region co-segregating with FCMD, we analyzed recombination events in FCMD families. Haplotypes were constructed assuming the most parsimonious linkage phase. Seven families exhibited recombination between FCMD and some marker loci. Fig. 3 shows examples of recombination events detected in the FCMD pedigrees. Crossing-over was evident between D9S127 and more centromeric loci in family 30. Recombinations at a more distal locus, D9S58, were observed in family 26. The observed recombination events in these families place the FCMD gene distal to D9S127 and proximal to D9S58 [7].

In autosomal recessive disorders, affected individuals from consanguineous families may be "homozygous by descent" at the region surrounding the disease locus, as mentioned. We examined affected members of the inbred FCMD families for homozygosity at seven 9q31–33 microsatellite loci (Fig. 4). Most of the patients were homozygous at the mfd220 locus, in spite of the remarkably high heterozygosity in the general population. The patients in families 2, 7, 19 and 21 were heterozygous at D9S176, and those in families 1, 7 and 14 were heterozygous at CA246. The results of the homozygosity mapping suggest that the FCMD gene lies within a region distal to D9S176 and proximal to CA246 [7]. Recombination mapping showed that the target region was between D9S127 and D9S58. Taking the

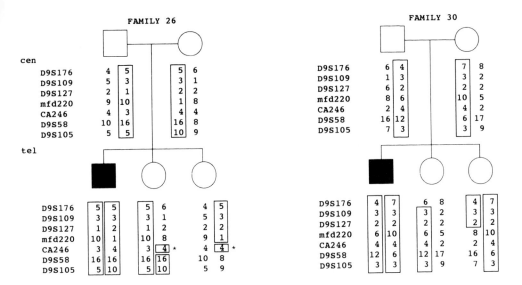

Fig. 3. Recombination mapping. Genotypes are indicated for 7 polymorphic microsatellite loci in families demonstrating crossovers near the FCMD gene. The haplotype carrying the FCMD allele is boxed. Asterisks under pedigree 26 indicate uncertainty with respect to the precise positions of crossovers because of the uninformativeness of CA246 in the mother of this family. The observed recombination events in these families place the FCMD gene proximal to D9S58 and distal to D9S127.

results of both analyses into consideration, we concluded that the most likely location of the FCMD gene is between the two loci, D9S127 and CA246. This candidate region includes mfd220 which showed no recombination.

Linkage disequilibrium

We also found evidence for strong linkage disequilibrium between FCMD and this marker, mfd220. A "111-bp" allele for the mfd220 locus was observed in 22 (34%) of 64

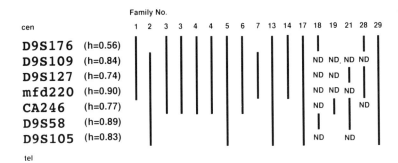

Fig. 4. Homozygosity mapping. Solid lines denote portions of the chromosomes that are homozygous in each inbred patient. ND indicates 'not determined' because of PCR failure in formalin-fixed samples. 'h' denotes observed heterozygosity. The results of this procedure support placement of the FCMD gene distal to D9S176 and proximal to CA246.

Table 2

Linkage disequilibrium of FCMD with mfd220

PCR product size (bp)	Control observed	FCMD observed
129	1	1
127	4	0
125	3	0
123	4	2
121	5	0
119	24	11
117	8	0
115	11	1
113	34	18
111	1	22
103	3	2
101	22	7
Total	120	64

$\chi^2 = 50.7$; 6d.f.; $P < 0.0001$

FCMD chromosomes (one patient from each family), but this allele was present in only one of 120 normal chromosomes (Table 2). This allelic association with FCMD was highly significant ($\chi 2 = 50.7$, $P < 0.0001$). No other marker locus yielded evidence for linkage disequilibrium. This suggests the possibility of a founder effect, i.e., a common origin of most affected alleles. Since the carrier frequency for FCMD is estimated to be about 1% in the Japanese population, the majority of the "111-bp" chromosomes in the normal population might reflect FCMD carriers. On the basis of evidence in cystic fibrosis and Huntington's disease, we suspect that the FCMD gene lies within a few hundred kilobases of mfd220 located on 9q31 [7].

Discussion

Dystrophin is known to be associated with a large oligomeric complex of sarcolemmal glycoproteins (dystrophin-associated proteins, DAPs) [16]. It has been reported that expression of DAPs, especially 43DAG, is abnormally low in FCMD muscles [17], and others have noted a significant reduction in immunostaining of a laminin isoform (merosin), an extracellular matrix component linked with DAPs [18]. Genes encoding these proteins are located on chromosomes 3p21 [19] and 6q22–23 [20], respectively. However, it was around mfd220 on chromosome 9q31(-33) that we localized the FCMD locus. Since there are few known proteins located on 9q31–33, we consider that the FCMD gene product could be an unknown protein. It may be (1) an unknown adhesion molecule related to neuronal migration, or (2) an unknown protein linked with the dystrophin-dystroglycan-laminin complex, because immunostaining against the constituents of this complex is reduced.

Homozygosity mapping is considered to be effective in linkage analyses of autosomal recessive disorders for which large families including multiple affected individuals are seldom observed. The linked markers reported here can be used for prenatal and carrier diagnosis in FCMD families. At present, prenatal diagnosis in FCMD families is feasible. Experiences of prenatal diagnoses are presented in another section of this issue [21].

It has been discussed whether FCMD and Walker-Warburg syndrome (WWS) [22], and muscle-eye-brain-disease (MEB) [23] belong to the same disease entity or not. These markers may also be useful for evaluating whether these similar disorders may be allelic to each other. Pihko et al. performed a linkage study on 7 families carrying MEB in Finland and excluded MEB from 9q31–33 [24]. The genetic homogeneity of the isolated Finnish population will make genetic analysis of MEB more accurate. Yoshioka and Kuroki [25] and Toda et al. [26] reported a family in which 3 siblings were affected with either FCMD or WWS. A genetic study using these flanking markers showed that both FCMD and WWS patients carried an identical combination of mutations on either allele of the FCMD locus. Therefore, we consider that these clinical conditions are caused by mutations in the same gene. The difference in clinical manifestations between FCMD and WWS may reflect variation of expressivity or variation in mutations. However, Dobyns analyzed 2 highly inbred families carrying WWS without muscle involvement and excluded the 9q31–33 region as the WWS locus. Analyses on WWS with muscle involvement are underway [27]. We presume that WWS could be genetically heterogeneous, since the spectrum of manifestations of WWS is broader (e.g., with or without muscle involvement), and WWS patients are of various ethnic origins. Some could be caused by the same gene as that for FCMD, and others by another gene whose chromosomal location is unknown.

The isolation of a disease gene is often compared to the search for one criminal among the entire population of the world. Through our initial linkage analysis of the FCMD gene, which localized it to chromosome 9q31–33, we have chased the criminal into an area with a population of only ten million. This time, with the evidence of strong linkage disequilibrium, the target area has been narrowed to a region whose population is about one million. We are now analyzing yeast artificial chromosome (YAC) clones containing the closest marker. Intensive efforts are being made in our laboratory at present.

Acknowledgments

We are grateful to the family members who participated in this study, and Drs. K. Masuda, T. Ishihara, M. Sakai, I. Tomita, Y. Origuchi, K. Ohno, N. Misugi, Y. Sasaki, K. Takada, M. Kawai, K. Otani, T. Murakami, T. Kumagai and K. Suzumori for their contributions. This work was supported in part by a Research Grant for Nervous and Mental Disorders (5A-2), and one for Pediatric Research from the Ministry of Health and Welfare, and also by a grant from the Ministry of Education, Science and Culture.

References

1. Hoffman EP, Brown RH, Kunkel LM. Dystrophin: the protein product of the Duchenne muscular dystrophy locus. Cell 1987; 51: 919–928.
2. Fukuyama Y, Kawazura M, Haruna H. A peculiar form of congenital progressive muscular dystrophy. Report of fifteen cases. Paediatr Univ Tokyo (Tokyo) 1960; 4: 5–8.
3. Fukuyama Y, Osawa M, Suzuki H. Congenital muscular dystrophy of the Fukuyama type -clinical, genetic and pathological considerations. Brain Dev (Tokyo) 1981; 3: 1–29.
4. Fukuyama Y, Ohsawa M. A genetic study of the Fukuyama type congenital muscular dystrophy. Brain Dev (Tokyo) 1984; 6: 373–390.
5. Lander ES, Botstein D. Homozygosity mapping: a way to map human recessive traits with the DNA of inbred children. Science 1987; 236: 1567–1570.

6. Toda T, Segawa M, Nomura Y, et al. Localization of a gene for Fukuyama type congenital muscular dystrophy to chromosome 9q31–33. Nat Genet 1993; 5: 283–286.

7. Toda T, Ikegawa S, Okui K, et al. Refined mapping of a gene responsible for Fukuyama type congenital muscular dystrophy: evidence for strong linkage disequilibrium. Am J Hum Genet 1994; 55: 946–950.

8. Weber JL, May PE. Abundant class of human DNA polymorphisms which can be typed using the polymerase chain reaction. Am J Hum Genet 1989; 44: 388–396.

9. Gyapay G, Morissette J, Vignal A, et al. The 1993–94 Genethon human genetic linkage map. Nat Genet 1994; 7: 246–339.

10. Lathrop GM, Lalouel JM, Julier C, Ott J. Strategies for multi-point linkage analysis in humans. Proc Natl Acad Sci USA 1984; 81: 3443–3446.

11. Weber JL. Genome Data Base (GDB) version 4.1, Welch WH Medical Library, Baltimore, MD.

12. Blumenfeld A, Slaugenhaupt SA, Axelrod FB, et al. Localization of the gene for familial dysautonomia on chromosome 9 and definition of DNA markers for genetic diagnosis. Nat Genet 1993; 4: 160–164.

13. Kwiatkowski DJ, Armour J, Bale AE, et al. Report on the second international workshop on human chromosome 9. Cytogenet Cell Genet 1993; 64: 93–121.

14. Attwood J, Chiano M, Collins A, et al. CEPH consortium map of chromosome 9. Genomics 1994; 19: 203–214.

15. Buetow KH, Weber JL, Ludwigsen S, et al. Integrated human genome-wide maps constructed using the CEPH reference panel. Nat Genet 1994; 6: 391–393.

16. Ervasti JM, Campbell KP. Membrane organization of the dystrophin-glycoprotein complex. Cell 1991; 66: 1121–1131.

17. Matsumura K, Nonaka I, Campbell KP. Abnormal expression of dystrophin-associated proteins in Fukuyama-type congenital muscular dystrophy. Lancet 1993; 341: 521–522.

18. Hayashi KY, Engvall E, Arikawa-Hirasawa E, et al. Abnormal localization of laminin subunits in muscular dystrophies. J Neurol Sci 1993; 119: 53–64.

19. Ibraghimov-Beskrovnaya O, Milatovich A, Ozcelik T, et al. Human dystroglycan: skeletal muscle cDNA, genomic structure, origin of tissue specific isoforms and chromosomal localization. Hum Mol Genet 1993; 2: 1651–1657.

20. Tryggvason K. The laminin family. Curr Opin Cell Biol 1993; 5: 877–882.

21. Kondo E, Saito K, Toda T, et al. Reconfirmation of the Fukuyama congenital muscular dystrophy (FCMD) gene locus at chromosome 9q31, and a successful prenatal diagnosis of FCMD in two families. In: Fukuyama Y, Osawa M, Saito K, eds. Congenital muscular dystrophies. Amsterdam: Elsevier, 1997: 309–319.

22. Dobyns WB, Pagon RA, Armstrong D, et al. Diagnostic criteria for Walker-Warburg syndrome. Am J Med Genet 1989; 32: 195–210.

23. Santavuori P, Somer H, Sainio K, et al. Muscle-eye-brain disease (MEB). Brain Dev (Tokyo) 1989; 11: 147–153.

24. Pihko H, Santavuori P. Muscle-eye-brain (MEB) disease – a review. In: Fukuyama Y, Osawa M, Saito K, eds. Congenital muscular dystrophies. Amsterdam: Elsevier, 1997: 99–104.

25. Yoshioka M, Kuroki S. Clinical spectrum and genetic studies of Fukuyama congenital muscular dystrophy. Am J Med Genet 1994; 53: 245–250.

26. Toda T, Yoshioka M, Nakahori Y, Kanazawa I, Nakamura Y, Nakagome Y. Genetic identity of Fukuyama type congenital muscular dystrophy and Walker-Warburg syndrome. Ann Neurol 1995; 37: 99–101.

27. Dobyns WB. Walker–Warburg and other cobblestone lissencephaly syndromes: 1995 update. In: Fukuyama Y, Osawa M, Saito K, eds. Congenital muscular dystrophies. Amsterdam: Elsevier, 1997: 89–98.

Y. Fukuyama, M. Osawa and K. Saito (Eds.), *Congenital Muscular Dystrophies*
© 1997 Elsevier Science B.V. All rights reserved

Reconfirmation of the Fukuyama congenital muscular dystrophy (FCMD) gene locus at chromosome 9q31, and a successful prenatal diagnosis of FCMD in two families

ERI KONDO[1], KAYOKO SAITO[1], TATSUSHI TODA[2], MAKIKO OSAWA[1], HAJIME TANAKA[3], SHOJI TSUJI[3], TOMOKO YAMAMOTO[4], MAKIO KOBAYASHI[4], YUSUKE NAKAMURA[5] and YUKIO FUKUYAMA[1]

[1]*Department of Pediatrics, Tokyo Women's Medical College, Tokyo, Japan*
[2]*Department of Human Genetics, University of Tokyo, Tokyo, Japan*
[3]*Department of Neurology, Brain Research Institute, Niigata University, Niigata, Japan*
[4]*Department of Pathology, Tokyo Women's Medical College, Tokyo, Japan*
[5]*Institute of Medical Science, University of Tokyo, Tokyo, Japan*

Introduction

Fukuyama-type congenital muscular dystrophy (FCMD), first described by Fukuyama et al. in 1960 [1], and designated by number 253800 in McKusick's catalog [2], is an autosomal recessively inherited disorder, characterized by brain malformation, principally cerebral and cerebellar cortical dysplasia, in addition to primary dystrophic changes in skeletal muscle [3,4].

Clinical features of the disease are unique; generalized hypotonia and weakness are present in early infancy, followed by marked muscle atrophy, multiple joint contractures and psychomotor developmental delay in childhood. The highest motor function acquired by most patients is sliding while sitting on the buttocks. Upright ambulation, even with support, is attained only rarely, in exceptional cases. Intellectual, cognitive and communicative functions are moderately delayed without exception, while febrile and/or non-febrile seizures occur in about half of cases.

The overall clinical course is slowly progressive and inexorable, with 16 years being the average age at death. No effective treatment is available at present. Not surprisingly, the parents of an afflicted child are generally extremely anxious about attempting another pregnancy, because the sib recurrence rate of this incurable devastating condition is known to be high (25%) [5,6].

In 1993 and 1994, however, Toda et al. [7,8] succeeded in mapping the FCMD gene locus to chromosome 9q31 using genetic linkage analysis and homozygous mapping. This discovery opened the door to the long-awaited possibility of prenatal diagnosis for FCMD families. It should be noted, however, that there are no reports on the same subject in the literature afterwards which can proves or disprove the findings of Toda et al.

Thus, the authors undertook here the same type of linkage analysis study as that of Toda et al. in a new series of 20 FCMD families, and a significant LOD score with mfd220 was found, confirming the legitimacy of Toda's report [7,8]. Furthermore, the authors conducted the first successful prenatal diagnosis of 2 families using genetic polymorphism analysis with the same markers.

Materials and methods

Linkage analysis of FCMD families

Twenty FCMD pedigrees recruited for genetic linkage analysis are shown in Fig. 1. Parental consanguinity (second cousins) was noticed in only one pedigree. Ten families were multiplex pedigrees having recurrent affection of 2 siblings, while the other 10 families included only one affected. Five out of 20 families have also served as the study subjects in the work of Toda et al. [7,8] (pedigree numbers 1,2,11–13). Pedigree numbers 3 and 7 are family 1 and family 2, respectively, in the following prenatal diagnosis section of this article. DNA samples from 20 FCMD families, with a total of 86 family members including 30 affected subjects, were used for linkage analysis. All 30 FCMD cases were examined by experienced pediatric neurologists, and the diagnosis was confirmed with a uniform clinical, as well as laboratory diagnostic, criteria [4]. Individuals were studied with 3 polymorphic microsatellite DNA markers, D9S 127 [9], mfd220 [10] and CA246 [11], which are demonstrated as significant markers for FCMD by previous studies [7,8]. Genotyping methods are identical to those mentioned in the prenatal diagnosis section below. LOD scores were calculated using the computer programs MLINK (LINKAGE version 5.20) [12].

Prenatal diagnosis in two FCMD families: clinical aspects of the probands

Neither parental marriage was consanguineous and no family members, other than the probands, were affected.

The proband of family 1, their second child, was floppy at birth. At age 10 months, a diagnosis of FCMD was made at another hospital based on a high serum CK value (13 970 mU/ml; normal < 140) and muscle biopsy findings of necrotic and regenerating fibers and markedly increased endo- and peri-mysial connective tissue. When the patient was 4 years 6 months old, the family visited our hospital with the aim of possibly obtaining a prenatal diagnosis. The patient was profoundly retarded in psychomotor development; he could slide while sitting, but could not stand or speak any meaningful words. Facial muscle involvement, multiple joint contractures, and absent deep tendon reflexes were noted. Brain MRI at 4 years 2 months (Fig. 2a) had revealed pachygyric frontal lobes, polymicrogyric occipital lobes and a delay of myelination in the same regions.

The proband of family 2 was recognized to be hypotonic and weak at 5 months of age. At age 1 year, a diagnosis of FCMD was made at another hospital based on clinical findings including high CK value (4 015 mU/ml) and dystrophic muscle changes in a biopsied specimen. A febrile convulsion occurred at 20 months of age. At age 2 years, the family visited our hospital for the first time, at which time the patient was able to maintain a sitting posture and to play with toys but could not slide while sitting or stand. Generalized hypotonia and weakness, a myopathic face and mild knee contractures were noted. The patient had no vocabulary. Brain MRI at 2 years 1 month (Fig. 2b) demonstrated decreased undulation of the subcortical white matter in frontal and occipital lobes (pachygyria), widely dilated

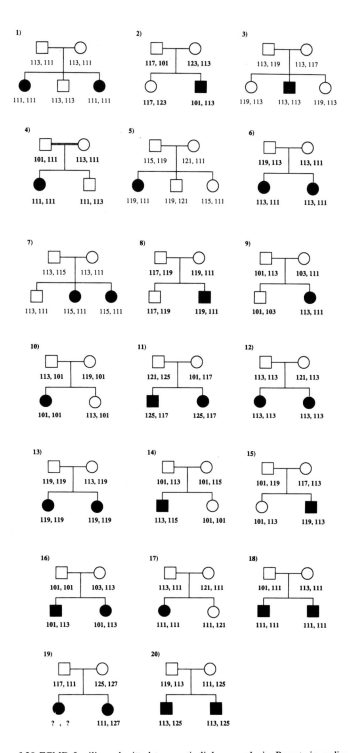

Fig. 1. Pedigrees of 20 FCMD families submitted to genetic linkage analysis. Parents in pedigree number 4 are second cousins. The allele size of mfd220 are shown under each individual.

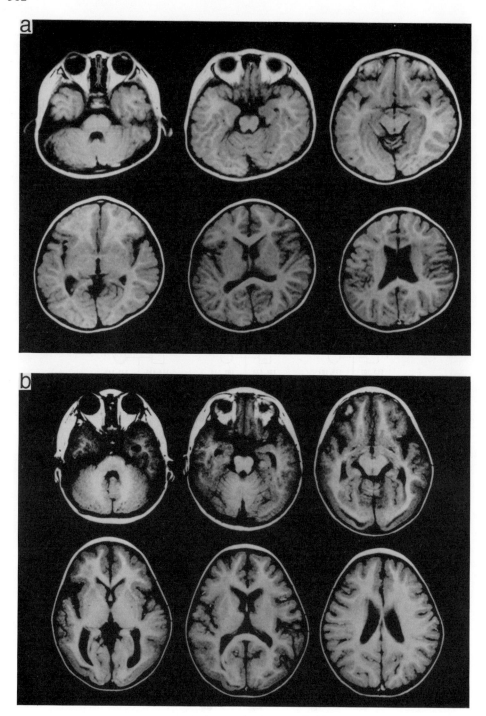

Fig. 2. Brain MRI of the probands. (a) Proband of family 1 at the age of 4 years 2 months. (b) Proband of family 2 at the age of 2 years 1 month. T1-weighted inversion-recovery images. Delayed myelination, mild ventricular enlargement, dilated Sylvian fissures (operculum dysgenesis) and pachygyria are apparent.

Sylvian fissures (operculum dysplasia), mild dilatation of the posterior horns of the lateral ventricles and delayed myelination in the centro-temporal subcortical regions.

We were consulted by both couples regarding prenatal diagnosis after a third child was conceived in family 1, and a fourth in family 2. Family 1 came to us specifically because the parents were under a great deal of pressure, from the paternal grandparents, to abort the pregnancy. They saw prenatal diagnosis as the only hope of avoiding this unwanted termination of the pregnancy. After the practical procedure, as well as the safety and risks of examination, had been explained and the confidentiality of all results guaranteed, both sets of parents expressed their eagerness to utilize prenatal diagnosis. At the time of amniocentesis for the fetal diagnosis, the probands in families 1 and 2 were 4 years 6 months and 2 years 2 months old, respectively.

Procedures in prenatal diagnosis

DNA was extracted from the whole blood of parents and siblings according to standard techniques [13]. Amniocentesis was performed under ultrasonography, at 17 gestational weeks in family 1 and at 16 weeks in family 2. The amniotic fluid was then divided in half. DNA was extracted directly from one half, as well as from cultured amniotic cells grown from the other half, to confirm the reproducibility of the results.

Haplotypes of all samples from family members and both fetuses were analyzed with polymorphic microsatellite markers flanking the 9q31-33 locus, as described below.

Genotyping

We used 9 polymorphic microsatellite CA repeat markers, previously described as being on chromosome 9q31-33 [14–20]. The markers used were D9S176 [16], D9S109 [17], D9S127 [9], mfd220 [10], CA246 [11], D9S58 [18], D9S105 [19], D9S59 [18] and HXB [20].

The locations of the markers used for this study are illustrated in Fig. 3. The FCMD gene is considered to lie within a few hundred kilobases of the mfd220 locus [8].

PCR and electrophoresis conditions were as previously described [7,8]. To reveal simple sequence repeat polymorphisms, 20 ng of genomic DNA from each subject was amplified by polymerase chain reaction (PCR) using 20 pmol of an unlabelled primer and 20 pmol of a primer end-labeled with 1.0 mCi [γ-^{32}P]ATP using T4 polynucleotide kinase; 1 × PCR buffer (16.6 Mm NH_4SO_4, 67 mM Tris-HCI pH 8.8, 10 mM β-mercaptoethanol, 6.7 mM EDTA); 10% (v/v) dimethyl sulfoxide; 1.5 mM of each dDTP; 5 mM $MgCl_2$ and 1.25 units Taq DNA polymerase. Samples were incubated in a DNA thermocycler (Perkin elmer thetus) for 35 cycles under the following conditions: 94°C for 1.5 min, 55°C for 2 min and 72°C for 1.5 min. After PCR, the products were analyzed on 6% polyacrylamide gels, and visualized by autoradiography.

Polymorphism analysis and fetal phenotype possibility calculation

Based on the genotypic data, haplotypes were constructed, assuming the most likely linkage phase, and the fetal phenotypes were analyzed.

Furthermore, fetal phenotype probability was calculated using the LINKAGE computer package [12]. For the calculation, we chose the genotypic data from D9S127, mfd220 and D9S58, all of which are known to be close to the FCMD locus and have been identified as reliable loci [7,8]. The calculation was carried out using two distinct possibilities for the FCMD locus. The order of these markers and FCMD gene loci were arranged in two ways, as follows: <1> centromere – D9S127 – 1 cM – FCMD – 1 cM – mfd220 – 7 cM – D9S58 – telomere; <2> centromere – D9S127 – 2 cM – mfd220 – 1 cM – FCMD – 6 cM – D9S58 – telomere (Fig. 4).

Results

Linkage analysis of FCMD families

The results of two point linkage analyses in FCMD families, with each of the 3 markers (D9S127, mfd220 and CA246), are presented in Table 1. The order of these loci was estimated as follows; centromere – D9S127 – 1.7 cM – mfd220 – 3 cM – CA246 – telomere. Significant lod scores to the FCMD locus were obtained at all 3 loci examined. The locus without obligate recombinations between FCMD and obtaining the highest LOD score (7.37), was mfd220, a result in accord with those of previous studies [6]. In addition, the LOD score of D9S127 was 5.20 and that of CA246 was 3.10, both of which were also significant.

Prenatal diagnosis in two FCMD families

The results of genetic polymorphism analysis are shown in Fig. 3.

In family 1, the fetus inherited an allele which does not carry the FCMD gene from the father while the other allele, from the mother, had a crossover. In the maternal allele, the markers on the telomere side of D9S127, including mfd220, showed haplotypes identical to those of the affected second child.

In family 2, the fetus had inherited an allele carrying the FCMD gene from the father. In the maternal allele, a crossover was identified between loci mfd220 and CA246. The centromere side of mfd220 had haplotypes identical to those of the proband.

According to the calculation of fetal phenotype probability, the fetus in family 1 was an FCMD carrier with a certainty of at least 99% for both assumption modes, while in family 2, the fetus had a high probability of being affected, that is, 99.9% under the assumption that the FCMD gene locates on the centromere side of mfd220, and 86.2% under the assumption that it locates on the telomere side (Fig. 4).

The parents were informed of the above results around 19 gestational weeks. The parents

Table 1

Two point linkage result between FCMD and flanking loci

Locus	θ_{max}	Z_{max}	θ							
			0.00	0.01	0.05	0.10	0.15	0.20	0.30	0.40
D9S127	0.00	5.20	5.20	5.06	4.49	3.38	3.08	2.41	1.22	0.39
mfd220	0.00	7.37	7.37	7.16	6.30	5.24	4.24	3.30	1.68	0.54
CA246	0.05	3.10	$-\infty$	2.36	3.10	2.89	2.45	1.96	1.03	0.34

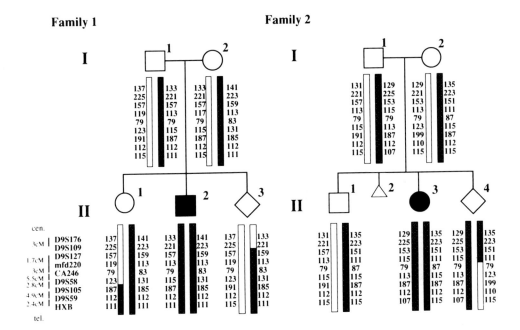

Fig. 3. Genotypes of the 2 pedigrees studied. (Genotypes are indicated for 9 polymorphic microsatellite loci. The FCMD gene is presumed to lie within a region between D9S127 and CA246. Mfd220 is the closest marker. The values shown as haplotypes are the sizes of PCR products obtained with each marker. The haplotype carrying the FCMD gene is shaded. Family 1: the fetus (II-3) had inherited a non-shaded allele from the father while in the maternal allele which had a crossover, the markers on the telomere side from D9S127 showed a shaded allele. Family 2: the fetus (II-4) had inherited a shaded allele from the father. In the maternal allele, a crossover was identified between loci mfd220 and CA246. The centromere side of mfd220 showed a shaded allele.

in family 1 decided to continue the pregnancy and a healthy girl was born, who has shown no signs suggestive of FCMD to date (she is currently 10 months old). Her serum CK level is 120 mU/ml.

In family 2, the parents opted for a therapeutic abortion at 20 gestational weeks. On macroscopic observation of the fetal brain, small multiple granular protrusions over the cerebral surface were noted (Fig. 5), which is a characteristic feature of the FCMD fetal brain [21].

Discussion

FCMD, which was first described by Fukuyama et al. in 1960, is now recognized as an independent subtype of progressive muscular dystrophy (McKusick's No. 253800). Judging from the high incidence of consanguineous parental marriage and sib recurrence, and the absence of sexual preference and vertical transmission, a simple autosomal recessive heredity was proposed as the most likely mode of inheritance of this disorder [1]. This idea was supported by detailed pedigree analyses conducted by Osawa [5] and Fukuyama and Osawa [6] which demonstrated that the segregation ratio in sibships of 153 FCMD families do not deviate significantly from 0.25.

316

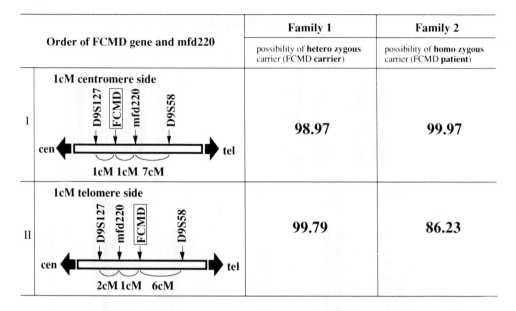

Order of FCMD gene and mfd220		Family 1	Family 2
		possibility of **hetero zygous** carrier (FCMD **carrier**)	possibility of **homo zygous** carrier (FCMD **patient**)
I	**1cM centromere side**	98.97	99.97
II	**1cM telomere side**	99.79	86.23

Fig. 4. Calculation of fetal phenotype probability by computer program. The calculation was established by hypothesizing two different location orders of the FCMD gene. <1> centromere – D9S127 – 1 cM – FCMD – 1 cM – mfd220 – 7 cM – D9S58 – telomere; <2> centromere – D9S127 – 2 cM – mfd220 – 1 cM – FCMD – 6 cM – D9S58 – telomere.

FCMD, which is seldom reported outside of Japan, is second in prevalence only to Duchenne type (DMD) among all subtypes of childhood progressive muscular dystrophy (PMD) in Japan. In the cohort of 337 cases of PMD followed at our pediatric neuromuscular clinic over the last 23 years (1971–1993), DMD and CMD accounted for 50.2% (169 cases) and 35.3% (177 cases), respectively [22]. Based on data obtained from the most recent nationwide multi-institutional collaborative study, the annual incidence of FCMD in Japan was estimated to be in the range of 1.92×10^5 to 3.68×10^{-5} live births [23].

FCMD patients suffer from profound mental and physical handicaps. Muscle impairment involves the entire body. There are also multiple joint contractures and skeletal deformities, as well as moderate to severe mental retardation. The majority of patients never acquire the ability to stand or walk independently, with 17 years being the average age at death. Neither curative measures nor means of arresting the progressive course are available, at present. Neither has there been any reliable method of prenatal diagnosis, until recently.

In 1993, for the first time ever, Toda et al. mapped the FCMD gene locus to chromosome 9q31-33 [7]. In addition, in 1994, this group further narrowed the locus to an area very close to mfd220 [8]. We also studied, at this time, 20 FCMD families providing DNA for our study of genetic linkage analysis based on previously reported methods. Our results were in agreement with those of previous studies [7,8].

In addition, these new findings have made prenatal diagnosis of FCMD, by polymorphism analysis, possible. In this article, the authors described 2 families in which prenatal diagnosis of FCMD was successfully carried out for the first time in the world.

Based on the haplotype results, the fetus in family 1 was considered to be a carrier who had inherited the FCMD mutation only from her mother. In the case of family 2, the fetus,

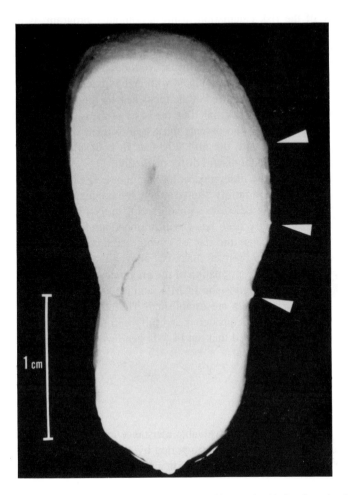

Fig. 5. Autopsied brain of the family 2 fetus. Sagittal section of a frontoparietal lesion from the right hemisphere. Small multiple granular protrusions, up to 0.5 mm in diameter, can be seen over the cerebral surface (arrowheads).

like the proband, had inherited an identical mfd220 haplotype from both parents. As mfd220 is the marker nearest the FCMD gene, the likelihood of the fetus in family 2 being affected was considered to be extremely high.

Considering the possibility, however, that significantly more recombination may have occurred at random in the parental alleles, genotypic data from the D9S127, mfd220 and D9S58 were entered into a computer and the calculation of fetal phenotype probability was performed. We did not use the CA246 data, as CA246 was a provisional locus obtained from the recombination fraction. This process was thought to be necessary to evaluate the case of family 2 in which the maternal allele might have eliminated the FCMD gene through recombination between mfd220 and CA246, in which case the fetus would have been a carrier. The calculation was carried out by hypothesizing two possibilities (Fig. 4). In one, the FCMD gene locates on the centromere side of mfd220, and in the other, on the telomere side of mfd220.

318

The reliability of the risk calculation, using a computer program, is tremendously enhanced when the parental haplotype of mfd220 shows homozygosity, indicating that the haplotype is non-informative, or when a recombination occurs near the mfd220 locus in the fetus. In family 1, the recombination site was far from the mfd220 locus, such that there was no difference between probabilities calculated with and without the risk inference. However, in family 2, the recombination occurred at the locus nearest the mfd220, such that there was a difference between the results calculated on the basis of the two hypothesized possibilities (Fig. 4). In the latter situation, the parents must be informed of both risk calculations. If recombination occurs adjacent to the mfd220 locus in both alleles, the results calculated from the two hypothetical situations will differ markedly.

After being informed of the likelihood of having another FCMD child, family 1 decided to continue the pregnancy, and family 2 to terminate the pregnancy. The eventual outcomes confirmed that both prenatal predictions were correct. Family 1 represents a special situation in that the parents had initially been faced with tremendous familial pressure to terminate the pregnancy, basically because the risk of having another affected child was 25%. The very low risk demonstrated by prenatal diagnosis allayed the concerns of the grandparents, allowing the parents to opt for continuation of the pregnancy.

The demand for prenatal diagnosis in FCMD families will certainly continue to increase until effective treatment measures are established. The ethical issues inherent to prenatal diagnosis should, of course, be considered carefully before the widespread application of prenatal diagnosis. It is also hoped that the FCMD gene will be cloned in the very near future.

Acknowledgments

We thank Ms. Y Kawakita for her invaluable assistance and Prof. M. Nakabayashi for performing amniocentesis. This work was supported by a Research Grant (SA-2) for Nervous and Mental Disorders from the Japanese Ministry of Health and Welfare.

References

1. Fukuyama Y, Kawazura M, Haruna H. A peculiar form of congenital progressive muscular dystrophy. Report of fifteen cases. Paediatr Univ Tokyo (Tokyo) 1960; 4: 5–8.
2. McKusick VA, ed. Mendelian inheritance in man. A catalog of human genetics and genetic disorders. 11th edn. Baltimore, MD: Johns Hopkins University Press, 1994.
3. Nonaka I, Chou SM. Congenital muscular dystrophy. In: Vinken PJ, Bruyn GW, eds. Handbook of clinical neurology, Vol 41. Amsterdam: North Holland, 1979: 27–50.
4. Fukuyama Y, Osawa M, Suzuki H. Congenital progressive muscular dystrophy of Fukuyama type – clinical, genetic and pathological considerations. Brain Dev (Tokyo) 1981; 3: 1–29.
5. Osawa M. A genetical and epidemiological study on congenital progressive muscular dystrophy (Fukuyama type) (in Japanese). Tokyo Joshi Ikadaigaku Zasshi (Tokyo) 1978; 48: 112–149.
6. Fukuyama Y, Osawa M. A genetic study of the Fukuyama type congenital muscular dystrophy. Brain Dev (Tokyo) 1984; 6: 373–390.
7. Toda T, Segawa M, Nomura Y, et al. Localization of a gene for Fukuyama type congenital muscular dystrophy to chromosome 9q31-33. Nat Genet 1993; 5: 283–286.
8. Toda T, Ikegawa S, Okui K, et al. Refined mapping of a gene responsible for Fukuyama type congenital muscular dystrophy: evidence for strong linkage disequilibrium. Am J Hum Genet 1994; 55: 946–950.

9. Lyall JEW, Forlong RA, Yuille MAR, et al. A dinucleotide repeat polymorphism at the D9S127 locus. Nucleic Acids Res 1992; 20: 925.

10. Weber JL. Genome Data Base (GDB) version 4.1. Baltimore, MD: Welch WH Medical Library: 21205.

11. Toda T, Ikegawa S, Miyake M, Nakaboti Y, Nakamura Y. Dinucleotide repeat polymorphism on chromosome 9q32. Jpn J Hum Genet 1995; 40: 333–334.

12. Lathrop GM, Lalouel JM, Julier C, Ott J. Strategies for multipoint linkage analysis in humans. Proc Natl Acad Sci USA 1984; 81: 3443–3446.

13. Sambrook J, Fritsch EF, Maniatis T. Molecular cloning: a laboratory manual, 2nd edn. Cold Spring Harbor, NY: Cold Spring Harbor Laboratory Press, 1989: 9.16–9.19.

14. Feener CA, Boyce FM, Kunkel LM. Rapid detection of CA polymorphisms in cloned DNA: application to the 5' region of the dystrophin gene. Am J Hum Genet 1991; 48: 621–627.

15. NIH/CEPH Collaborative Mapping Group. A comprehensive genetic linkage map of the human genome. Science 1992; 258: 67–86.

16. Weissenbach J, Gyapay G, Dib C, et al. A second-generation linkage map of the human genome. Nature 1992; 359: 794–801.

17. Furlong RA, Lyall JEW, Goudie DR, et al. A dinucleotide repeat polymorphism at the D9S109 locus. Nucleic Acids Res 1992; 20: 925.

18. Kwiatkowski DJ, Henske EP, Weimer K, Ozelius L, Gusella JF, Haines J. Construction of a GT polymorphism map of human 9q. Genomics 1992; 12: 229–240.

19. Wilkie PJ, Krizman DB, Weber JL. Linkage map of human chromosome 9 microsatellite polymorphisms. Genomics 1992; 12: 607–609.

20. Ozelius L, Schubach DE, Stefansson K, Slaugenhaupt S, Gusella JF, Breakfield XO. Dinucleotide repeat polymorphism for the hexabrachion gene (HXB) on chromosome 9q32-34. Hum Mol Genet 1992; 1: 141.

21. Takada K, Nakamura H, Suzumori K, IshikawaT, Sugiyama N. Cortical dysplasia in a 23-week fetus with Fukuyama congenital muscular dystrophy (FCMD). Acta Neuropathol 1987; 74: 300–306.

22. Fukuyama Y. Floppy infant syndrome and child neurology – a retrospective review of 27 years at Tokyo Women' s Medical College (in Japanese). Shoni Naika (Tokyo) 1994; 26: 2085–2097.

23. Osawa M, Suzuki N, Shiraiwa Y, Muto J, Fukuyama Y, Yoshioka M. Recent advances and epidemiological data in the research of congenital muscular dystrophy (in Japanese). In: Takahashi K, ed. The 1994–1995 annual report of the research committee of clinics, epidemiology and genetic counseling of progressive muscular dystrophy, sponsored by the Ministy of Health and Welfare. Hyogo, 1996: 93–95.

Y. Fukuyama, M. Osawa and K. Saito (Eds.), *Congenital Muscular Dystrophies*
© 1997 Elsevier Science B.V. All rights reserved

CHAPTER 27

Tubular aggregates myopathy

GEORGES SERRATRICE[1] and JEAN-FRANÇOIS PELLISSIER[2]

[1]*Professeur de Neurologie, Clinique des Maladies du Système Nerveux et de l'Appareil Locomoteur,*
Timone, Marseille, France
[2]*Professeur de Neuropathologie Service d'Anatomie Pathologique et de Neuropathologie,*
Timone, Marseille, France

Introduction

Tubular aggregates (TA) myopathy is usually classified among congenital myopathies. However, many questions can be raised. TA are nonspecific morphological changes, and can be observed in several neuromuscular diseases. On the other hand, TA are unusually frequent in the exercise intolerance syndrome [1] and in some congenital myopathies. In these cases, TA within the muscle fibers constitute the major and often the unique structural alteration.

TA were first described in 1964 by light microscopy [2] and in 1966 by electron microscopy [3]. In 1970, W.K. Engel et al. [4] published the main morphological data: focal aggregates with material stained by NADH but negative with myofibrillar ATPase or SDH; TA distribution in type II muscle fibers only; and contiguity with sarcoplasmic reticulum. They proposed a sequence formation from lateral sacs thought to be a massive proliferation of the sacs. With this description the morphological aspects of TA are well known. By light microscopy, TA appear as a basophilic material with hematoxylin and eosin staining, subsarcolemmal and intermyofibrillar. TA are red stained with the modified Gomori trichrome technique, accentuated when using NADH-TR and myoadenylate deaminase. Conversely they do not react with myofibrillar ATPase, SDH, or menadione linked alpha glycerophosphate dehydrogenase (GPDH). Electron microscopy shows that TA are localized under the plasma membrane or are intermyofibrillar. TA tubules are double walled with a second tubule of 50–70 nm in diameter and one or several inner tubules of 20–30 nm in diameter. Tubules are orientated parallel, perpendicular or oblique to the long axis of the fiber.

In a recent meeting considering 3 categories of rare neuromuscular diseases [5], TA myopathy was listed in category II. Category I was devoted to myopathies in which a genetic study has to be developed, for instance central core disease. In category III, the disease entity or heredity remained to be determined. Category II included the diseases for which criteria require further clarification, for instance familial inclusion body myositis. As regards TA myopathy, criteria appear to be mainly morphological if we take into account the unusual characteristics of this condition.

Patients

Patients with definite neuromuscular diseases such as periodic paralysis, congenital myasthenia, are not discussed in this paper. The following cases only have been considered. (1) Three cases of exercise intolerance with myalgia and cramps illustrated by a 39-year-old man with myalgias and cramps, mainly in the forearms, and difficulty in writing since the age of 34. Neurological examination was normal as well as serum creatine kinase, EMG, magnetic resonance spectroscopy, and muscle CT scan. A flexor carpi radialis biopsy was performed. The other 2 cases complained of cramps and myalgias, proximal and distal. Ancillary laboratory tests were normal. Serum creatine kinase, muscle CT scan and MRI were normal. (2) In 4 cases the clinical diagnosis was polymyositis or polyarteritis nodosa (Table 1). They were 52- to 72-year-old men and all complained of myalgias without cramps. There were biological inflammatory signs with high erythrocyte sedimentation rate. EMG was myogenic in 2 cases, and both neurogenic and myogenic in 2 cases. Corticotherapy was ineffective in all 4 patients. (3) Finally, 3 cases were classified as congenital TA myopathy, one of whom had experienced gait disturbances since the age of 2. During childhood, he had a waddling gait with frequent falls. He complained of post-exercise myalgias. At 22, the waddling gait was prominent with proximal and distal weakness. Myalgias lasted sometimes for a week after exercise. Serum creatine kinase level was 1150 IU/l (normal 130). EMG was myogenic with normal nerve conduction velocities. Muscle CT scan was normal as well as magnetic resonance spectroscopy. Therapeutic trials with nifedipine (35 mg/day) and spironolactone (100 mg/day) were ineffective. Myalgias were improved by diltiazem (120 mg/day). A second muscle biopsy, 6 months later showed the same alterations (Table 2).

Materials and methods

Open muscle biopsies were performed under local anesthesia. Specimens were frozen in liquid nitrogen. Sections of 5 μm were stained using modified Gomori trichrome, NADH-

Table 1

Tubular aggregates and pseudopolymyositic or pseudoinflammatory cases

Sex	Age	Chronic myalgias	ESR inflammation	EMG	Clinical diagnosis	Muscle biopsy		Cortico-therapy
						necrosis inflammation	TA	
M	57	++	++	Myo Neuro	PM		++	0
M	52	++	++	Myo	PM PAN		++	0
M	61	+	++	Myo Neuro	PM PAN	0	++	0
M	72	++	++	Myo	PM	0	++	0

M, male; EMG, electromyography; Myo, myogenic; Neuro, neurogenic; ESR, erythrocyte sedimentation rate; PM, polymyositis; PAN, polyarteritis nodosa.

Table 2

Congenital(?) myopathies with tubular aggregates

Sex	Age	Onset	Proximal weakness	Distal weakness	Exercise intolerance	CK	Myogenic EMG	Fiber type	Genetics
M	22	2	UL + LL	+	Myalgias	+	+	II > I	0
F	15	10	UL + LL	−	Myalgias	−	+	II	Translocation 4q.12 p
M	26	15	UL + LL	−	Cramps Myalgias	−	+	II > I	0

M, male; F, female; UL, upper limbs; LL, lower limbs; CK, creatine kinase

TR, myofibrillar ATPase (pH 9.5, 4.6, 4.2), SDH, myoadenylate deaminase, menadione-linked alpha GPDH, phosphatase and periodic acid Schiff.

A quantitative study of intramuscular calcium content revealed by the Von Kossa method has been done by SAMBA 2000 Alcatel TITN.

An immunohistochemical study with polyclonal antibody directed against Ca^{2+} SR AT-Pase was carried out.

An electron microscopic study was performed in each muscle specimen according to the method previously described [6].

Results

All muscle biopsies showed typical TA. They corresponded to basophilic zones with hematoxylin and eosin, and exhibited red masses with modified Gomori trichrome. They were strongly stained with NADH-TR and myoadenylate deaminase, but negative with myofibrillar ATPases, SDH and menadione linked-alpha GPDH. TA were localized in type II fibers in group I and in both type I and type II fibers in group 3. Electron microscopy showed intermyofibrillar or subsarcolemmal TA with 50–70 nm diameter tubules. There were no inflammatory changes and no fiber necrosis in muscle biopsies of patients from group II. As regards patients from group III, quadriceps muscle biopsy showed only TA in type I and type II muscle fibers.

Calcium quantitative study was expressed in density per area unit. The density was constant in TA (mean: 0, 118-SD 0, 038). Conversely the density was variable in the fiber (mean: 0, 223-SD: 0, 132). The calcium content of TA was lower than the normal sarcoplasma. Calcium content was statistically different from that of normal sarcoplasma (Student's t-test: $P < 0.02$). TA binding by anti-CA^{2+} SR ATPase was constant in the same area as AMP deaminase staining.

Discussion

Clinical correlations are difficult to assess in the field of TA myopathies. TA have been reported in several well defined neuromuscular diseases. The most frequent are periodic paralysis in which TA are associated with vacuoles. TA have also been described in various disorders (Table 3). The finding of TA in the muscles of patients with a wide variety of dis-

Table 3

Diseases associated with tubular aggregates

Periodic paralysis	Grüner, 1966 [3]
Congenital myotonia	Schröder and Becker, 1972 [27]
Paramyotonia	Julien et al., 1971 [28]
Myotonic dystrophy	Schotland, 1968 [29]
FSH dystrophy	Hurwitz et al., 1967 [30]
Myasthenia gravis	Bergman et al., 1971 [31]
Type 2 glycogenosis	Engel and Dale, 1968 [32]
Inflammatory myopathy	Rosenberg et al., 1985 [18]
Malignant hyperthermia	Reske-Nielsen et al., 1975 [33]
Acromegalia	Mastaglia, 1973 [34]
Hyperaldosteronism	Gallai, 1977 [35]
Osteomalacia	Doriguzzi et al., 1984 [36]
Denervation	Shafiq et al., 1967 [37]
Porphyria	Engel et al., 1970 [4]
Infarction	Lewis et al., 1971 [12]
Hyperornithinemia	Sipila et al., 1979 [38]
Ophthalmoplegia with melanosis	Sahashi et al., 1981 [39]
Diabetes	Chokroverty et al., 1977 [40]
Alcoholic myopathy	Chui et al., 1975 [41]
Drugs	Engel et al., 1970 [4]
Drug addiction	Richter et al., 1973 [42]
Normal people	Reske-Nielsen et al., 1975 [33]
Tetanic botulism	Duchen, 1971, 1973 [43,44]
Anoxia	Schiaffino et al., 1977 [45]
Perhexiline	Fardeau et al., 1979 [46]

orders suggest that they represent only a non-specific reaction in muscle. This lack of specificity is also supported by some personal observations [1] of familial cases of hyperkalemic periodic paralysis with SNC4A mutations (Thr 704 Met) with the presence of TA in one patient but the absence of TA in his brother and daughter. Likewise TA have been observed in several congenital myasthenic syndromes [8–10] including 2 personal cases. TA were randomly distributed and probably non-specific except in 5 cases of prolonged open time of the acetylcholine-induced ion channel [11], in which TA were observed close to the post-synaptic portion of motor end plates. However, it seems difficult to establish a relationship between TA and myasthenic symptoms.

In other groups of patients, TA constitute the major structural alterations. These 3 groups are: exercise-intolerance syndrome, pseudo-inflammatory cases and congenital myopathies.

Exercise-induced cramps and myalgias in which TA are the only morphological abnormality are well documented with the description of Morgan-Hughes et al. [1] reporting the case of a 54-year-old man complaining of myalgias without cramps but with a 6 year history of exercise intolerance. Muscle biopsy showed TA in type II muscle fibers. Other similar cases have also been published [12–18]. Our 3 cases are similar. All patients were men, adults or young adults. Myalgias were predominant in the lower limbs, sometimes in the upper limbs ([15] and 1 of our cases), absent only in one patient [16]. Cramps were frequently reported [12,13,16,18] (our cases). Exercise intolerance was constant but is not mentioned in the case of Lewis et al. [12]. The course lasted from 1 year [16] to 16 years [14]. The most constant feature was the localization of the changes. TA were confined to type II fibers in all the patients. There is no accurate explanation for this selectivity nor for the male predominance. In animals, in a strain of normal MRL mice of male sex, Kuncl et al. [19] observed TA in the absence of any other muscle abnormalities. Interestingly, TA were confined to type II fibers. Moreover, the development of TA was nearly completely prevented by castration. These data suggest hormonal factors associated to genetic predisposition. How gonadal hormones might induce the expression of TA confined to type II muscle fibers remains unknown. Muscle androgen receptors acting as target is unclear. This finding fits into a general pattern of hormonal influences on the skeletal muscle. The effects of androgenic hormones, related to testosterone, have been reported. Testicular androgenic steroids enhance type II fibers denervation atrophy [20]. Such effects are thought to be mediated through intracellular androgen receptors that are present in the skeletal muscle. However, the molecular basis of this phenomenon remains to be elucidated.

Such cases of exercise intolerance are sometimes not so clearly individualized. For instance, in one personal unpublished case, a 2 phase course was observed: from the ages of 13 to 20, exercise intolerance with only cramps and myalgias; after the age of 20, episodes of normokalemic periodic paralysis. The diagnosis was exercise-induced pain before aged 20 and periodic paralysis after 20. TA were present in both type I and type II fibers.

In the second group including 4 adult male patients (Table 1), the clinical diagnosis was inflammatory myopathy being either polymyositis or periarteritis nodosa. The main features were myalgias with biological signs of inflammation such as highly raised erythrocyte sedimentation rate. However, there was no inflammation or necrosis within muscle biopsy and corticotherapy was ineffective. Muscle changes were TA only. Are TA the expression of a non-specific inflammatory reaction? Are they strictly non specific and coincidental? There is no clear explanation.

A tentative approach can be suggested. TA proliferation could be induced by a general inflammation as a non-specific phenomenon. The following fact is in favor of this hypothesis: in 2 patients (case 2 and case 4) a second muscle biopsy was performed 6 months later; in both cases TA were absent. However, TA have never been reported in our cases of inflammatory neuromuscular diseases or in the cases in the literature, with the exception of the three cases of Rosenberg et al. [18]: a 52 year-old-man with dermatomyositis without pain, with perifascicular atrophy and two other men, 67 and 62 years old respectively, with inflammatory myopathy, demyelinating neuropathy and perivascular inflammation. In these cases, TA coexist with inflammatory changes. In contrast TA are the only changes in our 4 cases.

Congenital myopathies with TA are rare. There are 14 cases published which could belong to this group [21–24]. The inheritance is rarely autosomal recessive [21], more frequently autosomal dominant [22–24]. Proximal weakness is constant, sometimes confined to the lower limbs. Distal weakness is less frequent [21,22] (1 of our cases). Myalgias and cramps have been observed [23] (our cases). In some cases, serum CK level is higher than normal. EMG is myogenic. In muscle biopsy, TA are not confined to type II fibers but are randomly distributed to type II and type I fibers. On the whole, TA myopathy, although usually classified among congenital myopathies, is different. Its nosological place has to be discussed. Firstly, the onset of the disease is not congenital (except in our case 1 in which proximal weakness was present as from the age of 2). Earliest cases begin at the age of 4 [24], 6 [21], 10 and 15 (2 of our cases). The onset is frequently in young adults. Secondly, it is a painful myopathy whereas congenital myopathies are constantly painless. Moreover, amyotrophy is absent or moderate. CK level is variable. Muscle CT scan is normal in our 3 cases. The course is chronic and very slowly progressive (more than one decade in the majority of cases). These facts raise a question: is TA myopathy a congenital or a metabolic myopathy? It is difficult to answer. It must be pointed out that, in contrast to pseudoinflammatory cases, in our congenital case 1, repeated biopsy showed the persistence of TA in muscle. This fact indicates that TA were a constant change. In a family observed by Mahon et al. [24], proximal and distal weakness were associated with a thrombocytopenia, suggesting a primary defect involving several membranous systems.

TA correspond to extensions of the sarcoplasmic reticulum sacs as shown by electron microscopy [4]. More recent immunohistochemical studies [25,26] with a polyclonal antibody against Ca^{2+} SR ATPase showed an immunoreactivity of TA for this antibody. Release of calcium from the sarcoplasmic reticulum during the muscle contraction is determined by Ca^{2+} transport ATPase, as well as during relaxation by active pumping of calcium ions through the sarcoplasmic reticulum. Is there a calcium storage in TA? This is a controversial subject. Salviati et al. [25] incubated skinned muscle fibers in a calcium-oxalate medium and the ability of TA to store calcium was investigated by electron microscopy. They observed the formation of intraluminal Ca-oxalate deposits both in the terminal cisterns of the sarcoplasmic reticulum and in TA. Different results were obtained in our series [26]. A quantitative analysis (SAMBA 2000 Alcatel TITN) was carried out on frozen sections stained from calcium using the Von Kossa method. Twenty fibers with TA and 20 normal fibers were studied with this cytometric technique. The calcium content density was lower in TA: 0.118 (±0.38), than in normal sarcoplasm: 0.23 (±0.132). These results were obtained in physiologic conditions in contrast with the experimental conditions of the study of Salviati et al. [25]. Our study suggests that TA are not liable to increase calcium uptake.

There is no treatment to TA myopathy, particularly in exercise-induced cramps and myalgias. Dantrolene sodium which allows the release of calcium from the sarcoplasmic reticulum is ineffective as well as calcium channel blockers. In one patient with TA myopathy (case 1), nifedipine was ineffective. However, myalgias were improved with diltiazem (120 mg/day).

Finally, many questions remain. Are there non-specific and specific TA syndromes? Probably yes. Is exercise-intolerance with TA a sex-related syndrome? Undoubtedly yes. Why are TA present only in type II fibers in exercise-intolerance? The reason is unclear. Is the inflammatory syndrome with TA an entity? Probably not. Further studies are necessary for an assessment. Is TA myopathy a congenital myopathy? Probably so, but very different from other congenital myopathies. Are there effective calcium channel blockers on calcium homeostasis? Usually not.

References

1. Morgan-Hughes JA, Mair WGP, Lascelles PT. A disorder of skeletal muscle associated with tubular aggregates. Brain 1970; 93: 873–880.
2. Engel WK. Mitochondrial aggregates in muscle disease. J Histochem Cytochem 1964; 12: 46–48.
3. Grüner JE. Anomalies du reticulum sarcoplasmique et prolifération de tubules dans le muscle d'une paralysie périodique familiale. CR Soc Biol 1966; 160: 193.
4. Engel WK, Bishop DW, Cunningham GG. Tubular aggregates in type II muscle fibers: ultrastructural and histochemical correlation. J Ultrastructure Res 1970; 31: 507–505.
5. Middleton LT, Moser H. Twenty-third ENMC workshop on rare neuromuscular diseases. Neuromusc Disord 1994; 4: 273–275.
6. Pellissier JF, Pouget J, Charpin C, Figarella D. Myopathy associated with desmin intermediate filaments. An immunoelectron-microscopic study. J Neurol Sci 1989; 89: 49–61.

7. Plassart E, Reboul J, Rime CS, et al. Mutations in the muscle sodium channel gene (SCN4A) in 13 French families with hyperkalemic periodic paralysis and paramyotonia congenita: phenotype to genotype correlations and demonstration of the predominance of two mutations. Eur J Hum Genet 1994; 2: 110–124.

8. Johns TR, Campa JF, Adelman LS. Familial myasthenia with "tubular aggregates" treated with prednisone. Neurology 1973; 23: 426 (Abstr).

9. Dobkin BH, Verity MA. Familial neuromuscular disease with type I fiber hypoplasia, tubular aggregates, cardiomyopathy and myasthenic features. Neurology 1978; 28: 1135–1140.

10. Morgan-Hughes JA, Lecky BRF, Landon DN, Murray NMF. Alteration in the number and affinity of junctional acetylcholine receptors in myopathy with tubular aggregates: a newly recognized receptor defect. Brain 1981; 104: 279–295.

11. Engel AG, Lambert EH, Mulder DM, et al. A newly recognized congenital myasthenic syndrome attributed to a prolonged open time of the acetylcholine-induced ion channel. Ann Neurol 1982; 11: 553–569.

12. Lewis PD, Pallis C, Pearse AGE. Myopathy with tubular aggregates. J Neurol 1971; 13: 381–388.

13. Lazaro J, Fenichel GM, Kilroy AW, Saito A, Fleischer S. Cramps, muscle pain and tubular aggregates. Arch Neurol 1980; 37: 715–717.

14. Brumback RA, Staton RD, Susag M. Exercise-induced pain, stiffness, and tubular aggregation in skeletal muscle. J Neurol Neurosurg Psychiatry 1981; 44: 250–254.

15. Roullet E, Fardeau M, Collin H, Marteau R. Myopathies avec agrégats tubulaires. Etude clinique, biologique et histologique de 2 cas. Rev Neurol 1985; 10: 655–662.

16. Orimo S, Araki M, Ishii H, et al. A case of "myopathy with tubular aggregates" with increased muscle fiber sensitivity to caffeine. J Neurol 1987; 234: 424–426.

17. Niakan E, Harati Y, Danon MJ. Tubular aggregates: their association with myalgia. J Neurol Neurosurg Psychiatry 1985; 48: 882–886.

18. Rosenberg NL, Neville HE, Ringel MD. Tubular aggregates. Their association with neuromuscular diseases including the syndrome of myalgias/cramps. Arch Neurol 1985; 42: 973–976.

19. Kuncl RW, Pestronk A, Lane J, Alexander E. The MRL +/+ mouse: a new model of tubular aggregates which are gender- and age- related. Acta Neuropathol 1989; 78: 615–620.

20. Karpati G, Hilton-Jones D, Prescott S, Carpenter S. Castration reduces the rate of denervation atrophy of skeletal muscle fibers in rat solei and plantares. Ann Neurol 1987; 22: 169 (Abstr).

21. De Groot JG, Arts WF. Familial myopathy with tubular aggregates. J Neurol 1982; 227: 35–41.

22. Rohkamm R, Boxler K, Ricker K, Jerusalem F. A dominantly inherited myopathy with excessive tubular aggregates. Neurology 1983; 33: 331–336.

23. Pierobon-Bormioli S, Armani M, Ringel SP, et al. Familial neuromuscular disease with tubular aggregates. Muscle Nerve 1985; 8: 291–298.

24. Mahon M, Cumming WJK, Kristmundsdottir F, Evans Dik, Carrington PA. Familial myopathy associated with thrombocytopenia: a clinical and histomorphometric study. J Neurol Sci 1988; 88: 55–67.

25. Salviati G, Pierobon-Bormioli S, Betto R, et al. Tubular aggregates: sarcoplasmic reticulum oligin, calcium storage ability, and functional implications. Muscle Nerve 1985; 8: 299–306.

26. Figarella-Branger D, Pellissier JF, Perez-Castillo AM, Desnuelle C, Pouget J, Serratrice G. Myopathie lentement progressive avec accumulation d'agrégats tubulaires. Rev Neurol (Paris) 1991; 147: 586–594.

27. Schröder JM, Becker PE. Anomalies des T-systems und des sarkoplasmatischen Reticulum bei der Myotonie, Paramyotonie und Adynamie. Virchows Arch Abt A Pathol Anat 1972; 357: 319–344.

28. Julien J, Vital C, Vallat JM, Martin F. Paramyotonie d'Eulenburg. J Neurol Sci 1971; 13: 447–452.

29. Schotland D. Ultrastructural abnormalities in myotonic dystrophy including an unusual T system alteration. J Neuropathol Exp Neurol 1968; 27: 109–110.

30. Hurwitz LJ, Carson NAJ, Allen IV, Fannin TF, Lyttle JA, Neill DW. Clinical, biochemical and histopathological findings in a family with muscular dystrophy. Brain 1967; 40: 799–816.

31. Bergman RA, Johns RJ, Afifi AK. Ultrastructural alterations in muscle from patients with myasthenia and Eaton–Lambert syndrome. Ann N Y Acad Sci 1971; 183: 88–120.

32. Engel AG, Dale AJD. Autophagic glycogenosis of late onset with mitochondrial abnormalities: light and electron microscopic observations. Mayo Clin Proc 1968; 43: 233–279.

33. Reske-Nielsen E, Haase J, Kelstrup J. Malignant hyperthermia in a family: the ultrastructure of muscle biopsies of healthy members. Acta Pathol Microbiol Scand (A) 1975; 83: 651–662.

34. Mastaglia FL. Pathological changes in skeletal muscle in acromegaly. Acta Neuropathol 1973; 24: 273–286.

35. Gallai M. Myopathy with hyperaldosteronism. J Neurol Sci 1977; 32: 337–345.

36. Doriguzzi C, Mongini T, Jeantet A, Monga G. Tubular aggregates in a case of osteomalacic myopathy due to anticonvulsant drugs. Clin Neuropathol 1984; 3: 42–45.

37. Shafiq SA, Milhorat AT, Gorycki MA. Fine structure of human muscle in neurogenic atrophy. Neurology 1967; 17: 934–948.

38. Sipila I, Simell O, Rapola J, Sainio K, Tuteri L. Gyrate atrophy of the choroid and retina with hyperornithinemia: tubular aggregates and type II fiber atrophy in muscle. Neurology 1979; 29: 996–1005.

39. Sahashi K, Hirose K, Uono M. Recurrent ophthalmoplegia, internuclear ophthalmoplegia, amyotrophy, melanosis, apnea and tubular aggregates in muscle fibers: a case report and pathogenesis of tubular aggregates (in Japanese). Rinsho Shinkeigaku (Clin Neurol) (Tokyo) 1981; 21: 23–36.

40. Chokroverty S, Reyes MG, Rubino FA, Tonaki H. The syndrome of diabetic amyotrophy. Ann Neurol 1977; 2: 181–184.

41. Chui LA, Neustein H, Munsat TL. Tubular aggregates in subclinical alcoholic myopathy. Neurology 1975; 25: 405–412.

42. Richter RW, Person J, Bruun B. Neurological complications of addiction to heroin. Bull N Y Acad Med 1973; 49: 3–21.

43. Duchen LW. Changes in the electron microscopic structure of slow and fast skeletal muscle fibers of the mouse after the local injection of botulinisation toxin. J Neurol Sci 1971; 16: 61–74.

44. Duchen LW. The local effect of tetanus toxin on the electron microscopic structure of skeletal muscle fibers of the mouse. J Neurol Sci 1973; 19: 169–177.

45. Schiaffino S, Severin E, Cantini M, Sartore S. Tubular aggregates induced by anoxia in isolated rat skeletal muscle. Lab Invest 1977; 37: 223–228.

46. Fardeau M, Tome FMS, Simon P. Muscle and nerve changes induced by perhexiline maleate in man and mice. Muscle Nerve 1979; 2: 24–36.

Y. Fukuyama, M. Osawa and K. Saito (Eds.), *Congenital Muscular Dystrophies*
© 1997 Elsevier Science B.V. All rights reserved

Cerebral cortical gyration abnormality and denervation muscular atrophy: a case report

GIOVANNI LANZI[1], ANGELA BERARDINELLI[1], ELISA FAZZI[1], CARLA UGGETTI[2] and PIERANGELO VEGGIOTTI[1]

[1]*Department of Child Neuropsychiatry IRCCS "C. Mondino", University of Pavia, Pavia, Italy*
[2]*Neuroradiological Department IRCCS "C. Mondino", University of Pavia, Pavia, Italy*

Introduction

It is well known that gyration abnormalities can be associated with neuromuscular diseases. Fukuyama et al. [1] first described the association between CNS abnormalities and congenital muscular dystrophy in 1960. Subsequently, there were reports of further cases with different kinds of clinical features [1–7], both neurogenic and myopathic, and cortical abnormalities.

Other authors, on the other hand, have discussed the influence of the CNS (and its abnormalities) on the development of skeletal muscle [8]. Adding to the number of such possible associations, we report the case of an infant born at term, to healthy, non-consanguineous parents, with frontal-parietal-temporal pachygyria and a typical picture of denervation atrophy in the skeletal muscle and on neurogenic EMG.

Personal history

The patient was referred to us at the age of 11 months because of seizures. The baby is a male, born at term to healthy, non-consanguineous parents. The pregnancy was uneventful. Active fetal movements began at 3 months gestational age, and were reported to be normal throughout the pregnancy. He was born by means of cesarean section due to breech presentation and acute perinatal distress with decreased cardiac rhythm.

At birth, he had a clubfoot equinovarus deformity, congenital hip dislocation and inguinal hernia, all on the right side. He never had any difficulty in sucking, swallowing or breathing. He was able to control his head at 3 months, but he is still unable to sit independently. His parents also noticed very poor spontaneous motility of the lower limbs as early as the first days of life.

The child has been having spasms in both flexion and extension (up to 25 per day) since he was 10 months old. Standard EEG did not show typical hypsarrythmia, but general slowing of the background activity, and the presence of alpha-like activity, multifocal abnormalities of spike-waves or spikes. During the EEG we recorded asymmetrical flexor spasms, which triggered partial seizures characterized by: deviation of the head and eyes to the left, and loss of responsiveness, crying and breathing alterations. Treatment with sodium valproate (VPA) and benzodiazepine (BZ) reduced the number of these episodes; in the following 4 months the child had 5–6 flexor spasms per week. Four months after beginning the treatment, he had an erratic myoclonic status for about 3 h, which stopped on endorectal administration of clobazam (CLB). Since then, the child has not had further epileptic status, but only 1–2 generalized tonic seizures per week.

Clinical features on admission

Neurological examination performed at 11 months of age showed: microcephaly (head circumference 43.5 cm, <10th centile), the splanchnocranium being bigger than the neurocranium, and a flat occiput, short forehead and a flat nose bridge. He showed normal facial motility. There was poor spontaneous motility of the upper limbs (he did have antigravity power, however, in the upper limbs and was able to reach his mouth with both hands), his lower limbs, on the other hand, were completely still, in a frog-like position; muscle tone was decreased everywhere, especially on the left side. There were no tendon reflexes. He was able to control his head for a while, sit supported and roll with some help. During the examination, the child was alert and from time to time he seemed to be interested in what was happening around him. He failed to react, however, to a sonorous stimulus.

Laboratory findings

Normal results were obtained for: routine serum analysis, serum CK, serum pyruvic and lactic acids, long chain fatty acids, visual evoked potentials and auditory brainstem evoked potentials. ERG was normal in the left eye and of low amplitude in the right eye (1/5 with respect to the contralateral one).

Brain magnetic resonance imaging showed bilateral, fronto-parieto-temporal pachygyria (Figs. 1–3).

EMG showed rich spontaneous fibrillation-like activity; amplitude and duration of motor unit potentials above the normal mean. Normal sensory and motor conduction velocities.

Muscle biopsy showed a well preserved general architecture, marked increase in perimysial connective tissue and fat, round, atrophic fibers, in most of the fascicles, hypertrophic fibers in a few other fascicles, peripheral nuclei and no necrosis or cellular reaction. ATPase showed type grouping (Figs. 4–6). In conclusion, the biopsy findings represented a typical picture of denervation atrophy.

The spine MRI was normal.

EEG showed general slowing of the background activity and alpha-like activity, multifocal abnormalities of spikes-waves or spikes.

Ictal examination showed numerous spasms which triggered partial seizures.

Chromosome analysis showed 46 XY. Analysis performed by fluorescence in situ hybridization, with a specific probe for the Miller Dieker region (17p13.3) showed a normal hybridization signal on both alleles of chromosome 17.

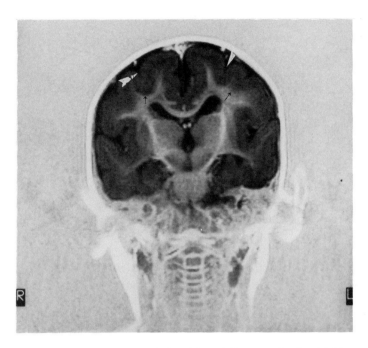

Fig. 1. MR, 0.5 T, I.R (TR 1500, TI 300), coronal slice. A few, shallow convoluted gyri (white arrow-heads) are seen. The frontal cortex is thickened, with smooth grey-white interface (arrows).

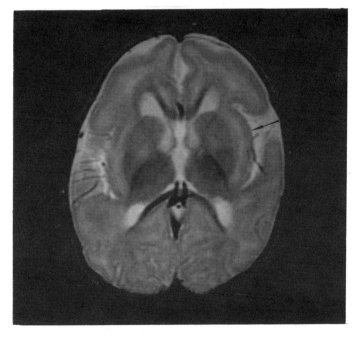

Fig. 2. MR, 0.5 T, SE, T2-weighted (TR 3000, TE 100), axial image. The cortex of frontal and temporal lobes is thickened and smooth, while occipital lobes are quite normal. Note the underopercularization of the sylvian fissures, with exposition of the insula (arrow).

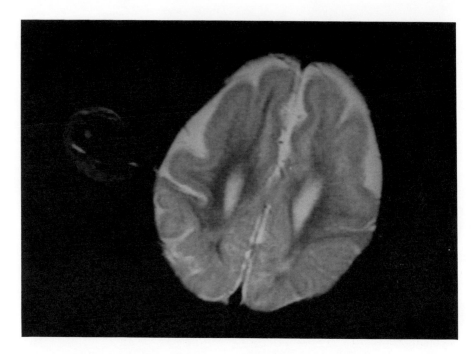

Fig. 3. MR, 0.5 T, SE, T2-weighted (TR 3000, TE 100), axial image. Smooth appearance of frontal cortex. Convexity subarachnoid spaces are widened.

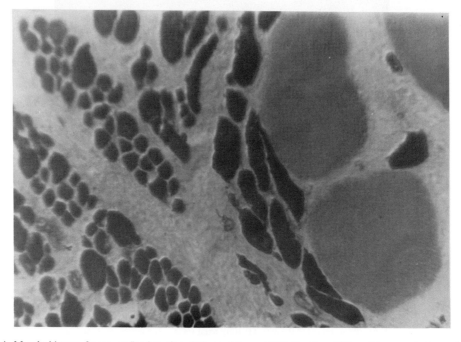

Fig. 4. Muscle biopsy: frozen, unfixed section. Left quadriceps. ×400. Routine ATPase. Two populations of fibers: all of the largest fibers are type 1, all of the smallest are type 2 fibers.

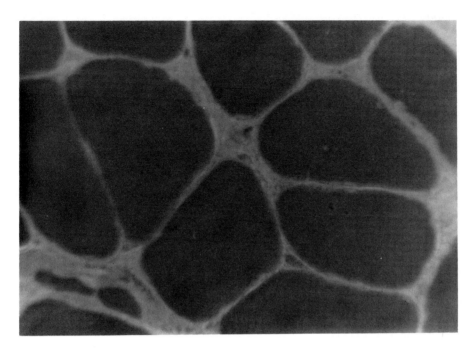

Fig. 5. Muscle biopsy: frozen, unfixed section. Left quadriceps. ×400. **ATPase pH 4.6.** A group of large type 1 fibers.

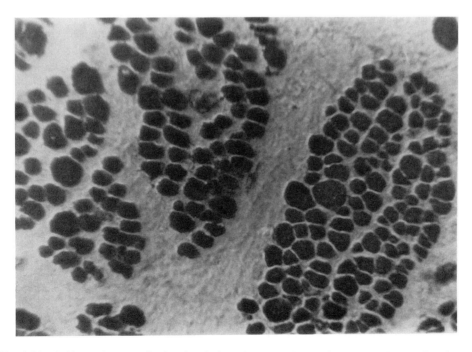

Fig. 6. Muscle biopsy: frozen, unfixed section. Left quadriceps. ×400. Routine ATPase. Groups of small type 2 fibers.

Discussion

The peculiar case we have just described prompted us to review the literature regarding CNS abnormalities and their association with neuromuscular disorders.

These have been described in the literature for long time. The best known is the so-called Fukuyama congenital muscular dystrophy (FCMD) characterized by: an autosomal recessive inheritance, onset before 8 months, facial involvement, joint contractures, mental retardation, high serum CK level and histologic evidence of dystrophic muscle, with a marked increase in connective tissue, polymicrogyria and loss of normal cerebral cytoarchitecture [1,2]. Subsequently, other syndromes with CNS and brain dysplasia were described [9–11]: the Walker–Warburg syndrome (WWS), characterized by lissencephaly and marked hydrocephaly, a hypoplastic corpus callosum, small basal ganglia and thalami, severely hypoplastic cerebellum, and no pyramidal tracts; the so-called muscle-eye-brain (MEB) disease or Santavuori disease, with type two lissencephaly (although with pachygyria or polymycrogyria rather than agyria), and vermis hypoplasia and retinal changes, but less severe than in WWS, the occidental type of congenital muscular dystrophy (OCMD), which can be associated with CNS involvement and also with a normal intellectual level; some malformative syndromes also involving the kidneys and eyes (Lowe syndrome), the congenital multiple arthrogryposis group [12–14], both myogenic and neurogenic, including the Pena–Shokeir syndrome [15,16], and even a neonatal adrenoleukodystrophy referred to as infantile spinal muscular atrophy (SMA) [17].

In the majority of these syndromes, a muscle biopsy shows typical dystrophic features, even when autopsy fails to reveal pyramidal tracts. Only the neurogenic cases of congenital multiple arthrogryposis [12,14,18–20], the Pena–Shokeir syndrome [15,16], and a case of neonatal adrenoleukodystrophy muscle biopsies have neurogenic features.

Other authors [21] have attempted to determine the relation, if any, between cerebral and muscle development. Different patterns of histological muscular findings have been reported, associated with cerebral damage, i.e., congenital fiber type disproportion associated with Krabbe leukodystrophy, delayed muscle maturation, fiber type predominance, selective type 1 or type 2 atrophy, and so on. Normal muscle development has even been found in two children with a severely dysplastic CNS and hypoplastic brainstem.

However, our patient differs from all the cases described so far. He cannot be classified as having classical SMA because of his CNS abnormalities and seizures, he cannot be labelled as FCMD, WWS or MEB, simply because muscle biopsy did not show dystrophic features and he has no eye abnormalities. While he had congenital multiple arthrogryposis (at birth, he had dislocated hips and an equinovarus clubfoot, which is enough for CMA), he had no pulmonary abnormalities, so he cannot be defined as having the Pena–Shokeir syndrome (although this syndrome is quite heterogeneous and it is not currently known what it depends on). He does not have adrenoleukodystrophy.

As far as we know, an association between denervation atrophy in muscle and CNS abnormality has been described in Lowe syndrome, but the patient we describe does not have the typical features of the Lowe syndrome (no cataracts, no glaucoma, no renal tubular dysfunction, etc.). In 1988, Horoupian et al. [22] reported denervation atrophy in muscle associated with CNS abnormality in a female full-term infant, the twin of a macerated stillborn, with a monochorionic and monoamniotic placenta. This newborn, who died at 7 months of age, had renal hypoplasia, double aortic arch and foci of myocardial calcification. The pattern of brain convolution was very irregular and there was polymicrogyria. The authors hypothesized that an ischemic insult could have caused both the cerebral dysplasia and the denervation atrophy in the muscle, because it occurred at a critical stage of muscle innervation. As far as our patient is concerned, we have no evidence of ischemic insult during pregnancy and we have not found any other report in the literature, supporting this hypothesis.

On the other hand, the only SNC abnormality described in association with SMA is olivo-ponto-cerebellar atrophy [23,24], which our patient does not have. We are therefore unable to explain this peculiar association, but we believe that it could be of considerable clinical significance as well as being a useful addition to the possible associations between CNS abnormalities and muscle development.

References

1. Fukuyama Y, Kawazura M, Haruna H. A peculiar form of congenital progressive muscular dystrophy. Report of 15 cases. Paediatr Univ Tokyo (Tokyo) 1960; 4: 5–8.
2. Fukuyama Y, Osawa M, Suzuki H. Congenital progressive muscular dystrophy of the Fukuyama type – clinical, genetic and pathological considerations. Brain Dev (Tokyo) 1981; 3: 1–29.
3. Warburg M. Hydrocephaly, congenital retinal non attachment and congenital falciform fold. Am J Ophthalmol 1978; 85: 88–94.
4. Dobyns WB, Kirkpatrick JB, Hittner HM, Robert RM, Kretzer FL. Syndrome with lissencephaly type II. Walker–Warburg and cerebro-oculo-muscular syndromes and a new syndrome with type II lissencephaly. Am J Med Genet 1985; 22: 157–195.
5. Santavuori P, Somer H, Sainio K, et al. Muscle-eye-brain disease (MEB). Brain Dev (Tokyo) 1989; 11: 147–153.
6. Chou SM, Gilbert EF, Chun RWM, et al. Infantile olivopontocerebellar atrophy with spinal muscular atrophy. Neuropathology 1990; 9 : 21–32.
7. Moerman Ph, Barth PG. Olivo-ponto-cerebellar atrophy with muscular atrophy, joint contractures and pulmonary hypoplasia of prenatal onset. Virchows Arch A 1987; 410: 339–345.
8. Yamanouchi H., Ikuya N., Kaga M, Hirayama Y, Kurokawa T. Congenital focal muscle dysplasia in the lower extremities from probable abnormal innervation: a case report. Brain Dev (Tokyo) 1992; 14: 118–121.
9. Sarnat HB. Cerebral dysgeneses and their influence on fetal muscle development. Brain Dev (Tokyo) 1986; 8: 495–499.
10. Dobyns WB. Classification of the cerebro-oculo-muscular syndrome(s). Commentary to Kimura's paper (pp. 182–191). Brain Dev (Tokyo) 1993; 15: 242–244.
11. Takada K. Fukuyama-type congenital muscular dystrophy and the Walker–Warburg syndrome. Commentary to Kimura's paper (pp. 182–191). Brain Dev (Tokyo) 1993; 15: 244–245.
12. Kimura S, Sasaki Y, Kobayashi T, et al. Fukuyama-type congenital muscular dystrophy and the Walker–Warburg syndrome. Brain Dev (Tokyo) 1993; 15: 182–191.
13. Boylan KB, Ferriero DM, Greco CM, Sheldon RA, Dew M. Congenital hypomyelination neuropathy with arthrogryposis multiplex congenita. Ann Neurol 1992; 31: 337–340.
14. Krugliak L, Gadoth N, Behar AJ. Neuropathic form of arthrogryposis multiplex congenita. J Neurol Sci 1978, 37: 179–185.
15. Drachman DB, Banker BQ. Arthrogryposis multiplex congenita. Case due to disease of the anterior horn cells. Arch Neurol 1961; 5: 89–93.
16. Abe J, Nemoto K, Ohnishi Y, Kimura K, Honda T, Yoshizawa H. Case report: Pena–Shokeir I syndrome: a comparative pathological study. Am J Med Sci 1989; 297: 123–127.
17. Hageman G, Willemse J. The heterogeneity of the Pena–Shokeir syndrome. Neuropediatrics 1987, 18: 45–50.
18. Paul DA, Goldsmith LS, Miles DK, Moser AB, Spiro AJ, Grover WD. Neonatal adrenoleukodystrophy presenting as infantile progressive spinal muscular atrophy. Pediatr Neurol 1993; 9: 496–497.
19. Quinn CM, Wigglesworth JS, Heckmatt J. Lethal arthrogryposis multiplex congenita: a pathological study of 21 cases. Histopathology 1991; 19: 155–162.

336

20. Hageman G, Willemse J. The pathogenesis of fetal hypokinesia. A neurological study of 75 cases of congenital contractures with emphasis on cerebral lesions. Neuropediatrics 1987; 18: 22–23.
21. Vogel H, Halpert D, Horoupian DS. Hypoplasia of posterior spinal roots and dorsal spinal tracts with arthrogryposis multiplex congenita. Acta Neuropathol 1990; 79: 692–669.
22. Horoupian DS, Yoon JJ. Neuropathic arthrogryposis multiplex congenita and intrauterine ischemia of anterior horn cells: a hypothesis. Clin Neuropathol 1988; 7: 285–293.

Y. Fukuyama, M. Osawa and K. Saito (Eds.), *Congenital Muscular Dystrophies*

CHAPTER 29

Congenital muscular dystrophy and brain malformation in two sibs: a pathological and neuroradiological comparison

KARIN EDEBOL EEG-OLOFSSON[1], ORVAR EEG-OLOFSSON[2] and YNGVE OLSSON[3]

[1]*Department of Clinical Neurophysiology, University Hospital, Uppsala, Sweden*
[2]*Department of Pediatrics, University Hospital, Uppsala, Sweden*
[3]*Department of Neuropathology, University Hospital, Uppsala, Sweden*

Introduction

Congenital muscular dystrophy (CMD) is a phenotypically heterogeneous autosomal recessive myopathy described in several reports over the years, and recently reviewed by Cook et al. [1]. An extensive bibliography on CMD has been compiled by Fukuyama [2]. The classification of CMD has been a matter of debate, and has changed several times mainly due to new information obtained in neuroimaging and molecular studies. The classification adopted in 1993 [3] is now slightly changed according to Dobyns and Parano (Table 1). Most reported cases of CMD with normal intelligence do not show involvement of the central nervous system. However, there have been about 20 cases described which showed diffuse low density in the central white matter [4]. The purpose of this report is to present a sib pair with pure CMD and normal mental development, but with localized cortical and subcortical malformations.

Case 1

This girl was the first child of healthy unrelated parents, born at term without complications after an uneventful pregnancy. The birth weight was 2960 g, length 50 cm, and head circumference 34 cm. On examination at day 1, she was extremely hypotonic (arms > legs) with weak tendon reflexes. Serum CK was 91 μkat/l (reference value <2.5; 1 unit = $16.67 \times 10^{-3}\,\mu$kat/l). EMG on day 4 showed suspected myopathy. A muscle biopsy on day 11 was typical for CMD (Fig. 1). ECG, echocardiography, metabolic screening and chromosomes were normal. At the age of 3 weeks, EMG was myopathic and serum CK 20 μkat/l. At 15 months of age, the girl was generally hypotonic with muscle atrophy, foot contractures bilaterally, areflexia of the upper limbs, and weak reflexes of the lower limbs. There were no fasciculations.

Between the ages of 18 months and 6 years she was lost to follow-up. However, she attended a rehabilitation center in another Swedish region. She was wheelchair bound. Now and then the girl had shown transitory respiratory difficulty. She was mentally normal and could read with a weak voice at the age of 6 years. A clinical examination at that age re-

Table 1

1994 CMD classification (Dobyns and Parano, personal communication)

A. Pure CMD (with normal intelligence)
  1. CMD with merosin deficiency
  2. CMD without merosin deficiency
B. CMD with brain malformations/mental retardation
  1. Cobblestone lissencephaly syndromes
    (a) Fukuyama congenital muscular dystrophy
    (b) Muscle-eye-brain disease
    (c) Walker–Warburg syndrome
  2. CMD with occipital agyria
  3. CMD with mental retardation (NOC)

vealed generalized hypotonia, muscle atrophy, no fasciculations, joint contractures, and areflexia. Serum CK was 0.7 μkat/l, and a muscle biopsy showed a "burnt out" picture. She suddenly died due to pneumonia.

There was a healthy brother of 2 years.

Autopsy findings

The brain was enlarged, with a weight of 1700 g and moderate generalized swelling with flattening of the gyri, but no evidence of herniations at the base of the brain. The ventricles were somewhat compressed, presumably due to edema. Extensive changes were present in

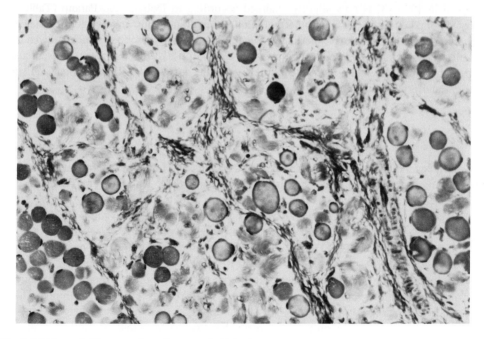

Fig. 1. Initial muscle biopsy specimen from case 1 obtained at age 11 days. This specimen shows marked changes with multiple degenerating and regenerating muscle fibers. There is marked variation in fiber diameter and many of the fibers are totally atrophic. Pronounced fibrosis is present; the vessels are normal and there is no inflammation (hematoxylin and eosin).

the occipital poles of both hemispheres. On the dorsolateral surface, regions measuring up to 8 cm in diameter with pachygyria-like abnormalities were seen. Similar but less extensive cortical lesions were present in a few parts of the frontal, parietal and temporal lobes. The occipital lesions thus consisted of a cortical malformation with a lack of normal gyral configurations and rudimentary sulci. In the subcortical white matter there was a narrow band of grey matter, i.e., the occipital changes gave an impression of a double cortex (Fig. 2). The cerebral white matter within the centrum semiovale was widened but the corpus callosum was thinner than normal. The basal ganglia were normal. No changes were seen in the brain stem including the cerebellum. The vessels were normal. The spinal cord had an abnormal configuration, with reduced cervical and lumbar enlargements. Microscopy, however, did not show any clear-cut lesions of the cord. Macroscopy of the spinal nerve roots did not show any gross changes, but microscopy revealed obvious lesions with reduced myelin staining, and increased numbers of Schwann cells and fibroblast nuclei.

Case 2

This brother of case 1 was born at term 2 years after her death. The pregnancy as well as the delivery were uneventful. The birth weight was 3605 g, length 51 cm, and head circumference 36.5 cm. On examination he was extremely hypotonic with weak tendon reflexes. Serum CK was 1280 μkat/l. On day 4 EMG was normal, while a muscle biopsy showed a picture typical for CMD. Serum CK had decreased to 255 μkat/l. Metabolic screening, ECG, echocardiography and chromosomes were normal.

At the age of 3 months, the boy was generally hypotonic with areflexia of the upper limbs. The tendon reflexes of the lower limbs were brisk and he had bilateral foot contractures. No fasciculations were noticed. Serum CK was 26 μkat/l and EMG was myopathic. Ophthalmological examination showed alternating esotropia, and VEP was normal but with high amplitudes. Metabolic screening showed aminoaciduria, but the plasma aminogram was normal. MRI of the spine was normal, while MRI of the brain showed occipital pachygyria (Fig. 3) with a high intensity subcortical laminar structure, "double cortex" (Fig. 4).

At the age of 6 months, the boy was generally hypotonic, laying in frog position with areflexia, except for a weak knee response, and with bilateral foot contractures. There were no fasciculations. Serum CK was 30 μkat/l. His mental development seemed to be normal.

Biopsy findings

A biopsy specimen was obtained from the quadriceps muscle on day 4. Severe pathological changes were present with numerous regenerating muscle fibers, marked variation of fiber diameters, numerous atrophic fibers and an increase in endomysial collagen. The blood vessels were normal and there was no evidence of inflammatory disease. The changes were very similar to those in the initial biopsy specimen from the sister (case 1).

Immunohistochemistry revealed a normal dystrophin pattern [5] with the exception of the regenerating fibers, in which there was no detectable amount of dystrophin antigen. Merosin immunohistochemistry [6] with a monoclonal primary antibody (Chemicon MAB 1922) showed abnormal staining with the absence of immunoreactive material at the position of the basal lamina surrounding the muscle fibers.

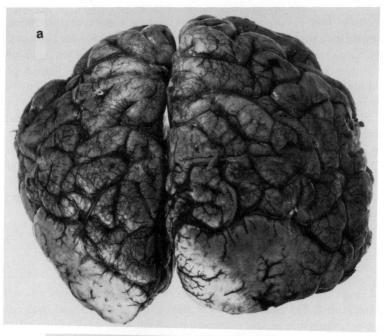

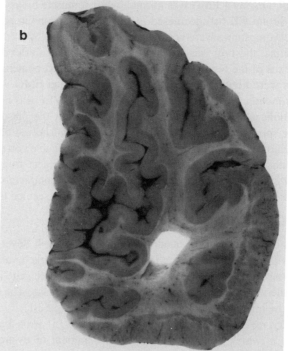

Fig. 2. (a) The brain of case 1, showing each of the occipital poles. Note the extensive white regions in which the normal gyral pattern is lacking. (b) A transverse section of the occipital lobe of case 1. An extensive cortical malformation is present. The normal gyral pattern is absent, and there is a double layer of grey matter forming a "double cortex".

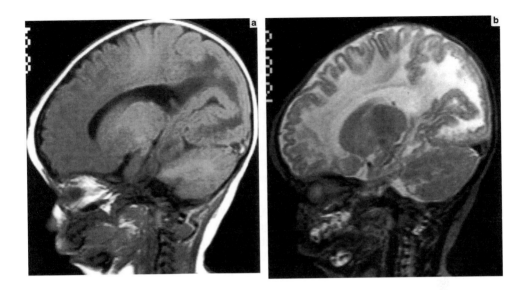

Fig. 3. MRI, T1- (a) and T2-weighted (b) images, of the brain of case 2. Note the lack of a gyral pattern of the occipital area.

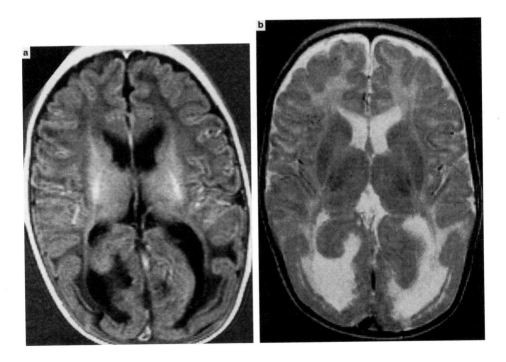

Fig. 4. MRI, axial T1- (a) and T2-weighted (b) images, of the brain of case 2. Note the double cortex layer of the occipital poles.

Discussion

According to the classification of CMD (Table 1) these children with obviously normal mental development should belong to the category "pure CMD".

Immunohistochemical staining for merosin in the muscle biopsy specimen from the boy was negative. Both children showed brain malformations. Thus, they do not actually fit into the mentioned classification. In the classification proposed by Lenard [7], a subdivision according to whether or not there is CNS involvement was used. Our cases should probably then be classified as classical CMD with hypomyelination or the so-called "occidental type" [8]. However, even this would not be correct. We consider that the children belong to a category of "pure CMD" with merosin deficiency and brain malformations, an entity apparently not previously delineated.

Of utmost interest was the autopsy findings in the girl with CNS pachygyria and a double cortical layer. Similar abnormalities were seen in the boy on neuroimaging, representing signs of a neuronal migration disorder. Such subcortical laminar heterotopias have been found in another type of CMD, the Walker–Warburg syndrome [9]. The so-called "double cortex" has been described as a specific syndrome in girls [10]. Of interest is the similarity between the last-mentioned cases and cases of CMD with brain malformations and mental retardation. Merosin studies on brain tissue, however, have not been performed. The question is whether merosin is a matrix protein in muscle and brain of importance for both muscle development and neuronal migration.

The inheritance of CMD is autosomal recessive. Genetically, Fukuyama CMD has been mapped to chromosome 9q31-33 [11]. It is naturally important to perform genetic studies also on families with "pure CMD" in order to improve the classification and to facilitate prenatal counselling.

Addendum

Since the investigation of these two sibs, a national survey of congenital muscular dystrophy in Sweden has begun. To date, 19 cases are known, of whom 3 patients have died. The 16 living children, of whom 6 are girls, were born between 1981 and 1995 (mean age 7.5 years, median 7.5 years). Seven children present with a quite severe form of muscle weakness; one of these is a boy with Walker–Warburg's syndrome. Three of the children with severe weakness are deficient in laminin M (merosin), two have normal findings of merosin, and two children are under investigation. There is no Fukuyama type CMD among the children. Six of the children with moderate-slight muscular weakness have normal findings for merosin and two have not yet been investigated for immunohistochemistry. Neuroradiology shows cerebellar hypotrophy in three children with moderate muscular weakness, speech difficulties and merosin-positive muscles. One child has severe muscle weakness and marked pseudohypertrophy of calf muscles, intact cognitive function and cerebellar cysts at MRI. Twin sisters present with a MEB like picture but do not fulfil the criteria for the eye abnormalities described in MEB. Some newly reported cases of CMD not included here are to be further investigated. There might be under-reporting of the condition since it is rare and quite heterogeneous clinically so that suspicion of the condition might not arise in all cases. Results of this national survey are to be published as soon as the study is finished.

Acknowledgments

Dr. K.G. Henriksson, University Hospital, Linköping, Sweden, kindly evaluated the original muscle biopsy specimen of case 1 and provided material for one of our illustrations (Fig. 1).

References

1. Cook JD, Gascon GG, Haider MD, et al. Congenital muscular dystrophy with abnormal radiographic myelin pattern. J Child Neurol 1992; 7(Suppl): S51–63.
2. Fukuyama Y. Bibliography of congenital muscular dystrophies. Tokyo, 1994.
3. Dubowitz V. 22nd ENMC sponsored workshop on congenital muscular dystrophy, Baarn, the Netherlands, 1993. Neuromusc Disord 1994; 4: 75–81.
4. Tanaka J, Mimaki T, Okada Sh, Fujimura H. Changes in cerebral white matter in a case of congenital muscular dystrophy (non-Fukuyama type). Neuropediatrics 1990; 21: 183–186.
5. Hsu S, Raine L, Fanger H. Use of avidin-biotin-peroxidase complex (ABC) in immunoperoxidase techniques: a comparison between ABC and unlabelled antibody (PAP) procedures. J Histochem Cytochem 1981; 29: 577–580.
6. Tomé FMS, Evangelista T, Leclerc A, et al. Congenital muscular dystrophy with merosin deficiency. C R Acad Sci Paris, Life Sci, Genet 1994; 317: 351–357.
7. Lenard H. Congenital muscular dystrophies. Problems of classification. Acta Pediatr Jpn (Tokyo) 1991; 33: 256–260.
8. Topaloglu H, Yalaz K, Renda Y, et al. Occidental type cerebromuscular dystrophy. A report of eleven cases. J Neurol Neurosurg Psychiatry 1991; 54: 226–229.
9. Yamaguchi E, Hayashi T, Kondoh H, et al. A case of Walker–Warburg syndrome with uncommon findings. Double cortical layer, temporal cyst and increased serum IgM. Brain Dev 1993; 15: 61–66.
10. Palmini A, Andermann F, Aicardi J, et al. Diffuse cortical dysplasia, or the "double cortex" syndrome: the clinical and epileptic spectrum in 10 patients. Neurology 1991; 41: 1656–1662.
11. Toda T, Segawa M, Nomura Y, et al. Localization of a gene for Fukuyama type congenital muscular dystrophy to chromosome 9q31-33. Nat Genet 1993; 5: 283–286.

Y. Fukuyama, M. Osawa and K. Saito (Eds.), *Congenital Muscular Dystrophies*
345

CHAPTER 30

A milder form of Walker–Warburg syndrome

KAYOKO SAITO, HARUKO SUZUKI, KEIKO SHISHIKURA,
MAKIKO OSAWA AND YUKIO FUKUYAMA

Department of Pediatrics, Tokyo Women's Medical College, Shinjuku-ku, Tokyo, Japan

Introduction

Congenital muscular dystrophy with cerebral involvement of the Fukuyama type (FCMD) was originally described in 1960 [1]. To date, FCMD reports have been almost entirely confined to Japan, where it is not uncommon. In a multi-center collaborative survey carried out in 1975, the ratio of Duchenne muscular dystrophy to FCMD in Japan was found to be 2.1:1 [2]. The Walker–Warburg syndrome (WWS) [3,4] is a rare disease characterized by type II lissencephaly with progressive hydrocephalus, agyria and ocular abnormalities. Few patients survive beyond 4 months in classic cases [5]. Only in recent years has the involvement of muscle in WWS been appreciated [6]. The muscle-eye-brain syndrome (MEBS), first reported by Santavuori et al. [7] and Raitta et al. [8], is also a rare disorder characterized by severe mental retardation, hypotonia and visual failure. Most patients have come from a small, geographically isolated population in Finland, with a few exceptions. Death occurs between 6 and 16 years of age. Inheritance of these 3 diseases is autosomal-recessive. The relationship between FCMD, WWS and MEBS has not been adequately clarified. The lingering question is whether these diseases are allelic, that is, expressing mutations in the same gene, or whether they represent 3 separate diseases. We report a case with congenital muscular dystrophy in association with cerebral and ocular involvement, which was considered to exemplify an atypical mild form of WWS rather than FCMD. This case presented two important observations; first, that WWS has a broad clinical spectrum including a relatively mild form as in the case here reported, and second, that milder WWS cases are distinguishable from FCMD on clinical grounds.

Case report

A 7-month-old girl was admitted to our hospital for investigation of psychomotor retardation, muscle weakness and nystagmoid eye movements in 1978. She was the only child of a Japanese mother and an American father of Scandinavian descent. Neither family has any history of a similar disease nor any neurological problems. The mother was 35 years old at the time of the patient's birth. She had developed glucosuria and proteinuria, at 32 and 36 weeks of gestation, respectively. The delivery was normal, birth weight 3.510 g, but weak cry and moderate flaccidity were noted. The girl was breast fed for several months and her diet was then supplemented with soybean formula. Developmental history revealed good weight gain but inability to lift her head at 2 months of age. At 3 months of age, she smiled spontaneously, responded to sounds, and followed a light with her eyes: however, the parents were concerned about her hypotonicity, frog leg posture and the lack of active limb movement. Only occasionally did she show social responses such as smiling, and she sometimes appeared apathetic. At 4 months of age she could no longer move her hands to the midline or roll over. These signs and symptoms, suggestive of developmental delay, prompted the parents to bring the baby to a physician for the first time, who pointed out poor head control and constant nystagmus. At 6 months of age, she was seen at another hospital where abnormalities of the ocular fundi were pointed out. She was admitted to our hospital at 7 months of age.

On examination, the child's length was 72.3 cm (+1.7 SD), weight 9.3 kg (+1.4 SD), and the head circumference 44.5 cm (+0.8 SD). She was a well-nourished, moderate sized baby with no particular findings except for the neurological status. The most remarkable findings were the extreme paucity or lack of spontaneous movement of the trunk and all limbs (Fig. 1a). She was not able to control her head, and was unable to roll, sit or crawl; no visual following was noted. Generalized, but proximal dominant, muscle hypotonia and weakness were noted. Deep tendon reflexes were absent. However, such primitive reflexes as Moro, Galant, and grasp (both palmar and plantar) were clearly present. The optico-facial and acoustico-facial reflexes were also positive. The plantar response was of the plantar flexion type. She responded promptly to painful stimulation applied to every part of the body. Ophthalmological study revealed internal strabismus (Fig. 1b), pendular or rotatory nystagmus, no limitation of eye movement and no anterior chamber malformation. Funduscopic examination revealed slightly pale optic discs and retinal dysplasia bilaterally (Fig. 2).

The serum creatine kinase (CK) value was consistently high (621–1923 U/l). EMG showed a myogenic pattern. Motor nerve conduction velocity was slightly decreased. EEG revealed scattered spikes arising from both occipital and right occipito-temporal regions of the brain. Cranial CT scan was performed at 8 months and at 3 years, and both showed diffuse low density of the white matter (Fig. 3), ventricular dilatation, cortical dysplasia (pachygyria), and hypoplasia of the cerebellar vermis and pons. In the needle biopsied muscle specimen obtained at 8 months of age, the most conspicuous finding was the presence of numerous large groups of fibers with basophilic staining, representing regenerating fibers which distribute widely within the muscle (Fig. 4a,b). An increase in fibers with central nuclei, marked variation in fiber sizes and connective tissue proliferation were noted. Modified ATPase staining revealed no fiber type grouping or predominance. No accumulation of glycogen or lipids was observed in muscle. Electron microscopic changes such as dilatation of the intermyofibrillar space, increased glycogen granules and scattered disarrangement of the Z-zone were noted. Basic striation structure is rather well preserved (Fig. 5). Serum and urinary organic acids, lysosomal enzyme activities and serum amino acids were within normal limits.

After discharge from our hospital at 8 months, the child became significantly more active, but was still unable to crawl. Whenever she caught a cold, the physical activity decreased dramatically. At 1 year old, she was admitted to the University of California, San Diego where an extensive work-up was carried out, including a brain biopsy. According to Dr. Lampert's pathological reports, examination of the biopsy material from the right frontal lobe revealed chronic edema and gliosis of the white matter. The cortex was well preserved, and there was no evidence of neuronal storage disease, although there was striking gliosis in the subcortical white matter, as well as sponginess in the deeper white matter. Electron mi-

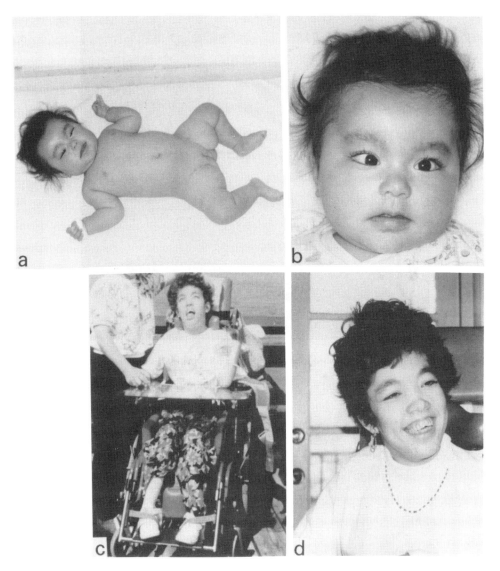

Fig. 1. General appearance. (a) At 7 months, frog leg posture and lack of spontaneous trunk and extremity movements were noticed. (b) Lack of visual following was noted. She did not show the facial muscle involvement characteristic of FCMD. (c) At 15 years, she was wheelchair bound, had never walked, was hypotonic, could not sit by herself, and had myopia and cataracts. (d) Her facial expressions were, at times, quite lively, reflecting the absence of facial muscle involvement characteristic of FCMD.

croscopy of the cerebral cortex was unremarkable except for some swollen astrocytic processes containing unusually large mitochondria. Nerve cells and synapses showed no changes. The white matter showed very wide extracellular spaces (Fig. 6a). Oligodendrocytes were normal or showed proliferative changes, i.e. an increased amount of cytoplasm containing granular endoplasmic reticulum (Fig. 6b). Microglial cells, or macrophages, were filled with granular lysosomes as well as large electron dense masses presumably derived

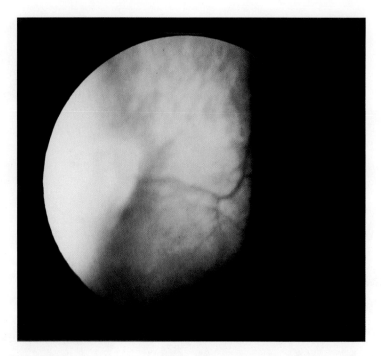

Fig. 2. Funduscopic examination revealed slightly pale optic discs and retinal dysplasia.

from the phagocytosis of red cells (Fig. 6c). No intramyelinic vacuoles were detected. Degenerating cells with large watery nuclei suggestive of Alzheimer's glia were noted. Unusually large mitochondria with few or no cristae but filled with a granular matrix were seen in clear astrocytic processes (Fig. 6d). Viral and bacterial cultures of the brain biopsy were negative.

At 1 year 3 months, the motor function was improved compared to the status on the initial examination. She could bring fingers to the mouth, place hands so as to cross the midline, and had slightly more steady head control. However, she was still unable to roll, crawl or sit. Continuous nystagmoid eye movements, pendular or rotatory, were still present, but visual following was consistently noted. She had had acupuncture treatment at the mother's request. Head control became steady up to 2 years of age.

At 10 years of age, the patient revisited our hospital. She was wheelchair bound, had never attended school, was hypotonic and had never been able to sit by herself. Joint contractures were noted at the wrist, elbow, ankle, knee and hip, bilaterally. She had myopia (−9 diopters) and bilateral cataracts. The CK titer was 798 U/l. A second needle biopsy carried out at age 10 years (the femoral muscle) revealed peri- and endomysial connective tissue proliferation, mildly increased fatty cells, variation in fiber diameters ranging from 25 to 110 μm (normal mean for age; 40 μm), numerous internal nuclei and fiber necrosis, as well as mild to moderate phagocytosis (Fig. 4c,d). The patient is now 16 years old (Fig. 1c,d) and lives in the USA. She indicates 'yes' and 'no' with gestures. Occasionally generalized seizures continue to occur despite valproic acid medication. She has bilateral cataracts and is nearly blind.

a

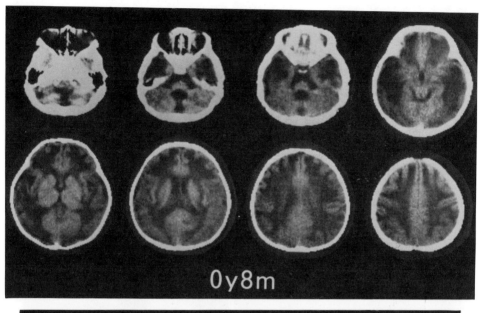

b

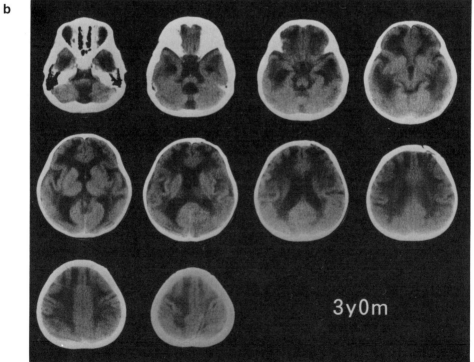

Fig. 3. Cranial CT scan of the present case. (a) 0 year 8 months: diffuse white matter low density, ventricular dilatation, pachygyria and hypoplasia of the cerebeller vermis and pons. (b) 3 years 0 months: white matter low density in the occipital area is markedly reduced.

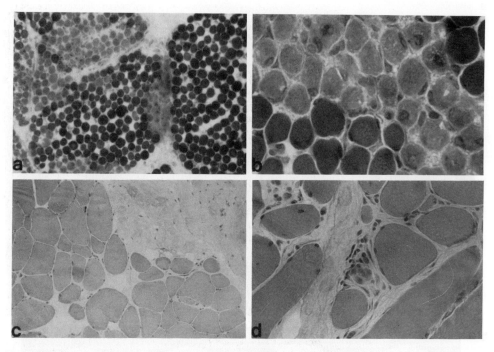

Fig. 4. Histopathological study of biopsied rectus femoris muscle specimens. (a,b) 0 year 8 months: numerous large groups of fibers with phagocytosis and basophilic staining, representing regenerating fibers, can be seen as faint stained fibers. An increase in fibers with central nuclei, variation in fiber sizes and connective tissue proliferation are also apparent. Small, rounded darkly stained fibers resemble fetal muscle fibers. Gomori-trichrome staining. (a), ×100; (b), ×400. (c,d) 10 years: perimysial connective tissues and moderately increased fatty cells, focal endomysial connective tissues proliferation, variation in fiber diameters ranging from 25 to 110 μm (normal mean for age; 40 μm), numerous internal nuclei and fiber necrosis, as well as mild to moderate phagocytosis can be seen. Hematoxylin-eosin staining. (c), ×200; (d), ×400.

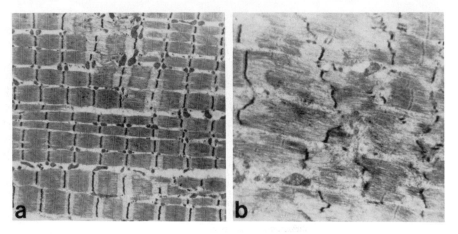

Fig. 5. Electron microscopic study of biopsied muscles at the age of 8 months. (a) Dilatation of the intermyofibrillar space, increased glycogen granules and partial tortuosity of the Z-zone are apparent. ×5000. (b) Partial tortuosity of the Z-zone is illustrated. ×10 000

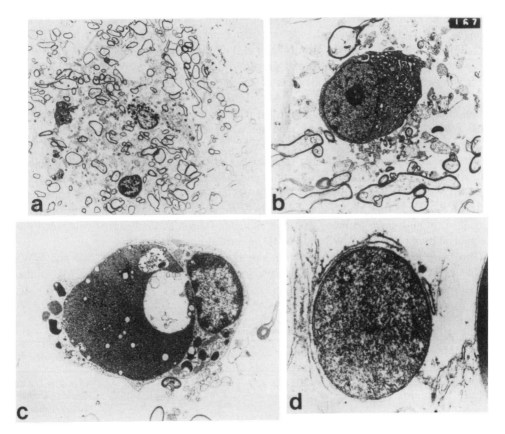

Fig. 6. Electron microscopic study of biopsied brain obtained from the right frontal lobe showed the following findings: (a) edematous subcortical white matter; (b) preservation of oligodendrocytes in the edematous white matter; (c) phagocytosed red cells within the edematous white matter; and (d) abnormal mitochondria in swollen astrocytes.

Discussion

According to Fenichel [9], congenital muscular dystrophy (CMD) is classified into CMD without cerebral involvement, CMD with cerebral involvement and CMD with autosomal dominant inheritance. CMD with cerebral involvement consists of FCMD [1,2], CMD with hypomyelination and CMD with cerebro-ocular anomalies. CMD with hypomyelination has now been designated CMD with merosin deficiency [10], and CMD with cerebro-ocular anomalies includes WWS [3–6] and MEBS [7,8]. FCMD is the most common type of CMD in Japan. The characteristic neuropathological feature of FCMD is a disturbance of cellular migration to the cortex expressed as cortical dysplasia, including polymicrogyria, lissencephaly and heterotopia [11]. Hypodensity of the white matter is demonstrated by CT in 50% of FCMD cases. Recently, the FCMD gene was localized to 9q31 by Toda et al. [12]. WWS is a rare autosomal recessive disorder characterized by type II lissencephaly, cerebellar and ocular malformations, and muscular changes consistent with CMD. It is a lethal syndrome and patients rarely survive beyond 4 months; most die of aspiration in the first year [5]. Dystrophic muscular change was first reported in patients with type II lissencephaly by Krijgsman et al. [6]. Dambska et al. [13,14] designated this condition cerebro-oculo-muscular syndrome (COMS) and suggested that COMS is a severe form of FCMD, but it is now widely considered identical to WWS. MEBS, first reported by Santavuori et al. [7] and Raitta et al. [8], is also a rare disorder characterized by severe mental retardation, hypotonia and visual failure. Most patients have come from a small, geographically isolated population in Finland, with a few exceptions. Death occurs between 6 and 16 years of age.

While FCMD shows considerable resemblance to WWS, both clinically and pathologically, the lack of severe ocular abnormalities and the rarity of major cerebellar abnormalities in FCMD clearly distinguish FCMD from WWS and MEBS [15,16]. Dobyns considered that WWS, COMS and MEBS are caused by different alleles of the same developmental gene [16]. From a neuropathological point of view, Takada and colleagues concluded that the genetic background of WWS and FCMD are probably different [17].

The characteristic features of this case were compared with those of FCMD and WWS (Table 1). Clinical features in this case have some resemblance to those of FCMD in that

Table 1

The characteristic features of this case are summarized, in comparison with those of FCMD and WWS [4]

Features	FCMD	WWS	This case
Age of death	1-35 years	<1 year	Alive at 16
Ethnic	Japanese	Caucasian	Father, Caucasian
			Mother, Japanese
Mental retardation	Moderate	Severe	Moderate
Type II lissencephaly	+++	+++	✓
Predominate agyria	–	++	✓
Predominate polymicrogyria	++	+	?
White matter lucency	50%	++	✓
Cerebellar malformation	+++	+++	✓
Cortical dysplasia	+++	+++	✓
Vermis hypoplasia	–	+++	✓
Dandy–Walker malformation	–	++	–
Posterior cephalocele	–	+	–
Eye malformation	?	+++	✓
Typical retinal dysplasia	–	++	✓
Optic nerve pallor	33%	++	✓
Other retinal abnormality	+	+	–
Microphthalmia	–	+	–
Muscle disease			
Congenital muscular dystrophy	+++	+++	✓
Calf pseudohypertrophy	+	–	–
Associated abnormalities			
Ventricular dilatation	++	++	✓
Hypoplastic corpus callosum	+	++	–
Congenital macrocephaly	–	++	–
Congenital microcephaly	++	+	–
Anterior chamber malformation	–	++	✓

+++, constant; ++, frequent; +, occasional; –, rare/not observed; ✓, observed.

she showed severe hypotonia with a very early onset, consistently high serum CK values, concomitant involvement of both CNS and the muscle system, and characteristic white matter low density on CT scan which is common for FCMD, WWS and merosin-negative CMD cases. However, her facial expressions were, at times, quite lively, reflecting the absence of the facial muscle involvement characteristic of FCMD. The findings of needle biopsied muscle, which were examined twice, at 8 months and again at 10 years, were markedly different from those of FCMD. Perimysial connective tissues and fatty cell infiltration were far less prominent and basic structures of muscle bundles as well as muscle fibers were relatively well preserved compared with a typical FCMD case of the same age.

The authors believe that the present case represents a relatively mild form of WWS, rather than FCMD, because the degree of muscle involvement is milder, the elevation of serum CK activities was consistently moderate, in spite of a rather early onset of clinical manifestations (hypotonia and weakness), while CNS and eye abnormalities were not only more severe in degree than those seen in FCMD, but also included such specific findings as cerebellar vermis hypoplasia, retinal dysplasia and cataracts which are common in WWS but rare in FCMD.

The racial specificity of both diseases is, however, interesting. FCMD is the most common type of CMD in Japan, whereas WWS is unusual. The patient was born to a Japanese mother and an American father of Scandinavian descent. Interestingly, MEBS cases have been described almost exclusively in Finland. It is possible that the father is a carrier of MEBS.

Recently, Yoshioka and colleagues [18] reported a family in which one child was diagnosed as FCMD and the other as WWS. Toda et al. [19] showed that the FCMD case and the WWS case in the above family had the same haplotype using microsatellite polymorphism analysis of DNA. They considered WWS and FCMD to be allelic diseases, the relationship between the two being similar to that between Duchenne and Becker muscular dystrophies. However, the case presented herein showed substantial differences from FCMD on clinical grounds, described above. The lingering question is whether FCMD and WWS are expressions of the same disease or whether they represent separate diseases. The answer to this question will come ultimately with identification of the gene(s) and gene product(s) and with analysis of the genetic mutation(s) responsible for these diseases.

The present case also suggests that the clinical spectrum of WWS is wider than previously believed. WWS is the most severe of the 3 diseases. It has long been assumed that few patients survive beyond 4 months [5], and virtually all WWS patients die within the first year of life. As Raitta and colleagues [8] reported an adult MEB patient aged 40 years, Dobyns [16] concluded that MEB may represent a mild form of WWS, with the oldest WWS case in his experience being 10 years of age [4]. As for FCMD, most cases survive beyond the infantile period and the average age at death was found to be 18 (range: 1–35) years old in the 1981 survey [2]. The present case is now 16 years old, which suggests the existence of relatively mild cases of WWS with a longer life-expectancy.

References

1. Fukuyama Y, Kawazura M, Haruna H. A peculiar form of congenital progressive muscular dystrophy: Report of fifteen cases. Pediatr Univ Tokyo (Tokyo) 1960; 4: 5–8.
2. Fukuyama Y, Ohsawa M. A genetic study of the Fukuyama type congenital muscular dystrophy. Brain Dev (Tokyo) 1984; 6: 373–390.

3. Dobyns WB, Kirkpatrick JB, Hittner HM, Roberts RM, Kretzer FL. Syndrome with lissencephaly. II: Walker–Warburg and cerebro-oculo-muscular syndromes and a new syndrome with type II lissencephaly. Am J Med Genet 1985; 22: 157–195.

4. Dobyns WB, Pagon RA, Armstrong D, et al. Diagnostic criteria for Walker–Warburg syndrome. Am J Med Genet 1989; 32: 195–210.

5. Williams RS, Swisher CN, Jennings M, Ambler M, Caviness VS. Cerebro-ocular dysgenesis (Walker–Warburg syndrome): neuropathologic and etiologic analysis. Neurology 1984; 34: 1531–1541.

6. Krijgsman JB, Barth PG, Stam FC, Slooff JL, Jasper HHJ. Congenital muscular dystrophy and cerebral dysgenesis in a Dutch family. Neuropaediatrie 1980; 11: 108–120.

7. Santavuori P, Leisti J. Muscle, eye and brain disease: a new syndrome. Neuropaediatrie 1977; 8 (Suppl): 553–558.

8. Raitta C, Lamminen M, Santavuori P, Leisti J. Ophthalmological findings in a new syndrome with muscle, eye and brain involvement. Acta Ophthalmol 1978; 56: 465–472.

9. Fenichel GM. Congenital muscular dystrophies. Neurol Clin 1988; 6: 519–528.

10. Tomé FMS, Evangelista T, Leclerc S, et al. Congenital muscular dystrophy with merosin deficiency. C R Acad Sci Paris 1994; 317: 351–357.

11. Takada K, Nakamura H, Tanaka J. Cortical dysplasia in congenital muscular dystrophy with central nervous system involvement (Fukuyama type). J Neuropathol Exp Neurol 1984; 43: 395–407.

12. Toda T, Ikegawa S, Okui K, et al. Refined mapping of a gene responsible for Fukuyama-type congenital muscular dystrophy: evidence for strong linkage disequilibrium. Am J Hum Genet 1994; 55: 946–950.

13. Dambska M, Wisniewski K, Sher J, Solish G. Cerebro-oculo-muscular syndrome: a variant of Fukuyama congenital cerebromuscular dystrophy. Clin Neuropathol 1982; 1: 93–98.

14. Dambska M, Wisniewski K, Sher J. Lissencephaly: two distinct clinico-pathologic types. Brain Dev (Tokyo) 1983; 5: 302–310.

15. Kimura S, Sasaki Y, Kobayashi T, et al. Fukuyama-type congenital muscular dystrophy and the Walker–Warburg syndrome. Brain Dev (Tokyo) 1993; 15: 182–191.

16. Dobyns WB. Classification of the cerebro-oculo-muscular syndrome(s). Brain Dev (Tokyo) 1993; 15: 242–244.

17. Takada K, Becker LE, Takashima S. Walker–Warburg syndrome with skeletal muscle involvement. Pediatr Neurosci 1987; 13: 202–209.

18. Yoshioka M, Kuroki S, Nigami H, Kawai T, Nakamura H. Clinical variation within sibships in Fukuyama-type congenital muscular dystrophy. Brain Dev (Tokyo) 1992; 14: 334–337.

19. Toda T, Yoshioka M, Nakahori Y, Kanazawa I, Nakamura Y, Nakagome Y. Genetic identity of Fukuyama-type congenital muscular dystrophy and Walker–Warburg syndrome. Ann Neurol 1995; 37: 99–101.

Y. Fukuyama, M. Osawa and K. Saito (Eds.), *Congenital Muscular Dystrophies*

Bibliography of congenital muscular dystrophies: the up-dated, second edition (February, 1997)

COMPILED BY YUKIO FUKUYAMA

Child Neurology Institute, Tokyo, Japan

Introduction

This is a comprehensive collection of the world literature contributing specifically to the subject of congenital muscular dystrophy.

The first edition of "Bibliography of Congenital Muscular Dystrophies", as of March 31, 1994, was printed in Tokyo with the support of a Grant-in-aid (A-024046) from the Ministry of Education, Science and Culture. It listed 836 pertinent articles, including 554 by Japanese authors, and 282 by non-Japanese authors, which were published during the period extending from 1898 through March 1994. However, the booklet was printed rather privately and never put on the market; in addition, articles written in Japanese were printed in Japanese, as they were. These circumstances prevented a wider circulation of the first edition.

In the second edition, relevant information on Japanese articles was translated into English, significantly enhancing the accessibility of the Japanese literature to non-Japanese investigators. Furthermore, a considerable number of abstracts listed in the first edition was omitted from the second edition, because original articles were known to have subsequently been published.

In addition, approximately 150 new articles/abstracts have been included in this edition, the great majority of which appeared very recently, that is, during the period from April 1994 through March 1996.

Thus, the up-dated second edition of the Bibliography lists 623 original articles, 60 books, 207 Proceedings reports, and 157 abstracts, for a total of 1047 items (see Table 1).

In Fig. 1, original articles were broken down chronologically and by the nationalities of the authors (Japanese versus non-Japanese). Japanese authors contributed 280 original articles (45%), non-Japanese authors 343 (55%). These proportions approach equality, if 60 classic articles published before 1959 are excluded from the list, taking into consideration non-specificity of the content, that is, 276/563 (49%) versus 287/563 (51%), respectively.

Editorial policy

1.   The aim is to collect publications on congenital muscular dystrophies (CMD) as exhaustively and as accurately, as possible.

Table 1

World literature on congenital muscular dystrophies listed in the Bibliography

Year	Original articles	Books[b]	Proceedings[c] of research committees	Abstracts[d]	Total
1890–1909	10[a]	0	0	0	10
1910–1919	7[a]	0	0	0	7
1920–1929	5[a]	0	0	0	5
1930–1939	6[a]	0	0	0	6
1940–1949	5[a]	0	0	0	5
1950–1909	27[a]	1	0	1	29
1960–1969	34	3	0	3	40
1970	6	3	0	3	12
1971	6	0	0	0	6
1972	10	0	0	0	10
1973	6	3	1	1	11
1974	9	0	3	2	14
1975	14	0	0	0	14
1976	7	0	2	2	10
1977	8	1	3	2	14
1978	19	1	6	0	27
1979	10	1	8	5	24
1980	23	1	8	5	34
1981	15	2	10	3	30
1982	23	3	14	7	48
1983	27	3	13	6	49
1984	19	2	14	2	37
1985	24	3	22	4	53
1986	27	4	15	3	49
1987	26	2	16	6	50
1988	28	0	8	3	39
1989	23	1	9	1	34
1990	25	3	8	10	46
1991	24	3	13	4	44
1992	31	2	5	7	46
1993	47	2	12	7	68
1994	25	8	9	32	74
1995	43	5	8	29	85
1996	6	1	0	7	14
Total	623	60	207	157	1047

[a]The vast majority of these classic articles did not deal with congenital muscular dystrophy (CMD) specifically, but rather, dealt with floppy infant syndrome in general.

[b]Books counted in this column include 16 Japanese and 44 non-Japanese (mostly English) books. Non-Japanese books, especially textbooks, were intentionally sought on the basis of whether or not they included any description of CMD. This was not the case with Japanese books, as Japanese textbooks published in Japan commonly contain a section on CMD.

[c]This category includes almost exclusively Japanese articles published as the annual reports of various research committees, sponsored by the Ministry of Health and Welfare of Japan.

[d]Only abstracts which had never been published as an original article were included under this category.

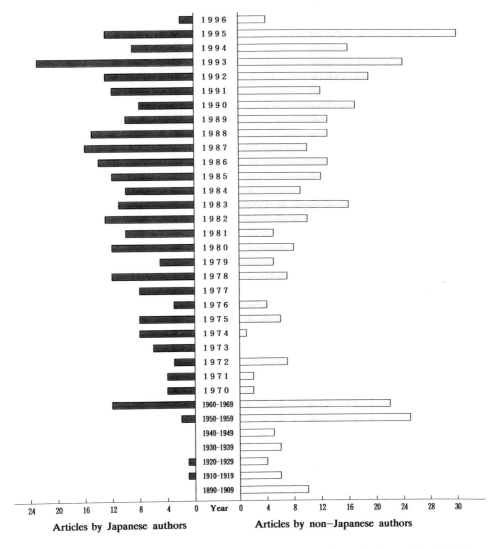

Fig. 1. Chronological trend of publications of original articles on congenital muscular dystrophies. In the figure, original articles, review articles and case reports which appeared in various journals were included, but books (or chapters), proceedings of research committees and abstracts were all excluded from the count.

2. Congenital muscular dystrophy is defined here rather strictly as a primary, systemic and essentially progressive muscle fiber degeneration with clinical manifestation either in the neonatal period or in early infancy, most likely occurring on a genetic basis.

3. Literature on the Walker–Warburg syndrome, muscle–eye–brain disease and Ullrich type CMD was also sought out systematically, but not necessarily exhaustively. Only a few articles on congenital multiple arthrogryposis, especially on its myopathic form, were included, while articles on congenital non-progressive myopathies, with or without structural abnormalities, were carefully excluded from the list.

4.   The period covered extends from the dawning of modern medicine (Haushalter, 1898) through March 31, 1996.

5.   Some articles were included in the Bibliography although they did not carry the word CMD in the title, in cases in which CMD patients were found to constitute part of the study subjects.

6.   Most abstracts in the proceedings of meetings were omitted, except for those which were not yet published in any other form.

7.   The style of the literature in the Bibliography follows the recommendation issued by the International Committee of Medical Journal Editors (Uniform requirements for manuscripts submitted to medical journals. Philadelphia: American College of Physicians, 1993).

8.   The list is arranged in alphabetical order, starting with the first author's family name. In the event of a particular first author having published multiple articles, the publications were arranged chronologically.

9.   Articles written in Japanese are indicated as such in parentheses at the end of the title. Papers written in English are not denoted by parentheses even when contributed by Japanese authors.

Supplement to the Bibliography at the time of proofreading (March 1997)

At the time of proofreading, the Bibliography was updated further by adding 147 new items, the majority of which are new papers which appeared in 1996 (118/147, 79.6%). The distribution of new items according to the year and kind of publication is shown in Table 2. Sixty-five papers (44.2%) were contributed by Japanese authors, while 82 (55.8%) were by non-Japanese authors.

The updated Bibliography in its final form contains 1194 items in total. All other figures expressed in the introduction, Table 1 and Fig. 1 should be read accordingly, by taking the Supplement into consideration.

Table 2

Additional literature on CMD supplemented to the Bibliography at the time of proofreading

Year	Original articles	Books[a]	Proceedings[a] of research committees	Abstracts[a]	Total
1900s	2	0	0	0	2
1950s–1960s	3	0	0	0	3
1970s–1980s	2	0	0	0	2
1990–1993	1	1	0	0	2
1994	3	0	0	3	6
1995	7	1	0	0	7
1996	43	7	2	66	118
1997	7	3	0	3	7
Total	68	8	2	69	147

[a]The same inclusion criteria as those explained in the footnotes of Table 1 were applied to these categories.

Y. Fukuyama, M. Osawa and K. Saito (Eds.), *Congenital Muscular Dystrophies*
© 1997 Elsevier Science B.V. All rights reserved

Bibliography

Afifi A, Zellweger H, McCormick WF, Mergner W. Congenital muscular dystrophy: light and electron microscopic observations. J Neurol Neurosurg Psychiatry 1969; 32: 273–279.

Aicardi J. The agyria-pachygyria complex. A spectrum of cortical malformation. Brain Dev (Tokyo) 1991; 13: 1–8.

Aicardi J. Congenital muscular dystrophy. In: Aicardi J, ed. Diseases of the nervous system in childhood. Clinics in developmental medicine, Nos. 115/118. London: MacKeith Press, 1992: 1182–1185.

Aida N, Yagishita A, Takada K, Katsumata Y. Cerebellar MR in Fukuyama congenital muscular dystrophy: polymicrogyria with cystic lesions. Am J Neuroradiol 1994; 15: 1755–1759.

Aida N, Yagishita A, Tamagawa K, Kobayashi N, Chikumaru K, Morimatsu Y. MR imaging appearance of Fukuyama congenital muscular dystrophy: pathologic correlation (abstract). Radiology 1994; Suppl to vol 193:214.

Aida N, Kobayashi N, Chikumaru K, Iwamoto H, Tamagawa K, Yagishita A, Takada K. Brain MRI findings in Fukuyama congenital muscular dystrophy – Neuroradiological assessment and a review of literature (in Japanese). Med Rev (Tokyo) 1995; 58: 1–9.

Aida N, Tamagawa K, Takada K, Yagishita A, Kobayashi N, Chikumaru K, Iwamoto H. Brain MR in Fukuyama congenital muscular dystrophy. Am J Neuroradiol 1996; 17: 605–613.

Aihara M, Iai M, Takeuchi A, Tamai K, Tanabe Y, Saitoh Y, Goto M, Nakajima H. Magnetic resonance imaging in children with neurological disorders – T_1,T_2-weighted images. On Fukuyama type congenital muscular dystrophy, acute recurrent disseminated encephalomyelitis and tuberous sclerosis (in Japanese). No To Hattatsu (Brain Dev) (Tokyo) 1987; 19(1): 29–36.

Aihara M, Tanabe Y, Kato K. Serial MRI in Fukuyama type congenital muscular dystrophy. Neuroradiology 1992; 34: 396–398.

Allamand V, Sunada Y, Ozo CO, Al-Turaike HS, Akbar M, Kolo T, Salih MAM, Campbell KP. Congenital muscular dystrophy with partial laminin α2-chain caused by an inframe deletion leading to a truncated protein (abstract no. 1201). Am J Hum Genet 1996; 59(4)(Suppl): A210.

Allen RJ, Wong P, Rothenberg SP, DiMauro S, Headington JT. Progressive neonatal leukoencephalomyopathy due to absent methylenetetrahydrofolate reductase responsive to treatment (abstract). Ann Neurol 1980; 8: 211.

Al-Shehab A, Morling P, Kakulas BA. The ultrastructural features of skeletal muscle in congenital progressive ovine muscular dystrophy including studies of the transverse tubular system. Acta Cardiomiol 1993; 5(2): 259–286.

Ando T, Shimizu T, Kato T, Osawa M, Fukuyama Y. Myoglobinemia in children with progressive muscular dystrophy. Clin Chim Acta 1978; 85: 17–22.

Ando T, Shimizu T, Kato T, Osawa M, Fukuyama Y. Clinical significance of serum myoglobin determination in progressive muscular dystrophy (in Japanese). No To Hattatsu (Brain Dev) (Tokyo) 1978; 10: 25–29.

Ando T, Osawa M, Fukuyama Y. Myoglobinemia in Duchenne muscular dystrophy carriers. Brain Dev (Tokyo) 1980; 2: 87–88.

Angelini C, Trevisan CP, Isaya G, Segallo P. Follow-up di 93 casi di ipotonia muscolare neonatale: dati preliminari sull'ipotonia congenita benigna e sulla distiofia muscolare congenita. XI Congresso Nazionale, Società Italiana di Neuropsychiatria Infantile, Urbino, 1984: 536–539.

Aoyagi A, Ishihara T, Yotsukura M, Gifu S, Hantani M. Causes of death in Fukuyama type congenital muscular dystrophy (in Japanese). In: Sobue I, ed. The 1983 annual report of the research committee on clinics, epidemiology and management of progressive muscular dystrophy, sponsored by the Ministry of Health and Welfare of Japan. Nagoya, 1984; 202–207.

Aoyama M, Izumi T, Fukuyama Y, Kodama K, Mineshima N, Miyaji S. On the ictal electroencephalogram of symptomatic infantile spasms occurred in a case of congenital muscular dystrophy (Fukuyama type) (in Japanese). Tokyo Joshi Ikadaigaku Zasshi (J Tokyo Women's Med Coll) (Tokyo) 1977; 47: 638–643.

Arahata K, Arikawa E, Kaido M, Ishiura S, Nonaka I. A study on dystrophin in Fukuyama type congenital muscular dystrophy (in Japanese). In: Araki S, ed. The 1990 annual report of the research committee on pathogenesis and treatment exploration of progressive muscular dystrophy and related disorders, sponsored by the Ministry of Health and Welfare of Japan. Kumamoto. 1991; 75–77.

Arahata K, Hayashi YK, Koga R, Goto K, Lee JH, Miyagoe Y, Ishii H, Tsukahara T, Takeda S, Woo M, Nonaka I, Matsuzaki T, Sugita H. Laminin in animal models for muscular dystrophy. Defect of laminin M in skeletal and cardiac muscles and peripheral nerves of the homozygous dystrophic *dy/dy* mice. Proc Jpn Acad 1993; 69 Ser B (10): 259–264.

Arahata K, Hayashi YS, Mizuno Y, Yoshida M, Ozawa E. Dystrophin-associated glycoprotein and dystrophin co-localisation at sarcolemma. Lancet 1993; 342: 623–624.

Arahata K, Hayashi Y, Koga R, Nagano A, Tsukahara T, Ishii H, Engvall E, Nonaka I. Merosin submit (laminin M chain) deficiency and congenital muscular dystrophy (in Japanese). In: National Center of Neurology and Psychiatry (Planning Division), ed. Annual report of the research on nervous and mental disorders, 1994. Kodaira: National Center of Neurology and Psychiatry, 1995; 30.

Arahata K, Hayashi Y, Kaido M, Nonaka I. Fukuyama type congenital muscular dystrophy and non-Fukuyama type congenital muscular dystrophy – morphological aspects (in Japanese). In: Sugita H, Ozawa E, Nonaka I, eds. Principle of myology. Tokyo: Nankodo 1995; 482–483.

Arahata K, Ishii H, Hayashi YK. Congenital muscular dystrophies. Curr Opin Neurol 1995; 8: 385–390.

Arahata K, Hayashi Y, Takemitsu M, Ishii H, Matsuda C, Matsuzaki T. A trial of myoblast infusion transplantation into *dy* mice muscles (abstract in Japanese). In: Takagi A, chairman. Abstracts for the 1996 annual meeting of the research committee on pathogenesis and treatment of progressive muscular dystrophy and related disorders, sponsored by the Ministry of Health and Welfare of Japan. Tokyo, 1996; 52.

Arahata K, Ishii H, Hayashi Y, Nonaka I. Electron microscopic changes of muscle cell basement membrane in Fukuyama congenital muscular dystrophy (abstract in Japanese). In: Takagi A, chairman. Abstracts for the 1996 annual meeting of the research committee on pathogenesis and treatment of progressive muscular dystrophy and related disorders, sponsored by the Ministry of Health and Welfare of Japan. Tokyo, 1996; 8.

Arahata K, Ishii H, Hayashi YK, Nonaka I. Muscular dystrophy as a disease of cell adhesion molecules (abstract). Abstracts of the 5th Asian and Oceanian Congress of Child Neurology, Istanbul, Turkey, 1996; 20.

Arai Y. Characteristics of muscle involvement evaluated by CT scans in early stages of progressive muscular dystrophy: comparison between Duchenne and Fukuyama types (in Japanese). Tokyo Joshi Ikadaigaku Zasshi (J Tokyo Women's Med Coll) (Tokyo) 1993; 63(10): 1089–1103.

Arai Y, Shishikura K, Sumida S, Osawa M. Neuroimaging findings in Fukuyama type congenital muscular dystrophy (in Japanese). Shoni Naika (Jpn J Pediatr Med) (Tokyo) 1995; 27 Suppl: 703–708.

Araki S, Saida K, Hirose K, Matsuoka Y, Sato H. A questionnaire survey concerning the CNS and immunological abnormalities in progressive muscular dystrophy (in Japanese). In: Nishitani H, ed. The 1984 annual report of the research committee on genetics, epidemiology, clinics and treatment of progressive muscular dystrophy, sponsored by the Ministry of Health and Welfare of Japan. Kyoto, 1985; 251–257.

Araki S, Saida K, Hirose K, Matsuoka Y, Sato I, Sato H. CNS and immunological abnormalities in progressive muscular dystrophy. A review of literatures (in Japanese). In: Nishitani H, ed. The 1985 annual report of the research committee on genetics, epidemiology, clinics and treatment of progressive muscular dystrophy, sponsored by the Ministry of Health and Welfare of Japan. Kyoto, 1986; 255–260.

Araki S, Arai S, Kohyama J, Murakami N, Nonaka I. A case of congenital muscular dystrophy manifesting distinct CNS symptoms (abstract in Japanese). No To Hattatsu (Tokyo) 1994; 26(Suppl): S281.

Arancio O, Bongiovanni LG, Bonadonna G, Tomalleri G, DeGrandis D. Congenital muscular dystrophy and cerebellar vermis agenesis in two brothers. Ital J Neurol Sci 1988; 9: 483–487.

Arikawa E, Arahata K, Nonaka I, Sugita H. Dystrophin analysis in Fukuyama type congenital muscular dystrophy (in Japanese). Igaku No Ayumi (Tokyo) 1989; 150: 747–748.

Arikawa E, Arahata K, Nonaka I, Sugita H. Dystrophin analysis in congenital muscular dystrophy (abstract). Neurology 1990; 40(Suppl 1): 206.

Arikawa E, Arahata K, Nonaka I, Sugita H. Immunohistochemical analysis of dystrophin in congenital muscular dystrophy (CMD) (abstract). J Neurol Sci 1990, 98(Suppl): 438.

Arikawa E, Arahata K, Sunohara N, Ishiura S, Nonaka I, Sugita H. Immunocytochemical analysis of dystrophin in muscular dystrophy. In: Kakulas BA, Howell JM, Roses AD, eds. Duchenne muscular dystrophy. Animal models and genetic manipulation. New York: Raven Press, 1992; 81–88.

Arikawa-Hirasawa E, Hayashi YK, Nonaka I, Arahata K. Membrane instability of skeletal muscle in Fukuyama congenital muscular dystrophy (abstract). Muscle Nerve 1994; (Suppl 1): S53.

Attia MFD, Burn J, McCarthy JH, Purohit DP, Milligan DWA. Warburg (HARD ± E) syndrome without retinal dysplasia. Case report and review. Br J Ophthalmol 1986; 70: 742–747.

Awaya A, Ishikawa T, Shimizu K, Fujikake M, Nonaka I. A female case of Ullrich disease (congenital atonic sclerotic muscular dystrophy) (abstract in Japanese). Nihon Shonika Gakkai Zasshi (J Jpn Pediatr Soc) (Tokyo) 1982; 86: 1849.

Aymé S, Mattei J-F. HARD (± E) syndrome: report of a sixth family with support for autosomal-recessive inheritance. Am J Med Genet 1983; 14: 759–766.

Bado M, Cordone G, Veneselli E, Doria Lamba L, Celle ME, Balestri P, Toti P. Ultra-structural study of muscle basal lamina in congenital muscular dystrophies (CMDs) (abstract). Neuromusc Disord 1996; (Suppl): S28.

Baker N, Houston R, Linder S, Iannaccone ST. Merosin deficiency and CNS abnormalities (abstract). Neuromusc Disord 1996; (Suppl): S26–S27.

Balestrini MR, Mora M, Daniel S. Congenital muscular dystrophy with central nervous system involvement (Fukuyama disease) (abstract) Acta Neurol (Napoli) 1982; 37: 256.

Bando K, Wachi A, Okudaira Y, Sato K, Osawa M. Complicated hydrocephalus in Fukuyama type congenital muscular dystrophy – on the evaluation of abnormal CSF dynamics and surgical treatment (abstract in Japanese). No To Hattatsu (Brain Dev) (Tokyo) 1991; 23S: S262.

Banker BQ, Victor M, Adams RD. Arthrogryposis multiplex due to congenital muscular dystrophy. Brain 1957; 80: 319–334.

Banker BQ. The congenital muscular dystrophies. In: Engel AG, Franzini-Armstrong C, eds. Myology: basic and clinical, 2nd edn. Vol 2. New York: McGraw-Hill, 1994; 1275–1289.

Baraitser M. Congenital muscular dystrophy. In: Baraitser M, ed. The genetics of neurological disorders. 2nd edn. Oxford: Oxford University Press, 1990; 397–399.

Barkovich AJ. Imaging of the cobblestone lissencephalies. Am J Neuroradiol 1996; 17: 615–618.

Barth RA, Pagon RA, Hunt-Milan AH. "Leopard spot" retinopathy in Warburg syndrome. Ophthalmol Pediatr Genet (Amsterdam) 1986; 7: 91–96.

Bassöe HH. Familial congenital muscular dystrophy with gonadal dysgenesis. J Clin Endocrinol 1956; 16: 1614–1624.

Batten FE. Myositis fibrosa. Br Med J 1903; 2: 1333.

Batten FE. Three cases of myopathy, infantile type. Brain 1903; 26: 147–148.

Batten FE. Case of myositis fibrosa with pathological examination. Trans Clin Soc London 1903; 37: 12.

Batten FE. The myopathies or muscular dystrophies (critical review). Q J Med 1909–1910; 3: 313–328.

Batten FE. Simple atrophic type of myopathy: so-called "myatonia congenita" or "amyotonia congenita". Proc R Soc Med 1911; 4: 100–103.

Batten FE. Myopathy. Simple atrophic type. Proc R Soc Med (Neurol) 1915; 8: 69–70.

Batten FE. Case of amyotonia congenita. Proc R Soc Med (Neurol) 1917; 10(2): 47.

Beckmann R, Pernice W, Lensing-Hebben D, Hoffmann M. Cerebro-muskuläre Erkrankung mit klinischer Symptomatik der kongenitale Muskeldystrophie vom Typ Fukuyama. Kinderarzt 1985; 16: 796–800.

Beggs AH, Neumann PE, Arahata K, Arikawa E, Nonaka I, Anderson MDS, Kunkel LM. Possible influences on the expression of X chromosome-linked dystrophin abnormalities by heterozygosity for autosomal recessive Fukuyama congenital muscular dystrophy. Proc Natl Acad Sci USA 1992; 89: 623–627.

Berg G, Scheiffarth F, Bulitta A. Morphologische Untersuchungen bei Dystrophia musculorum progressiva mit fibrillären Zuckungen. Nervenarzt 1955; 26(6): 240–242.

Bernier JP, Brooke MH, Naidich TP, Carroll JE. Myoencephalopathy: cerebral hypomyelination revealed by CT scan of the head in a muscle disease. Trans Am Neurol Ass 1979; 104: 244–246.

Bertrand I, Gruner J. The status verrucosus of the cerebral cortex. J Neuropathol Exp Neurol 1955; 14: 331–347.

Bethlem J. Congenital muscular dystrophy. In: Bethlem J, ed. Myopathies. Amsterdam: North Holland, 1977; 91–92.

Bharucha EP, Pandya SS, Dastur DK. Arthrogryposis multiplex congenita. Part 1. Clinical and electromyographic aspects. J Neurol Neurosurg Psychiatry 1972; 35: 425–434.

Biscoe TJ, Caddy KWT, Pallot DJ, Pehrson UMM, Stirling CA. The neurological lesion in the dystrophic mouse. Brain Res 1974; 76: 534–536.

Biscoe TJ, Caddy KWT, Pallot DJ, Pehrson UMM. Investigation of cranial and other nerves in the mouse with muscular dystrophy. J Neurol Neurosurg Psychiatry 1975; 38: 391–403.

Bode H, Bubl R. EEG-Veränderungen bei Typ I und Typ II Lissenzephalien. Klin Paediatr 1994; 206: 12–17.

Bömelburg T, Kurlemann G, Schuierer G, Palm DG. Ultrasonography in muscle disease (abstract). Childs Nerv Syst 1993; 9: 127.

Bordarier C, Aicardi J, Goutières H. Congenital hydrocephalus and eye abnormalities with severe developmental brain defects: Warburg syndrome. Ann Neurol 1984; 16: 60–65.

Bornemann A, Aigner T, Schlicker U, Meyermann R, Kirchner T. Glio-mesenchymal interrelationship in cortical dysplasia of type II lissencephaly (abstract). Clin Neuropathol 1995; 14(5): 252.

Bornemann A, Aigner T, Kirchner T. Spatial and temporal development of the gliovascular tissue in type II lissencephaly. Acta Neuropathol 1997; 93: 173–177.

Bove KE, Iannaccone ST, Ball W. Case 6. Infantile myositis with leukoencephalopathy. Pediatr Pathol 1992; 12: 289–298.

Bradley WG, Jenkinson M. Neural abnormalities in the dystrophic mouse. J Neurol Sci 1975; 25: 249–255.

Bradley WG. Involvement of peripheral and central nerves in murine dystrophy. Ann N Y Acad Sci 1979; 317: 132–142.

Brandt S. Werdnig–Hoffmann's infantile progressive muscular atrophy. Clinical aspects, pathology, heredity and relation to Oppenheim's amyotonia congenita and other morbid conditions with laxity of joints or muscles in infants. Copenhagen: Munksgaard, 1950.

Brett EM, Lake BD. The congenital muscular dystrophies. In: Brett EM, ed. Paediatric neurology, 3rd edn. Edinburgh: Churchill Livingstone, 1997; 54–57.

Brooke MH. Congenital muscular dystrophy. In: Brooke MH, ed. A clinician's view of neuromuscular diseases, 2nd edn. Baltimore, MD: Williams and Wilkins, 1986; 345–354.

Brooke MH, Cwik VE. Congenital muscular diseases. In: Bradley WG, Daroff RB, Fenichel GM, Marsden CD, eds. Neurology in clinical practice, Vol II, 2nd edn. Boston, MA: Butterworth-Heinemann, 1996; 2043–2046.

Burgeson RE, Chiquet M, Deutzmann R, Ekblom P, Engel J, Kleinman H, Martin GR, Meneguzzi G, Paulsson M, Sanes J, Timpl R, Tryggvason K, Yamada Y, Yurchenco PD. A new nomenclature for the laminins. Matrix Biol 1994; 14: 209–211.

364

Burton BK, Dillard RG, Weaver RG. Brief clinical report: Walker–Warburg syndrome with cleft lip and cleft palate in two sibs. Am J Med Genet 1987; 27: 537–541.

Byrd SE, Bohan TP, Osborn BE, Naidich TP. The CT and MR evaluation of lissencephaly. Am J Neuroradiol 1988; 9: 923–927.

Campbell KP. Three muscular dystrophies: loss of cytoskeleton – extracellular matrix linkage. Cell 1995; 80: 675–679.

Carpenter S, Karpati G. Congenital muscular dystrophy. In: Carpenter S, Karpati G, eds. Pathology of skeletal muscle. New York: Churchill Livingstone, 1984; 453, 511.

Castro de Castro P, Pascual-Castroviejo I, Lopez-Terradas JM, Gutierrez-Molina M. Distrofia muscular con participacion del sistema nervioso central. A proposito de dos casos espanoles. An Esp Pediatr 1983; 19: 111–117.

Castro-Gago M, Cervilla JR, Curros MC, Ugarte J, Becerra P, Durán JV, Alonso A. Distrofia musucular congénita associada a meningocele occipital, hidrocefalia y malformaciones oculares. Rev Esp Pediatr 1983; 39: 57–62.

Castro-Gago M, Diaz-Cardama I, Monasterio L, Fuster M, Perez-Becerra E, Peña J. Congenital muscular dystrophy with central nervous system involvement: an intermediate form? The Annals (Houston, TX) 1985; 7: 5–12.

Castro-Gago M, Pena-Guitian J. Congenital muscular dystrophy of non-Fukuyama type with characteristic CT images (letter). Brain Dev (Tokyo) 1988; 10: 60.

Chakova LD, Genev E, Zaprianov Z, Christov G, Ivanov I. Congenital muscular dystrophy – a report of four cases. Poster at the 1st Congress of the European Pediatric Neurology Society, Eilat, Israel, 1995.

Chan CC, Egbert PR, Herrick MK, Urich H. Oculocerebral malformations – a reappraisal of Walker's 'lissencephaly'. Arch Neurol 1980; 31: 104–108.

Chemke J, Czernobilsky B, Mundel G, Barishak YR. A familial syndrome of central nervous system and ocular malformations. Clin Genet 1975; 7: 1–7.

Chijiiwa T, Nishimura M, Ushijima H, Yamana Y, Inomata H, Fung KC, Kurokawa T. Ocular manifestations of congenital muscular dystrophy (Fukuyama type) in two cases (in Japanese). Rinsho Ganka (Clin Ophthalmol) (Tokyo) 1982; 36(1): 21–25.

Chijiiwa T, Nishimura M, Inomata H, Yamana T, Narazaki O, Kurokawa T. Ocular manifestations of congenital muscular dystrophy (Fukuyama type). Ann Ophthalmol 1983; 15: 921–928.

Chitayat D, Toi A, Babul R, Levin A, Michaud J, Summers A, Rutka J, Blaser S, Becker LE. Prenatal diagnosis of retinal non-attachment in the Walker–Warburg syndrome. Am J Med Genet 1995; 56: 351–358.

Choi BH, Matthias SC. Cortical dysplasia associated with massive ectopias of neurons and glia within the subarachnoid space. Acta Neuropathol (Berlin) 1987; 73: 105–109.

Chou SM. Reappraisal of the neuropathology of Fukuyama type progressive muscular dystrophy. A special report presented at the 1976 annual meeting of the muscular dystrophy research group, sponsored by the Ministry of Health and Welfare of Japan. Tokyo, 1976.

Claes C, Smets J, Jacobs K. La myopathie précocissime – étude électroclinique et pathologique d'une entité clinique particulière. J Neurol Sci 1968; 6: 141–154.

Cohn RD, Herrmann R, Wewer U, Voit T. Expression of laminin β2 chain in congenital muscular dystrophies (abstract). Neuromusc Disord 1996; (Suppl): S28–S29.

Cole AJ, Kuzniecky R, Karpati G, Carpenter S, Andermann E, Andermann F. Familial myopathy with changes resembling inclusion body myositis and periventricular leucoencephalopathy. Brain 1988; 111: 1025–1037.

Collier J, Holmes G. The pathological examination of two cases of amyotonia congenita with the clinical description of a fresh case. Brain 1909; 32: 269–284.

Comi GP, Ciafaloni E, Bardoni A, Bresolin N, Moggio M, Messina S, Fortunato F, Motta F, Felsari G, Garghentino R, Scarlato G. Absence of muscle and nerve specific dystrophin isoforms in a congenital myopathy patient (abstract). Clin Neuropathol 1994; 3: 148.

Connolly AM, Pestronk A. Congenital muscular dystrophy distinguished pathologically by specific patterns of alkaline phosphatase and acid phosphatase staining (abstract). Ann Neurol 1994; 36(3): 521.

Connolly AM, Pestronk A, Planes GJ, Yue J, Mehta S, Choksi R. Congenital muscular dystrophy syndromes distinguished by alkaline and acid phosphatase, merosin, and dystrophin straining. Neurology 1996; 46: 810–814.

Cook J, Haider A, Banna M, Stigsby B, Gascon G, Ozand P, Buyco C. Occidental congenital muscular dystrophy in Saudi Arabia; clinical, muscle pathology, and neuroradiological aspects. Abstracts of 8th Asian and Oceanian Congress of Neurology, Tokyo, 1991.

Cook J, Gascon G, Haider A, Adra C, Kunkel L, Ozand P, Stigsby B, Banna M, Brismar J, Coates R. Congenital muscular dystrophy (CMD) with CNS myelin involvement in Saudi Arabia (abstract). In: Angelini C, Danieli GA, Fontanari D, eds. Muscular dystrophy research: from molecular diagnosis toward therapy. Amsterdam: Excerpta Medica, 1991; 201.

Cook JD, Gascon GG, Haider A, Coates R, Stigsby B, Ozand PT, Banna M. Congenital muscular dystrophy with abnormal radiographic myelin pattern. J Child Neurol 1992; 7(Suppl): S51–S63.

Cook JD. Are progressive encephalopathic and leukoencephalopathic congenital muscular dystrophies the same syndrome? In: Fukuyama Y, Osawa M, Comp. Program and abstracts of the International Symposium on Congenital Muscular Dystrophies, Tokyo: Tokyo Women's Medical College, 1994: 45.

Cordone G, Bado M, Morreale G, Pedemonte M, Minetti C. Severe dystrophinopathy in a patient with congenital hypotonia. Childs Nerv Syst 1996; 12:466–469.

Cordone G, Bado M, Prigione P, Minetti C. Le distrofie muscolari congenite (abstract). Atti de XXII Congresso Nazionale della Societa Italiana di Neuropediatria, Pietrasanta (Lucca), 1996; 74–76.

Councilman WT, Dunn CH. Myatonia congenita: a report of a case with autopsy. Am J Dis Child 1911; 2: 340–355.

Crowe C, Jassani M, Dickerman L. The prenatal diagnosis of the Walker–Warburg syndrome. Prenat Diag 1986; 6: 177–185.

Cullen KM, Walsh J, Roberds SL, Campbell KP. Ultrastructural localization of adhalin, γ-dystroglycan and merosin in normal and dystrophic mice. Neuropathol Appl Neurobiol 1996; 22: 30–37.

D'Alessandro M, Ferlini A, Sewry C, Naom I, Dubowitz V, Muntoni F. Search for rearrangements in the laminin $\alpha2$ chain gene in merosin deficient congenital muscular dystrophy (abstract). Neuromusc Disord 1996; (Suppl): S26.

Dambska M, Wisniewski K, Sher J, Solish G. Cerebro-oculo-muscular syndrome: a variant of Fukuyama congenital cerebromuscular dystrophy. Clin Neuropathol 1982; 1: 93–98.

Dambska M, Wisniewski K, Sher JH. Lissencephaly: two distinct clinico-pathological types. Brain Dev (Tokyo) 1983; 5: 302–310.

Dastur DK, Razzak ZA, Bharucha EP. Arthrogryposis multiplex congenita. Part II. Muscle pathology and pathogenesis. J Neurol Neurosurg Psychiatry 1972; 35: 435–450.

de Lange C. Studien über angeborene Lähmungen bzw angeborene Hypotonie. II. Über die angeborene oder frühinfantile Form der Dystrophia musculorum progressiva (Erb). Acta Paediatr (Uppsala) 1938; 20(Suppl 33): 1–51.

De Paillette L, Aicardi J, Goutières F. Ullrich's congenital atonic sclerotic muscular dystrophy. A case report. J Neurol 1989; 236: 108–110.

De Stefano N, Dotti MT, Villanova M, Scarano G, Federico A. Merosin positive congenital muscular dystrophy with severe involvement of the central nervous system. Brain Dev (Tokyo) 1996; 18(4): 323–326.

Defféminis Rospidi HA, Vincent O, Silva Gaudin E, Scarabino R, Médici M. Distrofia muscular congenital pura. Ubicación nosologica, frecuencia, aspectos clinicos y evolutivos y classificación. Acta Neurol Latinoamer 1972; 18: 20–36.

Dent AC, Richards RB, Nairn ME. Congenital progressive ovine muscular dystrophy in Western Australia. Aust Vet J 1979; 55: 297.

Di Ricco M, Leveratto L, Cama A, Bado M, Tortori Donati P, Andreussi L, Borrone C. Report on a patient with congenital muscular dystrophy, hydrocephalus, Dandy–Walker malformation and leukodystrophy. Genet Couns 1993; 4: 295–298.

Dobyns WB, Stratton RF, Greenberg F. Syndromes with lissencephaly. I: Miller–Dieker and Norman–Roberts syndromes and isolated lissencephaly. Am J Med Genet 1984; 18: 509–526.

Dobyns WB, McCluggage CW. Computed tomographic appearance of lissencephaly syndromes. Am J Neuroradiol 1985; 6: 544–550.

Dobyns WB, Kirkpatrick JB, Hittner HM, Roberts RM, Kretzer FL. Syndromes with lissencephaly. II: Walker–Warburg and cerebro-oculo-muscular syndromes and a new syndrome with type II lissencephaly. Am J Med Genet 1985; 22: 157–195.

Dobyns WB, Gilbert EF, Opitz JM. Further comments on the lissencephaly syndrome (letter to the editor). Am J Med Genet 1985; 22: 197–211.

Dobyns WB. Walker–Warburg syndrome (letter to the editor). Neurology 1985; 35: 1082.

Dobyns WB. Developmental aspects of lissencephaly and the lissencephaly syndromes. In: Gilbert EF, Opitz JM, eds. Genetic aspects of developmental pathology. New York: Alan R Liss, 1987: 225–241.

Dobyns WB. The neurogenetics of lissencephaly. Neurol Clin 1989; 7: 89–105.

Dobyns WB, Pagon RA, Armstrong D, Curry CJR, Greenberg F, Grix A, Holmes LB, Laxova R, Michele VV, Robinow M, Zimmerman RL. Diagnostic criteria for Walker–Warburg syndrome. Am J Med Genet 1989; 32: 195–2l0.

Dobyns WB, Pagon RA, Curry CJR, Greenberg R. Response to Santavuori et al., regarding Walker–Warburg syndrome and muscle-eye-brain disease (letter). Am J Med Genet 1990; 36: 373–374.

Dobyns WB. Classification of the cerebro-oculo-muscular syndrome(s). Commentary to Kimura's paper. Brain Dev (Tokyo) 1993; 15: 242–244.

Dobyns WB. Walker–Warburg syndrome: clinical characteristics and diagnostic criteria for CMD with congenital brain and eye malformations (abstract). Muscle Nerve 1994; (Suppl 1): S53.

Dobyns WB, Truwit CL. Lissencephaly and other malformations of cortical development: 1995 update. Neuropediatrics 1995; 26(3): 132–147.

Dobyns WB, Patton MA, Stratton RF, Mastrobattista JM, Bianton SH, Northrup H. Cobblestone lissencephaly only (CLO) syndrome: exclusion from chromosome 9q31-32 (abstract #476). Am J Hum Genet 1995; 57(4): A87.

Dobyns WB, Patton MA, Stratton JM. Cobblestone lissencephaly with normal eyes and muscle. Neuropediatrics 1996; 2: 70–75.

Donnai D, Frandon PA. Walker–Warburg syndrome (Warburg syndrome, HARD ± E syndrome). J Med Genet 1986; 23: 200–203.

Donner M, Rapola J, Somer H. Congenital muscular dystrophy: a clinico-pathological and follow-up study of 15 patients. Neuropaediatrie 1975; 6: 239–258.

Doriguzzi C, Palmucci L, Mongini T, Bertolotto A, Maniscalco M, Chiado-Piat L, Zina AM, Bundino S. Congenital muscular dystrophy associated with familial junctional epidermolysis bullosa letalis. Eur Neurol 1993; 33: 454–460.

Drachman DB, Weiner LP, Price DL. Experimental arthrogryposis caused by viral myopathy. Arch Neurol 1976; 33: 362–367.

Dubois R, Graffar M, Ley R. Forme précoce de myopathie infantile simulant la maladie de Werdnig–Hoffmann. Acta Paediatr Belg 1946; 1: 1–8.

Dubowitz V. The floppy infant, 2nd edn. London: William Heinemann, 1980.

Dubowitz V, Brooke MH. Congenital muscular dystrophy. In: Dubowitz V, Brooke MH, eds. Muscle biopsy: a practical approach. 2nd edn. London: Saunders, 1985; 370–380.

Dubowitz V. Congenital muscular dystrophy. In: Dubowitz V, ed. Muscle disorders in childhood. 2nd edn. London: Saunders, 1995: 93–105.

Dubowitz V. Congenital muscular dystrophy. In: Dubowitz V, ed. A color atlas of muscle disorders in childhood. London: Wolfe Medical Publishers, 1989; 52–65.

Dubowitz V. 22nd ENMC sponsored workshop on congenital muscular dystrophy held in Baarn, The Netherlands, 14–16 May, 1993. Neuromusc Disord 1994; 4(1): 75–81.

Dubowitz V, Fardeau M. Proceedings of the 27th ENMC sponsored workshop on congenital muscular dystrophy, 22-24 April, 1994, The Netherlands (workshop report). Neuromusc Disord 1995; 5(3): 253–258.

Dubowitz V. Exciting new developments in congenital muscular dystrophy (abstract). Dev Med Child Neurol 1995; 37(Suppl 72): 36.

Dubowitz V. The clinical phenotype in congenital muscular dystrophy (abstract). Neuromusc Disord 1996; 6(2): S17.

Dubowitz V. New developments in congenital muscular dystrophy (annotation). Neuromusc Disord 1996; 6: 228.

Dubowitz V. 41st ENMC international workshop on congenital muscular dystrophy. 8-10 March, 1996, Naarden, The Netherlands. Neuromusc Disord 1996; 6: 295–306.

Echenne B, Pages M, Marty-Double C, Pages AM, Astruc J, Brunel D. Progressive muscular dystrophy with central nervous system involvement; an original variant of congenital neuromuscular disease (abstract). Proceedings of the 5th International Congress of Neuromuscular Diseases, Marseille, France, 1982.

Echenne B, Astruc J, Brunel D, Pages M, Baldet P, Martinazzo G. Congenital muscular dystrophy and rigid spine syndrome. Neuropediatrics 1983; 14: 97–101.

Echenne B, Pages M, Marty-Double C. Congenital muscular dystrophy with cerebral white matter spongiosis. Brain Dev (Tokyo) 1984; 6: 491–495.

Echenne B, Arthuis M, Billard C, Campos-Castello J, Castel Y, Dulac O, Fontan D, Gauthier A, Kulakowski S, De Meuron G, Moore JR, Nieto-Barrera M, Pages M, Parain D, Pavone L, Ponsot G. Congenital muscular dystrophy and cerebral CT scan anomalies. Results of a collaborative study of the Société de Neurologie Infantile. J Neurol Sci 1986; 75: 7–22.

Echenne B. Congenital muscular dystrophy of a non-Fukuyama type (letter). Brain Dev (Tokyo) 1988; 10: 397.

Echenne B. Congenital muscular dystrophy. A reappraisal (abstract). J Neurol Sci 1990; 98(Suppl): 436.

Echenne B, Chevron M-P, Pons F, Amram D, Chaustres M, Léger J-J, Demaille J. Congenital muscular dystrophy with absence of dystrophin (abstract). Abstract No 111, 6th Congress of the International Child Neurology Association, Buenos Aires, 1992.

Echenne B. Congenital muscular dystrophies. In: Lane RJM, ed. Handbook of muscle disease. New York: Marcel Dekker, 1996: 139–150.

Echenne B, Rivier F, Azais M, Pons F. Occidental-type, merosin positive CMD with mental deficiency, epilepsy and MRI changes in the cerebral white matter: another form of CMD. Neuromusc Disord 1996; (Suppl): S24–S25.

Eda I, Takashima S, Ohno K, Takeshita K. Lipid composition of the cerebral grey and white matter in a case with Fukuyama type congenital muscular dystrophy. Brain Dev (Tokyo) 1985; 7: 523–525.

Edgar TS, Lotz BP, Campbell KP, Rust RS. Role of dystrophin-associated glycoprotein/laminin complex in congenital muscular dystrophies (abstract). Muscle Nerve 1994; (Suppl 1): S180.

Edgar TS, Connolly A, Rust RS, Lotz BP. Normal peripheral nerve myelination in merosin (−) congenital muscular dystrophy (abstract #165). Ann Neurol 1996; 40: 329.

[Editorial] Benign congenital hypotonia. Br Med J 1957; ii: 931–932.

Eeg-Olofsson O, Eeg-Olofsson KE, Olsson Y. Congenital muscular dystrophy and neuronal organization disorder of cerebrum in two sibs (abstract). Pediatr Neurol 1994; 11(4): 172.

Egawa S, Fumita M, Takazawa N. Cranial CT findings in female patients with progressive muscular dystrophy (in Japanese). In: Sobue I, ed. The 1978 annual report of the research committee on clinic, epidemiology and management of progressive muscular dystrophy sponsored by the Ministry of Health and Welfare of Japan. Nagoya, 1979: 193–196.

Egger J, Kendall BE, Erdohazi M, Lake BD, Wilson J, Brett EM. Involvement of the central nervous system in congenital muscular dystrophies. Dev Med Child Neurol 1983; 25: 32–42.

Emery AEH. The congenital muscular dystrophies. In: Emery AEH. Duchenne muscular dystrophy, Rev. edn. Oxford: Oxford University Press, 1987: 70–71.

Engvall E, Vachon P, Loechel F, Xu H, Wewer U. Merosin is necessary for the survival of differentiated muscle cell *in vitro* and *in vivo* (abstract). Neuromusc Disord 1996; Suppl: S20–21.

Engvall E, Wewer UM. The domains of laminin. J Cell Biochem 1996.

Endo C, Tsuneyoshi N, Gejo M, Takashima H, Matsui M, Yukitake M, Matsuda Y, Kuroda Y. Two adult sisters with non-Fukuyama type congenital muscular dystrophy associated with diffuse cerebral white matter lesion (abstract in Japanese). Rinsho Shinkeigaku (Clin Neurol) (Tokyo) 1994; 34(6): 649.

Estournet-Mathiaud B, Barois A, Chouchane C, Leclair-Richard D. Merosin positive congenital muscular dystrophies (CMD): a heterogeneous group (abstract). Neuromusc Disord 1996; Suppl: S25.

Farber S, Craig JM, eds. Muscular dystrophy of the congenital type. Clinical pathological conference, the Children's Medical Center, Boston, MA. J Pediatr 1958; 53: 744–750.

Fardeau M. The congenital muscular dystrophies. In: Mastaglia FL, Walton J, eds. Skeletal muscle pathology. 2nd edn. Edinburgh: Churchill-Livingstone, 1992: 262–266.

Fardeau M, Tomé FMS, Evangelista T, Barois A, Estrounet B, Campbell KP. Clinical, histopathological and immunocytochemical data in congenital muscular dystrophies in France (abstract). Muscle Nerve 1994: Suppl 1: S52.

Fardeau M, Tomé FMS, Helbling-Leclerc A, Evangelista T, Ottolini A, Chevallay M, Barois A, Estournet B, Harpey JP, Faure S, Guicheney P, Hillaire D. Dystrophie musculaire congénitale avec déficience en mérosine : Analyse clinique, histocytochimique et génétique. Rev Neurol 1996; 152: 11–19.

Farrell SA, Toi A, Leadman ML, Davidson RG, Caco C. Prenatal diagnosis of retinal detachment in Walker–Warburg syndrome. Am J Med Genet 1987; 28: 619–624.

Federico A, Dotti MT, Malandrini A, Guazzi GC, Hayek G, Simonati A, Rizzuto N, Toti P. Cerebro-ocular dysplasia and muscular dystrophy: report of two cases. Neuropediatrics 1988; 19: 109–112.

Felisari G, Turconi AC, Bresolin N, Comi GP, Rigoletto C, Prelle A, Piccinini L, Garghentino RR, Scarlato G. Atypical features in a case of congenital muscular dystrophy (CMD) with partial merosin deficiency (abstract). Neuromusc Disord 1996; Suppl: S24.

Fenichel GM, Bazelon M. Myopathies in search of a name; benign congenital forms. Dev Med Child Neurol 1966; 8: 532–548.

Fenichel GM. Congenital muscular dystrophies. Neurol Clin 1988; 6: 519–528.

Fernandez Martinez MD, Rodriguez Sanchez F, Martinez-Lage JF, Costa TR, Puche A, Casas C, Almagro MJ. Walker–Warburg syndrome: experience at the Virgen de la Arrixaca Hospital (in Spanish). An Esp Pediatr 1992; 36: 213–217.

Fidzianska A, Goebel HH, Lenard HG, Heckmann C. Congenital muscular dystrophy (CMD) – a collagen formative disease? J Neurol Sci 1982; 55: 79–90.

Finkelnburg. Anatomischer Befund bei progressiver Muskeldystrophie in den ersten Lebensjahren. Dtsch Z Nervenheilk 1908; 35: 453–460.

Fiore G. Contributo allo studio delle miopatie della prima infanzia. Riv Clin Pediatr 1924; 22: 606–636.

Fontaine J-L, Graveleau D, Houllemare L, Laplane R. Les myopathies congénitales. A propos de 2 observations. Ann Pédiatr (Paris) 1965; 12: 1563–1568.

Fowler M, Manson JI. Congenital muscular dystrophy with malformation of central nervous system. In: Kakulas BA, ed. Clinical studies in myology. Proceedings of the 2nd International Congress on Muscle Diseases, Perth, 1971. Amsterdam: Excerpta Medica, 1973: 192–197.

Fujii S, Yakabe K, Eguchi K. Development of painting skill through practices in Fukuyama type congenital muscular dystrophy children (in Japanese). In: Nakajima T, ed. The 1978 annual report of the research committee: on clinico-sociological study of nursing care of progressive muscular dystrophy, sponsored by the Ministry of Health and Welfare of Japan, Matsue. 1979: 91–93.

Fukuyama Y, Kawazura M, Haruna H. A peculiar form of congenital progressive muscular dystrophy. Report of fifteen cases. Paediatr Univ Toyko (Tokyo) 1960; 4: 5–8.

Fukuyama Y. Progressive muscular dystrophy and related conditions (in Japanese). Naika (Intern Med) (Tokyo) 1960; 5: 1082–1089.

Fukuyama Y, Kawazura M, Haruna H. A report on fifteen cases of congenital muscular dystrophy with early onset in infancy and frequently accompanying intellectual impairment (abstract in Japanese). Shonika Shinryo (J Pediatr Pract) (Tokyo) 1960; 23(2): 279.

Fukuyama Y, Nagahata M, Shima N, Maruyama H, Kawazura M. Congenital progressive muscular dystrophy with onset in infancy and frequent accompaniment of intellectual im-

370

pairment – 18 cases (abstract in Japanese). Seishin Shinkeigaku Zasshi (J Jpn Soc Neuropsychiatry) (Tokyo) 1960; 62(8): 1366–1367.

Fukuyama Y. Shima N, Kawazura M, Sugita H. On the value of the determination of serum enzyme activities in the differential diagnosis of various neuromuscular diseases in children. Its correlation with the clinical, electromyographic, histologic and metabolic findings (in Japanese). No To Shinkei (Brain Nerve) (Tokyo) 1960; 12(9): 783–795.

Fukuyama Y. Muscle diseases in pediatric practice (in Japanese). Rinsho Shinkeigaku (Clin Neurol) (Tokyo) 1961; 1(5): 409–416.

Fukuyama Y, Kawazura M. On the nature of so-called amyotonia congenita Oppenheim, Critical review of literature and all reported Japanese cases (in Japanese). Shinkei Kenkyu No Shinpo (Adv Neurol Sci) (Tokyo) 1962; 6(2): 419–468.

Fukuyama Y, Segawa M. Clinical features and genetics of congenital muscular dystrophy (abstract In Japanese). Jinrui Idengaku Zasshi (Jpn J Hum Genet) (Tokyo) 1974; 19: 42–43.

Fukuyama Y, Hirayama Y, Suzuki H, Suzuki M, Yokota J, Osawa M. Clinico-genetic, epidemiologic and nosological studies of congenital progressive muscular dystrophy (CMD). I. Clinico-genetic study of CMD. II. Investigations by questionnaire on incidence of patients with CMD at the main hospitals throughout Japan. III. On the classification of PMD with onset in the early infancy period (in Japanese). In: Okinaka S, ed. The 1975 annual report of the research group on the etiology of progressive muscular dystrophy, sponsored by the Ministry of Health and Welfare, Tokyo. 1976: 123–129.

Fukuyama Y, Maruyama H, Hirayama Y, Suzuki H, Harada J, Nakane A, Osawa M, Tsukamoto A, Goto T, Miyata A, Ogawa K. A neuroradiological study on CNS abnormalities in congenital muscular dystrophy (in Japanese). In: Okinaka S, ed. The 1976 annual report of the research group on the etiology of muscular dystrophy, sponsored by the Ministry of Health and Welfare, Tokyo. 1977: 116–118.

Fukuyama Y. Congenital muscular dystrophy (in Japanese). Shinkei Kenkyu No Shinpo (Adv Neurol Sci) (Tokyo) 1978; 22: 828–829.

Fukuyama Y, Mori H, Osawa M, Harada J, Suzuki H, Hirayama Y. Sibling cases of Fukuyama type congenital muscular dystrophy-like disease with diffuse white matter hypodensity and atypical muscle biopsy findings (in Japanese). In: Sobue I, ed. The 1978 annual report of the research group on the clinical and epidemiologic study of muscular dystrophy, sponsored by the Ministry of Health and Welfare of Japan. Nagoya, 1979: 214–218.

Fukuyama Y, Ogawa K, Osawa M, Suzuki H, Hirayama Y, Ogata T, Yoneyama E, Ohya A. Serum anti-viral antibody titers in congenital muscular dystrophy (Fukuyama type) (in Japanese). In: Sobue I, ed. The 1978 annual report of the research group on the clinical and epidemiologic study of muscular dystrophy, sponsored by the Ministry of Health and Welfare of Japan. Nagoya, 1979: 225–229.

Fukuyama Y, Saito K, Osawa M, Suzuki H, Hirayama Y, Ogata T, Ohya A. Muscular changes in intrauterine Akabane virus infection (in Japanese). In: Sobue I, ed. The 1979 annual report of the research group on the clinical and epidemiologic study of muscular dystrophy, sponsored by the Ministry of Health and Welfare of Japan. Nagoya, 1980: 396–402.

Fukuyama Y, Osawa M, Adachi K, Nakada E, Suzuki H, Hirayama Y. Natural history of congenital muscular dystrophy (in Japanese). In: Sobue I, ed. The 1980 annual report of the research group on clinical pathology and epidemiology of muscular dystrophy sponsored by the Ministry of Health and Welfare of Japan. Nagoya, 1981: 36–42.

Fukuyama Y, Osawa M, Nakada E, Suzuki H, Hirayama Y, Mauyama H, Shishikura K, Saito K. Cranial computed tomography in progressive muscular dystrophy (in Japanese). In: Sobue I, ed. The 1980 annual report of the research group on clinical pathology and epidemiology of muscular dystrophy, sponsored by the Ministry of Health and Welfare of Japan. Nagoya, 1981: 176–183.

Fukuyama Y. Central nervous system manifestations in congenital muscular dystrophy of Fukuyama type (in Japanese). In: Kinoshita M, Saito T, ed. Internal medicine Q and A – Neurology. Tokyo: Kanehara Shuppan, 1981: 225–227.

Fukuyama Y, Osawa M, Suzuki H. Congenital progressive muscular dystrophy of the Fukuyama type. Clinical, genetic and pathological considerations. Brain Dev (Tokyo) 1981; 3: 1–29.

Fukuyama Y, Osawa M. Congenital muscular dystrophy; clinico-nosological aspects. In: Ebashi S, ed. Muscular dystrophy. Proceedings of the International Symposium of Muscular Dystrophy, 1980, Tokyo. Tokyo: University of Tokyo Press, 1982: 399–424.

Fukuyama Y. Congenital muscular dystrophy (Fukuyama type) (in Japanese). Taisha (Metabolism) (Osaka) 1982; 19S: 804–806.

Fukuyama Y, Osawa M, Tsubaki T, Nishitani H, Miyao M, Shinoda M, Miyoshino S. An epidemiologic and genetic study on congenital muscular dystrophy (preliminary report) (in Japanese). In: Sobue I, ed. The 1981 annual report of the research committee on epidemiology, clinics, and treatment of progressive muscular dystrophy, sponsored by the Ministry of Health and Welfare of Japan. Nagoya, 1982: 10–17.

Fukuyama Y, Saito K, Osawa M, Suzuki H, Hirayama Y, Shishikura K, Ogata T. A trial of virus isolation from autopsy materials of congenital muscular dystrophy (in Japanese). In: Sobue I, ed. The 1981 annual report of the research committee on epidemiology, clinics, and treatment of progressive muscular dystrophy, sponsored by the Ministry of Health and Welfare of Japan. Nagoya, 1982: 77–83.

Fukuyama Y, Suzuki H, Hirayama Y, Osawa M, Shishikura K, Saito K, Nakada E. Reevaluation of muscle histology in the Fukuyama type congenital muscular dystrophy (in Japanese). In: Sobue I, ed. The 1981 annual report of the research committee on epidemiology, clinics, and treatment of progressive muscular dystrophy, sponsored by the Ministry of Health and Welfare of Japan. Nagoya, 1982: 256–264.

Fukuyama Y, Shishikura K, Osawa M, Saito K, Suzuki H, Hirayama Y. An autopsy case of Fukuyama type congenital muscular dystrophy (in Japanese). In: Sobue I, ed. The 1981 annual report of the research committee on epidemiology, clinics and treatment of progressive muscular dystrophy, sponsored by the Ministry of Health and Welfare of Japan. Nagoya, 1982: 301–306.

Fukuyama Y, Tsubaki T, Nishitani H, Miyao M, Miyoshino S, Osawa M. An epidemiological and genetic study on congenital muscular dystrophies (in Japanese). In: Sobue I, ed. The 1982 annual report of the research committee on epidemiology, clinics, and treatment of progressive muscular dystrophy, sponsored by the Ministry of Health and Welfare of Japan. Nagoya, 1983: 16–24.

Fukuyama Y, Ashida E, Osawa M, Miyazawa Y, Shishikura K, Suzuki H, Hirayama Y, Oguni H, Monma K, Toyota Y, Imai M. An evaluation of cardiac function in congenital and Duchenne muscular dystrophies (in Japanese). In: Sobue I, ed. The 1982 annual report of the research committee on epidemiology, clinics, and treatment of progressive muscular dystrophy, sponsored by the Ministry of Health and Welfare of Japan. Nagoya, 1983: 160–165.

Fukuyama Y, Osawa M. A genetic study of the Fukuyama type congenital muscular dystrophy. Brain Dev (Tokyo) 1984; 6: 373–390.

Fukuyama Y, Nishitani Y, Miyao M, Shinoda M, Miyoshino S, Osawa M. Epidemiological and genetic studies on congenital muscular dystrophies (in Japanese). In: Sobue I, ed. The 1983 annual report of the research committee on epidemiology, clinics, and treatment of progressive muscular dystrophy, sponsored by the Ministry of Health and Welfare of Japan. Nagoya, 1984: 92–100.

Fukuyama Y, Suyama A, Yabe K, Sugie H, Sugie Y, Osawa M, Suzuki H. Calcium-staining study of biopsied muscle in the Duchenne type and the Fukuyama type progressive muscular dystrophy (in Japanese). In: Sobue I, ed. The 1983 annual report of the research committee on epidemiology, clinics, and treatment of progressive muscular dystrophy, sponsored by the Ministry of Health and Welfare of Japan. Nagoya, 1984: 490–495.

Fukuyama Y. Fukuyama type congenital muscular dystrophy (in Japanese). Medicina (Tokyo) 1985; 22: 244–245.

Fukuyama Y. Fukuyama type congenital muscular dystrophy (in Japanese). Clin Neurosci (Tokyo) 1985; 3: 320–321.

Fukuyama Y, Nishitani H, Miyao M, Shinoda M, Miyoshino S, Osawa M, Tsutsumi A, Uchida S. Epidemiological and genetic study of congenital muscular dystrophy (in Japanese). In: Nishitani H, ed. The 1984 annual report of the research committee on epidemiology, pathophysiology and treatment of progressive muscular dystrophy, sponsored by the Ministry of Health and Welfare of Japan. Kyoto, 1985: 51–54.

Fukuyama Y, Osawa M, Nakada E, Suzuki H, Shishikura K, Hirayama Y, Morimoto T. Physical growth of patients with congenital muscular dystrophy (in Japanese). In: Nishitani H, ed. The 1984 annual report of the research committee on epidemiology, pathophysiology and treatment of progressive muscular dystrophy, sponsored by the Ministry of Health and Welfare of Japan. Kyoto, 1985: 198–204.

Fukuyama Y, Suyama A, Osawa M, Nishitani H, Miyao M, Miyoshino S, Yoshioka M. Ophthalmological findings in the Fukuyama type congenital muscular dystrophy based upon the material obtained by the 1983 national survey (in Japanese). In: Nishitani H, ed. The 1985 annual report of the research committee on epidemiology, pathogenesis and therapeutic exploration of progressive muscular dystrophy, sponsored by the Ministry of Health and Welfare of Japan. Kyoto, 1986: 69–73.

Fukuyama Y, Osawa M, Okada R, Suzuki H, Shishikura K, Nakada E, Saito K, Hirayama Y, Tsutsumi A, Oi I, Oto K, Uchida Y. Eye findings in our personal cases with the Fukuyama type congenital muscular dystrophy (in Japanese). In: Nishitani H, ed. The 1985 annual report of the research committee on epidemiology, pathogenesis and therapeutic exploration of progressive muscular dystrophy, sponsored by the Ministry of Health and Welfare of Japan. Kyoto, 1986: 74–79.

Fukuyama Y, Mitsuishi Y, Osawa M, Shishikura K, Kono A, Maki M. Evaluation of apparently hydrocephalic CT findings in patients with the Fukuyama type congenital muscular dystrophy by means of RI cisternography and serial CT examinations (in Japanese). In: Matsumoto S, ed. The 1986 annual report of the research committee on intractable hydrocephalus, sponsored by the Ministry of Health and Welfare of Japan. Kobe, 1987: 8.

Fukuyama Y, Mitsuishi Y, Osawa M, Maki M. A RI-cisternographic study on hydrocephalic state in patients with the Fukuyama type congenital muscular dystrophy (in Japanese). In: Nishitani H, ed. The 1986 annual report of the research committee on epidemiology, pathophysiology and treatment of progressive muscular dystrophy, sponsored by the Ministry of Health and Welfare of Japan. Kyoto, 1987: 19–24.

Fukuyama Y, Suyama A, Osawa M, Yoshioka M, Miyoshino S. National survey on congenital muscular dystrophy in Japan – with emphasis on the comparison of clinical pictures between the Fukuyama type and the non-Fukuyama type cases – (in Japanese). In: Nishitani H, ed. The 1986 annual report of the research committee on epidemiology, pathophysiology and treatment of progressive muscular dystrophy, sponsored by the Ministry of Health and Welfare of Japan. Kyoto, 1987: 65–69.

Fukuyama Y, Osawa M, Sumida S, Kawai M, Okada N, Hirasawa K, Suzuki H, Hirayama Y, Shishikura K, Saito K. Evaluation of skeletal muscle changes by CT scan in progressive muscular dystrophy, especially in congenital muscular dystrophy (in Japanese). In: Nishitani H, ed. The 1987 annual report of the research committee on genetics, epidemiology, clinics and treatment of progressive muscular dystrophy, sponsored by the Ministry of Health and Welfare of Japan. Kyoto, 1988: 131–136.

Fukuyama Y, Okada N, Osawa M, Suzuki H, Shishikura K, Saito K, Kasajima T. Immunohistochemical study of skeletal muscles in Fukuyama type congenital muscular dystrophy (in Japanese). In: Nishitani H, ed. The 1987 annual report of the research committee on genetics, epidemiology, clinics and treatment of progressive muscular dystrophy, sponsored by the Ministry of Health and Welfare of Japan. Kyoto, 1988: 329–332.

Fukuyama Y, Arai Y, Sumida S, Osawa M, Okada N, Hirasawa K, Kawai M, Shishikura K, Suzuki H, Hirayama Y, Nakada E, Saito K. CT scans of skeletal muscles in Fukuyama type congenital muscular dystrophy (in Japanese). In: Nishitani H, ed. The 1988 annual report of the research committee on genetics, epidemiology, clinics and treatment of progressive muscular dystrophy, sponsored by the Ministry of Health and Welfare of Japan. Kyoto, 1989: 127–133.

Fukuyama Y, Osawa M, Sumida S, Ikenaka H, Sugawara N, Hirasawa K, Arai Y, Suzuki H, Shishikura K, Saito K, Hirayama Y. Elements of congenital anomalies in congenital muscular dystrophy. Report 1. On physical minor anomalies (in Japanese). In: Nishitani H, ed. The 1989 annual report of the research committee on genetics, epidemiology, clinics and treatment of progressive muscular dystrophy, sponsored by the Ministry of Health and Welfare of Japan. Kyoto, 1990: 227–230.

Fukuyama Y, Murasugi H, Osawa M, Sumida S, Arai Y, Ikenaka H, Hirasawa K, Suzuki H, Shishikura K, Mitsuishi Y, Kohno A, Kobayashi N. Cranial MRI findings in Fukuyama type congenital muscular dystrophy (preliminary report) (in Japanese). In: Nishitani H, ed. The 1989 annual report of the research committee on genetics, epidemiology, clinics and treatment of progressive muscular dystrophy, sponsored by the Ministry of Health and Welfare of Japan. Kyoto, 1990: 235–238.

Fukuyama Y, Osawa M, Sumida S, Okada N, Hirasawa K, Shishikura K, Suzuki H, Ikenaka H. Evaluation of skeletal muscle changes by CT scans in progressive muscular dystrophy, especially in congenital muscular dystrophy (in Japanese). In: Nishitani H, ed. The 1989 annual report of the research committee on genetics, epidemiology, clinics and treatment of progressive muscular dystrophy, sponsored by the Ministry of Health and Welfare of Japan. Kyoto, 1990: 247–250.

Fukuyama Y. Fukuyama type congenital muscular dystrophy (in Japanese). Clin Neurosci (Tokyo) 1991; 9: 72–73.

Fukuyama Y, Sumida S, Osawa M, Ikenaka H, Sugawara N, Murasugi H, Hirasawa K, Arai Y, Suzuki H, Shishikura K, Saito K, Hirayama Y. Elements of congenital anomalies in congenital muscular dystrophy. Part 2. Dermatoglyphic analysis (in Japanese). In: Takahashi K, ed. The 1990 annual report of the research committee on clinics, genetic counselling and epidemiology of progressive muscular dystrophy, sponsored by the Ministry of Health and Welfare of Japan. Hyogo, 1991: 217–221.

Fukuyama Y, Ikenaka H, Osawa M, Sumida S, Hirasawa K, Arai Y, Okada N, Shishikura K, Suzuki H, Hirayama Y. Natural course of serum CK, GOT, GPT and LDH values in congenital muscular dystrophy patients (in Japanese). In: Takahashi K, ed. The 1990 annual report of the research committee on clinics, genetic counselling and epidemiology of progressive muscular dystrophy, sponsored by the Ministry of Health and Welfare of Japan. Hyogo, 1991: 222–226.

Fukuyama Y, Arai Y, Osawa M, Sumida S, Shishikura K, Suzuki H, Hirasawa K, Sugawara N, Ikenaka H, Saito K, Hirayama Y. Evolution of CT values of thigh muscles in congenital muscular dystrophy, especially in its early stage (in Japanese). In: Takahashi K, ed. The 1990 annual report of the research committee on clinics, genetic counselling and epidemiology of progressive muscular dystrophy. sponsored by the Ministry of Health and Welfare of Japan. Hyogo, 1991: 227–230.

Fukuyama Y, Sumida S, Osawa M, Suzuki H, Hirasawa K, Arai Y, Murasugi H. Convulsive seizures in congenital muscular dystrophy patients (in Japanese). In: Takahashi K, ed. The 1991 annual report of the research committee on clinics, genetic counselling and epidemiology of progressive muscular dystrophy, sponsored by the Ministry of Health and Welfare of Japan. Hyogo, 1992: 229–231.

Fukuyama Y, Ikeya K, Saito K, Yamauchi A, Ikenaka H, Ishii H, Kondo E, Sakauchi Y, Mishima M, Takahashi R, Harada T, Osawa M. Dystrophin in skeletal muscles of congenital muscular dystrophy patients (in Japanese). In: Takahashi K, ed. The 1991 annual report of the research committee on clinics, genetic counselling and epidemiology of progressive muscular dystrophy, sponsored by the Ministry of Health and Welfare of Japan. Hyogo, 1992: 281–285.

Fukuyama Y, Osawa M, Saito K, Sakauchi Y, Kondo E. Congenital muscular dystrophy (in Japanese). In: Takahashi K, ed. The 1992 annual report of the research committee on clinics, genetic counselling and epidemiology of progressive muscular dystrophy, sponsored by the Ministry of Health and Welfare of Japan. Hyogo, 1993: 231–234.

Fukuyama Y, Osawa M, Saito K, Sumida S, Arai Y, Shishikura K, Suzuki H, Yamauchi A, Hirayama Y. An unusual case of Duchenne muscular dystrophy with verified dystrophin DNA deletion which had been suspected clinically to be a case of congenital muscular dystrophy of unclassified type characterized by stereotypic behavior and autistic tendency (in Japanese). In: Takahashi K, ed. The 1992 annual report of the research committee on clinics, genetic counselling and epidemiology of progressive muscular dystrophy, sponsored by the Ministry of Health and Welfare of Japan. Hyogo, 1993: 235–237.

Fukuyama Y, Saito K, Osawa M, Harada T, Yamauchi A, Ikeya K, Kondo E, Umii H. Dystrophin gene deletion in congenital muscular dystrophy (in Japanese). In: Takahashi K, ed. The 1992 annual report of the research committee on clinics, genetic counselling and epidemiology of progressive muscular dystrophy, sponsored by the Ministry of Health and Welfare of Japan. Hyogo, 1993: 238–242.

Fukuyama Y, Osawa M, Shishikura K, Suzuki H, Hirayama Y, Sumida S, Arai Y, Saito K. Congenital muscular dystrophy with normal intelligence and diffuse white matter hyperlucency (in Japanese). In: Takahashi K, ed. The 1992 annual report of the research committee on clinics, genetic counselling and epidemiology of progressive muscular dystrophy, sponsored by the Ministry of Health and Welfare of Japan. Hyogo, 1993: 243–246.

Fukuyama Y, Osawa M, Ikeya K, Sumida S, Shishikura K, Suzuki H, Hirayama Y, Arai Y, Saito K, Kondo E, Morikawa T, Toyota C, Kobayashi M. A case study: intra vitam diagnosis of severe Duchenne muscular dystrophy was disproved by the demonstration of positive immunostaining of muscle dystrophin and cerebral polymicrogyria at autopsy (in Japanese). In: Takahashi K, ed. The 1992 annual report of the research committee on clinics, genetic counselling and epidemiology of progressive muscular dystrophy, sponsored by the Ministry of Health and Welfare of Japan. Hyogo, 1993: 247–251.

Fukuyama Y, Osawa M, comp. Program and abstracts of the International Symposium on Congenital Muscular Dystrophies, Tokyo. Tokyo: Tokyo Women's Medical College, 1994: 45 pp.

Fukuyama Y, Osawa M, Saito K. Congenital muscular dystrophies: an overview. In: Arzimanoglou A, Goutières F, eds. Trends in child neurology. A Festschrift for Jean Aicardi. Paris: John Libbey Eurotext, 1996: 107–135.

Fukuyama Y. Fukuyama type congenital muscular dystrophy (in Japanese). Shonika Shinryo (J Pediatr Pract) (Tokyo) 1997; 60(2): 284–287.

Fumita M, Tokiguchi S. Brain computed tomography of congenital muscular dystrophy (Fukuyama type) with discussion on possible pathogenesis of Mycoplasma infection (in Japanese). Shinkei Naika (Neurol Med) (Tokyo) 1978; 9(1): 49–53.

Furtado D. L'évolution de l'amyotrophie spinale infantile. Rev Neurol 1958; 98: 742–749.

Furukawa T, Toyokura Y. Congenital hypotonic-sclerotic muscular dystrophy. In: Okinaka S, ed. Current research in muscular dystrophy, Japan. The proceedings of the annual meeting of muscular dystrophy research group. Tokyo; 1977: 100–101.

Furukawa T, Toyokura Y. Congenital hypotonic-sclerotic muscular dystrophy. J Med Genet 1977; 14: 426–429.

Furusho T, Fukuyama Y, Osawa M, Ogawa K, Tsukamoto A, Kondo K. Genetic analysis of congenital progressive muscular dystrophy (in Japanese). In: Okinaka S, ed. The 1976 annual report of the research group on the etiology of muscular dystrophy, sponsored by the Ministry of Health and Welfare of Japan. Tokyo, 1977: 91–94.

Gardner-Medwin D, Walton J. The congenital muscular dystrophies. In: Walton J, Karpati G, Hilton-Jones D, eds. Disorders of voluntary muscle. 6th edn. Edinburgh: Churchill Livingstone, 1994: 572–576.

Gelot A, Billette de Villemeur T, Bordarier C, Ruchoux MM, Moraine C, Ponsot G. Developmental aspects of type II lissencephaly. Comparative study of dysplastic lesions in fetal and post-natal brains. Acta Neuropathol 1995; 89: 72–84.

Gerding H, Gullotta E, Kuchelmeister K, Busse H. Ocular findings in Walker–Warburg syndrome. Childs Nerv Syst 1993; 9: 418–420.

Gerhard JP, Brini A, Willard D, Rohmer A, Messer J. Le syndrome de dysplasie retinienne familiale associé á une hydrocephalie. Klin Monatsbl Augenheilk 1978; 172: 546–548.

Gershoni-Baruch R, Mandel H, Miller B, Sujow P, Braun J. Walker–Warburg syndrome with microtia and absent auditory canals. Am J Med Genet 1990; 37: 87–91.

Gobernado JM, Gimeno A. Changes in cerebral white matter in a case of congenital muscular dystrophy. Pediatr Radiol 1982; 12: 201–203.

Goebel HH, Lenard HG, Langenbeck U, Mehl B. A form of congenital muscular dystrophy. Brain Dev (Tokyo) 1980; 2: 387–400.

Goebel HH, Fidzianska A, Heckmann C. Recent enzyme histochemical and ultrastructural observations in congenital myopathies and congenital muscular dystrophy. Wiss Ztsch Friedrich-Schiller Univ Jena, Math Naturwiss R 1983; 32: 759–769.

Goebel HH, Fidzianska A, Lenard HG, Osse G, Hori A. A morphological study of non-Japanese congenital muscular dystrophy associated with cerebral lesions. Brain Dev (Tokyo) 1983; 5: 292–301.

Goebel HH. Congenital myopathies. Acta Paediatr Jpn (Tokyo) 1991; 33: 247–255.

Goebel HH. Neuropathology of congenital muscular dystrophies (abstract). Muscle Nerve 1994; Suppl 1: S53.

Goemans N, Lemmens M, Casaer P. Congenital muscular dystrophy: clinical, pathological and neuroradiological review of 12 patients (abstract). Dev Med Child Neurol 1995; 37(2)(Suppl 72): 49.

Gordon N, Muscle and brain disease: an update. Child Care Health Dev 1994; 20:279-287.

Goto A, Ishida A, Kobayashi Y, Takada G. A case of Ullrich disease with distinct dystrophic changes of muscles (in Japanese). No To Hattatsu (Brain Dev) (Tokyo) 1991; 23: 289–293.

Goto Y, Kobayashi O, Nonaka I. Clinical and pathological study of merosin-positive, non-Fukuyama type congenital muscular dystrophy (classical form) (abstract in Japanese). In: National Center of Neurology and Psychiatry (Planning Division), ed. Annual Report of the Research on Nervous and Mental Disorders, 1994. Kodaira: National Center of Neurology and Psychiatry, 1995: 29.

Goto Y, Nishino I, Kobayashi O, Nonaka I, Kurihara M, Kumagai K, Fujita T, Hashimoto K, Horai S. Congenital muscular dystrophy associated with mitochondrial dysgenesis (abstract in Japanese). In: Takagi A, chairman. Abstracts for the 1996 annual meeting of the research committee on pathogenesis and treatment of progressive muscular dystrophy and related disorders, sponsored by the Ministry of Health and Welfare of Japan. Tokyo; 1996: 40.

Gött H, Josten EA. Beitrag zur kongenitalen atonisch-sklerotischen Muskeldystrophie (Typ Ullrich). Z Kinderheilk 1954; 75: 105–118.

Granata C, Merlini R, Govoni E. Distrofia muscolare congenita tipo Fukuyama (abstract). Riv Ital EEG Neurofisiol Clin 1983; Suppl 1: 491.

Granata C, Franzoni E, Moscano FC, Malaspina E, Gobbi G, Pini A, Mora M, Morandi L, Maraldi NM, Sabatelli P, Donzelli O. Clinical and laboratory data of 63 CMD patients and delineation of a peculiar mild phenotype with axial-distal weakness and proximal-axial contractures(abstract). Neuromusc Disord 1996; Suppl: S19.

Greenberg GR, Jacobs HK, Nylen TE, Gibb M, Chodirker BN, Moffatt M, Lacson A, Halliday W, Bernier F, El-Husseini A, Cameron A, Wrogemann K. Congenital hydrocephalus secondary to Walker–Warburg syndrome identified on the Manitoba Neonatal Screening Programme for Duchenne muscular dystrophy. J Med Genet 1992; 29: 583–585.

Greenfield JG. The anatomical identity of the Werdnig-Hoffmann and Oppenheim forms of infantile muscular dystrophy. Brain 1927; 50: 652–686.

Greenfield JG, Cornman T, Shy GM. The prognostic value of the muscle biopsy in the "floppy infant". Brain 1958; 81: 461–484.

Gubbay SS, Walton JN, Pearce GW. Clinical and pathological study of a case of congenital muscular dystrophy. J Neurol Neurosurg Psychiatry 1966; 29: 500–508.

Guibaud P, Carrier H, Mathieu M, Dorche C, Parchoux B, Béthenod M, Larbre F. Observation familiale de dystrophie musculaire congénitale par déficit en phosphofructokinase. Arch Fr Pédiatr 1978; 35: 1105–1115.

Guicheney P, Helbling-Leclerc A, Vignier N, Zhang X, Tome F, Cruaud C, Topaloglu H, Merlini L, Weissenbach J, Schwartz K, Fryggvason K, Fardeau M. Mutations in the laminin α2-chain gene (LAMA2) cause merosin-deficient congenital muscular dystrophy (abstract). Eur J Hum Genet 1996; 4 Suppl 1: 94.

Gunther A, Stoltenburg-Didinger G, Vogel M. Cerebro-ocular dysplasia in a 20-week-old fetus (abstract). Childs Nerv Syst 1993; 9: 124.

Hahn JS, Ela T, Nespeca M. Arthrogryposis multiplex congenita associated with neuronal migrational abnormalities and open opercular sign (abstract). Ann Neurol 1990; 28: 430–431.

Haltia M, Leivo I, Somer H, Pihko H, Paetau A, Kivelä T, Tarkkanen A, Tomé F, Engvall E, Santavouri P. Muscle-eye-brain disease – a neuropathological study. Ann Neurol 1997; 41: 173–180.

Hamazaki Y, Ishii M, Togo Y, Kamiya S, Yamagiwa Y. Three cases of congenital muscular dystrophy (in Japanese). Shonika (Tokyo) 1971; 12: 165–169.

Hanaka S, Nakamoto N, Kobayashi M, Tajima T, Ohmi K, Abe T, Nonaka I. Two female siblings affected with Fukuyama type congenital muscular dystrophy (abstract in Japanese). No To Hattatsu (Brain Dev) (Tokyo) 1994; 26 Suppl: S281.

Hansson O, Kristensson K, Lycke E, Solymar L, Sourander P. Generalized myopathy and cerebral malformations possibly related to an enteroviral infection. Acta Paediatr Scand 1975; 64: 881–885.

Hantai D, Labat-Robert J, Grimaud J-A, Fardeau M. Fibronectin, laminin, type I, III and IV collagens in Duchenne's muscular dystrophy, congenital muscular dystrophies and congenital myopathies; an immunocytochemical study. Connect Tissue Res 1985; 13: 273–281.

Hara M, Murasugi H, Osawa M, Shishikura K, Fukuyama Y. Neuroradiological study of Fukuyama type congenital muscular dystrophy brain (type II lissencephaly) (in Japanese). In: Takeshita K, ed. The 1992 annual report of the research committee on the pathogenesis and epidemiology of brain dysplasia, sponsored by the Ministry of Health and Welfare of Japan. Yonago, 1993: 50–63.

Harding BN. Cerebro-ocular dysplasia with muscular involvement (abstract). Neuropathol Appl Neurobiol 1988; l4: 258.

Harris JG, Wallace C, Wing J. Myelinated nerve fiber counts in the nerves of normal and dystrophic mouse muscle. J Neurol Sci 1972; 15: 245–249.

Hart MN, Malamud N, Ellis WG. The Dandy–Walker syndrome: a clinicopathological study based on 28 cases. Neurology 1972; 22: 771–780.

Hatano E, Kameo H, Masuda K, Hiraki Y, Miyoshi K, Jo K, Murata H. Flexibility of shoulder joints in various types of progressive muscular dystrophy (in Japanese). In: Nishitani H, ed. The 1984 annual report of the research committee on genetics, epidemiology, clinics and treatment of progressive muscular dystrophy, sponsored by the Ministry of Health and Welfare of Japan. Kyoto, 1985: 172–176.

Hatano E, Masuda K, Miyoshi K, Jo K, Karakawa T, Kameo H. Bone fractures in progressive muscular diseases (in Japanese). In: Nishitani H, ed. The 1986 annual report of the research committee on genetics, epidemiology, clinics and treatment of progressive muscular dystrophy, sponsored by the Ministry of Health and Welfare of Japan. Kyoto, 1987: 204–209.

378

Haushalter P. Trois nouveaux cas d'amyotrophie primitive progressive dans l'enfance. Rev Méd 1898; 18: 445–460.

Haushalter P. Sur la myatonie congénitale (maladie d'Oppenheim). Arch Méd Enfants 1920; 23(3): 133–144.

Hayashi H, Awaya Y, Iwamoto H, Komiya K, Misugi N. Clinical study of congenital muscular dystrophy (Fukuyama type) (abstract). Brain Dev (Tokyo) 1981; 3: 239.

Hayashi K, Ota M, Sakate M, Ota K, Mori F, Itagaki Y, Nishitani H. On polymorphism of creatine phosphokinase. In: Nishitani H, ed. The 1984 annual report of the research committee on genetics, epidemiology, clinics and treatment of progressive muscular dystrophy, sponsored by the Ministry of Health and Welfare of Japan. Kyoto, 1985: 238–241.

Hayashi M, Yamashita S, Miyake S, Iwamoto H, Misugi N, Hayashi N. Congenital muscular dystrophy: two sibling cases with different clinical courses (abstract). Brain Dev (Tokyo) 1986; 8: 220.

Hayashi Y, Arikawa E, Nonaka I, Sugita H, Arahata K. Changes in extracellular matrix, laminin and collagen IV in Fukuyama congenital muscular dystrophy (abstract). Brain Pathol 1992; 2: 257.

Hayashi YK, Engvall E, Arikawa-Hirasawa E, Goto K, Koga R, Nonaka I, Sugita H, Arahata K. Abnormal localization of laminin subunits in muscular dystrophies. J Neurol Sci 1993; 119: 53–64.

Hayashi YK, Koga R, Tsukahara T, Ishii H, Matsuishi T, Yamashita Y, Nonaka I, Arahata K. Deficiency of laminin α2-chain mRNA in muscle in a patient with merosin-negative congenital muscular dystrophy. Muscle Nerve 1995; 18(9): 1027–1030.

Hayashi YK, Ishihara T, Domen K, Arahata K. Unusual type of laminin α2-chain deficient muscular dystrophy (abstract). Neuromusc Disord 1996; Suppl: S22.

Heffner RR Jr. Congenital muscular dystrophy. In: Nelson JS, Parisi JE, Schochet SS Jr, eds. Principles and practice of neuropathology. St Louis, MO: Mosby, 1993: 528.

Heggie P, Grossniklaus HE, Roessmann U, Chou SH, Cruse RP. Cerebro-ocular dysplasia-muscular dystrophy syndrome. Report of two cases. Arch Ophthalmol 1987; 105: 520–524.

Helbling-Leclerc A, Topaloğlu K, Tomé FMS, Sewry C, Cyapay G, Naom I, Muntoni F, Dubowitz V, Barois A, Estournet B, Urtizberea JA, Weissenbach J, Schwartz K, Fardeau M. Guicheney P. Readjusting the localization of merosin (laminin α2-chain) deficient congenital muscular dystrophy locus on chromosome 6q2. CR Acad Sci Paris, Sci Vie 1995; 318: 1245–1252.

Helbling-Leclerc A, Zhang X, Topaloğlu H, Cruaud C, Tesson F, Weissenbach J, Tomé FMS, Schwartz K, Fardeau M, Tryggvason K, Guichency P. Mutations in the laminin α2-chain gene (LAMA 2) cause merosin-deficient congenital muscular dystrophy. Nat Genet 1995; 11(2): 216–218.

Helbling-Leclerc A, Vignier N, Topaloğlu H, Tomé FMS, Sewry C, Gyapay G, Muntoni F, Barois A, Estournei B, Weissenbach J, Dubowitz V, Schwartz K, Fardeau M, Guicheney P. Readjusting the localization of merosin (α 2-chain) deficient congenital muscular dystrophy on chromosome 6q2: application to prenatal diagnosis (abstract). Eur J Hum Genet 1996; 4(Suppl 1): 146.

Hermann R, Straub V, Meyer K, Kahn T, Wagner M, Voit T. Congenital muscular dystrophy with laminin α 2-chain deficiency: correlation of clinical findings and muscle immunocytochemistry and characterisation of a new milder phenotype. Eur J Pediatr 1996; 155: 968–976.

Herva R, von Wendt L, von Wendt G, Saukkonen A-L, Leisti J, Dubowitz V. A syndrome with juvenile cataract, cerebellar atrophy, mental retardation and myopathy. Neuropediatrics 1987; 18: 164–169.

Heyck H, Laudahn G. Die kongenitalen und mit besonderen morphologischen Veränderungen der Muskulatur einhergehende Myopathien. In: Heyck H, Laudahn G, eds. Die progressiv-dystrophischen Myopathien. Berlin: Springer, 1969: 307–313.

Heyer R, Ehrich H, Goebel H, Brewitt W. Cerebro-oculo-muskuläres Syndrom. Monatssch Kinderheilk 1983; 142: 64–68.

Heyer R, Ehrich J, Goebel HH, Christen H-J, Hanefeld F. Congenital muscular dystrophy with cerebral and ocular malformations (cerebro-oculo-muscular syndrome). Brain Dev (Tokyo) 1986; 8: 614–618.

Hillaire D, Leclerc A, Faure S, Topaloglu H, Chiannilkulchai N, Guicheney P, Grinas L, Legos P, Philpot J, Evangelista T, Routon M-C, Mayer M, Pellissier J-F, Estournet B, Barrois A, Hentati F, Feingold N, Beckmann JS, Dubowitz V, Tomé FMS, Fardeau M. Localization of merosin-negative congenital muscular dystrophy to chromosome 6q2 by homozygosity mapping. Hum Genet 1994; 3(9); 1657–1661.

Hilton-Jones D, Squier MV. Muscular dystrophy. Dystrophin associated protein complex: clinical implications. Lancet 1993; 341: 528–529.

Hirase T, Uchino M, Yoshida S, Ide M, Araki S, Teramoto J. A study of CNS lesions in progressive muscular dystrophy. The 3rd report (abstract in Japanese). Rinsho Shinkeigaku (Clin Neurol) (Tokyo) 1983; 23: 1192–1193.

Hirase T, Kawasaki S, Ide M, Imamura S, Araki S, Okamoto H. Cranial CT and CSF proteins in progressive muscular dystrophy (in Japanese). Saishin Igaku (Modern Med) (Osaka) 1983; 38: 1178–1183.

Hirase T, Araki S. Cerebrospinal fluid proteins in muscular dystrophy patients. Brain Dev (Tokyo) 1984; 6: 10–16.

Hirata H, Mishima H, Shimizu K, Shirabeeda K, Kimura T, Nishi M, Fukuda K. A case of congenital muscular dystrophy associated with a peculiar eyeground abnormality (in Japanese). Rinsho Ganka Iho (Jpn Rev Clin Ophthalmol) (Tokyo) 1984; 38: 1241–1244.

Hirayama Y, Osawa M, Fukuyama Y. EEG findings in progressive muscular dystrophy (in Japanese). Rinsho Noha (Clin Electroenceph) (Osaka) 1977; 19: 714–722.

Hirayama Y, Fukuyama Y. Diagnosis of congenital myopathy (in Japanese). Chiryo (J Ther) (Tokyo) 1978; 59: 1495–1500.

Hirayama Y, Suzuki F, Arima M. Survey of Fukuyama type congenital muscular dystrophy in Tokyo (in Japanese). No To Hattatsu (Brain Dev) (Tokyo) 1992; 24(1): 27–31.

Hizawa K, Hayashi K, Minato J. Autopsy studies of progressive muscular dystrophy – a registration system of autopsies – (in Japanese). In: Sobue I, ed. The 1978 annual report of the research committee on clinics, epidemiology and management of progressive muscular dystrophy, sponsored by the Ministry of Health and Welfare of Japan. Nagoya, 1979: 35–36.

Hizawa K, Hayashi K. Histopathological study of autopsied cases (in Japanese). In: Sobue I, ed. The 1981 annual report of the research committee on clinics, epidemiology and management of progressive muscular dystrophy, sponsored by the Ministry of Health and Welfare of Japan. Nagoya, 1982: 51–53.

Hizawa K, Ii K, Fujii Y, Moriuchi M, Miike T, Nonaka I. Localization of dystrophin in muscle cells in various neuromuscular disorders (in Japanese). In: Sobue I, ed. The 1988 annual report of the research committee on clinics, epidemiology and management of progressive muscular dystrophy, sponsored by the Ministry of Health and Welfare of Japan. Nagoya, 1989: 323–326.

Hizawa K, Ichimura S, Tamura K, Moriuchi M, Mukoyana M. Autopsy registration of progressive muscular dystrophy, and a histopathological study of laryngeal muscles (in Japanese). In: Takahashi K, ed. The 1990 annual report of the research committee on clinics, genetic counselling and epidemiology of progressive muscular dystrophy, sponsored by the Ministry of Health and Welfare of Japan. Hyogo, 1991: 243–246.

Holmes G. On the spinal changes in a case of muscular dystrophy. Rev Neurol Psychiatry (Edinburgh) 1908; 6(2): 137–149.

Holzgreve W, Feil R, Louwen F, Miny P. Prenatal diagnosis and management of fetal hydrocephaly and lissencephaly. Childs Nerve Syst 1993; 9: 408–412.

Homma A, Ishii R, Samoto T, Suzuki S, Owashi K, Kanauchi Y, Hayasaka K, Nonaka I. A 14 year old boy with non-Fukuyama type congenital muscular dystrophy (abstract in Japanese). Nihon Shonika Gakkai Zasshi (J Jpn Pediatr Soc) (Tokyo) 1994; 98(10): 1932.

Honda Y, Yoshioka M. Eye findings in muscular dystrophies (in Japanese). Ganka Rinsho Iho (Jpn J Clin Ophthalmol) (Tokyo) 1978; 72: 1483–1485.

Honda Y, Yoshioka M. Ophthalmological findings of muscular dystrophies: a survey of 53 cases. J Pediatr Ophthalmol Strab 1978; 15: 236–238.

Hori A, Bardosi A, Goebel HH, Roessmann U. Muscular alteration in agyria with pyramidal tract anomaly. Brain Dev (Tokyo) 1986; 8: 625–629.

Horikawa H, Konishi T, Konagaya M, Mano Y, Takayanagi T. A case of Fukuyama type congenital muscular dystrophy associated with Fallot's tetralogy (letter in Japanese). Shinkei Naika (Neurol Med) (Tokyo) 1986: 24: 99.

Horikawa H, Konishi T, Konagaya M, Mano Y, Takayanagi T. Cranial X-ray CT and MRI in congenital muscular dystrophy (in Japanese). Rinsho Shinkeigaku (Clin Neurol) (Tokyo) 1988; 28(1): 102–106.

Howard R. A case of congenital defect of the muscular system (dystrophia muscularis congenita) and its association with congenital talipes equino-varus. Proc R Soc Med 1908; 1(3) pathol section: 157–166.

Huh J, Kim KJ, Ko TS, Kim DW, Hwang SH, Hwang YS. A case of Fukuyama congenital muscular dystrophy (in Korean). Korean J Neurol (Seoul) 1992; 10(3): 388–394.

Hund E, Jansen O, Koch MC, Ricker K, Fogel W, Niedermaier N, Otto M, Kuhn E, Meinck H-M. Proximal myotonic myopathy with MRI white matter abnormalities of the brain. Neurology 1997; 48:33-37.

Igarashi K, Otake S, Kudo M, Kuronuma T, Koide N, Akimoto Y, Takase H. Spine deformity in congenital muscular dystrophy (in Japanese). In: Takahashi K, ed. The 1991 annual report of the research committee on clinics, genetic counselling and epidemiology of progressive muscular dystrophy, sponsored by the Ministry of Health and Welfare of Japan. Hyogo, 1992: 307–310.

Igarashi K, Otake S, Nakajima K, Kawahara R, Sasaki M, Kuronuma T, Koide N, Shioya M. A case of congenital muscular dystrophy manifesting nocturnal hypoxemia (in Japanese). In: Takahashi K, ed. The 1992 annual report of the research committee on clinics, genetic counselling and epidemiology of progressive muscular dystrophy, sponsored by the Ministry of Health and Welfare of Japan. Hyogo, 1993: 252–255.

Iida M, Harada K, Kurizaki H, Kamakura K. A histopathological study of congenital muscular dystrophy (in Japanese). In: Sobue I, ed. The 1978 annual report of the research committee on clinics, epidemiology and management of progressive muscular dystrophy, sponsored by the Ministry of Health and Welfare of Japan. Nagoya, 1979: 238–242.

Iida M, Iwata H, Bando M, Kurizaki H. A pathogenetic consideration of brain pathology in Fukuyama type congenital muscular dystrophy (in Japanese). In: Sobue I, ed. The 1979 annual report of the research committee on clinics, epidemiology and management of progressive muscular dystrophy, sponsored by the Ministry of Health and Welfare of Japan. Nagoya, 1980: 385–387.

Iida M, Kurizaki H, Takatsu S. A pathological study of spinal anterior horns and anterior roots in Duchenne and congenital muscular dystrophies (in Japanese). In: Sobue I, ed. The 1980 annual report of the research committee on clinics, epidemiology and management of progressive muscular dystrophy, sponsored by the Ministry of Health and Welfare of Japan. Nagoya, 1981: 279–285.

Iida M, Ito S, Yamazaki M, Matsubayashi M, Sakai F, Ogi M. Care of low grade school children with congenital muscular dystrophy (in Japanese). In: Inoue M, ed. The 1983 annual report of the research committee on comprehensive study of nursing care of progressive muscular dystrophy, sponsored by the Ministry of Health and Welfare of Japan. 1984: 54–56.

Iida M, Kobayashi C, Sakurai Y, and others. Elementary care for congenital muscular dystrophy patients – sphincter control (in Japanese). In: Inoue M, ed. The 1983 annual report of the research committee on comprehensive study of nursing care of progressive muscular dystrophy, sponsored by the Ministry of Health and Welfare of Japan. 1984: 316–320.

Iida M, Hosoda Y, Kobayashi C, et al. Urination training for congenital muscular dystrophy children (in Japanese). In: Inoue M, ed. The 1984 annual report of the research committee on comprehensive study of nursing care of progressive muscular dystrophy, sponsored by the Ministry of Health and Welfare of Japan. 1985: 33–36.

Iida K, Takashima S, Miyahara S. Formation of leptomeningeal glioneuronal heterotopia: its developmental aspects in trisomy 13 children (abstract in Japanese). Abstract of the 32nd annual meeting of the Japanese Society for Congenital Anomalies, Tokyo, 1992.

Iinuma K, Ohnuma A, Tanabe M, Takamatsu T. CNS disturbances in congenital muscular dystrophy (in Japanese). No To Hattatsu (Brain Dev) (Tokyo) 1974; 6: 340–348.

Ikenaka H. Serum enzyme activities in progressive muscular dystrophies. Part 2. Serial changes of serum GOT, GPT, LDH and CK activities in congenital muscular dystrophy (in Japanese). Tokyo Joshi Ikadaigaku Zasshi (J Tokyo Women's Med Coll) (Tokyo) 1992; 62: 1185–1196.

Ikeya K, Saito K, Komine S, Kondo E, Yamauchi A, Mishima M, Takahashi R, Harada H, Osawa M, Shishikura K, Suzuki H, Fukuyama Y. An immunocytochemical study of skeletal muscle in Fukuyama type congenital muscular dystrophy (in Japanese). Shonika Rinsho (Jpn J Pediatr) (Tokyo) 1994; 47(9): 1996–2002.

Ikeya K, Saito K, Komine S, Ishii N, Mishima M, Takahasi R, Osawa M. Cytoskeletal protein in muscle tissues of muscular dystrophies with onset in childhood (abstract in Japanese). No To Hattatsu (Brain Dev) (Tokyo) 1995; 27 Suppl: S141.

Ikeya K, Saito K, Miyagawa M, Osawa M, Fukuyama Y. An immunohistological analysis of cytoskeletal proteins of skeletal muscle in a FCMD fetus (abstract in Japanese). No To Hattatsu (Brain Dev) (Tokyo) 1996; 28 Suppl: S329.

Imamura A, Yamauchi H, Kurokawa T. Epileptic seizures evidenced by continuous respiratory monitoring in a case of Fukuyama type congenital muscular dystrophy (in Japanese). Shonika Rinsho (Jpn J Pediatr) (Tokyo) 1993; 46: 327–331.

Inaba Y, Kurogi H, Omori T. Akabane disease: epizootic abortion, premature birth, still-birth and congenital arthrogryposis-hydroencephaly in cattle, sheep and goats caused by Akabane virus. Aust Vet J 1975; 51: 584–585.

Indo K, Miyaji T. An autopsy case of congenital muscular dystrophy (abstract in Japanese). Nihon Byori Gakkai Zasshi (J Jpn Pathol Soc) (Tokyo) 1970; 59: 194–195.

Inoue K, Toshimori K, Kitano S, Tsuruta K, Kurihara T. Short latency SEP in muscular dystrophies (in Japanese). In: Sobue I, ed. The 1982 annual report of the research committee on clinics, epidemiology and management of progressive muscular dystrophy, sponsored by the Ministry of Health and Welfare of Japan. Nagoya, 1983: 331-336.

Ishihara T, Yoshimura M, Inoue M, Nonaka I. A case of Ullrich disease – with emphasis on histochemical findings (abstract in Japanese). Rinsho Shinkeigaku (Clin Neurol) (Tokyo) 1980; 20: 302.

Ishihara T, Yoshitake S, Aoyagi T, Nonaka I, Sugita H. Causes of death in Fukuyama type congenital muscular dystrophy (in Japanese). Rinsho Shinkeigaku (Clin Neurol) (Tokyo) 1984; 24: 968–974.

Ishihara T, Tsuya T, Miyagawa M, Yoshitake S, Aoyagi T. Histopathological study of respiratory muscles in Fukuyama type congenital muscular dystrophy (in Japanese). Iryo (Jpn J Natl Med) (Tokyo) 1987; 41(10): 862–866.

Ishihara T, Miyagawa M, Yoshitake S, Aoyagi T, Fukuda J. A probable case of congenital muscular dystrophy presenting pulmonary hypoplasia since young age (in Japanese). In: Nishitani H, ed. The 1986 annual report of the research committee on genetics, epidemiology, clinics and treatment of progressive muscular dystrophy, sponsored by the Ministry of Health and Welfare of Japan. Kyoto, 1987: 340–343.

Ishihara T, Kawamura J, Tamura T, Kawashiro T, Fukuda J. Cause of death among adolescent patients with Fukuyama congenital muscular dystrophy (abstract). Neuromusc Disord 1996; Suppl: S29.

Ishikawa A. Fukuyama type congenital muscular dystrophy (letter). Arch Neurol 1982; 39: 671.

Ishikawa A, Shinoda M, Murayama T, Sakuma N, Saito Y, Oishi T, Kajii N. A case of congenital muscular dystrophy (Fukuyama type) showing improvement of abnormal CT findings including white matter hypodensity on sequential CT scan (in Japanese). Nihon Shonika Gakkai Zasshi (J Jpn Pediatr Soc) (Tokyo) 1982; 86(1): 13–16.

Ishikawa T, Shimizu K, Awaya A, Inoue Y. A 6-year-old girl of congenital muscular dystrophy – a typical Fukuyama type congenital muscular dystrophy type 4? (in Japanese). No To Hattatsu (Brain Dev) (Tokyo) 1982; 16(1): 38–46.

Itagaki Y, Sakamoto Y, Nishitani H. Peculiar type of congenital muscular dystrophy (Fukuyama type) (in Japanese). Rinsho Shinkeigaku (Clin Neurol) (Tokyo) 1980: 20: 897–903.

Itagaki Y, Sakamoto Y, Yoshioka M, Nishitani H, Haebara H. An autopsy case of severe congenital muscular dystrophy with arthrogryposis multiplex (in Japanese). Rinsho Shinkeigaku (Clin Neurol) (Tokyo) 1982; 22: 896–900.

Itagaki Y, Saida K, Sakamoto Y. Light and electron microscopic study on the benign type of CMD with central nervous system involvement (abstract). Brain Dev (Tokyo) 1986; 8: 216.

Itagaki Y, Saida K, Nishitani H. Immunohistochemical studies of dystrophin and desmin in Fukuyama type congenital muscular dystrophy and various neuromuscular disorders (in Japanese). Shinkei Naika (Neurol Med) (Tokyo) 1992; 36: 492–497.

Itahara K, Sato H. A survey of the present status of progressive muscular dystrophy patients staying at the institutions for multiply handicapped children (in Japanese). In: Sobue I, ed. The 1981 annual report of the research committee on clinics, epidemiology and management of progressive muscular dystrophy, sponsored by the Ministry of Health and Welfare of Japan. Nagoya, 1982: 61–62.

Itahara K, Sato H. A continued survey of the present status of progressive muscular dystrophy patients staying at the institutions for multiply handicapped children. The 2nd report (in Japanese). In: Sobue I, ed. The 1982 annual report of the research committee on clinics, epidemiology and management of progressive muscular dystrophy, sponsored by the Ministry of Health and Welfare of Japan. Nagoya, 1983: 92.

Itoh K, Kiribuchi K, Nakagawa H, Uchida Y, Osawa M. Vitreoretinal involvement in Fukuyama type congenital muscular dystrophy (in Japanese). Ganka Rinsho Iho (Jpn Rev Clin Ophthamol) (Tokyo) 1990; 84(3): 526–529.

Itoh M, Kawahara H, Houdou S, Ohama E. A neuropathological study of brainstem lesions in Fukuyama type congenital muscular dystrophy (abstract in Japanese). No To Hattatsu (Brain Dev) (Tokyo) 1995; 27 Suppl: S277.

Ito Y. Amyotonia congenita (clinical lecture) (in Japanese). Fukuoka Ikadaigaku Zasshi (J Fukuoka Medical School), (Fukuoka). 1911; 5: 406–409.

Itoga E, Kito S, Aoki Y, Masuda K. An autopsy case of Fukuyama type congenital muscular dystrophy (abstract in Japanese). Shinkei Kenkyu No Shinpo (Adv Neurol Sci) (Tokyo) 1977; 21: 602–603.

Itoh M, Houdou S, Kawahara H, Ohama E. Morphological study of the brainstem in Fukuyama type congenital muscular dystrophy. Pediatr Neurol 1996; 15(4): 327–331.

Iwasaki N, Hamano K, Kawashima K, Terauchi M. A case of Fukuyama type congenital muscular dystrophy (in Japanese). Shoni Naika (Jpn J Pediatr Med) (Tokyo) 1988; 20: 309–312.

Iwasaki N, Hamano K, Takeya T, Honmura S, Takita H. A case of Fukuyama congenital muscular dystrophy with ocular abnormalities. In: Fukuyama Y, Osawa M, eds. Program and abstracts of the International Symposium on Congenital Muscular Dystrophies, Tokyo. Tokyo: Tokyo Women's Medical College, 1994: 33.

Iwase K, Watanabe K, Sato I. A case of congenital muscular dystrophy (in Japanese). Shonika (Pediatrics Japan) (Tokyo) 1971; 12: 363–367.

Iwashita H, Antoku Y, Mawatari S, Koga M, Miyoshino S. An autopsy case of atypical Fukuyama type congenital muscular dystrophy with milder cerebral symptoms (in Japanese). In: Sobue I, ed. The 1982 annual report of the research committee on clinics, epidemiology and management of progressive muscular dystrophy, sponsored by the Ministry of Health and Welfare of Japan. Nagoya, 1983: 407–413.

Iwata S, Shibuya N, Takahashi Y, Iida Y. Relation of progressive muscular dystrophy and ABO blood typing (in Japanese). In: Sobue I, ed. The 1979 annual report of the research committee on clinics, epidemiology and management of progressive muscular dystrophy, sponsored by the Ministry of Health and Welfare of Japan. Nagoya, 1980: 358–361.

Izumi T, Novo MLP, Osawa M, Saito K, Fukuyama Y. Analysis of cerebral gangliosides in a patient with Fukuyama type congenital muscular dystrophy (FCMD) (in Japanese). Tokyo Joshi Ikadaigaku Zasshi (J Tokyo Wom Med Coll) (Tokyo) 1993; 63: 22–25.

Izumi T, Hara K, Ogawa T, Osawa M, Saito K, Novo MLP, Fukuyama Y, Takashima S. Abnormality of cerebral gangliosides in Fukuyama type congenital muscular dystrophy. Brain Dev (Tokyo) 1995; 17(1): 33–37.

Jaatoul NY, Haddad NE, Khoury LA, Afifi AK, Bahuth NB, Deeb ME, Mikati MA, Der Kaloustian VM. The Marden-Walker syndrome. Am J Med Genet 1982; 11: 259–271.

Jellinger K, Rett A. Agyria-pachygyria (lissencephaly syndrome). Neuropaediatrie 1976; 7: 66–91.

Jervis GA. Progressive muscular dystrophy with extensive demyelination of the brain. J Neuropathol Exp Neurol 1955; 14: 376–386.

Johnson EW. Examination for muscle weakness in infants and small children. JAMA 1958; 168: 1306–1313.

Jones R, Khan R, Hughes S, Dubowitz V. Congenital muscular dystrophy: the importance of early diagnosis and orthopedic management in the long-term prognosis. J Bone Joint Surg 1979; 61-B: 13–17.

Jong Y-J, Liu G-C, Chiang C-H, Wang P-J, Shen Y-Z. Fukuyama type congenital muscular dystrophy – two Chinese families. In: Fukuyama Y, Osawa M, eds. Program and abstracts of the International Symposium on Congenital Muscular Dystrophies, Tokyo. Tokyo: Tokyo Women's Medical College, 1994: 36.

Joseph R, Pellerin D, Job JC. L'arthrogrypose multiple congénitale. Sem Hôp Paris 1958; 34: 525–536.

Juchler H. Über die Myatonia congenita Oppenheim (Inaugural-Dissertation) Schwarzenburg: Gerber-Buchdruck, 1952: 23pp.

Kaciński M, Bándo B, Kroczka S, Malinowska-Matuszewska MM. A case of congenital muscular dystrophy with changes in the white matter of the brain (in Polish). Neurol Neurochir Pol 1992; 26: 383–387.

Kakulas BA, Adams RD. Congenital muscular dystrophies. In: Kakulas BA, Adams RD. eds. Diseases of muscle. Pathological foundations of clinical myology, 4th edn. Philadelphia, PA: Harper and Row, 1985: 329–332.

Kaloustian VM, Afifi AK, Mire J. The myopathic variety of arthrogryposis multiplex congenita: a disorder with autosomal recessive inheritance. J Pediatr 1972; 81: 76–82.

Kalyanaraman K, Kalyanaraman UP, Lee RH. Autosomal dominant congenital muscular dystrophy (CMD) with possible central nervous system (CNS) involvement (abstract). J Neuropathol Exp Neurol 1980; 39: 366.

Kalyanaraman K, Kalyanaraman UP. Myopathic arthrogryposis with seizures and abnormal electroencephalogram. J Pediatr 1982; 100: 247–250.

Kameo H, Miyoshi T, Masuda K, Hiraki Y, Jo K, Marubayashi S, Ochi C, Yamada K, Kawasaki H. Determination of serum co-enzyme Q10 in progressive muscular dystrophy (in Japanese). In: Nishitani H, ed. The 1984 annual report of the research committee on genetics, epidemiology, clinics and treatment of progressive muscular dystrophy, sponsored by the Ministry of Health and Welfare of Japan. Kyoto, 1985: 246–249.

Kameo H, Jo K, Karakawa T. Measurement of respiratory compliance in progressive muscular dystrophy patients (in Japanese). In: Nishitani H, ed. The 1987 annual report of the research committee on genetics, epidemiology, clinics and treatment of progressive muscular dystrophy, sponsored by the Ministry of Health and Welfare of Japan. Kyoto, 1988: 252–253.

Kamoshita S, Konishi Y, Segawa M, Fukuyama Y. Congenital muscular dystrophy as a disease of the central nervous system. Arch Neurol 1975; 33: 513–516.

Kamoshita S. Pathogenesis of congenital muscular dystrophy (Fukuyama type) (in Japanese). Nihon Rinsho (Jpn J Clin Med) (Osaka) 1977; 35: 3929–3935.

Kamoshita S. Pathology of congenital muscular dystrophy: suggestive evidence of intrauterine infection. In: Ebashi S, ed. Muscular dystrophy. Tokyo: University of Tokyo Press, 1982: 425–439.

Kanazawa I, Toda T. Search for Fukuyama congenital muscular dystrophy gene (abstract in Japanese). Planning Division, National Center of Neurology and Psychiatry, ed. Annual report of research committees on mental and nervous diseases, sponsored by the Ministry of Health and Welfare of Japan. Kodaira, 1996: 225.

Kanazawa O, Ohgiya A, Kawai I. Atypical absence status associated with Fukuyama type congenital muscular dystrophy – a trial of rectal VPA administration (in Japanese). Tenkan Kenkyu (J Jpn Epil Soc) (Tokyo) 1985; 3: 141–150.

Kanazawa O, Naruto T. Ictal EEG findings in 2 cases of Fukuyama type congenital muscular dystrophy associated with epilepsy. Shonika Kiyo (Ann Paediatr Jpn) (Kyoto) 1987; 33: 61–68.

Kao K-P, Lin K-P. Congenital muscular dystrophy of a non-Fukuyama type with white matter hyperlucency on CT scan. Brain Dev (Tokyo) 1992; 14: 420–422.

Kasagi S, Kawahara H, Takakura H. Electrophysiological study of peripheral nerves in progressive muscular dystrophy. Especially on motor nerve conduction velocity study. In Nishitani H, ed. The 1984 annual report of the research committee on genetics, epidemiology, clinics and treatment of progressive muscular dystrophy, sponsored by the Ministry of Health and Welfare of Japan. Kyoto, 1985: 278–281.

Kasagi S, Ando M, Shioda M, Ishii S. Urinary free amino acids in muscular atrophic diseases. In: Nishitami H, ed. The 1985 annual report of the research committee on genetics, epidemiology, clinics and treatment of progressive muscular dystrophy, sponsored by the Ministry of Health and Welfare of Japan. Kyoto, 1986: 225–228.

Kasagi S, Takakura H, Shioda M, Ando M. Clinical significance of T-wave and M-wave in muscular disorders (in Japanese). In: Nishitani H, ed. The 1987 annual report of the research committee on genetics, epidemiology, clinics and treatment of progressive muscular dystrophy, sponsored by the Ministry of Health and Welfare of Japan. Kyoto, 1988: 238–242.

Kasubuchi Y, Haneba S, Wakaizumi S, Shimada M. An autopsy case of congenital muscular dystrophy associated with hydrocephalus (in Japanese). No To Hattatsu (Brain Dev) (Tokyo) 1974; 6: 36–41.

Kato E. Three cases of congenital amyotonia (in Japanese). Shonika Rinsho (Jpn J Pediatr) (Tokyo) 1952; 5: 26–28.

Kato T, Funahashi M, Matsui S, Suzuki Y, Iwasaki A, Kato S, Nonaka I. FLAIR-MR imaging study of Fukuyama type congenital muscular dystrophy (abstract in Japanese). No To Hattatsu (Brain Dev) (Tokyo) 1994; 26 Suppl: S279.

Kawahara H, Hodo S, Ohama E. Pathological study of heart in 5 autopsied cases of Fukuyama type congenital muscular dystrophy (in Japanese). In: Takahashi K, ed. The 1993 annual report of the research committee on clinics, genetic counselling and epidemiology of progressive muscular dystrophy, sponsored by the Ministry of Health and Welfare of Japan. Hyogo, 1994: 188–190.

Kawahara H, Ito M, Ohama E. Neuropathological basis of sudden death in Fukuyama type congenital muscular dystrophy (in Japanese). In: Takahashi K, chairman. The 1995 annual report of the research committee on clinics, genetic counselling and epidemiology of progressive muscular dystrophy, sponsored by the Ministry of Health and Welfare of Japan. Hyogo, 1996; 314-316.

Kawahara H, Ito M, Ohama E. A pathological study of brainstem lesions in FCMD – the

386

second report (abstract in Japanese). In: Ishihara T, chairman. Abstracts for the 1996 annual meeting of the research committee on genetic counselling and comprehensive understanding and management of progressive muscular dystrophy, sponsored by the Ministry of Health and Welfare of Japan. Saitama, 1996: 41.

Kawahira M, Inoue S, Osame M, Igata A. Amyotrophic diseases in Okinawa prefecture (in Japanese). In: Sobue I, ed. The 1981 annual report of the research committee on clinics, epidemiology and management of progressive muscular dystrophy, sponsored by the Ministry of Health and Welfare of Japan. Nagoya, 1982: 59–60.

Kawahira M, Nakahara T, Osame M, Igata A. Amyotrophic diseases in Okinawa prefecture (in Japanese). In: Sobue I, ed. The 1982 annual report of the research committee on clinics, epidemiology and management of progressive muscular dystrophy, sponsored by the Ministry of Health and Welfare of Japan. Nagoya, 1983: 92–93.

Kawai M. A computed tomographic study of calf pseudohypertrophy in the three types of progressive muscular dystrophy (Duchenne, Becker and Fukuyama) (abstract). Brain Dev (Tokyo) 1985; 7: 241.

Ketelsen UP, Freund-Mölbert E, Beckmann R. Klinische und ultrastrukturelle Befunde bei kongenitaler Muskeldystrophie. Msch Kinderheilk 1971; 119: 586–592.

Khan Y, Heckmatt JZ, Dubowitz V. Sleep studies and supportive ventilatory treatment in patients with congenital muscle disorders. Arch Dis Child 1996; 74: 195–200.

Kihira S, Nonaka I. Congenital muscular dystrophy. A histochemical study with morphometric analysis on biopsied muscles. J Neurol Sci 1985; 70: 139–149.

Kikuchi N. On the course of so-called atypical congenital muscular dystrophy children to the stage at which they will loose the capacity of ambulation (in Japanese). Rigaku Ryoho To Sagyo Ryoho (Jpn J Phys Ther Occup Ther) (Tokyo) 1974; 8: 749–754.

Kikuchi N. Motor exercise therapy for congenital muscular dystrophy (in Japanese). Rigaku Ryoho To Sagyo Ryoho (Jpn J Phys Ther Occup Ther) (Tokyo) 1978; 12: 383–391.

Kimura S, Kobayashi T, Amemiya F, Sasaki Y, Misugi N. Diaphragm muscle pathology in Fukuyama type congenital muscular dystrophy. Brain Dev (Tokyo) 1990; 12: 779–783.

Kimura S, Kobayashi T, Sasaki Y, Hara M, Nishino T, Miyake S, Iwamoto H, Misugi N. Congenital polyneuropathy in Walker–Warburg syndrome. Neuropediatrics 1992; 23: 14–17.

Kimura S, Sasaki Y, Kobayashi T, Ohtsuki N, Tanaka Y, Hara M, Miyake S, Yamada M, Iwamoto H, Misugi N. Fukuyama type congenital muscular dystrophy and the Walker–Warburg syndrome. Brain Dev (Tokyo) 1993; 15: 182–191.

Kimura S, Kobayashi T, Nezu A, Osaka H. Cranial MRI of Fukuyama type congenital muscular dystrophy (abstract). Pediatr Neurol 1994; 11(2): 143.

Kinoshita M, Iwasaki Y, Ishizuka Y, Segawa M. On the etiology of congenital muscular dystrophy – a study on two cases. In: Miyoshi K, ed. The 1978 annual report of the research committee on clinical study on pathogenesis of progressive muscular dystrophy, sponsored by the Ministry of Health and Welfare of Japan. Tokushima, 1979: 86–90.

Kinoshita M, Iwasaki Y, Wada F, Segawa M. A case of congenital polymyositis – a possible pathogenesis of Fukuyama type congenital muscular dystrophy (in Japanese). Rinsho Shinkeigaku (Clin Neurol) (Tokyo) 1980; 20(11): 911–916.

Kinoshita M, Iwasaki Y, Wada F, Seki T. Infantile polymyositis with mental retardation and peculiar muscle pathology (in Japanese). No To Hattatsu (Brain Dev) (Tokyo) 1981; 13(5): 435–440.

Kinoshita M, Nishina M, Koya N. Ten years follow-up study of steroid therapy for congenital encephalomyopathy. Brain Dev (Tokyo) 1986; 8: 281–284.

Kirchhof JKJ, Müller F. Über Nachuntersuchungen an Kindern mit spinaler Muskelatrophie vom Typus Werdnig-Hoffmann (zugleich ein kritischer Beitrag zum Problem der Amyotonia congenita Oppenheim). Nervenarzt 1958; 29: 158–167.

Klee GD, Smith CE. Progressive spinal muscular atrophy: report of a case with onset in infancy and survival to adulthood. J Nerv Ment Dis 1958; 127: 466–468.

Kletter G, Evans OB, Lee JA, Melvin B, Yates AB, Bock H-GO. Congenital muscular dystrophy and epidermolysis bullosa simplex. J Pediatr 1989; 114: 104–107.

Knubley WA, Bertorini T. Congenital muscular dystrophy with cerebellar atrophy. Dev Med Child Neurol 1988; 30: 378–390.

Kobayashi N, Segawa M, Mizuno Y, Hosaka A, Ishikawa N, Nagashima K. Visual evoked potentials in congenital muscular dystrophy (Fukuyama type) (in Japanese). In: Okinaka S, ed. The 1975 annual report of the research committee on the pathogenesis of muscular dystrophy, sponsored by the Ministry and Welfare, Japan. Tokyo. 1976: 230–233.

Kobayashi O, Murakami N, Goto Y, Nonaka I. A clinical study of non-Fukuyama type congenital muscular dystrophy (abstract in Japanese). Nihon Shonika Gakkai Zasshi (J Jpn Pediatr Soc) (Tokyo) 1994; 98(3): 560.

Kobayashi O, Hayashi Y, Arahata K, Ozawa E, Nonaka I. Congenital muscular dystrophy: Clinical and pathological study of 50 patients with the classical (occidental) merosin-positive form. Neurology 1996; 46: 815–818.

Kobayashi C, Miyake M, Tokunaga K, Nakahori Y, Toda T. Haplotype mapping of FCMD gene (abstract in Japanese). In: Kondo K, ed. Abstracts for the 41st annual meeting of the Japanese Society of Human Genetics, Sapporo, 1996: 136.

Koga M, Abe M, Tateishi J, Antoku Y, Iwashita H, Miyoshino S. Two autopsy cases of congenital muscular dystrophy of Fukuyama type – a typical and an atypical case (in Japanese). No To Shinkei (Brain Nerve) (Tokyo) 1984; 36(11): 1103–1108.

Kohrman MH, Picchietti DL, Wollmann R, Chelmicka-Schorr EE. A variant of Fukuyama congenital muscular dystrophy in a non-Japanese girl. Pediatr Neurol 1986; 2: 290–293.

Kohyama J, Nakano I, Iwakawa Y, Mori K. Polysomnographical examination on patients with congenital muscular dystrophy of the Fukuyama type (in Japanese). Rinsho Noha (Clin Electroenceph) (Osaka) 1987; 29: 318–322.

Koide N, Morikawa S, Ogawa Y, Morimatsu Y, Matsuyama H. Pathology of cerebellar polymicrogyria (abstract in Japanese). Abstracts of the 20th annual meeting of the Japan Society of Neuropathology, Maebashi, 1979.

Koide N, Shiotani M, Otake S, Nakajima K. Thiopental stone was found in the right atrium by autopsy, in a case with congenital muscular dystrophy (in Japanese). Tenkan Kenkyu (J Jpn Epil Soc) (Tokyo) 1996; 14(2): 142–146.

Komberg AJ, Dennett X, Shield LK, Phelan EM, Coleman LT, Kean MJ. A case of congenital muscular dystrophy without weakness presenting as a "leukodystrophy" (abstract). Neuromusc Disord 1996; Suppl: S25–S26.

Kondo E, Saito K, Ikeya K, Osawa M, Komine S, Shishikura K, Suzuki H, Fukuyama Y. Immunocytochemical analysis of dystrophin in muscle specimens of a brother with intravitam diagnosis of Duchenne muscular dystrophy and in his sister with congenital muscular dystrophy (in Japanese). Tokyo Joshi Ikadaigaku Zasshi (J Tokyo Wom Med Coll) (Tokyo) 1993; 63: S60–S69.

Kondo E, Saito K, Toda T, Osawa M, Fukuyama Y. Prenatal diagnosis of two families carrying Fukuyama type congenital muscular dystrophy by polymorphisms analysis (abstract). Jpn J Hum Genet (Toyko) 1995; 40(1): 86.

Kondo E, Saito K, Toda T, Nakamura Y, Osawa M, Fukuyama Y. Successful prenatal diagnosis in two families with Fukuyama type congenital muscular dystrophy by polymorphism analysis (in Japanese). Igaku No Ayumi (Tokyo) 1995; 173(9): 889–890.

Kondo E, Saito K, Toda T, Osawa M, Fukuyama Y. Prenatal diagnosis of Fukuyama type congenital muscular dystrophy by polymorphism analysis. Am J Med Genet 1996; 66: 169–174.

Kondo-Iida E, Saito K, Osawa M, Ishihara T, Toda T, Fukuyama Y. Polymorphism analysis of Fukuyama congenital muscular dystrophy (FCMD) siblings with different phenotypes. Brain Dev 1997; 19(3): 181–186.

Kondo-Iida E, Saito K, Tanaka H, Tsuji S, Ishihara T, Osawa M, Fukuyama Y, Toda T. Molecular genetic evidence of clinical heterogeneity in Fukuyama type congenital muscular dystrophy. Hum Genet 1997; 99: 427–432.

Kondo K, Segawa M, Fukuyama Y. Addendum to the genetic study of congenital muscular dystrophy (Fukuyama type) (abstract in Japanese). Abstracts of the 16th annual meeting of the Japanese Society of Child Neurology, Yonago, 1974.

Kondo K, Fumita M, Toshima I, Ishikawa K, Haraguchi M. Immunoglobulins and immune complexes in both serum and CSF of Fukuyama type congenital muscular dystrophy patients (in Japanese). In: Miyoshi K, ed. The 1980 annual report of the research committee on clinical study on pathogenesis of progressive muscular dystrophy, sponsored by the Ministry of Health and Welfare of Japan. Tokushima, 1981: 190–192.

Konishi Y, Aoyama M, Segawa M, Kamoshita S. An autopsy case of congenital muscular dystrophy (in Japanese). No To Hattatsu (Brain Dev) (Tokyo) 1974; 6: 320–327.

Korematsu S, Kobayashi O, Fukushima N, Sawaguchi H, Ishihara T, Izumi T. Non-Fukuyama type merosin-positive congenital muscular dystrophy with delayed muscle fibre type differentiation: a case report (in Japanese). No To Hattatsu (Brain Dev) (Tokyo) 1995; 27(4): 309–314.

Korényi-Both AL. Congenital muscular dystrophy. In: Korényi-Both AL, ed. Muscle pathology in neuromuscular disease. Springfield: CC Thomas, 1983: 299–302.

Korinthenberg R, Palm D, Schlake W, Klein J. Congenital muscular dystrophy, brain malformation and ocular problems (muscle, eye and brain disease), in two German families. Eur J Pediatr 1984; 142: 64–68.

Koshimizu T, Okamoto H, Yamamura Y. Pathophysiological study of congenital muscular dystrophy (II). Mental function, EEG, CT scan findings and their correlation (in Japanese). In: Sobue I, ed. The 1978 annual report of the research committee on clinics, epidemiology and management of progressive muscular dystrophy, sponsored by the Ministry of Health and Welfare of Japan. Nagoya, 1979: 230–231.

Krijgsman JB, Barth PG, Stam FC, Slooff JL, Jaspar HHJ. Congenital muscular dystrophy and cerebral dysgenesis in a Dutch family. Neuropaediatrie 1980; 11: 108–120.

Kryger MH, Steljes DG, Yee W-C, Mate E, Smith SA, Mahowald M. Central sleep apnoea in congenital muscular dystrophy. J Neurol Neurosurg Psychiatry 1991; 54: 710–712.

Kuchelmeister K, Bergmann M, Gullotta F. Lissencephalie – Spektrum der pathomorphologischen Befunde. Acta Histochem 1992; 42(Suppl): 251–255.

Kuchelmeister K, Bergmann M, Gullotta F. Neuropathology of lissencephalies. Childs Nerv Syst 1993; 9: 394–399.

Kühner S, Gürer Y, Saatçi I, Akçören Z, Topaloğlu H. Laminin α2-chain (merosin M) is preserved in the Walker–Warburg syndrome. Neuropediatrics 1996; 27(5): 279–280.

Kumabe H, Ukita J, Ueda T, Sato K, Shiraishi Y. An autopsy case of myatonia congenita Oppenheim (in Japanese). Kumamoto Domon Kaishi (J Kumamoto Alumni) (Kumamoto) 1960; 35: 346–349.

Kumagai T, Negoro T, Hashizume Y, Mukoyama M. Cerebral white matter lesions in Fukuyama type congenital muscular dystrophy (in Japanese). Shonika Rinsho (Jpn J Pediatr) (Tokyo) 1981; 34: 1713–1717.

Kumagai T, Mizutani A. Cranial CT scan and neuropathological findings in Fukuyama type congenital muscular dystrophy (abstract in Japanese). Shinkei Byorigaku (Neuropathology) (Kyoto) 1984; 5: 226.

Kurizaki H, Taketsu S, Inoue S, Iwata M, Toyokura Y, Harada K. Two autopsy cases of congenital muscular dystrophy (abstract in Japanese). Abstracts of the 20th annual meeting of the Japanese Society of Neuropathology, Maebashi, 1979: 43.

Kurizaki H, Toyokura Y. Myelination abnormality observed in nerve roots of congenital muscular dystrophy (Fukuyama type) (abstract in Japanese). Rinsho Shinkeigaku (Clin Neurol) (Tokyo) 1983; 23: 1158.

Kurlemann G, Schuierer G, Kuchelmeister K, Kleine M, Weglage J, Palm DG. Lissencephaly syndromes: clinical aspects. Childs Nerv Syst 1993; 9: 380–386.

Kurogi H, Inaba Y, Takahashi E, et al. Epizootic congenital arthrogryposis-hydroencephaly syndrome in cattle: isolation of Akabane virus from affected fetuses. Arch Virol 1976; 51: 67–74.

Kusuyama Y, Nakamine H, Nishihara T, Saito K, Kawamura H, Uemura S, Koike M. Immunofluorescent autopsy study of congenital muscular dystrophy. Dev Med Child Neurol 1982; 24: 194–199.

Kuwajima K, Misugi N, Komiya K. A case of progressive muscular dystrophy with multiple physical/mental handicaps and hydrocephalus (in Japanese). No To Hattatsu (Brain Dev) (Tokyo) 1974; 6: 29–35.

Kyriakides T, Gabriel G, Drousiotou A, Petrusa-Meznanic M, Middleton L. Dystrophinopathy presenting as congenital muscular dystrophy. Neuromusc Disord 1994; 4: 387–392.

Lacson AG, Seshea SS, Sarnat HB, Anderson J, De Groot WR, Chudley A, Adams C, Darwish HZ, Lowry RB, Kuhn S, Lowry NJ, Ang LC, Gibbings E, Trevenen CL, Johnson ES, Hoogstratten J. Autosomal recessive, fatal infantile hypertonic muscular dystrophy among Canadian natives. Can J Neurol Sci 1994, 21(3): 203–212.

Lake BD. Congenital muscular dystrophy (CMD). In: Wigglesworth JS, Singer DB, eds. Textbook of fetal and perinatal pathology. Boston: Blackwell, 1991: 1230–1232.

Lamy M, Jammet MI, Ajjan N. Arthrogrypose ou syndrome arthrogryposique? A propos de dix observations. Ann Pediat (Paris) 1965; 12: 591–602.

Larroche JCI, Razavi-Encha F, Squier W. The lissencephalies: a large spectrum of morphological abnormalities. Proceedings of XIth International Congress of Neuropathology, Kyoto, 1990. Neuropathology (Kyoto) 1991; Suppl 4: 434–437.

Larroche J-C, Nessmann C. Focal cerebral anomalies and retinal dysplasia in a 23/24-week-old fetus. Brain Dev (Tokyo) 1993; 15: 51–56.

Laverda AM, Battaglia MA, Drigo P, Battistella PA, Casara GL, Suppiej A, Castellato R. Congenital muscular dystrophy, brain and eye abnormalities; one or more clinical entities? Childs Nerv Syst 1993; 9: 84–87.

Lazaro RP, Fenichel GM, Kilroy AW. Congenital muscular dystrophy: case reports and reappraisal. Muscle Nerve 1979; 2: 349–355.

[Leading article] Amyotonia congenita (leading article). Lancet 1957; ii: 82–83.

[Leading article] The floppy infant (leading article). Lancet 1959; i: 294–295.

Lebenthal E, Schochet SB, Adam A, Seelenfreund M, Fried A, Najenson T, Sandbank U, Matoth Y. Arthrogryposis multiplex congenita – 23 cases in an Arab kindred. Pediatrics 1970; 46: 891–899.

Lebenthal E, Ben-Bassat M, Reisner SH, Seelenfreund X. Arthrogryposis multiplex congenita – myopathic type. Isr J Med Sci 1973; 9: 463–468.

Lee YE, Kim MH, Lee K. A case of Fukuyama type congenital muscular dystrophy (in Korean). J Korean Pediatr Assn (Seoul) 1992; 35(10): 1463–1468.

Leijten QH. Congenital muscular dystrophy. Clinical and morphological studies. (Proefschrift). Nijmegen: Kathelieke Universiteit, 1996: 1–255.

Leivo I, Engvall E. Merosin, a protein specific for basement membrane of Schwann cells, striated muscle, and trophoblast, is expressed late in nerve and muscle development. Proc Natl Acad Sci USA 1988; 85: 1544–1548.

Lelong M, Canlorbe P, Le Tan-Vinh, Cobbin JG, Vassal J. Myopathie chez une fille de 9 ans révélée à la naissance par une hypotonie musculaire géneralisée. Arch Fr Pediatr 1962; 19: 581–596.

Lenard H-G, Goebel HH, Langenbeck U. A form of congenital muscular dystrophy (abstract). Dev Med Child Neurol 1980; 22: 256–257.

Lenard H-G, Goebel HH. Congenital muscular dystrophies and unstructured congenital myopathies. Brain Dev (Tokyo) 1980; 2: 119–126.

Lenard H-G, Goebel HH. Kongenitale Myopathien und Dystrophien. In: Hirt HR, ed. Aktuelle Neuropaediatrie III. Stuttgart: Georg Thieme, 1981: 106–121.

Lenard H-G. Congenital muscular dystrophies – problems of classification. Acta Paediatr Jpn (Tokyo) 1991; 33: 256–260.

Lereboullet P, Baudouin A. Un cas de myatonia congénitale avec autopsie. Bull Soc Méd Hôp Paris 1909; 27: 1162.

Levesque J, Lepage F, Boeswillwald M, Grüner J. Deux cas de dystrophie musculaire familiale congénitale simulant une maladie de Werdnig-Hoffmann-Oppenheim. Arch Fr Pédiatr 1956; 13: 202–207.

Levine RA, Gray DL, Gould N, Pergament E, Stillerman ML. Warburg syndrome. Ophthalmology 1983; 90: 1600–1603.

Lewis AJ, Besant DF. Muscular dystrophy in infancy. Report of 2 cases in siblings with diaphragmatic weakness. J Pediatr 1962; 60: 376–384.

Leyten QH, Gabreëls FJM, Joosten EMG, Renier WO, Ter Laak HJ, Ter Haar BGA, Stadhouders AM. An autosomal dominant type of congenital muscular dystrophy. Brain Dev (Tokyo) 1986; 8: 533–537.

Leyten QH, Gabreëls FJM, Renier WO, ter Laak HJ, Sengers RCA, Mullaart RA. Congenital muscular dystrophy. J Pediatr 1989; 115; 214–221.

Leyten QH, Gabreëls FJM, Renier WO. Reply (to the correspondence of Topaloğlu et al.)(letter). J Pediatr 1990; 117: 166–167.

Leyten QH, Renkawek K, Renier WO, Gabreels FJM, Mooy CM, Ter Laak HJ, Mullaart RA. Neuropathological findings in muscle-eye-brain disease (MEB-D). Neuropathological delineation of MEB-D from congenital muscular dystrophy of the Fukuyama type. Acta Neuropathol 1991; 83: 55–60.

Leyten QH, Gabreëls FJM, Renier WO, Renkawek K, ter Laak HJ, Mullart RA. Congenital muscular dystrophy with eye and brain malformations in six Dutch patients. Neuropediatrics 1992; 23: 316–320.

Leyten QH, Renier WO, Gabreëls FJM, ter Laak HJ, Hinkofer LHA. Dystrophic myopathy of the diaphragm in a neonate with severe respiratory failure during infectious episodes. Neuromusc Disord 1993; 3(1): 51–55.

Leyten QH, ter Laak HJ, Gabreëls FJM, Renier WO, Renkawek K, Sengers RCA. Congenital muscular dystrophy. A study of the variability of morphological changes and dystrophin distribution in muscle biopsies. Acta Neuropathol 1993; 86(4): 386–392.

Leyten QH, Gabreëls FJM, Renier WO, van Engelen BGM, Ter Laak HJ, Sengers RCA, Thijssen HOM. White matter abnormalities in congenital muscular dystrophy. J Neurol Sci 1995; 129: 162–169.

Leyten QH, Barth PG, Gabreëls FJM, Renkawek K, Renier WO, Gabreels-Festen AAWM, Ter Laak HJ, Smits MG. Congenital muscular dystrophy and severe central nervous system atrophy in two siblings. Acta Neuropathol 1995; 90: 650–656.

Leyten QH, Renier WO, Gabreëls FJM, Brunner HG, ter Laak HJ, Mullaart RA. Association of congenital muscular dystrophy with hypoplasia of the lateral abdominal wall musculature and hypoplasia of the external genitalia. Neuropediatrics 1996; 27(2): 108–110.

Leyten QH, Gabreëls FJM, Renier WO, ter Laak HJ. Congenital muscular dystrophy: a review of the literatures. Clin Neurol Neurosurg 1996; 98: 267–280.

Liang WH, Lin JT, Hsiao LC, Lin ST. Congenital muscular dystrophy: report of one case. Acta Paediatr Sin 1995; 36: 442–444.

Lichtig C, Ludatscher RM, Mandel H, Gershoni-Baruch R. Muscle involvement in Walker–Warburg syndrome: clinicopathologic features of four cases. Am J Clin Pathol 1993; 100(5): 493–496.

Lidge RT. Hypotonia. J Pediatr 1954; 45: 474–477.

Lipton EL, Morgenstein SH. Arthrogryposis multiplex congenita in identical twins. Am J Dis Child 1955; 89: 233-236.

Lubinsky MS, Kobayashi RH, Kader FJ, Adickes ED. Arthrogryposis multiplex congenita from an autoimmune disorder of prenatal onset. Pediatr Asthma Allergy Immunol 1990; 4: 57–63.

Lücking T, Otto HF. Kongenitale Muskeldystrophie. Z Kinderheilk 1971; 110: 59–73.

Lyon G, Raymond G, Mogami K, Gadisseux J-F, Giustina ED. Disorder of cerebellar foliation in Walker's lissencephaly and Neu-Laxova syndrome. J Neuropathol Exp Neurol 1993; 52(6): 633–639.

Macaya AT, Roig MQ, Sancho SO, Navarro CIV, Tallada MS, Marco MO. Walker–Warburg syndrome: cerebro-ocular dysgenesis and congenital muscular dystrophy (in Spanish). An Esp Pediatr 1989; 31: 465–469.

Mahjineh I, Marconi GP. Congenital muscular dystrophy: A clinico-pathological study of 10 patients belonging to a large Arab family (abstract). In: Angelini C, Danieli GA, Fontanari P, eds. Muscular dystrophy research. From molecular diagnosis toward therapy. Amsterdam: Excerpta Medica 1991: 230–231.

Mahjineh I, Bushby K, Johnson M, Bashir R, Pizzi A, Marconi G. Merosin-positive congenital muscular dystrophy: a large inbred family (abstract). Neuromusc Disord 1996; Suppl: S25.

Makifuchi T, Fukuhara N, Omori T. Correlation between neuropil threads and neurofibrillary changes in Fukuyama type congenital muscular dystrophy (abstract in Japanese). Shinkei Byorigaku (Neuropathology) (Kyoto) 1993; 13 Suppl: 34.

Malandrini A, Villanova M, Sabatelli P. Squarzoni S, Six J, Toti P, Guazzi G, Maraldi NM. Localization of the laminin $\alpha2$ chain in normal human skeletal muscle and peripheral nerve: an ultrastructural immunolabelling study. Acta Neuropathol 1997; 93: 166–172.

Malik S, Cruse RP, Chou SM, Chafel T. Non-Fukuyama congenital muscular dystrophy with central nervous system involvement: clinical, radiographic, and pathologic correlates (abstract). Ann Neurol 1990; 28: 430.

Mancias P, Mrak R, Rock L, Hoffman E. Merosin deficiency: Clinical presentation and progression in three patients with congenital muscular dystrophy (abstract). J Child Neurol 1996; 11: 154.

Mandel H, Brik R, Ludatscher R, Braun J, Berant M. Congenital muscular dystrophy with neurological abnormalities. Association with Hirschsprung disease. Am J Med Genet 1993; 47: 37–40.

Marchetti C, Merlini L, Bianchi A. Therapeutic challenges for facial malformations in congenital muscular dystrophy patients (abstract). Neuromusc Disord 1996; Suppl: S27–S28.

Martinelli P, Gabellini AS, Ciucci G, Govoni E, Vitali S, Gulli MR. Congenital muscular dystrophy with central nervous system involvement: case report. Eur Neurol 1987; 26: 17–22.

Martinello F, Fanin M, Freda MP, Pastoreelo E, Tormene AP, Angelini C, Trevisan CP. Congenital muscular dystrophy with partial merosin deficiency: Leukoencephalopathy and visual pathways findings. Brain Dev 1997; (in press).

Martinez-Lage JF, Poza M, Hidalgo F. In-utero diagnosis of cerebro-oculo-muscular syndrome (letter). Childs Nerv Syst 1991; 7: 118.

Martinez-Lage JF, Garcia Santos JM, Poza M, Puche A, Casas C, Costa TR. Neurosurgical management of Walker–Warburg syndrome. Childs Nerv Syst 1995; 11: 145–153.

Massa G, Casaer P, Ceulemans B, Van Eldere S. Arthrogryposis multiplex congenita associated with lissencephaly: a case report. Neuropediatrics 1988; 19:24-26.

Matsubara S, Mizuno Y, Yoshida M, Kitaguchi T, Isozaki E, Miyamoto K, Hirai S. An observation of muscle cell basement membrane by co-focusing laser microscope with special reference to Fukuyama congenital muscular dystrophy (abstract in Japanese). In: Takagi A, chairman. Abstracts for the 1996 annual meeting of the research committee on pathogenesis and treatment of progressive muscular dystrophy and related disorders, sponsored by the Ministry of Health and Welfare of Japan. Tokyo, 1996: 7.

Matsuda H, Morimoto T. Congenital muscular dystrophy (Fukuyama type) (a grand round) (in Japanese). Shonika Rinsho (J Pediatr Pract) (Tokyo) 1990; 53(1): 5–12.

Matsuishi T, Yano E, Ishihara O, Fujimoto T, Rititake N, Aoki N, Yamamoto M. A case presenting slight myopathic changes in muscle biopsy associated with central nervous system signs, facial muscle involvement and elevated serum CPK activity – a variant form of Fukuyama type congenital muscular dystrophy? (in Japanese). No To Hattatsu (Brain Dev) (Tokyo) 1982; 14(1): 65–70.

Matsuka Y, Hayata M, Kawai T, Nakanishi M, Watanabe Y. Formulation of daily activity evaluation criteria for congenital muscular dystrophy patients (in Japanese). In: Inoue M, ed. The 1980 annual report of the research committee on comprehensive study of nursing care of progressive muscular dystrophy, sponsored by the Ministry of Health and Welfare of Japan. 1981; 71–79.

Matsuka Y, Yagi S, Okumura T, Shirai Y. Exploring new types of apparatuses for treating spinal deformity in CMD children (in Japanese). In: Inoue M, ed. The 1980 annual report of the research committee on comprehensive study of nursing care of progressive muscular dystrophy, sponsored by the Ministry of Health and Welfare of Japan. Matsue, 1981: 158–160.

Matsumoto T. Myopathies in children (in Japanese). Shonika Shinryo (J Pediatr Pract) (Tokyo) 1961; 24: 1414–1418.

Matsumoto T, Takashima S. Recent advances and problems concerning myopathies in childhood. With emphasis on congenital hypotonia syndrome (in Japanese). Shonika (Pediatrics) (Tokyo) 1967; 8: 162–179.

Matsumoto T, Mitsudome A, Nagayama T. Progressive muscular dystrophy in infancy. Acta Paediatr Jpn (Tokyo) 1970; 12: 4–8.

Matsumura K, Shimizu T, Nonaka I, Mannen T. Immunochemical study of connectin (titin) in neuromuscular diseases using a monoclonal antibody: connectin is degraded extensively in Duchenne muscular dystrophy. J Neurol Sci 1989; 93: 147–156.

Matsumura K, Toda T, Watanabe T. Evaluation of CNS changes in Fukuyama type congenital muscular dystrophy by means of three-dimensional brain surface MRI (in Japanese). In: Nishitani H, ed. The 1989 annual report of the research committee on genetics, epidemiology, clinics and treatment of progressive muscular dystrophy, sponsored by the Ministry of Health and Welfare of Japan. Kyoto, 1990: 243–246.

Matsumura K, Shimizu T, Sunada Y, Mannen T, Nonaka I, Kimura S, Maruyama K. Degradation of connectin (titin) in Fukuyama type congenital muscular dystrophy: immunochemical study with monoclonal antibodies. J Neurol Sci 1990; 98: 155–162.

Matsumura K, Toda T, Hasegawa T, Kamei N, Imoto N, Shimizu I. A family in which both Duchenne muscular dystrophy patient and Fukuyama type congenital muscular dystrophy patient occurred: dystrophin test and gene analysis (in Japanese). In: Araki S, ed. The 1990 annual report of the research committee on pathogenesis and treatment exploration of progressive muscular dystrophy and related disorders, sponsored by the Ministry of Health and Welfare of Japan. Kumamoto, 1991: 78–80.

Matsumura K, Mannen T, Nonaka I, Maruyama K, Kimura S, Hori K, Sugiura H. Immunochemical analysis of connectin by means of mono- and bi-dimensional electrophoresis: especially on degeneration and degradation of connectin in Fukuyama type congenital muscular dystrophy (in Japanese). In: Araki S, ed. The 1990 annual report of the research committee on pathogenesis and treatment exploration of progressive muscular dystrophy and related disorders, sponsored by the Ministry of Health and Welfare of Japan. Kumamoto, 1991: 226–230.

Matsumura K, Toda T, Hasegawa T, Nakano I, Watanabe T. Assessment of CNS lesions in Fukuyama type congenital muscular dystrophy by means of three dimensional brain surface MRI. 2nd report. A correlation with autopsy finding (in Japanese). In: Takahashi K, ed. The 1990 annual report of the research committee on clinics, genetic counselling and epidemiology of progressive muscular dystrophy, sponsored by the Ministry of Health and Welfare of Japan. Hyogo, 1991: 236–241.

Matsumura K, Toda Y, Hasegawa T, Kamei M, Imoto N, Shimizu T. A Japanese family with two types of muscular dystrophy: DNA analysis and the dystrophin test. J Child Neurol 1991; 6: 251–256.

Matsumura K, Nonaka I, Campbell KP. Abnormal expression of dystrophin-associated proteins in Fukuyama-type congenital muscular dystrophy. Lancet 1993; 341: 521–2.

Matsumura K, Yamada H, Shimizu T, Campbell KP. Differential expression of dystrophin, utrophin and dystrophin-associated proteins in peripheral nerve. FEBS Lett 1993; 334: 281–285.

Matsumura K, Yamada H, Shimizu T. How does laminin-2 deficiency cause peripheral dysmyelination in congenital muscular dystrophy patients and *dy* mice? (abstract). Neuromusc Disord 1996; Suppl: S20.

Matsumura K, Yamada H, Saito F, Sunada Y, Shimizu T. Peripheral nerve involvement in merosin-deficient congenital muscular dystrophy and dy mouse. Neuromusc Disord 1997; 7(1) :7-12.

Matsuo M, Hirao C, Hotta S, Rikiishi T. Guidance for congenital muscular dystrophy (in Japanese). In: Inoue M, ed. The 1983 annual report of the research committee on comprehensive study of nursing care of progressive muscular dystrophy, sponsored by the Ministry of Health and Welfare of Japan. 1984: 64–65.

Matsuoka Y, Koga H, Kai S, Sobue I, Sato I. A quantitative study of central nuclei in pathologic muscles (in Japanese). In: Sobue I, ed. The 1983 annual report of the research committee on clinics, epidemiology and management of progressive muscular dystrophy, sponsored by the Ministry of Health and Welfare of Japan. Nagoya, 1984: 447–455.

Matsuoka Y, Mokuno K, Riku S, Iida M, Kato K. Serum carbonic anhydrase III activity in muscular dystrophies – a comparison with serum creatine kinase and muscle-specific enolase activities (in Japanese). In: Nishitani H, ed. The 1984 annual report of the research committee on genetics, epidemiology, clinics and treatment of progressive muscular dystrophy, sponsored by the Ministry of Health and Welfare of Japan. Kyoto, 1985: 230–234.

Matsuoka Y, Konagaya Y, Konagaya M, Honda H, Yoneyama S, Takahasi A, Sakai M, Iida M. Serum myosin light chain I in muscular dystrophies (in Japanese). In: Takahashi K, ed. The 1990 annual report of the research committee on clinics, genetic counselling and epidemiology of progressive muscular dystrophy, sponsored by the Ministry of Health and Welfare of Japan. Hyogo, 1991: 192–194.

Matsutani I, Okamoto M, Kita K. Electroencephalographic and brain CT findings in FCMD patients (in Japanese). In: Sobue I, ed. The 1982 annual report of the research committee on clinics, epidemiology and management of progressive muscular dystrophy, sponsored by the Ministry of Health and Welfare of Japan. Nagoya, 1983: 86–87.

Matsutani I, Ameya Y, Hosoki Y, Ohara T. Play goods for CMD children (in Japanese). In: Inoue M, ed. The 1983 annual report of the research committee on comprehensive study of nursing care of progressive muscular dystrophy, sponsored by the Ministry of Health and Welfare of Japan. 1984: 151–153.

Maynor CH, Hertzberg BS, Ellington KS. Antenatal sonographic features of Walker–Warburg syndrome. Value of endovaginal sonography. J Ultrasound Med 1992; 11: 301–303.

McGavin MD, Byrnes ID. A congenital progressive ovine muscular dystrophy. Pathol Vet 1969; 6: 513.

McKusick VA. 236670 Hydrocephalus, agyria, and retinal dysplaia (HARD syndrome, HARD ±E syndrome; Warburg syndrome; Chemke syndrome; Pagon syndrome; Walker–Warburg syndrome; cerebro-ocular dysgenesis; COD; cerebro-ocular-dysplasia-muscular dystrophy syndrome; COD-MD syndrome. In: McKusick VA, ed. Mendelian inheritance in man. 11th edn. Baltimore, MD: Johns Hopkins University Press, 1994: 1899–1900.

McKusick VA. 253280 Muscle-eye-brain disease (MEB disease). In: McKusick VA, ed.

Mendelian inheritance in man. 11th edn. Baltimore, MD: Johns Hopkins University Press, 1994: 2034.

McKusick VA. 253800 Muscular dystrophy, congenital progressive, with mental retardation (Muscular dystrophy, congenital, with central nervous system involvement; Fukuyama disease; cerebro-muscular dystrophy, Fukuyama type; FCMD; micropolygyria with muscular dystrophy). In: McKusick VA, ed. Mendelian inheritance in man, 11th edn. Baltimore, MD: Johns Hopkins University Press, 1994: 2040–2041.

McMenamin JB, Becker LE, Murphy EG. Congenital muscular dystrophy: a clinicopathologic report of 24 cases. J Pediatr 1982; 100: 692–697.

McMenamin JB, Becker LE, Murphy EG. Fukuyama type congenital muscular dystrophy. J Pediatr 1982; 101: 580–582.

Mendell JT, Feng B, Sahenk Z, Marzluf GA, Amato AA, Mendell JR. Novel laminin α 2 mutations in congenital muscular dystrophy (abst). Neurology 1997; 48(3) Suppl 2:A195.

Menges O. Ein Beitrag zur Pathologie der Myatonia congenita. Dtsch Z Nervenheilk 1931; 121: 240–254.

Mercuri E, Dubowitz L, Berardinelli A, Pennock J, Jongmans M, Henderson S, Muntoni E, Sewry C, Philpot J, Dubowitz V. Minor neurological and perceptuo-motor deficits in children with congenital muscular dystrophy: correlation with brain MRI changes. Neuropediatrics 1995; 26(3): 156–162.

Mercuri E, Muntoni F, Berardinelli A, Pennock J, Sewry C, Philpot J, Dubowitz V. Somatosensory and visual evoked potentials in congenital muscular dystrophy: correlation with MRI changes and muscle merosin status. Neuropediatrics 1995; 26(1): 3–5.

Mercuri E, Pennock J, Goodwin F, Sewry C, Cowan F, Dubowitz L, Dubowitz V, Muntoni F. Sequential study of central and peripheral nervous system involvement in an infant with merosin deficient congenital muscular dystrophy (abstract). Abstracts of the 5th Asian and Oceanian Congress of Child Neurology, Istanbul, Turkey, 1996: 217.

Mercuri E, Pennock J, Goodwin F, Sewry C, Cowan F, Dubowitz L, Dubowitz V, Muntoni F. Sequential study of central and peripheral nervous system involvement in an infant with merosin-deficient congenital muscular dystrophy. Neuromusc Disord 1996; 6: 425–429.

Merlini L, Granata C, Ballestrazzi A, Barile P, Mattutini P, De Santis U, Ciufici D, Cervellati S. Rigid spine in myopathies (abstract). J Neurol Sci 1990; 98(Suppl): 435.

Merton WL, Boya SG. Muscle-eye-brain disease (MEB) (letter). Brain Dev (Tokyo) 1990; 12: 274.

Middleton DS. Studies on prenatal lesions of striated muscle as a cause of congenital deformity. I. Congenital tibial kyphosis. II. Congenital high shoulder. III. Myodystrophia foetalis deformans. Edinburgh Med J 1934; 41: 401–442.

Mielke R, Lu JH, Kowalewski S. Zerebro-okulo-muskuläres Syndrom. Helv Paediatr Acta 1986; 41: 369–376.

Mielke R, Lu JH, Kochs G, Kowalewski S. Klinische und aetiopathogenetische Aspekte des Lissencephalie – Syndroms Typ II. Monatsschr Kinderheilk 1987; 135: 780–783.

Miike T, Ohtani Y, Matsuda I, Nonaka I. Electron microscopic observation of T-tubules in biopsied congenital muscular dystrophy muscles using lanthanum staining (in Japanese). In: Sobue I, ed. The 1982 annual report of the research committee on clinics, epidemiology and management of progressive muscular dystrophy, sponsored by the Ministry of Health and Welfare of Japan. Nagoya, 1983: 402–406.

Miike T. Maturational defect of regenerating muscle fibers in cases with Duchenne and congenital muscular dystrophies. Muscle Nerve 1983; 6: 545–552.

Miike T, Tamari H, Ohtani Y, Nakamura H, Matsuda I, Miyoshino S. A fluorescent microscopic study of biopsied muscles from infantile neuromuscular disorders. Acta Neuropathol 1983; 59: 48–52.

Miike T, Ohtani Y. A histochemical study of skeletal muscles of autopsied anencephalic babies (in Japanese). In: Sobue I, ed. The 1983 annual report of the research committee on epidemiology, clinics and treatment of progressive muscular dystrophy, sponsored by the Ministry of Health and Welfare of Japan. Nagoya, 1984: 501–507.

Miike T, Ohtani Y, Tamari H, Ishitsu T, Nonaka I. An electron microscopical study of the T-system in biopsied muscles from Fukuyama type congenital muscular dystrophy. Muscle Nerve 1984; 7: 629–635.

Miike T. Muscle pathology in progressive muscular dystrophy (in Japanese). Kumamoto Igakukai Zasshi (J Kumamoto Med Soc) (Kumamoto) 1987; 61(2): 63–78.

Miike T, Sugino S, Yoshioka T, Taku S. Blood vessels lesions in congenital muscular dystrophy (in Japanese). In: Nishitani H, ed. The 1987 annual report of the research committee on genetics, epidemiology, clinics and treatment of progressive muscular dystrophy, sponsored by the Ministry of Health and Welfare of Japan. Kyoto, 1988; 325–328.

Miike T, Yoshioka T, Zhao J, Nonaka I. Dystrophin in congenital myopathies (in Japanese). In: Takahashi K, ed. The 1991 annual report of the research committee on clinics, genetic counselling and epidemiology of progressive muscular dystrophy, sponsored by the Ministry of Health and Welfare of Japan. Hyogo, 1992: 276–280.

Mikawa H, Nakano S, Okuno T. Brainstem auditory evoked response in congenital muscular dystrophy (Fukuyama type) (in Japanese). In: Fukuyama Y, ed. The 1983 annual report of the research committee on etiology and treatment of brain damage of prenatal origin, sponsored by the Ministry of Health and Welfare of Japan. Tokyo, 1984: 147–149.

Miller G, Ladda RL, Towfighi J. Cerebro-ocular dysplasia-muscular dystrophy (Walker–Warburg) syndrome. Findings in a 20-week-old fetus. Acta Neuropathol 1991; 82: 234–238.

Mimaki T, Mino M. Non-Fukuyama type congenital muscular dystrophy (in Japanese). Shoni Naika (Jpn J Pediatr Med) (Tokyo) 1991; 23: 134–138.

Minami R, Noro H, Ishikawa Y, Okabe M, Nagaoka M, Ishikawa Y. Electrophysiological evaluation of myotonic dystrophy and congenital muscular dystrophy – an evaluation of brainstem function with blink reflex (in Japanese). In: Takahashi K, ed. The 1990 annual report of the research committee on clinics, genetic counselling and epidemiology of progressive muscular dystrophy, sponsored by the Ministry of Health and Welfare of Japan. Hyogo, 1991: 103–107.

Minato J, Takazawa H, Sugano M, Katakura Y, Endo M. Nursing of congenital muscular dystrophy children – an experience of urinary control training in a case (in Japanese). In: Nakajima T, ed. The 1978 annual report of the research committee on clinico-sociological study of nursing care of progressive muscular dystrophy, sponsored by the Ministry of Health and Welfare of Japan. Matsue, 1979: 248–249.

Minato J, Takazawa H. Nursing of congenital muscular dystrophy children – play together (in Japanese). In: Nakajima T, ed. The 1979 annual report of the research committee on clinico-sociological study of nursing care of progressive muscular dystrophy, sponsored by the Ministry of Health and Welfare of Japan. Matsue, 1980: 151–2.

Minetti G, Bado M, Morreale G, Pedemonte M, Cordone G. Disruption of muscle basal lamina in congenital muscular dystrophy with merosin deficiency. Neurology 1996; 46: 1354–1358.

Miny P, Holzgreve W, Horst J. Genetic aspects in lissencephaly syndromes: a review. Childs Nerv Syst 1993; 9: 413–417.

Mishima H, Hirata H, Ono H, Choshi K, Nishi Y, Fukuda K. A Fukuyama type of congenital muscular dystrophy associated with atypical gyrate atrophy of the choroid and retina. A case report. Acta Ophthalmol 1985; 63: 155–159.

Mishima K, Miyoshino S, Mitsune K, Nonaka I, Miike T. An autopsy case of Ullrich type congenital muscular dystrophy (in Japanese). No To Hattatsu (Brain Dev) (Tokyo) 1973; 5: 530–540.

Misugi N, Komiya K, Nishino T, Misugi K. A case of congenital muscular dystrophy in which tubular structure was found (in Japanese). No To Hattatsu (Brain Dev) (Tokyo) 1978; 10: 335–337.

Misugi N. Light and electron microscopic studies of congenital muscular dystrophy. Brain Dev (Tokyo) 1980; 2: 191–199.

Misugi N. Congenital muscular dystrophy (in Japanese). In: Misugi N, ed. Color atlas of neuromuscular diseases in childhood. Tokyo: Igaku Kyoiku Shuppan; 1985: 42–51.

Misugi N, Izawa T, Iwamoto H, Yamada M, Miyake S, Yamashita S. Observation on scoliosis secondary to neuromuscular diseases (abstract). Brain Dev (Tokyo) 1987; 9: 240.

Mitsudome T, Kuroki Y, Kurokawa T, Takeshita K. A case of progressive muscular dystrophy with unusual clinical course (in Japanese). Shonika Shinryo (J Pediatr Pract) (Tokyo) 1969; 32: 1461–1466.

Mitsuyoshi I, Hattori H, Higuchi Y, Yonekura Y. Cerebral glucose metabolism in Fukuyama type congenital muscular dystrophy (in Japanese). No To Hattatsu (Brain Dev) (Tokyo) 1995; 27 Suppl: S268.

Miura K, Shirasawa H. Congenital muscular dystrophy of the Fukuyama type (FCMD) with severe myocardial fibrosis. Acta Pathol Jpn (Tokyo) 1987; 37: 1823–1835.

Miyake S, Goto A, Tsuchida M, Misugi N, Komiya K. An autopsy case of congenital muscular dystrophy associated with hydrocephalus and occipital dermal sinus (in Japanese). No To Hattatsu (Brain Dev) (Tokyo) 1977; 9: 212–219.

Miyake S, Nishino T, Hayashi M, Iwamoto H, Misugi N, Hara M. Fukuyama-type congenital muscular dystrophy (FCMD) and Walker–Warburg syndrome (cerebro-ocular dysgenesis) (abstract). Brain Dev (Tokyo) 1986; 8: 218.

Miyake S, Yamashita S, Sugio Y, Yamada M, Iwamoto H, Misugi N. Cranial CT and ocular findings in Fukuyama type congenital muscular dystrophy (abstract in Japanese). No To Hattatsu (Brain Dev) (Tokyo) 1987; 19: S89.

Miyake M, Toda T, Mizuno K, Matsushita I, Nakagome Y, Nakahori Y. Physical map of Fukuyama-type congenital muscular dystrophy candidate region based on YACs and cosmids (abstract). Jpn J Hum Genet (Tokyo) 1996; 41: 42.

Miyake M, Nakahori Y, Matsushita I, Kobayashi K, Mizuno K, Hirai M, Kanazawa I, Nakagome Y, Tokunaga K, Toda T. YAC and cosmid contigs encompassing the Fukuyama-type congenital muscular dystrophy (FCMD) candidate region on 9q31. Genomics 1997; 40(2): 284–293.

Miyoshino S, Sato T, Kusumoto S, et al. Sphincter control training in congenital muscular dystrophy (Fukuyama type), Part 2. (in Japanese). In: Nakajima T, ed. The 1979 annual report of the research committee on clinico-sociological study of nursing care of progressive

398

muscular dystrophy, sponsored by the Ministry of Health and Welfare of Japan. Matsue, 1980: 265–267.

Miyoshino S, Sato Y, Kusumoto S, Sato N, Goto M, Tsuruoka M. Sphincter control training in congenital muscular dystrophy (Fukuyama type) (in Japanese). In: Inoue M, ed. The 1980 annual report of the research committee on comprehensive study of nursing care of progressive muscular dystrophy, sponsored by the Ministry of Health and Welfare of Japan. 1981: 296–301.

Miyoshino S, Miike T, Matsuda I. Fluorescent microscopic observation of biopsied muscles in various neuromuscular diseases in childhood using acridine orange staining (in Japanese). In: Sobue I, ed. The 1981 annual report of the research committee on clinics, epidemiology and management of progressive muscular dystrophy, sponsored by the Ministry of Health and Welfare of Japan. Nagoya, 1982: 310–313.

Miyoshino S, Miike T, Ohtani Y. On the grouping of regenerating fibers in muscular dystrophies (in Japanese). In: Nishitani H, ed. The 1984 annual report of the research committee on genetics, epidemiology, clinics and treatment of progressive muscular dystrophy, sponsored by the Ministry of Health and Welfare of Japan. Kyoto, 1985: 349–351.

Miyoshino S, Ikeda R, Yano K, Ohe S, Kawahara N. Various complications in congenital muscular dystrophy (in Japanese). In: Aoyagi A, ed. The 1984 annual report of the research committee on clinical and psychological study of care and nursing of progressive muscular dystrophy, sponsored by the Ministry of Health and Welfare of Japan. 1985: 28–32.

Miyoshino S, Kawahara N, Yano K, Ohe S, Ikeda R. Malocclusion in congenital muscular dystrophy (in Japanese). In: Aoyagi A, ed. The 1984 annual report of the research committee on clinical and psychological study of care and nursing of progressive muscular dystrophy, sponsored by the Ministry of Health and Welfare of Japan. 1985: 37–39.

Miyoshino S, Kira Y, Morita K. A study of sensation in Fukuyama type congenital muscular dystrophy (in Japanese). In: Aoyagi A, ed. The 1984 annual report of the research committee on clinical and psychological study of care and nursing of progressive muscular dystrophy, sponsored by the Ministry of Health and Welfare of Japan. 1985: 152–154.

Miyoshino S, Kawahara N, Yano K, Ikeda R, Kurosawa K. Malocclusion in congenital muscular dystrophy patients (in Japanese). In: Aoyagi A, ed. The 1985 annual report of the research committee on clinical and psychological study of care and nursing of progressive muscular dystrophy, sponsored by the Ministry of Health and Welfare of Japan. 1986: 29–33.

Miyoshino S, Eda I. Serum pipecolic acid in muscular dystrophies. In: Nishitani H, ed. The 1985 annual report of the research committee on genetics, epidemiology, clinics and treatment of progressive muscular dystrophy, sponsored by the Ministry of Health and Welfare of Japan. Kyoto, 1986: 223–224.

Miyoshino S, Mibuchi H, Eda I, Tanoue A, Matsuura K, Ohtsu T, Morisawa Y, Matsuura N. A study of pulmonary atelectasis in muscular dystrophies using bronchial fiberscope (in Japanese). In: Nishitani H, ed. The 1986 annual report of the research committee on genetics, epidemiology, clinics and treatment of progressive muscular dystrophy, sponsored by the Ministry of Health and Welfare of Japan. Kyoto, 1987: 156–159.

Miyoshino S, Eda I, Tanoue A, Mibuchi H. Serum ketone bodies in congenital muscular dystrophy (Fukuyama type) (in Japanese). In: Nishitani H, ed. The 1986 annual report of the research committee on genetics, epidemiology, clinics and treatment of progressive muscular dystrophy, sponsored by the Ministry of Health and Welfare of Japan. Kyoto, 1987: 236–238.

Miyoshino S, Kurosawa K, Yano K, Tanaka S, Kinoshita K, Eda I. Malocclusion in congenital muscular dystrophy (in Japanese). In: Aoyagi A, ed. The 1986 annual report of the research committee on clinical and psychological study of care and nursing of progressive muscular dystrophy, sponsored by the Ministry of Health and Welfare of Japan. 1987: 44–49.

Miyoshino S, Kira Y, Morita K. Intelligence in congenital muscular dystrophy (Fukuyama type and others) patients (in Japanese). In: Aoyagi A, ed. The 1986 annual report of the research committee on clinical and psychological study of care and nursing of progressive muscular dystrophy, sponsored by the Ministry of Health and Welfare of Japan. 1987: 78–82.

Miyoshino S, Eda I, Kusakabe T, Oyama H, Shimomura T. Cranial MRI findings in Fukuyama type congenital muscular dystrophy (in Japanese). In: Nishitani H, ed. The 1987 annual report of the research committee on genetics, epidemiology, clinics and treatment of progressive muscular dystrophy, sponsored by the Ministry of Health and Welfare of Japan. Kyoto, 1988: 101–103.

Miyoshino S, Eda I, Koga H, Yamada M. Clinical and epidemiological study on congenital muscular dystrophy (Fukuyama type) patients observed at our hospital (in Japanese). In: Nishitani H, ed. The 1989 annual report of the research committee on genetics, epidemiology, clinics and treatment of progressive muscular dystrophy, sponsored by the Ministry of Health and Welfare of Japan. Kyoto, 1990; 231–234.

Miyoshino S, Sannomiya K, Ogata T, Sakata A, Kohno T. Autonomic nervous system disturbances in muscular dystrophies (in Japanese). In: Takahashi K, ed. The 1990 annual report of the research committee on clinics, genetic counselling and epidemiology of progressive muscular dystrophy, sponsored by the Ministry of Health and Welfare of Japan. Hyogo, 1990: 117–119.

Moerman P, Fryns JP, van Dijck H, Lauweryns JM. Congenital muscular dystrophy associated with lethal arthrogryposis multiplex congenita. Virchows Arch Pathol Anat 1985; 408: 43–48.

Montgomery A, Swenarchuk L. Further observations on myelinated axon numbers in normal and dystrophic mice. J Neurol Sci 1978; 38: 77–82.

Moosa A, Habib Y, Bastaki L. Merosin deficiency in Arab children with the classical form of congenital muscular dystrophy (abstract). Neuromusc Disord 1996; Suppl: S23.

Mooy CM, Clark BJ, Lee WR. Posterior axial corneal malformation and uveoretinal angiodysgenesis: a neurocristopathy? Graefe's Arch Clin Exp Ophthalmol 1990; 228: 9–18.

Morandi L, Gussoni E, Mora M, Gebbia M, Merlini L, Cornelio F. Dystrophin analysis in congenital muscular dystrophies (abstract). J Neurol Sci 1990; 98(Suppl): 436.

Morandi L, Di Blasi C, Barresi R, Moroni I, Lanfossi M, Uziel G, Mora M. Mild clinical phenotype in partial merosin deficiency (abstract). Neuromusc Disord 1996; Suppl: S24.

Mori H, Oguni H, Osawa M, Suzuki H, Fukuyama Y. Fukuyama type congenital muscular dystrophy with unusual features – evidence for the hypothesis of an intrauterine infectious disease? (in Japanese). No To Hattatsu (Brain Dev) (Tokyo) 1980; 12: 544–553.

Mori K, Saijo T, Hamaguchi H, Tayama M, Kawano N, Hashimoto T, Miyao M. A case of Fukuyama type congenital muscular dystrophy with progressive changes of brain CT scanning (in Japanese). No To Hattatsu (Brain Dev) (Tokyo) 1988; 20: 418–422.

Morimatsu Y, Shinohara R, Koya T, Handa T, Murofushi K. An autopsy case of congenital muscular dystrophy with polymicrogyria (abstract in Japanese). Abstracts for the 15th annual meeting of the Japanese Society of Child Neurology, Osaka, 1973.

Morimatsu Y, Shinohara T, Matsuyama H, Funabashi M, Tamagawa K, Sasaki H. Developmental disturbance of the brain. Based on neuropathology of severe cerebral palsy (in Japanese). No To Hattatsu (Brain Dev) (Tokyo) 1975; 7: 190–201.

Morimatsu Y, Shinohara T, Tamagawa K, Sakamoto K, Satoh J, Nagashima T, Uono K, Oda M, Fukuyama Y. A neuropathological study of congenital muscular dystrophy (Fukuyama type) with mental retardation (abstract). Abstracts, IXth International Congress on Neuropathology, Vienna, 1982.

Morimatsu Y, Tamagawa K, Satoh J, Mizutani T, Shinohara T, Sakamoto K. A neuropathological study of severe mental retardation. Senten Ijo (Cong Anom) (Nagoya) 1983; 23: 445–459.

Morimatsu Y, Saito J, Mizutani T, Umezu R, Arai Y, Hayashi M, Tamagawa K. The lesions of white matter in mental retardation – investigation of the Fukuyama type congenital muscular dystrophy (in Japanese). In: Kamoshita S, ed. The 1985 annual meeting of the research committee on pathogenesis and prevention of mental retardation caused by disturbances to developing brain, sponsored by the Ministry of Health and Welfare of Japan. Tokyo, 1986: 164–166.

Morimoto A, Otani I, Ochi M, Yoshioka H, Sawada T. A case of Fukuyama type congenital muscular dystrophy with hydrocephalus and ophthalmic abnormalities (in Japanese). Nihon Shonika Gakkai Zasshi (J Jpn Pediatr Soc) (Tokyo) 1989; 93: 1881–1885.

Moriyoshi T, Morino Y, Kawai T, Matsumura K, Kaneko S. Elementary nursing for CMD children (in Japanese). In: Inoue M, ed. The 1983 annual report of the research committee on comprehensive study of nursing care of progressive muscular dystrophy, sponsored by the Ministry of Health and Welfare of Japan. 1984: 313–316.

Mortier W. Kongenitale Myopathien mit charakteristischen Strukturveränderungen. In: Mortier W, ed. Muskel- und Nervenerkrankungen im Kindesalter. Stuttgart: Georg Thieme, 1994: 222–236.

Mostacciuolo ML, Miorin M, Martinello F, Angelini C, Perini P, Trevisan CP. Genetic epidemiology of congenital muscular dystrophy in a sample from north-east Italy. Hum Genet 1996; 97: 277–279.

Mukoyama M, Takayanagi T, Sobue I, Kato T. Congenital neurogenic muscular atrophy. A relation to congenital PMD (in Japanese). In: Okinaka S, ed. Cumulative articles of the research committee on progressive muscular dystrophy, sponsored by the Ministry of Health and Welfare of Japan. Tokyo, 1974: 151–159.

Mukoyama M, Sobue I, Kumagai T, Negoro T, Iwase K. Fukuyama type congenital muscular dystrophy-autopsied brain and computed tomography. In: Okinaka S, ed. Current research in muscular dystrophy, Japan. The proceedings of the annual meeting of muscular dystrophy research group, 1977. Tokyo, 1978: 102–103.

Mukoyama M, Kohno K. On brain changes in Fukuyama type congenital muscular dystrophy (in Japanese). In: Yamada K, ed. The 1977 annual report of the research committee on the cause and therapy of progressive muscular dystrophy, sponsored by the Health and Welfare of Japan. Tokushima, 1978: 66–67.

Mukoyama M, Sobue I, Kumagai T, Negoro T, Iwase K. The brain pathology in Fukuyama type congenital muscular dystrophy. CT and autopsy findings. Jpn J Med (Tokyo) 1979; 18: 218–222.

Mukoyama M, Hizawa K, Hayashi K, and 12 other collaborators. A summary of autopsy registry for progressive muscular dystrophy (in Japanese). In: Sobue I, ed. The 1982 annual report of the research committee on clinics, epidemiology and management of progressive muscular dystrophy, sponsored by the Ministry of Health and Welfare of Japan. Nagoya, 1983; 61–67.

Mukoyama M, Hizawa K, Hayashi K. Pathological changes – Fukuyama type congenital muscular dystrophy (in Japanese). In: Sobue I, Nishitani H, eds. Clinics of progressive muscular dystrophy. Tokyo: Ishiyaku Shuppan, 1985: 53–55.

Mukoyama M, Fukuyama Y. Electroencephalograms and CT findings in congenital muscular dystrophy of the Fukuyama type (in Japanese). In: Sobue I, Nishitani H, eds. Clinics of progressive muscular dystrophy. Tokyo: Ishiyaku Shuppan, 1985: 228–232.

Mukoyama M, Hizawa K, Ishihara D, Fukuyama Y, Masuda K, Itagaki Y, Nojima M, Miike T, Miyoshino S, Iwashita H, Shibuya T, Minami R. National registry of autopsy cases with progressive muscular dystrophy and a neuropathological study of the Fukuyama type congenital muscular dystrophy (in Japanese). In: Nishitani H, ed. The 1985 annual report of the research committee on genetics, epidemiology, clinics and treatment of progressive muscular dystrophy, sponsored by the Ministry of Health and Welfare of Japan. Kyoto, 1986: 315–318.

Mukoyama M, Hizawa K, Ishihara T, Minami R, Fukuyama Y, Kameo H, Iwashita H, Shibuya T. Registration of autopsy cases with progressive muscular dystrophy in Japan and a neuropathological study of the Fukuyama type congenital muscular dystrophy (in Japanese). In: Nishitani H, ed. The 1986 annual report of the research committee on genetics, epidemiology, clinics and treatment of progressive muscular dystrophy, sponsored by the Ministry of Health and Welfare of Japan. Kyoto, 1987: 319–323.

Mukoyama M, Nashie A. Cerebral white matter pathology in Fukuyama type congenital muscular dystrophy (in Japanese). In: Nishitani H, ed. The 1988 annual report of the research committee on genetics, epidemiology, clinics and treatment of progressive muscular dystrophy, sponsored by the Ministry of Health and Welfare of Japan. Kyoto, 1989: 320–322.

Mukoyama M, Hizawa K, Kagawa N, Takahashi K. The life spans, cause of death and pathological findings of Fukuyama type congenital muscular dystrophy – analysis of 24 autopsy cases (in Japanese). Rinsho Shinkeigaku (Clin Neurol) (Tokyo) 1993; 33: 1154–1156.

Mukoyama M, Hizawa K, Kagawa N. A statistical study on the life spans, cause of death and autopsy findings in Fukuyama type congenital muscular dystrophy (in Japanese). In: Takahashi K, ed. The 1992 annual report of the research committee on clinics, genetic counselling and epidemiology of progressive muscular dystrophy, sponsored by the Ministry of Health and Welfare of Japan. Hyogo, 1993: 259–262.

Mukoyama M, Tamura T, Maehara M, Hashizume Y. An autopsy case of Fukuyama type congenital muscular dystrophy-with reference to factors relating to sudden death (in Japanese). In: Takahashi K, ed. The 1993 annual report of the research committee on clinics, genetic counselling and epidemiology of progressive muscular dystrophy, sponsored by the Ministry of Health and Welfare of Japan. Hyogo, 1994: 236–238.

Mukoyama M, Maehara M, Kinoshita S. Immunohistochemical study on Fukuyama type congenital muscular dystrophy brains (abstract in Japanese). In: National Center of Neurology and Psychiatry (Planning Division), ed. Annual report of the research on nervous and mental disorders, 1994. Kodaira: National Center of Neurology and Psychiatry, 1995: 124.

Mukoyama M, Maehara M, Kinoshita S. An immunohistochemical study of CNS lesions in Fukuyama type congenital muscular dystrophy (in Japanese). In: Takahashi K, ed. The

1994–1995 annual report of the research committee on clinics, genetic counselling and epidemiology of progressive muscular dystrophy, sponsored by the Ministry of Health and Welfare of Japan. Hyogo, 1996; 357-358.

Müller-Felber W, Toepfer M, Fischer P, Müller T, Pongratz D. Expression of tenascin, basic fibroblast growth factor (bFGF) and epidermal growth factor (EGF) in congenital muscular dystrophy (abstract). Neuromusc Disord 1996; Suppl: S27.

Muntoni E, Philpot J, Spyrou N, Camici P, Dubowitz V. Cardiac involvement in merosin-negative congenital muscular dystrophy (abstract). Dev Med Child Neurol 1995; 37(3) (Suppl 72): 90.

Muntoni F, Sewry C, Wilson L, Angelini C, Trevisan CP, Brambati B, Dubowitz V. Prenatal diagnosis in congenital muscular dystrophy. Lancet 1995; 345(8949): 591.

Murakami T, Konishi Y, Takamiya M, Tsukagoshi H. Congenital muscular dystrophy associated with micropolygyria – report of two cases. Acta Pathol Jpn (Tokyo) 1975; 25: 599–612.

Murakami T, Miyake T. Speech disorder in Fukuyama type congenital muscular dystrophy (in Japanese). In: Sobue I, ed. The 1978 annual report of the research committee on clinics, epidemiology and management of progressive muscular dystrophy, sponsored by the Ministry of Health and Welfare of Japan. Nagoya, 1979: 219–224.

Muramoto O, Sakuragawa N, Nonaka I, Arima M, Satoyoshi E. A syndrome presenting short stature, mental retardation, decreased adipose tissue, myopathy and chimpanzee-like face (in Japanese). Rinsho Shinkeigaku (Clin Neurol) (Tokyo) 1981; 21: 255–263.

Murasugi H. Neuroimaging study of Fukuyama type congenital muscular dystrophy (in Japanese). Tokyo Joshi Ikadaigaku Zasshi (J Tokyo Wom Med Coll) (Tokyo) 1992; 62: 1155–1174.

Murayama S, Beppu H, Tsubaki T. An adult case of benign congenital muscular dystrophy (non-Fukuyama type) (in Japanese). Rinsho Shinkeigaku (Clin Neurol) (Tokyo) 1986; 26: 419–424.

Murphy KJ, PeBenito R, Storm RL, Ferretti C, Liu DPC. Walker–Warburg syndrome. Case report and literature review. Ophthalmol Pediatr Genet 1990; 11; 103–108.

Mutoh K, Nakagawa Y, Hojo H. Computed tomography in neuromuscular diseases – myopathic diseases (abstract). Brain Dev (Tokyo) 1987; 9: 121.

Nagai T, Hasegawa T, Saito M, Hayashi S, Nonaka I. Infantile polymyositis: a case report. Brain Dev (Tokyo) 1992; 14: 167–169.

Nagao H, Habara S, Morimoto T, Sano N, Takahashi M, Kida K, Matsuda H. AMP deaminase activity of skeletal muscle in neuromuscular disorders in childhood. Histochemical and biochemical studies. Neuropediatrics 1986; 17: 193–198.

Nagao H, Takahashi M, Habara S, Nagai H, Matsuda H. Skeletal muscle computed tomography in neuromuscular diseases (in Japanese). Nihon Shonika Gakkai Zasshi (J Jpn Pediatr Soc) (Tokyo) 1986; 90: 140–147.

Nagao H, Sano N, Nagai H, Kusuda K, Habara S, Takahashi M, Morimoto T, Matsuda H. Three cases of congenital muscular dystrophy with partial epilepsy, West syndrome or Lennox syndrome (in Japanese). Nihon Shonika Gakkai Zasshi (J Jpn Pediatr Soc) (Tokyo) 1987; 91: 169–176.

Naide M, Nishimura K, Hase K, Kaya K. An experience of general anesthesia in congenital muscular dystrophy (in Japanese). Rinsho Masui (J Clin Anesth) (Tokyo) 1989; 13: 1421–1422.

Nakada K, Hirano A, Ota N. Duchenne muscular dystrophy phenotypically mimicking congenital muscular dystrophy – a case report (abstract in Japanese). Nippon Shonika Gakkai Zasshi (J Jpn Pediatr Soc) (Tokyo) 1997; 101(4): 868.

Nakajima T, Noda H, Obata C, and 10 other co-authors. Sphincter control training in CMD (Fukuyama type), Report I (in Japanese). In: Nakajima T, ed. The 1978 annual report of the research committee on clinico-sociological study of nursing care of progressive muscular dystrophy, sponsored by the Ministry of Health and Welfare of Japan. Matsue, 1979: 176–179.

Nakajima T, Iizuka H, Moriyama N. Guidance of congenital muscular dystrophy children (in Japanese). In: Nakajima T, ed. The 1979 annual report of the research committee on clinico-sociological study of nursing care of progressive muscular dystrophy, sponsored by the Ministry of Health and Welfare of Japan. Matsue, 1980: 73–75.

Nakajima T, Kasagi S, Takakura K, Takeshita K. A study of short latency SEP in congenital muscular dystrophy (Fukuyama type) (in Japanese). In: Sobue I, ed. The 1981 annual report of the research committee on clinics, epidemiology and management of progressive muscular dystrophy, sponsored by the Ministry of Health and Welfare of Japan. Nagoya, 1982: 338–341.

Nakajima T, Kasagi S, Takakura K. Brainstem function in Fukuyama type congenital muscular dystrophy (in Japanese). In: Sobue I, ed. The 1982 annual report of the research committee on clinics, epidemiology and management of progressive muscular dystrophy, sponsored by the Ministry of Health and Welfare of Japan. Nagoya, 1983: 337–344.

Nakagawa M, Nakamura A, Kubota R, Isashiki Y. Epidemiological and clinical features of muscular dystrophies in the Okinawa prefecture – mainly dealing with congenital muscular dystrophy (in Japanese). Kokuryo Okinawa Byoin Igaku Zasshi (J Natl Okin Hosp) (Naha) 1989; 10: 45–49.

Nakakura S, Itagaki Y. A study of body constituents in muscular dystrophy patients using radioactive 40K and measuring subcutaneous fatty tissue thickness (Especially in PMD-LG type, CMD-Fukuyama type and SPMA) (in Japanese). In: Aoyagi A, ed. The 1986 annual report of the research committee on clinical and psychological study of care and nursing of progressive muscular dystrophy, sponsored by the Ministry of Health and Welfare of Japan. 1987: 264–267.

Nakamigawa T, Shimoizumi H, Momoi M, Yamamoto Y, Yanagisawa H. Computed tomographic scans of skeletal muscles of various muscle diseases (abstract). Brain Dev (Tokyo) 1987; 9: 119.

Nakamoto N, Hanaka S, Tanaka M, Kobayashi M, Tajima T, Ohmi K, Kodama H, Abe T, Nonaka I. Female siblings with Fukuyama type congenital muscular dystrophy showed different brain anomalies. In: Fukuyama Y, Osawa M, eds. Program and abstracts of the International Symposium on Congenital Muscular Dystrophies, Tokyo. Tokyo: Tokyo Women's Medical College, 1994: 37.

Nakamura H, Takada K. Brain malformation in Fukuyama type congenital muscular dystrophy – characteristic changes of cerebellar polymicrogyria and its pathomechanism (in Japanese). In: Sugita H, ed. The 1987 annual report of the research committee on pathogenesis of progressive muscular dystrophy and related disorders, sponsored by the Ministry of Health and Welfare of Japan. Tokyo, 1988: 287–290.

Nakano I, Kawai M, Kunimoto M, Goto J. Application of muscle CT scanning to the diagnosis of muscle atrophic diseases – muscle CT findings in various muscle atrophies (in Japanese). In: Nishitani H, ed. The 1984 annual report of the research committee on genetics, epidemiology, clinics and treatment of progressive muscular dystrophy, sponsored by the Ministry of Health and Welfare of Japan. Kyoto, 1985: 177–180.

Nakano I, Goto J, Kurizaki H, Iwata M. Aberrant intraspinal course of pyramidal tract and related deformation of spinal cord under the level of medulla oblongata in Fukuyama type congenital muscular dystrophy (in Japanese). In: Nishitani H, ed. The 1985 annual report of the research committee on genetics, epidemiology, clinics and treatment of progressive muscular dystrophy, sponsored by the Ministry of Health and Welfare of Japan. Kyoto, 1986: 85–90.

Nakano I, Funahashi M, Takada K, Toda T. Are branches of the glia limitans the primary cause of the micropolygyria of Fukuyama type congenital muscular dystrophy (FCMD)? Pathological study of the cerebral cortex of a FCMD fetus. Acta Neuropathol 1996; 91: 313–321.

Nakano I, Toda T. An ultramicroscopic feature of cerebellum in a FCMD fetus – outflow of external granular cells through disrupted glia limitans basement membrane complex (abstract in Japanese). In: Takagi A, chairman. Abstracts for the 1996 annual meeting of the research committee on pathogenesis and treatment of progressive muscular dystrophy and related disorders, sponsored by the Ministry of Health and Welfare of Japan. Tokyo; 1996: 6.

Nakayama M, Sasaki Y, Misugi K, Misugi N, Iwamoto H. An autopsy case of congenital muscular dystrophy (Fukuyama type) (abstract). Brain Dev (Tokyo) 1979; 1: 237.

Nakayama H, Ando S. Tomi H, Sunohara N, Nonaka I, Eto K, Satoyoshi E. Myopathy, unique clinical features, and brain malformations mimicking Fukuyama congenital muscular dystrophy: a case report. Neuropathology 1993; 13(4): 253–258.

Namba Y, Maegaki Y, Maeoka Y, Yoshimura M, Houdou S, Ishii S, Takeshita K. Short somatosensory evoked potentials in patients with Fukuyama type congenital muscular dystrophy – a comparison with CT and MRI findings (in Japanese). No To Hattatsu (Brain Dev) (Tokyo) 1995; 27(5): 376–381.

Naom I, D'Alessandro M, Sewry C, Topaloğlu H, Ferlini A, Dubowitz V, Muntoni F. Prenatal diagnosis of merosin deficient CMD: The role of linkage and immunocytochemical analysis (abstract). Neuromusc Disord 1996; Suppl: S20.

Naom I, D'Alessandro M, Topaloğlu H, Sewry C, Helbling-Leclerc A, Guicheney P, Dubowitz V, Muntoni F. Linkage analysis to the $\alpha 2$ laminin locus on chromosome 6q2 in merosin-deficient congenital muscular dystrophy (abstract). Eur J Hum Genet 1996; 4 Suppl 1: 1.

Naom IS, D'Alessandro M, Topaloğlu H, Sewry C, Ferlini A, Helbling-Leclerc A, Guicheney P, Weissenbach J, Schwartz K, Ruchby K, Philpot J, Dubowitz V, Muntoni F. Refinement of the laminin α 2-chain locus to human chromosome 6q2 in severe and mild merosin deficient congenital muscular dystrophy. J Med Genet 1997; 34: 99–104.

Naom I, D'Alessandro M, Sewry C, Ferlini A, Topaloğlu H, Helbling-Leclerc A, Guicheney P, Schwartz K, Akcoren Z, Dubowitz V, et al. The role of immunohistochemistry and linkage analysis in the prenatal diagnosis of merosin-deficient congenital muscular dystrophy. Hum Genet 1997; 99(4): 535–540.

Nashef L, Lake BD, Schapira AHV. Congenital muscular dystrophy with severe retrocollis and mental retardation: a report of two siblings. J. Neurol Neurosurg Psychiatry 1997; 62:279-281.

Natori T, Sato H. A case of congenital muscular dystrophy associated with fragile X (abstract in Japanese). Rinsho Shinkeigaku (Clin Neurol) (Tokyo) 1985; 25: 1108–1109.

Natsume K, Mizutani A. Long-term observation of two institutionalized cases of Fukuyama type congenital muscular dystrophy (in Japanese). Shoni Naika (Jpn J Pediatr Med) (Tokyo) 1983; 15: 573–579.

Niemi KM, Somer H, Kero M, Kanerva L, Haltia Y. Epidermolysis bullosa simplex associated with muscular dystrophy with recessive inheritance. Arch Dermatol 1988; 124: 551–554.

Nihei K, Kamoshita S, Atsumi T. A case of Ullrich's disease (Kongenitale, atonisch-sklerotische Muskeldystrophie). Brain Dev (Tokyo) 1979; 1: 61–67.

Nihei K, Naito H, Koizumi N, Suzuki S. Three cases of congenital muscular dystrophy associated with congenital heart malformations (abstract). Brain Dev (Tokyo) 1981; 3: 241.

Nishikawa M, Ueda S, Ito T, Ohara T. Classification of muscular dystrophies (in Japanese). In: Okinaka S, ed. Cumulative articles of the research committee on progressive muscular dystrophy, sponsored by the Ministry of Health and Welfare of Japan. Tokyo, 1973: 50–60.

Nishimura A, Takashima S, Becker LE. Aberrant distribution of substance P and tyrosine hydroxylase in the brainstem of an infant with Walker–Warburg type lissencephaly (in Japanese). Nihon Shonika Gakkai Zasshi (J Jpn Pediatr Soc) (Tokyo) 1992; 96: 2541–2544.

Nishimura M. CT studies on the lower extremities in several neuromuscular diseases (abstract). Brain Dev (Tokyo) 1987; 9: 120.

Nishitani H. Congenital myopathy and neurogenic changes (in Japanese). No To Hattatsu (Brain Dev) (Tokyo) 1973; 5: 477–488.

Nishitani H, Itagaki Y, Sakamoto Y, Yoshikawa M. CNS disturbances in congenital muscular dystrophy (in Japanese). In: Sobue I, ed. The 1978 annual report of the research committee on clinics, epidemiology and management of progressive muscular dystrophy, sponsored by the Ministry of Health and Welfare of Japan. Nagoya, 1979: 232–234.

Nishitani H, Itagaki Y, Yoshioka M, Kohsaka T. Microdetermination of myoglobin in muscle diseases (in Japanese). In: Sobue I, ed. The 1979 annual report of the research committee on clinics, epidemiology and management of progressive muscular dystrophy, sponsored by the Ministry of Health and Welfare of Japan. Nagoya, 1980: 338–344.

Nishitani H, Itagaki Y, Yoshioka M, Otsuki H, Hayashi S. Two autopsy cases of congenital muscular dystrophy (Fukuyama type) (in Japanese). In: Sobue I, ed. The 1980 annual report of the research committee on clinics, epidemiology and management of progressive muscular dystrophy, sponsored by the Ministry of Health and Welfare of Japan. Nagoya, 1981: 303–308.

Nishitani H, Itagaki Y, Fujitake S, Yoshioka M, Haebara H. Autopsy findings in congenital muscular dystrophy (in Japanese). In: Sobue I, ed. The 1981 annual report of the research committee on clinics, epidemiology and management of progressive muscular dystrophy, sponsored by the Ministry of Health and Welfare of Japan. Nagoya, 1982: 306–309.

Nishitani H, Itagaki Y, Yoshioka M, Haebara H. Three autopsy cases of congenital muscular dystrophy (Fukuyama type) (in Japanese). In: Sobue I, ed. The 1983 annual report of the research committee on clinics, epidemiology and management of progressive muscular dystrophy, sponsored by the Ministry of Health and Welfare of Japan. Nagoya, 1984: 495–501.

Nishitani H, Mori F, Ota K, Itagaki M, Itagaki Y, Hayashi K. A comparative study of serum myoglobin, carbonic anhydrase III and creatine kinase in muscular dystrophies (in Japanese). In: Nishitani H, ed. The 1986 annual report of the research committee on genetics, epidemiology, clinics and treatment of progressive muscular dystrophy, sponsored by the Ministry of Health and Welfare of Japan. Kyoto, 1987: 232–235.

Nishitani H, Ota M, Ota K, Mori F, Ishimura T, Itagaki Y, Hayashi K. Serum-hANP in muscular dystrophies (in Japanese). In: Nishitani H, ed. The 1988 annual report of the research committee on genetics, epidemiology, clinics and treatment of progressive muscular dystrophy, sponsored by the Ministry of Health and Welfare of Japan. Kyoto, 1989: 187–189.

Nissinen M, Helbling-Leclerc A, Zhang X, Evangelista T, Topaloglu H, Cruaud C, Weissenbach C, Fardeau M, Tóme FMS, Schwartz K, Tryggvason K, Guicheney P. Substitution of a conserved cysteine-996 in a cysteine-rich motif of the laminin α2-chain in congenital muscular dystrophy. Am J Hum Genet 1996; 58: 1177–1184.

Nogen AG. Congenital muscle disease and abnormal findings on computerized tomography. Dev Med Child Neurol 1980; 22: 658–663.

Noguchi H, Yamanouchi S, Uchishiba M, Abe H, Tomiyama M, Tsunonami K, Awano F, Mayama K, Fukumoto Y. An infant with Fukuyama congenital muscular dystrophy (abstract in Japanese). Nihon Shonika Gakkai Zasshi (J Jpn Pediatr Soc) (Tokyo) 1996; 100(10): 1680.

Nojima M, Nagao H, Morimoto T, Sano N, Takahashi M, Habara S, Kida K, Matsuda H. AMP deaminase activity in biopsied muscles in various neuromuscular disorders in human (in Japanese) In: Sobue I, ed. The 1983 annual report of the research committee on clinics, epidemiology and management of progressive muscular dystrophy, sponsored by the Ministry of Health and Welfare of Japan. Nagoya, 1984: 586–590.

Nojima M, Nagao H, Habara S, Takahashi M, Nagai H, Matsuda H. AMP deaminase staining in neuromuscular disorders in children (in Japanese). In: Nishitani H, ed. The 1984 annual report of the research committee on genetics, epidemiology, clinics and treatment of progressive muscular dystrophy, sponsored by the Ministry of Health and Welfare of Japan. Kyoto, 1985: 343–348.

Nojima M, Nagao H, Morimoto T, Habara S, Takahashi M, Nagai H, Matsuda H. Muscle pathology in neuromuscular disorders in children – correlation of muscle CT and histological findings (in Japanese). In: Nishitani H, ed. The 1985 annual report of the research committee on genetics, epidemiology, clinics and treatment of progressive muscular dystrophy, sponsored by the Ministry of Health and Welfare of Japan. Kyoto, 1986: 31–36.

Nomura Y, Ehara M, Yamanaka T, Arahata K, Nonaka I, Segawa M. Heterogeneity of congenital muscular dystrophy (CMD) (abstract). J Neurol Sci 1990; 98(Suppl): 437.

Nonaka H, Tanaka K, Nagayama M, Kudo K, Akima M, Nakajima T, Sanada S, Kamio M. An autopsy case of Warburg syndrome (abstract in Japanese). Shinkei Byorigaku (Neuropathology) (Kyoto) 1985; 6: 186.

Nonaka I, Ueno T, Miyoshino S, Mitsune K, Miike T, Date E. Clinical and myopathological findings in congenital muscular dystrophy (Fukuyama type) (in Japanese). Shonika Shinryo (J Pediatr Pract) (Tokyo) 1972; 35: 964–970.

Nonaka I, Miike T, Ueno T, Miyoshino S. Benign congenital muscular dystrophy: a case report (in Japanese). No To Hattatsu (Brain Dev) (Tokyo) 1972; 4: 316–323.

Nonaka I, Miyoshino S, Miike T, Ueno T, Usuku G. An electron microscopical study of the muscle in congenital muscular dystrophy. Kumamoto Med J (Kumamoto) 1972; 25: 68–82.

Nonaka I, Miike T, Ueno T. Miyoshino S. An ultrastructural observation of satellite cells in biopsied muscles of congenital muscular dystrophy (in Japanese). No To Hattatsu (Brain Dev) (Tokyo) 1973; 5: 520–529.

Nonaka I, Ueno T, Miyoshino S, Miike T, Mishima K. Clinical and pathological study of Ullrich-type of congenital muscular dystrophy (in Japanese). No To Hattatsu (Brain Dev) (Tokyo) 1974; 6: 48–56.

Nonaka I, Uno K, Matsuishi T, Nagao H. The significance of type II C fibers in biopsied muscles in various infantile neuromuscular disorders (in Japanese). No To Hattatsu (Brain Dev) (Tokyo) 1978; 10: 439–445.

Nonaka I, Chou SM. Congenital muscular dystrophy. In: Vinken PJ, Bruyn GW, eds. Handbook of clinical neurology, Vol 41. Amsterdam: North Holland, 1979: 27–50.

Nonaka 1, Takada K. Comparative muscle histochemistry between Fukuyama type congenital muscular dystrophy (FCMD) and Duchenne muscular dystrophy (DMD) (abstract). Brain Dev (Tokyo) 1981; 3: 238.

Nonaka I, Une Y, Ishihara T, Miyoshino S, Nakashima T, Sugita H. A clinical and histological study of Ullrich's disease (congenital atonic-sclerotic muscular dystrophy). Neuropediatrics 1981; 12: 197–208.

Nonaka I, Sugita H, Takada K, Kumagai K. Muscle histochemistry in congenital muscular dystrophy with central nervous system involvement. Muscle Nerve 1982; 5: 102–106.

Nonaka I. Congenital muscular dystrophy (in Japanese). In: Nonaka I, ed. Introduction to muscle pathology for clinicians. Tokyo: Nihon Iji-Shuppan, 1992: 52–60.

Nonaka I, Kobayashi O, Osari S. Clinical and genetic nosology of non-Fukuyama type congenital muscular dystrophy (abstract in Japanese). Abstracts for the 40th annual meeting of the Japan Society of Human Genetics, Kumamoto; 1995: 5.

Nonaka I, Kobayashi O. Clinico-genetic analysis of non-Fukuyama (classical) form of congenital muscular dystrophy (abstract). Jpn J Hum Genet (Tokyo) 1996; 41: 26.

Nonaka I, Kobayashi O, Osari S. Non-dystrophinopathic muscular dystrophies including myotonic dystrophy. Sem Pediatr Neurol 1996; 3: 110–121.

Norman MG, McGillivray BC, Kalousek DK, Hill A, Poskitt KJ. Walker-Warburg syndrome. Fukuyama congenital muscular dystrophy (FCMD). Muscle-eye-brain disease of Santavuori. In: Norman MG, McGillivray BC, Kalousek DK, Hill, A, Poskitt KJ, eds. Congenital malformations of the brain. Pathologic, embryologic, clinical, radiologic and genetic aspects. New York: Oxford University Press. 1995: 236–242.

North KN, Beggs AH. Deficiency of a skeletal muscle isoform of α-actinin (α-actinin-3) in merosin-positive congenital muscular dystrophy. Neuromusc Disord 1996; 6(4): 229–235.

North KN, Specht LA, Sethi RK, Shapiro F, Beggs AT. Congenital muscular dystrophy associated with merosin deficiency. J Child Neurol 1996; 11: 291–295.

Nucci A, Queiroz LS, Piovezana AMG, Quagliato EMAB. Congenital muscular dystrophy (CHD) with cerebral anomalies, epilepsy and ocular dysfunction (abstract). Abstract No. 122, 6th Congress of the International Child Neurology Association, Buenos Aires, 1992.

Nucci A. Distrofia muscular congenita. Variações fenotípicas em 27 casos. Tese. Faculdade de Ciencias Medicas da Universidade Estadual de Campinas/SP, 1993.

Nucci A, Queiroz LS. Congenital muscular dystrophy (CMD), phenotypical analysis of twenty-seven cases (abstract). Muscle Nerve 1994, Suppl 1: S181.

O'Brien MD. An infantile muscular dystrophy: report of a case with autopsy findings. Guy's Hosp Rep 1962; 111: 98–106.

Ogasawara Y, Ito K, Murofushi K. Neuropathological studies on two cases of congenital muscular dystrophy with special reference to morphological characteristics of micropolygyria found in the cerebral and cerebellar cortex (in Japanese). No To Shinkei (Brain Nerve) (Tokyo) 1986; 28(5): 451–457.

Ogawa H, Komatsuyo M, Hirooka Y. A case of typical Fukuyama type congenital muscular dystrophy type IV (in Japanese). Shonika Rinsho (Jpn J Pediatr) (Tokyo) 1986; 39: 3216–3220.

Ogihara Y, Yagi Y, Sawai N, Nakazawa Y, Matsumura Y, Tsuno T, Kanda H, Ichikawa M, Koike K, Yano H, Momose Y. A case of Fukuyama type congenital muscular dystrophy associated with congenital anal atresia (in Japanese). No To Hattatsu (Brain Dev) (Tokyo) 1989; 21: 392–393.

Ogimi Y, Okuno M. Congenital arthrogryposis multiplex recurred in 3 siblings (in Japanese). Shonika Shinryo (J Pediatr Pract) (Tokyo) 1971; 34: 65–70.

Ohtake T, Nagashima Y, Tanabe H, Sato J, Oda M. Fukuyama type congenital muscular dystrophy with a long survival – an autopsy case report (in Japanese). Rinsho Shinkeigaku (Clin Neurol) (Tokyo) 1987; 27(6): 767–774.

Ohtani T, Ozaki R, Ishikawa N, Awaya A, Hashizume Y. An autopsied case of Fukuyama type congenital muscular dystrophy expired at the age of 20 years (abstract in Japanese). No To Hattatsu (Brain Dev) (Tokyo) 1988; 20 Suppl: S220.

Ohtani Y, Yoshioka T, Miike M, Ota J, Kai Y. Siblings with merosin (laminin M) deficiency – clinical features and myopathology (abstract in Japanese). No To Hattatsu (Brain Dev) (Tokyo) 1995; 27(Suppl): S266.

Oishi K, Kajiyama M, Ohtsuka H, Kubota H, Sugie H, Ohsawa M, Fukuyama Y. Serum carnitine in progressive muscular dystrophy (abstract). Brain Dev (Tokyo) 1985; 7: 240.

Oiwa N, Kato T, Ando T, Mori A, Yokoi K, Matsumoto H. Skeletal muscle CT findings in muscular dystrophies (in Japanese). No To Hattatsu (Brain Dev) (Tokyo) 1981; 13: 157–160.

Okada N, Osawa M, Jong YJ, Nakada E, Shishikura K, Suzuki H, Hirayama Y, Fukuyama Y. Physical growth of patients with the Fukuyama type congenital muscular dystrophy (in Japanese). Tokyo Joshi Ikadaigaku Zasshi (J Tokyo Wom Med Coll) (Tokyo) 1987; 57(Suppl): 532–539.

Okada N. Immunocytochemical study on muscular tissue of Fukuyama type congenital muscular dystrophy (in Japanese). Tokyo Joshi Ikadaigaku Zasshi (J Tokyo Wom Med Coll) (Tokyo) 1988; 58(4–5): 394–408.

Okamoto H, Hirase T, Yasutake T, Kawasaki S, Imamura S, Uekawa K, Tokuomi H. Brain CT and CSF proteins in muscular dystrophies (in Japanese). In: Sobue I, ed. The 1980 annual report of the research committee on clinics, epidemiology and management of progressive muscular dystrophy, sponsored by the Ministry of Health and Welfare of Japan. Nagoya, 1981: 183–189.

Okamoto K, Hirai S, Morimatsu M. Brain CT findings in Fukuyama type congenital muscular dystrophy (in Japanese). Shonika Shinryo (J Pediatr Pract) (Tokyo) 1983; 46: 2005–2007.

Okawa Y, Ueda S, Eto F, Kikuchi N. Clinical course of motor disturbances in Fukuyama type congenital muscular dystrophy (in Japanese). Rehabilitation Igaku (Rehab Med) (Tokyo) 1985; 22: 197–202.

Okudaira Y, Bando K, Wachi A, Sato K, Osawa M. A case of congenital muscular dystrophy associated with hydrocephalus – CSF dynamics and surgical treatment (in Japanese). No To Hattatsu (Brain Dev) (Tokyo) 1994; 26(1): 57–62.

Olive M, Sirvent J, Ferrer I. Congenital muscular dystrophy with distinct CNS involvement. Neuropediatrics 1994; 25(1): 48–50.

Oliveira ASB, Gabbai AA, Kiyomoto BH, Schmidt B. Distrofia muscular congênita. Apresentaçâo de oito casos com evidência de comprometimento do SNC. Rev Paul Med 1990; 108: 139–141.

Olney RK, Miller RG. Inflammatory infiltration in Fukuyama type congenital muscular dystrophy (letter). Muscle Nerve 1983; 6: 75–76.

Onuma A, Kobayashi Y, Soga T. A boy of lissencephaly type 2, spastic quadriplegia, severe myopia and dystrophic changes in muscle – a case of muscle-eye-brain syndrome? (abstract in Japanese). Presented at the 94th meeting of the Shikikai, Sendai, 1996.

Oppenheim H. Uber allgemeine und lokalisierte Atonie der Muskulatur (Myatonie) im frühen Kindesalter. Msch Psychiatr Neurol 1900; 8: 232.

Origuchi Y, Ikuta M, Miyoshino S. Histometric study of sural nerves in Fukuyama type congenital muscular dystrophy (in Japanese). In: Nakanishi T, ed. The 1981 annual report of the research committee on degeneration and regeneration of peripheral nerves, sponsored by the Ministry of Health and Welfare of Japan. Tsukuba, 1982: 41–44.

Osame M, Higuchi I, Nakagawa M, Usuki F, Fukunaga H, Arimura K, Nakahara K, Suehara M, Takenaga. Immunohistochemical study using anti-dystrophin antibody in various muscular dystrophies (in Japanese). In: Araki S, ed. The 1990 annual report of the research committee on pathogenesis and treatment exploration of progressive muscular dystrophy and related disorders, sponsored by the Ministry of Health and Welfare of Japan. Kumamoto, 1991: 60–63.

Osari S, Kobayashi O, Yamashita Y, Matsuishi T, Goto M, Tanabe Y, Migita T, Nonaka I. Basement membrane abnormality in merosin-negative congenital muscular dystrophy. Acta Neuropathol 1996; 91(4): 332–336.

Osawa M. A genetical and epidemiological study on congenital progressive muscular dystrophy (Fukuyama type) (in Japanese). Tokyo Joshi Ikadaigaku Zasshi (J Tokyo Wom Med Coll) (Tokyo) 1978; 48: 204–241.

Osawa M, Maruyama H, Hirayama Y, Suzuki H, Harada J, Goto T, Ogawa K, Miyata A, Fukuyama Y, Maruyama K. Computerized tomography in patients with progressive muscular dystrophy (abstract). Brain Dev (Old Series) (Tokyo) 1978; 3: 273.

Osawa M, Fukuyama Y, Nakada E, Adachi M. Congenital progressive muscular dystrophy (Fukuyama type) (in Japanese). Shoni Naika (Jpn J Pediatr Med) (Tokyo) 1980; 12: 2567–2574.

Osawa M, Maruyama H, Hirayama Y, Suzuki H, Harada J, Ogawa K, Ochiai E, Fukuyama Y. Computerized tomography (CT) in patients with progressive muscular dystrophy (PMD) (abstract). Dev Med Child Neurol 1980; 22: 262.

Osawa M, Ochiai E, Fukuyama Y. Congenital progressive muscular dystrophy (Fukuyama type) (in Japanese). Saishin-Igaku (Modern Medicine) (Osaka) 1980; 35: 988–998.

Osawa M, Suzuki H, Fukuyama Y. Congenital muscular dystrophy (in Japanese). Shinkei Kenkyu No Shinpo (Advances in Neurological Sciences) (Tokyo) 1980; 24: 702–717.

Osawa M, Suzuki H, Hirayama Y, Fukuyama Y. Congenital muscular dystrophy (in Japanese). In: Oda T et al., eds. Myopathies and neuropathies. Internal medicine seminar. PN 8. Osaka: Nagai Shoten, 1983: 159–173.

Osawa M, Suzuki H, Fukuyama Y. Congenital progressive muscular dystrophy of the

Fukuyama type. ZSZ – an extra issue (in Japanese). Tokyo: Japan Muscular Dystrophy Association, 1983: 56pp.

Osawa M, Fukuyama Y. Epidemiology and genetics of congenital muscular dystrophy (in Japanese). In: Sobue I, Nishitani H, eds. Clinics of progressive muscular dystrophy. Tokyo: Ishiyaku Shuppan, 1985: 20–31.

Osawa M, Shishikura K, Fukuyama Y. Congenital muscular dystrophy (in Japanese). In: Kobayashi N, supervisor. New encyclopedia of pediatrics. 15A. Pediatric diseases of motor apparatus, Vol 1. Tokyo: Nakayama Shoten, 1986: 266–273.

Osawa M. Congenital muscular dystrophy. In: Maekawa K, ed. Neurological diseases in children – case studies (in Japanese). Tokyo: Chugai Igakusha, 1986: 61–67.

Osawa M, Arai Y, Ikenaka H, Murasugi H, Sunahara N, Sumida S, Okada N, Shishikura K, Suzuki H, Hirayama Y, Hirasawa K, Fukuyama Y, Tsutsumi A, Ito K, Uchida Y. Fukuyama type congenital progressive muscular dystrophy. Acta Paediatr Jpn (Tokyo) 1991; 33: 261–269.

Osawa M, Suzuki S, Yanagaki S, Kobayashi M, Kaneda Y. Congenital muscular dystrophy of the Fukuyama type with severe scoliosis and horizontal nystagmus (in Japanese). Shonika Shinryo (J Pediatr Pract) (Tokyo) 1992; 55: 1317–1329.

Osawa M, Suzuki N, Arai Y, Ikenaka H, Sumida S, Shishikura K, Suzuki H, Fukuyama Y. Fukuyama type congenital progressive muscular dystrophy (FCMD) – special comment on the relationship between the case reported by Nakayama et al. and FCMD. Neuropathology (Tokyo) 1993; 13(4): 259–268.

Osawa M. Congenital progressive muscular dystrophy of the Fukuyama type (Syndrome in children) (in Japanese). Shonika Rinsho (Jpn J Pediatr) (Tokyo) 1993; 56: 148.

Osawa M, Sumida S. Management of congenital progressive muscular dystrophy of the Fukuyama type (in Japanese). Modern Physician (Tokyo) 1993; 13: 1062–1063.

Osawa M, Saito K, Suzuki N, Arai Y, Sumida S, Sakauchi M, Kondo E, Fukuyama Y, Yoshioka M. Congenital muscular dystrophy (in Japanese). In: Takahashi K, ed. The 1993 annual report of the research committee on clinics, genetic counselling and epidemiology of progressive muscular dystrophy, sponsored by the Ministry of Health and Welfare of Japan. Hyogo, 1994: 179–184.

Osawa M, Ikenaka H, Yanagaki S, Hirasawa K, Suzuki N, Arai Y, Suzuki H, Shishikura K, Saito K, Fukuyama Y. Transient aggravation of muscle weakness during intercurrent infection in congenital muscular dystrophy patients (in Japanese). In: Takahashi K, ed. The 1993 annual report of the research committee on clinics, genetic counselling and epidemiology of progressive muscular dystrophy, sponsored by the Ministry of Health and Welfare of Japan. Hyogo, 1994: 191–194.

Osawa M. Fukuyama type congenital muscular dystrophy (FCMD) – clinical, pathological and genetic approaches (abstract). Muscle Nerve 1994; Suppl 1: S53.

Osawa M, Sumida S, Murasugi H, Suzuki N, Arai Y, Shishikura K, Saito K, Wang ZP, Suzuki H, Hirayama Y, Fukuyama Y. Cerebral dysplasia and convulsions – a study in Fukuyama type congenital muscular dystrophy (in Japanese). In: Takeshita K, ed. The 1993 annual report of the research committee on the etiology and prevention of cerebral dysplasia, sponsored by the Ministry of Health and Welfare of Japan. Yonago, 1994: 66–71.

Osawa M. Congenital muscular dystrophy (in Japanese). In: Maekawa K, Imamura E, eds. Year book of pediatrics. Advances in pediatrics No. 15. Tokyo: Shindan to Chiryosha, 1995: 95–99.

Osawa M, Fukuyama Y. Congenital muscular dystrophy (in Japanese). In: Sugita H, Ozawa E, Nonaka I, eds. Principle in myology. Tokyo: Nankodo, 1995: 517–536.

Osawa M, Suzuki N, Shiraiwa Y, Muto J, Fukuyama Y, Yoshioka M. Recent advances and epidemiological data in the research of congenital muscular dystrophy (in Japanese). In: Takahashi K, ed. The 1994 - 1995 annual report of the research committee on the clinics, epidemiology and genetic counselling of progressive muscular dystrophy, sponsored by the Ministry of Health and Welfare of Japan. Hyogo, 1996: 93-95.

Osawa M, Sumida S, Suzuki N, Shiraiwa Y, Muto J, Yoshioka M. Non-Fukuyama type congenital muscular dystrophy (abstract in Japanese). In: Takahashi K, ed. The 1994 - 1995 annual report of the research committee on clinics, genetic counselling and epidemiology of progressive muscular dystrophy, sponsored by the Ministry of Health and Welfare of Japan, Hyogo 1996: 307 - 313.

Osawa M, Kondo E, Suzuki H, Hirayama Y, Harada J, Suzuki N, Saito K, Fukuyama Y, Ishihara T. A Japanese CMD case with diffuse white matter density on CT and normal mentality: a 16 year follow-up study. Tokyo Joshi Ikadaigaku Zasshi (J Tokyo Wom Med Coll) (Tokyo) 1996; 66(3): 95–109.

Osawa M, Suzuki N, Sumida S, Muto J, Yoshida M. A fact-finding survey of non-Fukuyama type CMD (abstract in Japanese). In: Ishihara T, chairman. Abstracts for the 1996 annual meeting of the research committee on genetic counselling and comprehensive understanding and management of progressive muscular dystrophy, sponsored by the Ministry of Health and Welfare of Japan. Saitama, 1996: 42.

Osawa M, Ikeya K, Saito K, Sumida S, Suzuki N, Shishikura K, Kobayashi M. An ambulant benign case of FCMD with polymicrogyria evidenced by autopsy (in Japanese). In: Ishihara T, chairman. Abstracts for the 1996 annual meeting of the research committee on genetic counselling and comprehensive understanding and management of progressive muscular dystrophy, sponsored by the Ministry of Health and Welfare of Japan. Saitama, 1996: 43.

Oshiro M, Nakagawa M, Nakamura A, Kubota R, Isashiki Y. Epidemiology and clinical features of congenital muscular dystrophy in Okinawa Prefecture (in Japanese). In: Nishitani H, ed. The 1988 annual report of the research committee on genetics, epidemiology, clinics, and treatment of progressive muscular dystrophy, sponsored by the Ministry of Health and Welfare of Japan. Kyoto, 1989: 23–26.

Pagon RA, Chandler JW, Collie WR, Clarren SK, Moon J, Minkin A, Hall JG. Hydrocephalus, agyria, retinal dysplasia, encephalocele (HARD±E) syndrome: an autosomal recessive condition. In: Summitt RL, Bergsma D, eds. Recent advances and new syndromes. New York: Alan R Liss, for the National Foundation – March of Dimes. BD: OAD 1978: XIV (6B): 232–241.

Pagon BA, Clarren S, Hard E. Warburg's syndrome. Arch Neurol 1981; 33: 66.

Pagon RA, Clarren S, Milan D Jr, Hendrickson AE. Autosomal recessive eye and brain anomalies: Warburg syndrome. J Pediatr 1983; 102: 542–546.

Palm DG, Bömelburg T, Kurlemann G, Korinthenberg R. Congenital muscular dystrophy and lissencephaly (abstract). Childs Nerv Syst 1993; 9: 127.

Parano E. Walker–Warburg syndrome (letter). Neuropediatrics 1990; 21: 224.

Parano E, Fiumara A, Falsaperla R, Vita G, Trifiletti RR. Congenital muscular dystrophy: correlation of muscle biopsy and clinical features. Pediatr Neurol 1994; 10: 233–236.

Parano E, Falsaperla R, Pavone V, Trifiletti RR. Congenital muscular dystrophy with syringomyelia. Pediatr Neurol 1994; 11(3): 263–265.

Parano E, Pavone L, Fiumara A, Falsaperla R, Trifiletti RR, Dobyns WB. Congenital muscular dystrophies: clinical review and proposed classification. Pediatr Neurol 1995; 13(2): 97–103.

Parker D, Root AW, Schimmel S, Andriola M, Di Mauro S. Encephalopathy and fatal myopathy in two siblings. Am J Dis Child 1982; 136: 598–601.

Pavone L, Gullotta F, Grasso S, Vannucchi C. Hydrocephalus, lissencephaly, ocular abnormalities and congenital muscular dystrophy. A Warburg syndrome variant? Neuropediatrics 1986; 17: 206–211.

Pearson CM, Fowler WG Jr. Hereditary non-progressive muscular dystrophy inducing arthrogryposis syndrome. Brain 1963; 86: 75–88.

Pegoraro E, Mancias P, Swerdlow SH, Raikow RB, Garcia C, Marks H, Crawford T, Carver V, Di Cianno B, Hoffman EP. Congenital muscular dystrophy with primary laminin α 2 (merosin) deficiency, presenting as inflammatory myopathy. Ann Neurol 1996; 40: 782–791.

Pegoraro E, Mancias P, Garcias C, Angelini C, Fanin M, Trevisan CP, Marks H, Crawford T, Connolly AM, Carver V, Hoffman EP. The genetic and phenotypic heterogeneity of merosin-negative congenital muscular dystrophy (abstract). Neurology 1997; 48(3) Suppl 2: A200.

Penisson-Besnier I, Tomé FMS, Echenne B, Dubas F, Dumez C, Chevallay M, Vignier N, Helbling-Leclerc A, Guicheney P, Fardeau M. Prolonged survival in a severe case of merosin deficient congenital muscular dystrophy (abstract). Neuromusc Disord 1996; Suppl: S29.

Peters ACB, Bots GTAM, Roos RAC, van Gelderen HH. Fukuyama type congenital muscular dystrophy – two Dutch siblings. Brain Dev (Tokyo) 1984; 6: 406–416.

Petrykowski WV, Beckmann R, Böhm N, Ketelsen UP, Ropers HH, Sauer M. Adrenal insufficiency, myopathic hypotonia, severe psychomotor retardation, failure to thrive, constipation and bladder ectasia in 2 brothers; adrenomyodystrophy. Helv Paediatr Acta 1982; 37: 387–400.

Philpot J, Zamir S, Francesco M, Dubowitz V. Peripheral nerve involvement in congenital muscular dystrophy (abstract). Dev Med Child Neurol 1995; Suppl No. 72: 37(3): 102.

Philpot J, Topaloğlu H, Pennock J. Dubowitz Y. Familial concordance of brain magnetic resonance imaging changes in congenital muscular dystrophy. Neuropediatrics 1995; 26(3): 227–231.

Philpot J, Sewry C, Pennock J, Dubowitz V. Clinical phenotype in congenital muscular dystrophy: correlation with expression of merosin in skeletal muscle. Neuromusc Disord 1995; 5(4): 301–305.

Philpot J, Dubowitz V. Congenital muscular dystrophies. In: Rimoin DL, Connor JM, Pyeritz RE, eds. Emery and Rimoin's principles and practice of medical genetics, 3rd edn. New York: Churchill Livingstone, 1996: 2325–2335.

Piantadosi C, Servidei S, Bertini E, Broccolini A, Ricci E, Spinazzola A, Silvestri G, Tonali P. Immunohistochemical studies of muscle and nerve in merosin-deficient congenital muscular dystrophy (abstract). Neuromusc Disord 1996; 6(2): S18.

Pihko H, Louhimo T, Valanne L, Donner H. CNS in congenital muscular dystrophy without mental retardation. Neuropediatrics 1992; 23: 116–122.

Pihko H, Lappi M, Raitta C, Sainio K, Valanne L, Somer H, Santavuori P. Ocular findings in muscle-eye-brain (MEB) disease: a follow-up study. Brain Dev 1995; 17(1): 57–61.

Pihko H, Santavuori P, Somer H, Rapola J. Muscle pathology in muscle-eye-brain (MEB) disease (abstract). Neuromusc Disord 1996; Suppl: S21.

Pike AC, Butcher JM, Kelsey A, Tarnoke C, Jardine P. Psychometric analysis and ocular involvement in congenital muscular dystrophy: correlation with muscle laminin 2 expression. Neuromusc Disord 1996; Suppl: S28.

Pike A, Butcher J, Kelsey A, Tarnoke C, Jardine P. Psychometric analysis and ocular involvement in congenital muscular dystrophy: correlation with muscle laminin 2 expression (abstract). J Med Genet 1996; 33(Suppl 1): S27.

Pillers DM, Weleber RG, Rash SM, Duncan NM, Woodward WR. The dark-adapted ERG is abnormal in the merosin-deficient dy/dy mouse model of muscular dystrophy (abstract No. 1612). Am J Hum Genet 1996; 59(Suppl): a278.

Pilz DT, Quarrell OWJ. Syndromes with lissencephaly. J Med Genet 1996; 33: 319–323.

Pini A, Baioni E, Zanotti S, Santucci M, Gobbi G, Granata C, Giovanardi Rossi P. Migratory disorders and muscular changes in infancy (abstract). Abstract No. 84, 6th Congress of the International Child Neurology Association, Buenos Aires, 1992.

Pini A, Gobbi G, Granata C, Merlini L, Ambrosetto P, Giovanardi Rossi P. Congenital muscular dystrophy, mental defect, partial epilepsy, white matter changes and focal pachygyria: report of a case (abstract). Muscle Nerve 1994; Suppl 1: S89.

Pini A, Merlini L, Tomé F, Chevallay M, Gobbi G. Merosin-negative congenital muscular dystrophy, cortical dysplasia and epilepsy: an association to investigate (abstract). Neuromusc Disord 1996; 6(2): SI7.

Pini A, Bertini E, Della Giustina E, Granata C, Merlini L, Mora M, Minetti C, Parano E, Gobbi G. Bilateral occipital cortical dysplasia (BOCD), leukoencephalopathy and epileptic spasms in merosin-negative CMD: a rare association? (abstract). Neuromusc Disord 1996; Suppl: S19–S20.

Pini A, Graziani E, Pines S, Merlini L, Gobbi G. Malocclusion in congenital muscular dystrophy (abstract). Neuromusc Disord 1996; Suppl: S22.

Pini A, Merlini L, Tomé FMS, Chevallay M, Gobbi G. Merosin-negative congenital muscular dystrophy, occipital epilepsy with periodic spasms and focal cortical dysplasia. Report of three Italian cases. Brain Dev (Tokyo) 1996; 18(4): 316–322.

Pollack MA, Kolbert GS. Congenital cataracts associated with agenesis of the corpus callosum and cerebral dysgenesis: a case report. J Pediatr Ophthalmol Strab 1981; 18: 6–8.

Prelle A, Medori R, Moggio M, Chan HW, Gallanti A, Scarlato G, Bonilla E. Dystrophin deficiency in a case of congenital myopathy. J Neurol 1992; 239: 76–78.

Quinn CM, Wigglesworth JS, Heckmatt J. Lethal arthrogryposis multiplex congenita. A pathological study of 21 cases. Histopathology 1991; 19: 155–62.

Rabe EF. The hypotonic infant. J Pediatr 1964; 64: 422–440.

Radu TNK, Deshpande DH, Desai AD. Congenital muscular dystrophy. In: Kakulas BA, ed. Clinical studies in myology. New York: Elsevier, 1973: 502–506.

Raitta C, Lamminen M, Santavuori P, Leisti J. Ophthalmological findings in a new syndrome with muscle, eye and brain involvement. Acta Ophthalmol 1978; 56: 465–472.

Ranta S, Pihko H, Santavuori P, Tahvanainen E, de la Chapelle A. Muscle-eye-brain disease and Fukuyama type congenital muscular dystrophy are not allelic. Neuromusc Disord 1995; 5(3): 221–225.

Rapisarda RH, Shorer Z, Muntoni F, Sewry C, Dubowitz V. Congenital myopia, ophthalmoplegia and ptosis, and congenital muscular dystrophy (abstract). Dev Med Child Neurol 1995; Suppl No. 72, 37(3): 105–106.

Reed UC, Marie SKN, Tsanaclis AMCB, Carvalho AAS, Roizenblatt J, Pedreira CC, Diament A, Levy JA. Congenital muscular dystrophy in two siblings with cataracts and slight cerebral involvement (abstract). Pediatr Neurol 1994; 11(2): 141.

Reed UC, Marie SKN, Carvalho AAS, Manreza MLG, Salum P, Diament A, Levy JA. Congenital muscular dystrophy: clinical and pathologic review of 24 patients (abstract). Pediatr Neurol 1994; 11(2): 141.

Reed UC, Marie SK, Vainzof M, Salum PB, Levy JA, Zatz M, Diament A. Congenital muscular dystrophy with cerebral white matter hypodensity. Correlation of clinical features and merosin deficiency. Brain Dev (Tokyo) 1996; 18(1): 53–58.

Rhodes RE, Hatten HP, Ellington KS. Walker–Warburg syndrome. Am J Neuroradiol 1992; 13: 123–126.

Ricci E, Bertini E, Boldrini R, Late onset scleroatonic familial myopathy (Ullrich disease). A study of two sibs. Am J Med Genet 1988; 31: 933–942.

Richards RB, Passmore IK, Bretag AH, Kubuler BA, McQuade NC. Ovine congenital progressive muscular dystrophy: clinical syndrome and distribution of lesions. Aust Vet J 1986; 63(12): 396–401.

Richards KB, Lewer RP, Passmore IK, McQuade NC. Ovine congenital progressive muscular dystrophy: mode of inheritance. Aust Vet J 1988; 65(3): 93–94.

Richards RB, Passmore IK, Dempsey EF. Skeletal muscle pathology in ovine congenital progressive muscular dystrophy. I. Histopathology and histochemistry. Acta Neuropathol 1988; 77: 161–167.

Richards RB, Passmore IK, Dempsey EF. Skeletal muscle pathology in ovine congenital progressive muscular dystrophy. 2. Myofiber morphometry. Acta Neuropathol 1988; 77: 95–99.

Richards RB, Passmore IK. Ultrastructural changes in skeletal muscle in ovine muscular dystrophy. Acta Neuropathol 1989; 79: 168–175.

Richter RB, Humphreys EM. Unusual myopathy: presentation of two cases with muscle biopsies. Am Med Assoc Arch Neurol Psychiatry 1955; 73: 574–575.

Riku S, Konagaya M, Ibi T, Sobue T. Unusual sibling cases of Fukuyama type congenital muscular dystrophy (in Japanese). Rinsho Shinkeigaku (Clin Neurol) (Tokyo) 1982; 22(3): 216–222.

Riku S, Kumagai T, Sobue I. Unusual familial occurrence of Fukuyama type congenital muscular dystrophy (in Japanese). Rinsho Shinkeigaku (Clin Neurol) (Tokyo) 1983; 23(8): 711–716.

Robain O, Dhermy P, Dufier JL, Blanck MF, Dulac O, Bursgtyn J. Les anomalies oculocérébrales au cours de la lissencéphalies de Walker. J Fr Ophthalmol 1985; 8: 59–72.

Roddy SM, Ashwal B, Peckham N, Nortensen S. Infantile myositis: a case diagnosed in the neonatal period. Pediatr Neurol 1986; 2: 241–244.

Rodgers BL, Vanner LV, Pai GS, Sens MA. Walker–Warburg syndrome: report of three affected sibs. Am J Med Genet 1994; 49: 198–201.

Rosman NP, Kakulas BA. Mental deficiency associated with muscular dystrophy: a neuropathological study. Brain 1966; 89: 769–788.

Rotthauwe HW, Kowalewski S, Mumenthaler M. Kongenitale Muskeldystrophie. Z Kinderheilk 1969; 106: 131–162.

Rotthauwe HW, Kowalewski S. Congenital muscular dystrophy. In: Walton JN, Canal N. Scarlato G, eds. Muscle diseases. Proceedings of an International Congress, Milano, 1969. International Congress Series, No 199. Amsterdam: Excerpta Medica 1970: 624–626.

Rudenskaya GE, Dadali EL, Sitnikov YH. Fukuyama type congenital muscular dystrophy: observations in Russia and Kazakhstan (abstract). Muscle Nerve 1994; Suppl 1: S181.

Saida K, Kyogoku M, Hojo H, Hirotani H, Nishitani H. Congenital muscular dystrophy (Fukuyama type). Quantitative histological study of distribution of affected muscles (in Japanese). Rinsho Shinkeigaku (Clin Neurol) (Tokyo) 1973; 10(10): 587–596.

Saida K, Nishitani H, Hirotani H, Hojo H, Kyoguku M, Fukase H. A quantitative histological study of biopsied muscles in congenital muscular dystrophy (in Japanese). In: Okinaka S, ed. Cumulative articles of the research committee on progressive muscular dystrophy, sponsored by the Ministry of Health and Welfare of Japan. Tokyo, 1974: 142–147.

Saida K, Itagaki Y, Iwamura K, Murayama H, Nishitani H. Dystrophin staining in Fukuyama type congenital muscular dystrophy and polymyositis (in Japanese). In: Takahashi K, ed. The 1990 annual report of the research committee on clinics, genetic counselling and epidemiology of progressive muscular dystrophy, sponsored by the Ministry of Health and Welfare of Japan. Hyogo, 1991: 292–295.

Saida K, Mitsuyoshi I, Hattori H, Higuchi Y, Yonekura Y, Konishi J. Cerebral glucose metabolism in FCMD revealed FDG-PET (in Japanese). In: Takahashi K, ed. The 1994–1995 annual report of the research committee on clinics, epidemiology and genetic counselling of progressive muscular dystrophy, sponsored by the Ministry of Health and Welfare of Japan. Hyogo, 1996: 101–102.

Saito K. Experimental intrauterine infection of Akabane virus – pathological studies of skeletal muscles and central nervous system of newborn hamsters (in Japanese). No To Hattatsu (Brain Dev) (Tokyo) 1980; l2: 519–534.

Saito K, Fukuyama Y, Ogata T, Oya A. Experimental intrauterine infection of Akabane virus: pathological studies of skeletal muscles and central nervous system of newborn hamsters – with relevance to the Fukuyama type muscular dystrophy. Brain Dev (Tokyo) 1981; 3: 65–80.

Saito A, Terai Y, Endo M, Suda H, Sasaki M, Nakamura T, Takano N, Terai K, Kon Y, Endo K, Nomura T. A case of Ullrich disease (in Japanese). Shonika Shinryo (J Pediatr Pract) (Tokyo) 1990; 53: 1472–1477.

Saito K, Osawa M, Kondo E, Ikeya K, Yamauchi A, Komine S, Sakuma I, Morita R, Shishikura K, Suzuki H, Harada T, Fukuyama Y. Genomic deletion study of the dystrophin gene in congenital muscular dystrophy (in Japanese). Tokyo Joshi Ikadaigaku Zasshi (J Tokyo Women's Med Coll) (Tokyo) 1993; 63(10, Suppl): E26–E35.

Saito K. A case of congenital muscular dystrophy presented a peculiar pattern in adhalin staining (abstract in Japanese). In: National Center of Neurology and Psychiatry (Planning Division), ed. Annual report of the research on nervous and mental disorders, 1994. Kodaira; National Center of Neurology and Psychiatry, 1995: 27.

Saito K. Recent advances in Fukuyama type congenital muscular dystrophy (in Japanese). No To Hattatsu (Brain Dev) (Tokyo) 1995; 27: 447–454.

Saito K, Yamamoto T, Shibata R, Kobayashi M, Kondo E, Kawakita Y, Ikeya K, Osawa M, Toda T. Cerebral cortical lesions in two Fukuyama type congenital muscular dystrophy fetuses aborted after prenatal diagnosis – a neuropathological consideration (in Japanese). In: Takagi A, ed. The 1994 - 1995 annual report of the research committee on pathogenesis and treatment of progressive muscular dystrophy and related disorders, sponsored by the Ministry of Health and Welfare of Japan. Tokyo, 1996: 80-81.

Saito K, Kondo E, Toda T, Tanaka H, Osawa M. Gene localization at 9q31 in clinically atypical (ambulant) Fukuyama type congenital muscular dystrophy patients (in Japanese).

In: Takagi A, ed. The 1994 - 1995 annual report of the research committee on pathogenesis and treatment of progressive muscular dystrophy and related disorders, sponsored by the Ministry of Health and Welfare of Japan. Tokyo, 1996: 82–83.

Saito K. Fukuyama type congenital muscular dystrophy (in Japanese). Hattatsu Shogai Kenkyu (J Dev Disabil Res) (Tokyo) 1996; 18(2): 122–127.

Saito K, Kondo E, Ikeya K, Shiraiwa Y, Osawa M, Fukuyama Y, Toda T, Yamamoto T, Kobayashi M. Prenatal diagnosis of Fukuyama type congenital muscular dystrophy by polymorphism analysis – the second report (abstract). Neuromusc Disord 1996; Suppl: S23.

Sakaino T. A case of amyotonia congenita (in Japanese). Rinsho Shoni Igaku (J Clin Pediatr) (Sapporo) 1957; 5: 42–45.

Sakamoto K, Shinohara T, Sumida K, Usui K, Sato J, Tamagawa K, Mizutani T, Morimatsu Y. Three autopsy cases of congenital muscular dystrophy (Fukuyama type) – especially on CNS findings (abstract in Japanese). Shinkei Byorigaku (Clin Neuropathol) (Kyoto) 1982; 3: 77.

Sakamoto Y, Itagaki Y, Yoshioka M. Treatment course of congenital muscular dystrophy with convulsive seizures (in Japanese). In: Kimura M, ed. The 1978 annual meeting of the research committee on child health and ecology for the prevention of physically/mentally disabled children, sponsored by the Ministry of Health and Welfare of Japan. Isehara; 1979: 66–67.

Salih MAM, Mahai AH, Al Jarallah AA, Jarallah AS, Al Saadi M, Hafeez MA, Aziz SA. Childhood neuromuscular disorders: decade's experience in Saudi Arabia (abstract). Abstracts of the 5th Asian and Oceanian Congress of Child Neurology 1996, Istanbul, Turkey: 51.

Sano N, Nagao H, Morimoto T, Takahashi M, Habara S, Matsumoto S, Matsuda H. A case of non-Fukuyama type congenital muscular dystrophy accompanied by CNS abnormalities (in Japanese). Shonika Shinryo (J Pediatr Pract) (Tokyo) 1984; 47: 2118–2122.

Santavuori P, Leisti J, Kruus S. Muscle, eye and brain disease: a new syndrome. Neuropaediatrie 1977; 8(Suppl): 553-558.

Santavuori P, Leisti J, Kruus S, Raitta C. Muscle, eye and brain disease: a new syndrome. Docum Ophthalmol Proc Ser 1978; 17: 393–396.

Santavuori P, Somer H, Sainio K, Rapola J, Kruus S, Nikitin T, Ketonen L, Leisti J. Muscle-eye-brain disease (MEB). Brain Dev (Tokyo) 1989; 11: 147–153.

Santavuori P, Pihko H, Sainio K, Lappi H, Somer H, Haltia M, Raitta C, Ketonen L, Leisti J. Muscle-eye-brain disease and Walker–Warburg syndrome (letter). Am J Med Genet 1990; 36: 371–372.

Santavuori P, Somer H, Haltia M, Pihko H, Sainio K. Reply to the letter of Merton et al. Brain Dev (Tokyo) 1990; 12: 274.

Sarala D, Gayathri N, Gouri Deri M. Variable histomorphology of muscle in congenital muscular dystrophy (abstract). J Neurol Sci 1990; 98(Suppl): 436.

Sarnat HB. Congenital muscular dystrophy. In: Sarnat HB, ed. Muscle pathology and histochemistry. Chicago, IL: American Society of Clinical Pathologists Press, 1983: 120–121.

Sarnat HB. Does the human fetal brain influence muscle development? Can J Neurol Sci 1985; 12: 111–120.

Sarnat HB. Cerebral dysgenesis and their influence on fetal muscle development. Brain Dev (Tokyo) 1986; 8: 494–499.

Sarnat HB. Vimentin/desmin immunoreactivity of myofibres in developmental myopathies. Acta Paediatr Jpn (Tokyo) 1991; 33: 238–246.

Sarnat HB, Darwish HZ, Barth PG, Trevenen CL, Pinto A, Kotagal S, Shishikura K, Osawa M, Korobkin R. Ependymal abnormalities in lissencephaly/pachygyria. J Neuropathol Exp Neurol 1993; 52: 525–541.

Sarnat HB. Disorders of neuroblast migration. In: Sarnat HB. Cerebral dysgenesis. Embryology and clinical expression. New York: Oxford University Press, 1992: 245–274.

Sasaki K, Shinoda M, Nakamura N. An autopsied case with Ullrich disease (in Japanese). Shonika Rinsho (Jpn J Pediatr) (Tokyo) 1985; 38: 411–416.

Sasaki K, Tachi N, Minagawa K, Yasunaka S, Minami R. A case of Ullrich disease. Clinical and muscle histopathological studies (in Japanese). Rinsho Shoni-igaku (J Clin Pediatr) (Sapporo) 1988; 36: 177–189.

Sasaki M, Yoshioka K, Yanagisawa T, Nemoto A, Takasago Y, Nagano T. Lissencephaly with congenital muscular dystrophy and ocular abnormalities: cerebro-oculo-muscular syndrome. Childs Nerv Syst 1989; 5: 35–37.

Sasaki Y, Iwamoto H, Kobayashi T. Case record: an 8 year 7 month old boy who had long been observed for muscular dystrophy and epilepsy and suddenly died (CPC No. 96; in Japanese). Kodomo Iryo Center Igakushi (J Kanagawa Children's Med Ctr) (Yokohama) 1991; 20: 123–128.

Sassani JW, Towfighi J, Laada RL. Ocular findings in patients with cerebromuscular dysplasia-muscular dystrophy syndrome. Ann Ophthalmol-Glaucomas 1994; 26: 225–235.

Sato A, Sannomiya Y. A case of Ullrich disease (in Japanese). Shonika Rinsho (Jpn J Pediatr) (Tokyo) 1970; 23(10): 1261–1263.

Sato H. Nakagawa K, Sakai K. Chromosomal abnormality in congenital muscular dystrophy (Fukuyama type) (in Japanese). In: Fukuyama Y. The 1981 annual report of the research committee on the cause and treatment of prenatal brain damage, sponsored by the Ministry of Health and Welfare of Japan. Tokyo; 1982: 65–69.

Sato J, Sakamoto K, Mizutani T, Tamagawa K, Shinohara T, Morimatsu Y. Congenital muscular dystrophy. Especially on Fukuyama type congenital muscular dystrophy (in Japanese). Byori To Rinsho (Pathology and Clinics) (Tokyo) 1985; 3: 962–966.

Sato J, Mizutani T, Morimatsu Y, Sakamoto K, Shinohara T, Fukuyama Y. Neuropathological study of white matter lesions in Fukuyama type congenital muscular dystrophy (abstract). Brain Dev (Tokyo) 1987; 9: 243.

Sato J. Neuropathology of lissencephalies – historical review of the nosology and the position of Fukuyama type congenital muscular dystrophy in the category (in Japanese). Tokyo Joshi Ikadaigaku Zasshi (J Tokyo Wom Med Coll) (Tokyo) 1992; 62(11, Extra): 1082–1087.

Sato M, Shimizu S, Tazawa M, Taguchi T, Sekiguchi E. A case of Fukuyama type congenital muscular dystrophy associated with cystinuria (in Japanese). No To Hattatsu (Brain Dev) (Tokyo) 1986; 18: 422–423.

Sato S, Shinoda M. Eight cases of congenital muscular dystrophy (in Japanese). Shonika Shinryo (J Pediatr Pract) (Tokyo) 1973; 36: 592–598.

Sato S, Mizutani M, Segawa K, Kumagai T, Aoki T, Arima M. Three cases of congenital muscular dystrophy (Fukuyama type) including one case which was detected in the neonatal period (abstract). Brain Dev (Tokyo) 1980; 2: 293.

Sato T, Oda S, Nabeya M, Honma H, Oya A. Arthrogryposis multiplex congenita caused by Akabane virus in calves and lower motor neuron degeneration in hamsters innoculated with virus. In: Okinaka S, ed. Current research in muscular dystrophy, Japan. The proceedings of the annual meeting of muscular dystrophy research group, 1977. Tokyo, 1978: 84–85.

Sato T, Oda S, Nabetani M, Homma H, Oya A. Congenital arthrogryposis multiplex of calves caused by arbovirus infection and animal inoculation experiments (in Japanese). In: Okinaka S, ed. Cumulative articles of the research committee on progressive muscular dystrophy, sponsored by the Ministry of Health and Welfare of Japan. (II). Tokyo, 1978; 188–193.

Sato T, Oda S, Nabetani M, Homma H, Oya A. Akabane virus-induced congenital multiple arthrogryposis in calves and an experimental inoculation to hamsters (in Japanese). Shinkei Kenkyu No Shinpo (Adv Neurol Sci) (Tokyo) 1979; 23: 461–471.

Sawada T, Sakamoto Y, Takahashi M, Kai Y, Miike T. A floppy infant with remarkable white matter abnormality on MRI (in Japanese). Nihon Shoni Hoshasen Kenkyukai Zasshi (J Jpn Pediatr Radiol) (Tokyo) 1989; 5: 82–83.

Schairer E. Fetale Myositis und ihre Folgen. Münch Med Wschr 1982; 14: 596–598.

Schlivek K. Report of a case of congenital muscular dystrophy. Arch Pediatr 1910; 27: 34–36.

Schmalbruch H, Kamieniecka Z, Fuglsang-Frederiksen A, Trojaborg W. Benign congenital muscular dystrophy with autosomal dominant heredity; problems of classification. J Neurol 1987; 234: 146–151.

Schmid PC. Beitrag zum Krankheitsbild der infantilen progressiven spinalen Muskelatrophie nach Werdnig–Hoffmann. Z Kinderheilk 1958; 81: 13–25.

Schmitt HP. Involvement of the larynx in a congenital myopathy, unilateral aplasia of the arytenoid, micrognathia and malformation of the brain – a new syndrome? Virchow's Arch A Pathol Anat Histol 1978; 381: 85–96.

Schneider H. Die atonisch-sklerotische Muskeldystrophie (Ullrich) im Rahmen mesodermalen Dysplasien. Z Orthop 1957; 88: 397–404.

Schochet SS Jr. Congenital muscular dystrophy. In: Schochet SS Jr, ed. Diagnostic pathology of skeletal muscle and nerve. Norwalk, CT: Appleton-Century-Crofts, 1986: 94–95.

Schuierer G, Kurlemann G, Lengerke H-J v. Neuroimaging in lissencephalies. Childs Nerv Syst 1993; 9: 391–393.

Segawa M. Clinical studies of congenital muscular dystrophy (arthrogrypotic type congenital muscular dystrophy with mental retardation and facial muscle involvement) (in Japanese). No To Hattatsu (Brain Dev) (Tokyo) 1970; 2(4): 439–451.

Segawa M. Histological, histochemical and electron microscopical studies of biopsied muscle of congenital muscular dystrophy (arthrogrypotic type congenital muscular dystrophy with mental retardation and facial muscle involvement) (in Japanese). No To Hattatsu (Brain Dev) (Tokyo) 1971; 3(1): 21–36.

Segawa M, Mizuno Y, Itoh K, Uono M. Neuropathic and myopathic arthrogryposis multiplex congenita. In: Kakulas BA, ed. Clinical studies in myology. Amsterdam: Excerpta Medica, 1973: 283–301.

Segawa M. Congenital muscular dystrophy (in Japanese). Shinkei Naika (Neurol Med) (Tokyo) 1975; 3: 199–208.

Segawa M. Congenital muscular dystrophy (in Japanese). Shinkei Kenkyu No Shinpo (Adv Neurol Sci) (Tokyo) 1976; 20: 68–80.

Segawa M, Nomura Y, Mizuno Y, Hosaka A, Hachimori K. Studies on pathogenesis of Fukuyama type congenital muscular dystrophy, Part 1. In: Okinaka S, ed. Current research in muscular dystrophy, Japan. The proceedings of the annual meeting of muscular dystrophy research group, 1977. Tokyo, 1978: 114–115.

Segawa M, Nomura Y, Hosaka A, Yamori K, Hara Y. Pathogenesis of Fukuyama type congenital muscular dystrophy (in Japanese). In: Okinaka S, ed. The 1977 annual report of the research committee on the pathogenesis of progressive muscular dystrophy, sponsored by the Ministry of Health and Welfare of Japan. Tokyo, 1978: 285–286.

Segawa M, Nomura Y, Hachimori N, Hosaka A, Mizuno A. Fukuyama type congenital muscular dystrophy as a natural model of childhood epilepsy. Brain Dev (Tokyo) 1979; 1: 113–120.

Segawa M, Nomura Y, Ogiso M, Shinomiya N, Honda K, Yoshihara S, Kinoshita M. Steroid therapy on Fukuyama type congenital muscular dystrophy is effective on the CNS pathology (abstract). Brain Dev (Tokyo) 1982; 4: 301.

Seidahmed MZ, Sunada Y, Ozo CO, Hamid F, Campbell KP, Salih MAM. Lethal congenital muscular dystrophy in two sibs with arthrogryposis multiplex: new entity or variant of cobblestone lissencephaly syndrome? Neuropediatrics 1996; 27: 305–310.

Serratrice G, Cros D, Pellissier J-F, Gastaut J-L, Pouget J. Dystrophie musculaire congénitale. Rev Neurol 1980; 136: 445–472.

Serratrice G, Pellissier JF. Une dystrophie musculaire oubliée: la maladie d'Ullrich. Rev Neurol 1983; 139: 523–525.

Sewry CA, Topaloğlu H, Dubowitz V. Myosin isoforms in congenital muscular dystrophy (abstract). Abstract No 264, 6th Congress of the International Child Neurology Association, Buenos Aires, 1992.

Sewry CA, Philpot J, Mahony D, Wilson LA, Muntoni F, Dubowitz V. Expression of laminin subunits in congenital muscular dystrophy. Neuromusc Disord 1995; 5(4): 307–316.

Sewry CA, Chevallay M, Tomé FMS. Expression of laminin subunits in human fetal skeletal muscle. Histochem J 1995; 27: 497–504.

Sewry CA, Philpot J, Sorokin LM, Wilson LA, Naom I, Goodwin F, D'Alessandro M, Dubowitz V, Muntoni F. Diagnosis of merosin (laminin-2) deficient congenital muscular dystrophy by skin biopsy. Lancet 1996; 347(9001): 582–584.

Sewry CA, D'Alessandro M, Ferlini A, Naom I, Dubowitz V, Muntoni F. Expression of laminin chains in skin in congenital muscular dystrophy (abstract). Neuromusc Disord 1996; Suppl: S26.

Sewry CA, Naom I, D'Alessandra M, Ferlini A, Bruno S, Dubowitz V, Muntoni F. Differential expression of the $\alpha2$ chain of laminin-2 (merosin) using two antibodies in patients with congenital muscular dystrophy (abstract). Neuromusc Disord 1996; Suppl: S19.

Sher JH. Congenital muscular dystrophy. In: Adachi M, Sher JH, eds. Neuromuscular disease. Tokyo: Igaku Shoin, 1990: 137–138.

Shevell M, Rosenblatt B, Silver K, Carpenter S, Karpati G. Congenital inflammatory myopathy. Neurology 1990; 40: 1111–1114.

Shevell MI, Rosenblatt B, Silver K. Inflammatory myopathy and Walker–Warburg syndrome – etiologic implications. Can J Neurol Sci 1993; 20: 227–229.

Shibuya O, Morooka K, Yasaka A. A female case of congenital muscular dystrophy associated with the West syndrome (in Japanese). Shonika Shinryo (J Pediatr Pract) (Tokyo) 1977; 30: 1701–1704.

Shimizu T, Sunada Y, Matsumura K, Saito S, Allamand V, Campbell KP, Salik MAM. Laminin $\alpha2$ chain deficiency associated with in-frame deletion (abstract in Japanese). In:

Takagi A, chairman. Abstracts for the 1996 annual meeting of the research committee on pathogenesis and treatment of progressive muscular dystrophy and related disorders, sponsored by the Ministry of Health and Welfare of Japan. Tokyo, 1996: 16.

Shinoda M, Jo M, Tachi N, Yoshimura H, Nagaoka M, Annaka T, Sato T, Fujuta M. An autopsy case of congenital muscular dystrophy (in Japanese). In: Sobue I, ed. The 1978 annual report of the research committee on clinics, epidemiology and management of progressive muscular dystrophy, sponsored by the Ministry of Health and Welfare of Japan. Nagoya, 1979: 235–237.

Shinoda M, Jo M, Nagaoka M, Fujita M, Sato T, Shinoda M. Three autopsy cases of congenital muscular dystrophy (Fukuyama type) (in Japanese). In: Sobue I, ed. The 1980 annual report of the research committee on clinics, epidemiology and management of progressive muscular dystrophy, sponsored by the Ministry of Health and Welfare of Japan. Nagoya, 1981: 308–313.

Shinoda M, Sasaki K, Onuma M, Nagaoka M, Nakamura N. Brain pathology of congenital muscular dystrophy – on cases with Fukuyama type congenital muscular dystrophy and Ullrich disease (in Japanese). In: Sobue I, ed. The 1982 annual report of the research committee on clinics, epidemiology and management of progressive muscular dystrophy, sponsored by the Ministry of Health and Welfare of Japan. Nagoya, 1983: 393–401.

Shinoda M, Sasaki K, Nagaoka M, Nakane K. Morphological and histological study of the tongue in muscular dystrophies (in Japanese). In: Sobue I, ed. The 1983 annual report of the research committee on clinics, epidemiology and management of progressive muscular dystrophy, sponsored by the Ministry of Health and Welfare of Japan. Nagoya, 1984: 434–441.

Shinoda M, Okuyama M, Kato K, Ueno I, Sasada H. Guidance for language comprehension in congenital muscular dystrophy children (in Japanese). In: Inoue M, ed. The 1983 annual report of the research committee on comprehensive study of nursing care of progressive muscular dystrophy, sponsored by the Ministry of Health and Welfare of Japan. 1984: 57–59.

Shinoda M, Nagaoka M, Wakai S, Nakane K, Amemiya Y. On tongue hypertrophy in Duchenne muscular dystrophy and congenital muscular dystrophy – relation between tongue hypertrophy and oral cavity morphology (in Japanese). In: Nishitani H, ed. The 1984 annual report of the research committee on genetics, epidemiology, clinics and treatment of progressive muscular dystrophy, sponsored by the Ministry of Health and Welfare of Japan. Kyoto, 1985: 25–29.

Shinoda M, Fujita M. Brain pathology in Fukuyama type congenital muscular dystrophy (in Japanese). In: Sobue I, Nishitani H, eds. Clinics of muscular dystrophies. Tokyo: Ishiyaku Shuppan, 1985: 79–82.

Shiraishi H, Okajima S, Hattori T, Sawada H, Ota Y, Nanbu H, Zenimaru T, Yamada K, Kashiwamura M. A case of Walker–Warburg syndrome (in Japanese). Rinsho Shoni Igaku (J Clin Pediatr) (Sapporo) 1994; 42(5): 232–233.

Shishikura K, Osawa M, Hirayama Y, Saito K, Okada H, Hayashi K, Fukuyama Y, Toyoda C, Kaneda Y, Inui M. A clinico-pathological study of congenital progressive muscular dystrophy (Fukuyama type) (in Japanese). Nihon Shonika Gakkai Zasshi (J Jpn Pediatr Soc) (Tokyo) 1988; 92(2): 215–224.

Shorer Z, Philpot J, Muntoni F, Sewry C, Dubowitz V. Demyelinating peripheral neuropathy in merosin-deficient congenital muscular dystrophy. J Child Neurol 1995; 10: 472–475.

Short JK. Congenital muscular dystrophy. A case report with autopsy findings. Neurology 1963; 13: 526–530.

Shu S, Cruse RP, Redmond GP. Hypoglycemia in a child with congenital muscular dystrophy. Brain Dev (Tokyo) 1989; 11: 62–65.

Silberberg M. Über die pathologische Anatomie der Myatonia congenita und die Muskeldystrophien im allgemeinen. Arch Pathol Anat Physiol 1923; 242: 42–57.

Silvestri T. Contributo allo studio della "Myatonia congenita" (malatteo di Oppenheim). Gazz Osp Clin 1909; 30: 577.

Simma B, Felber S, Maurer H, Gassner I, Krassnitzer S. MR and ultrasound findings in a case of cerebro-oculo-muscular-syndrome. Paediatr Radiol 1990; 20: 554–555.

Simonati A, Colamaria V, Federico A, Padovani GM, Rizzuto N. Cellular pathology of lissencephaly (abstract). Childs Nerv Syst 1993; 9: 124.

Smit LME, van Diik EI, Veldman H, Valk J. Congenital muscular dystrophy with white matter involvement; clinical, histological and MRI study (abstract). J Neurol Sci 1990; 98(Suppl): 437.

Smith SA, Mendelsohn NJ, Kriel RL. Walker–Warburg syndrome (abstract). J Child Neurol 1997; 17(2): 133.

Sobue I, Mukoyama M, Kumagai T, Negoro T, Iwase K. Brain CT scannings and brain pathology in Fukuyama type congenital muscular dystrophy (in Japanese). In: Okinaka S, ed. The 1977 annual report of the research committee on the pathogenesis of progressive muscular dystrophy, sponsored by the Ministry of Health and Welfare of Japan. Tokyo, 1978: 227–230.

Socol ML, Sabbagha RE, Elias S, Tamura RK, Simpson JL, Dooley SL, Depp R. Prenatal diagnosis of congenital muscular dystrophy producing arthrogryposis (correspondence). N Engl J Med 1985; 313: 1230.

Solish GI, Trisarnsri O. Autosomal recessive lissencephaly presenting with hydrocephalus. Birth Defects Conference. Chicago, 1979.

Sombekke BHF, Molenaar WM, van Essen AJ, Shoots CJF. Lethal congenital muscular dystrophy with arthrogryposis multiplex congenita. Three new cases and review of the literature. Pediatr Pathol 1994; 14: 277–285.

Sperner J, Stoltenburg CG. Migration disturbances in cerebral and cerebellar cortex and in retina as a salient feature of cerebro-oculo-muscular syndrome (COMS) (abstract). Childs Nerv Syst 1993; 9: 124.

Squarzoni S, Villanova M, Sabatelli P, Malandrini A, Toti P, Pini A. Intracellular detection of laminin $\alpha2$ chain in skin by electron microscopy immunocytochemistry: comparison between normal and laminin $\alpha2$ chain deficient subjects. Neuromusc Disord 1997; 7(2): 91–98.

Squier MV. Fetal type II lissencephaly: a case report. Childs Nerv Syst 1993; 9: 400–402.

Squier MV. Development of the cortical dysplasia of type II lissencephaly. Neuropathol Appl Neurobiol 1993; 19: 209–213.

Steinbrecher I, Stoltenburg-Diginger G. Developmental and migration disorders in lissencephaly type II (abstract). Clin Neuropathol 1995; 14(5): 288.

Stern LM, Albertyn L, Manson JI. Fukuyama congenital muscular dystrophy in two Australian female siblings. Dev Med Child Neurol 1990; 32: 808–813.

Stoeber E. Über atonisch-sklerotische Muskeldystrophie (Typ Ullrich). Z Kinderheilk 1930; 60: 279–284.

Storm RI, PeBenito R. Autosomal recessive lissencephaly presenting with hydrocephalus. Ann Ophthalmol 1984; 16: 988–992.

Streib EW, Lücking CH. Congenital muscular dystrophy with leukoencephalopathy. Eur Neurol 1989; 29: 211–215.

Stripathi N, Karpati G, Carpenter S. A distinctive type of infantile inflammatory myopathy with abnormal myonuclei. J Neurol Sci 1996; 136: 47–53.

Sugie H, Verity MA. A case of congenital muscular dystrophy with severe mental retardation and congenital glaucoma (abstract). Abstracts for the 5th International Congress of Neuromuscular Disease, Marseille, 1982.

Sugino S, Miyatake M, Ohtani Y, Yoshioka K, Miike T, Uchino M. Vascular alterations in Fukuyama type congenital muscular dystrophy. Brain Dev (Tokyo) 1991; 13: 77–81.

Sugita H, Arahata K, Tsukahara T, Ishiura S. Immunohistochemistry of dystrophin in various neuromuscular diseases. In: Kakulas BA, Mastaglia FL, eds. Pathogenesis and therapy of Duchenne and Becker muscular dystrophy. New York: Raven Press, 1990: 33–40.

Sugita H, Hayashi YK, Arikawa-Hirasawa E, Nonaka I, Arahata K. The molecular pathogenesis of Fukuyama type congenital muscular dystrophy. Acta Cardiomiol 1995; 7(1): 3–9.

Sumida S, Osawa M, Okada N, Kawai M, Arai Y, Hirasawa K, Shishikura K, Suzuki H, Hirayama Y, Fukuyama Y, Kono A, Miyake Y. Muscle CT findings in patients with Fukuyama type congenital muscular dystrophy (FCMD) (in Japanese). Nihon Shonika Gakkai Zasshi (J Jpn Pediatr Soc) (Tokyo) 1988; 92(11): 2389–2397.

Sumida S, Osawa M, Ikenaka H, Murasugi H, Hirasawa K, Arai Y, Shishikura K, Suzuki H, Hirayama Y, Fukuyama Y. Dermatoglyphic findings in children with congenital muscular dystrophy (in Japanese). Tokyo Joshi Ikadaigaku Zasshi (J Tokyo Wom Med Coll) (Tokyo) 1992; 62: 1197–1200.

Sumida S, Osawa M, Arai Y, Murasugi H, Suzuki N, Hirasawa K, Suzuki H, Hirayama Y, Saito K, Fukuyama Y. Clinical and electroencephalographic study on seizures in congenital muscular dystrophy (in Japanese). Tokyo Joshi Ikadaigaku Zasshi (J Tokyo Wom Med Coll) (Tokyo) 1993; 63: S36–S42.

Sumida S, Osawa M, Arai Y, Suzuki N, Shishikura K, Suzuki Y, Hirayama K, Saito K, Fukuyama Y. Congenital malformations other than central nervous system and ocular findings in Fukuyama type congenital muscular dystrophy. In: Fukuyama Y, Osawa M, eds. Program and abstracts of the International Symposium on Congenital Muscular Dystrophies, Tokyo. Tokyo: Tokyo Women's Medical College, 1994: 34.

Sunada Y, Bernier SM, Kozak CA, Yamada Y, Campbell KP. Deficiency of merosin in dystrophic dy mice and genetic linkage of laminin M chain gene to dy locus. J Biol Chem 1994; 269: 13729–13732.

Sunada Y, Bernier SM, Utani A, Yamada Y, Campbell KP. Identification of a novel mutant transcript of laminin α2 chain gene responsible for muscular dystrophy and dysmyelination in dy/dy mice. Hum Mol Genet 1995; 4(6): 1055–1061.

Sunada Y, Campbell KP. Dystrophin-glycoprotein complex: molecular organization and critical roles in skeletal muscle. Curr Opin Neurol 1995; 8: 379–384.

Sunada Y, Edgar TS, Lotz BP, Rust RS, Campbell KP. Merosin-negative congenital muscular dystrophy associated with extensive brain abnormalities. Neurology 1995; 45: 2084–2089.

Suzuki H. Histochemical study of biopsied muscle in floppy infant syndrome with special emphasis on the role of central neural influence in the pathogenesis (in Japanese). Nihon Shonika Gakkai Zasshi (J Jpn Pediatr Soc) (Tokyo) 1974; 78: 345–360.

Suzuki H, Osawa M, Shishikura K, Hirayama Y, Kawai M, Fukuyama Y. Histological changes of skeletal muscles in congenital muscular dystrophy of Fukuyama type (in Japanese). Nihon Shonika Gakkai Zasshi (J Jpn Pediatr Soc) (Tokyo) 1984; 88: 1763–1774.

Suzuki Y, Ueda S, Segawa M, Funayama M. A study of rehabilitation for CMD. Report 2. On articulation and speech (abstract in Japanese). Rehabilitation Igaku (Rehabilitation Med) (Tokyo) 1970; 7: 54–55.

Swaiman KF, Smith SA. Congenital muscular dystrophy. In: Swaiman KF, ed. Pediatric neurology. Principles and practice, 2nd edn, Vol II. St Louis/Baltimore/Toronto: CV Mosby, 1994: 1497–1498.

Swash M, Schwartz MS. Congenital muscular dystrophy. In: Swash M, Schwartz MS, eds. Biopsy pathology of muscle. London: Chapman and Hall, 1984; 130.

Tachi N, Tachi M, Sasaki K, Tanabe C, Minagawa M. Walker–Warburg syndrome in a Japanese patient. Pediatr Neurol 1988; 4: 236–240.

Tachi N, Tachi M, Sasaki K, Minagawa K, Tanabe C, Yamazaki H. Electroencephalographic findings of Walker–Warburg syndrome (in Japanese). Rinsho Shoni Igaku (J Clin Pediatr) (Sapporo) 1988; 36: 257–26l.

Tachi N, Nagata N, Wakai S, Chiba S. Congenital muscular dystrophy in Marinesco-Sjögren syndrome. Pediatr Neurol 1991; 7: 296–298.

Tachi N, Kozuka N, Ohya K, Chiba S, Matsuo M, Patria SY, Matsumura K. Deficiency of syntrophin, dystroglycan and merosin in a female infant with a congenital muscular dystrophy phenotype lacking cysteine-rich and C-terminal domains of dystrophin (abstract No. 1665). Am J Hum Genet 1996; 59(Suppl): a287.

Takada K, Nakamura H, Tanaka J. Cortical dysplasia in congenital muscular dystrophy with central nervous system involvement (Fukuyama type). J Neuropathol Exp Neurol 1984; 43: 395–407.

Takada K, Takashima S, Tanaka J. Is the Walker–Warburg syndrome a severe form of Fukuyama type congenital muscular dystrophy? (in Japanese). No To Hattatsu (Brain Dev) (Tokyo) 1985; 17: 269–271.

Takada K, Tanaka J. Cerebral cortical dysplasia. Some considerations of its morphogenesis as to the vascular architecture (abstract). Brain Dev (Tokyo) 1986; 8: 131.

Takada K, Kasagi S. Rin Y-S, Nakamura H. Fukuyama type congenital muscular dystrophy: Neurofibrillary changes in the locus ceruleus and nucleus basalis of Meynert in patients with a long survival (in Japanese). Shinkei Naika (Neurol Med) 1986; 25(4): 418–420.

Takada K, Rin Y-S, Kasagi S, Sato K, Nakamura H, Tanaka J. Long survival in Fukuyama congenital muscular dystrophy: occurrence of neurofibrillary tangles in the nucleus basalis of Meynert and locus ceruleus. Acta Neuropathol 1986; 71: 228–232.

Takada K, Becker LE, Takashima S. Walker–Warburg syndrome with skeletal muscle involvement. A report of three patients. Pediatr Neurosci 1987; 13: 202–209.

Takada K, Nakamura H, Suzumori K, Ishikawa T, Sugiyama N. Cortical dysplasia in a 23-week fetus with Fukuyama congenital muscular dystrophy (FCMD). Acta Neuropathol (Berlin) 1987; 74: 300–306.

Takada K. Fukuyama congenital muscular dystrophy as a unique disorder of neuronal migration: a neuropathological review and hypothesis. Yonago Acta Med (Yonago) 1988; 31: 1–16.

Takada K. Micropolygyria (in Japanese). Clin Neurosci (Tokyo) 1988; 6: 950–951.

Takada K, Nakamura H, Takashima S. Cortical dysplasia in Fukuyama congenital muscular dystrophy (FCMD): a Golgi and angioarchitectonic analysis. Acta Neuropathol 1988; 76; 170–178.

Takada K, Nakamura H. Cerebellar micropolygyria in Fukuyama congenital muscular dystrophy: Observations in fetal and pediatric cases. Brain Dev (Tokyo) 1990; 12: 774–778.

Takada K. Fukuyama-type congenital muscular dystrophy and the Walker–Walburg syndrome. Commentary to Kimura's paper. Brain Dev (Tokyo) 1993; 15: 244–245.

Takada K. Early appearance of Alzheimer neurofibrillary changes in brains with developmental disturbances (abstract in Japanese). Abstracts for the 34th annual meeting of the Japanese Society of Neuropathology. Tama-city, Tokyo, 1993: 20.

Takada K, Morimatsu Y, Arai N, Nakayama H, Oda M, Ohama E. Precocious appearance of Alzheimer's neurofibrillary tangles (NFT) in Fukuyama congenital muscular dystrophy (FCMD): a reappraisal (abstract). Brain Pathol 1994; 4: 578.

Takahashi T, Miyazaki Z, Sakaguchi M, Shimano O. A case of congenital muscular dystrophy presenting respiratory failure at birth (abstract in Japanese). Gunma Shonika Iho (Gunma Pediatrics Bull) (Maebashi) 1987; 108: 3.

Takanashi J, Uetani K, Iai M, Sugita K, Tanabe Y. A case of Fukuyama type congenital muscular dystrophy – brain MRI findings in pre-clinical stage (in Japanese). No To Hattatsu (Brain Dev) (Tokyo) 1989; 21: 588–589.

Takashima S, Becker LE, Chan F, Takada K. A Golgi study of the cerebral cortex in Fukuyama-type congenital muscular dystrophy, Walker-type "lissencephaly", and classical lissencephaly. Brain Dev (Tokyo) 1987; 9: 621–626.

Takashima S, Mito T. Lissencephalies (in Japanese) (photo). Clin Neurosci (Tokyo) 1989; 7.

Takayanagi T, Horikawa H, Konagaya M, Mano Y, Konishi T. Evaluation of CNS lesions in congenital muscular dystrophy patients with cranial X-ray CT and MRI (in Japanese). In: Nishitani H, ed. The 1987 annual report of the research committee on genetics, epidemiology, clinics and treatment of progressive muscular dystrophy, sponsored by the Ministry of Health and Welfare of Japan. Kyoto, 1988: 104–108.

Takayanagi T, Yanagimoto S, Mano Y, Iida M. Evoked potential study of diaphragm in muscular dystrophies (in Japanese). In: Nishitani H, ed. The 1989 annual report of the research committee on genetics, epidemiology, clinics and treatment of progressive muscular dystrophy, sponsored by the Ministry of Health and Welfare of Japan. Kyoto, 1990: 191–199.

Takazawa N, Watanabe K, Ayuzawa H, and 19 collaborators. A trial of improving toilet apparatuses for congenital muscular dystrophy patients (in Japanese). In: Inoue M, ed. The 1980 annual report of the research committee on comprehensive nursing care of progressive muscular dystrophy, sponsored by the Ministry of Health and Welfare of Japan. 1981: 290–292.

Takeda H, Fukui M, Kuroda K. Emotional stability in congenital muscular dystrophy children (in Japanese). In: Aoyagi A, ed. The 1985 annual report of the research committee on clinical and psychological study of care and nursing of progressive muscular dystrophies, sponsored by the Ministry of Health and Welfare of Japan. 1986: 33–39.

Takeshita K, Yoshino K, Kitahara T, Nakashima T, Kato N. Survey of Duchenne type and congenital type of muscular dystrophy in Shimane, Japan. Jpn J Hum Genet (Tokyo) 1977; 22: 43–47.

Takeshita K, Eda I. Cerebral lipid analysis in congenital muscular dystrophy (Fukuyama type). In: Fukuyama Y, ed. The 1983 annual report of the research committee on the cause and treatment of prenatal brain damage sponsored by the Ministry of Health and Welfare of Japan. Tokyo, 1983: 210–212.

Takeuchi S, Kajio M, Otsuka M, Higashio Y, Nagamatsu K, Matsumuro K, Kajima N, Osawa M, Umehara F. Two cases of congenital muscular dystrophy presented high serum CK values and muscle hypertonia in the neonatal period and diagnosed by muscle biopsy findings (in Japanese). Oita Kenritsu Byoin Igaku Zasshi (J Oita Prefect Hosp) (Oita) 1987; 16: 102–105.

Tamari H, Miike T, Miyoshino S, Nagatomi H. On cranial CT findings in congenital muscular dystrophy (in Japanese). Shoni Naika (Jpn J Pediatr Med) 1978; 10: 1038–1039.

Tamari H, Otani Y, Origuchi Y, Takagi T, Matsuda Y, Nonaka I, Miike T, Matsukura M, Miyoshino S. A case of Ullrich syndrome with congenital fibre type disproportion (in Japanese). No to Hattatsu (Brain Dev) (Tokyo) 1982; l4: 586–590.

Tan E, Topaloğlu H, Sewry C, Zorlu Y, Naom I, Erdem S, D'Allessandro M, Muntoni F, Dubowitz V. Late onset muscular dystrophy with cerebral white matter changes due to partial merosin deficiency. Neuromusc Disord 1997; 7: 85–89.

Tanabe H. Muscle biopsy in muscular dystrophies (in Japanese). Shinkei Naika (Neurol Med) (Tokyo) 1975; 3: 209–212.

Tanabe H, Nozawa T, Uchigata M, Shiozawa R, Hara M. Characteristic muscle changes in the respective form of muscular dystrophies (in Japanese). In: Miyoshi K, ed. The 1978 annual report of the research committee on clinical study on pathogenesis of progressive muscular dystrophy, sponsored by the Ministry of Health and Welfare of Japan. Tokushima, 1979: 97–101.

Tanabe H, Mizuno Y. Immunohistochemical study of extracellular matrix in Fukuyama type congenital muscular dystrophy (in Japanese). In: Takagi A, ed. The 1993 annual report of the research committee on pathogenesis and treatment of progressive muscular dystrophy and related disorders, sponsored by the Ministry of Health and Welfare of Japan. Tokyo, 1994: 35–37.

Tanaka J, Takada K, Nakamura H. Ectopic myelinated fiber bundles on cerebellar surface in Fukuyama type congenital muscular dystrophy (in Japanese). In: Fukuyama Y, ed. The 1982 annual report of the research committee on the cause and treatment of prenatal brain damage, sponsored by the Ministry of Health and Welfare of Japan. Tokyo, 1983: 169–172.

Tanaka J, Takada K, Kasagi S, Rin Y-S. Two autopsy cases of Fukuyama type congenital muscular dystrophy with long survival – with particular reference to neurofibrillary changes in Meynert nuclei and locus ceruleus (in Japanese). In: Kamoshita S, ed. The 1985 annual report of the research committee on the pathogenesis and prevention of mental retardation due to injuries of developing brain, sponsored by the Ministry of Health and Welfare of Japan. Tokyo, 1986: 167–170.

Tanaka J, Mimaki T, Okada S, Fujimura H. Changes in cerebral white matter in a case of congenital muscular dystrophy (non-Fukuyama type). Neuropediatrics 1990; 21: 183–186.

Tanaka K, Takeshita K, Takita M. Analysis of serum bile acids in various neuromuscular disorders (abstract in Japanese). Rinsho Shinkeigaku (Clin Neurol) (Tokyo) 1983; 23: 1194.

Tanaka S. A case of FCMD in which cerebral dysplasia was not verified on brain MRI (abstract in Japanese). Abstracts for the First Zao Seminar, Yamagata, 1996.

Tani J, Kagawa T, Shirakami K. Survey of current status of progressive muscular dystrophy patients at home in the Osaka area (in Japanese). In: Sobue I, ed. The 1978 annual report of the research committee on clinics, epidemiology and management of progressive muscular dystrophy, sponsored by the Ministry of Health and Welfare of Japan. Nagoya, 1979: 45–48.

Tanimura R. Ultrastructural study of skeletal muscle in floppy infant syndrome – with special emphasis on the cases of central nervous disorders with marked hypotonia (in Japanese). Nihon Shonika Gakkai Zasshi (J Jpn Pediatr Soc) (Tokyo) 1974; 78: 470–480.

Tatsuno M, Iwamoto H, Misugi N. A case of intrauterine infection with myopathy (abstract). Brain Dev (Tokyo) 1983; 5: 207.

Terasawa K. Muscle regeneration and satellite cells in Fukuyama type congenital muscular dystrophy. Muscle Nerve 1986; 9: 465–470.

Thieffry S, Arthuis M, Bargeton E. Quarante cas de maladie de Werdnig–Hoffmann avec onze examens anatomiques. Rev Neurol 1955; 93: 621–644.

Thompson CE. Infantile myositis. Dev Med Child Neurol 1982; 24: 307–313.

Toda T, Matsumura K, Watanabe T. Three-dimensional cerebral surface MRI of malformed brains in Fukuyama type congenital muscular dystrophy (in Japanese). No To Hattatsu (Brain Dev) (Tokyo) 1991; 23: 106–109.

Toda T, Watanabe T, Matsumura K, Shimizu T, Iwata M, Kanazawa I. Three-dimensional brain-surface MR images of brain anomalies in Fukuyama type congenital muscular dystrophy and its differentiation from Duchenne muscular dystrophy with severe mental retardation (in Japanese). CI Kenkyu (Prog Comput Imaging) (Tokyo) 1993; 15(2): 147–157.

Toda T. Three-dimensional brain-surface MRI in Fukuyama type congenital muscular dystrophy (in Japanese). Annual Review – Neurology 1993. Tokyo: Chugai Igakusha, 1993: 373–380.

Toda T, Segawa M, Nomura Y, Nonaka I, Masuda E, Ishihara T, Suzuki M, Tomita I, Origuchi Y, Ohno K, Misugi N, Sasaki Y, Takada K, Kawai M, Ohtani K, Murakami T, Saito K, Fukuyama Y, Shimizu T, Kanazawa I, Nakamura Y. Localization of a gene for Fukuyama type congenital muscular dystrophy to chromosome 9q 31-33. Nat Genet 1993; 5(3): 283–286.

Toda T, Ikegawa S, Okui K, Kondo E, Saito K, Fukuyama Y, Yoshioka M, Kumagai T, Suzumori K, Kanazawa I, Nakamura Y. Refined mapping of a gene responsible for Fukuyama-type congenital muscular dystrophy: evidence for strong linkage disequilibrium. Am J Hum Genet 1994; 55: 946–950.

Toda T, Kanazawa I, Nakamura Y, Takagi A. Fukuyama type congenital muscular dystrophy gene localizes on 9q31-33 (in Japanese). In: Takagi A, ed. The 1993 annual report of the research committee on pathogenesis and treatment of progressive muscular dystrophy and related disorders, sponsored by the Ministry of Health and Welfare of Japan. Tokyo, 1994: 58–61.

Toda T, Yoshioka M, Nakahori Y, Kanazawa I, Nakamura Y, Nakagome Y. Genetic identity of Fukuyama type congenital muscular dystrophy and Walker–Warburg syndrome. Ann Neurol 1995; 37(1): 99–101.

Toda T, Watanabe T, Matsumura K, Sunada Y, Yamada H, Nakano I, Mannen T, Kanazawa I, Shimizu T. Three dimensional MR imaging of brain surface anomalies in Fukuyama-type congenital muscular dystrophy. Muscle Nerve 1995; 18(5): 508–517.

Toda T, Miyake Y, Mizuno K, Nakagome Y, Nakahori Y. Linkage disequilibrium mapping of a gene for Fukuyama-type congenital muscular dystrophy (abstract). Jpn J Hum Genet (Tokyo) 1996; 41: 41.

Toda T. Fukuyama type congenital muscular dystrophy (in Japanese). In: Ozawa E, Ishihara T, Kaitani H, Nonaka I, eds. Muscular dystrophy '96. Advances in research. Tokyo: Zenkoku Shinshin Shogaiji Fukushi Zaidan, 1996: 31–35.

Toda T. Fukuyama type congenital muscular dystrophy (in Japanese). In: Nakamura S, ed. Molecular neurology. Tokyo: Nankodo, 1996: 126–128.

Toda T, Kobayashi C, Miyake M, Tokunaga K, Nakahori Y. Analysis of the founder chromosome and an aberrant insertion in FCMD gene (abstract in Japanese). In: Takagi A, chairman. Abstracts for the 1996 annual meeting of the research committee on pathogenesis and treatment of progressive muscular dystrophy and related disorders, sponsored by the Ministry of Health and Welfare of Japan. Tokyo, 1996: 1.

Toda T, Miyake M, Kobayashi K, Mizuno K, Saito K, Osawa M, Nakamura Y, Kanazawa I, Nakagome Y, Tokunaga K, Nakahori Y. Linkage disequilibrium mapping narrows the Fukuyama-type congenital muscular dystrophy (FCMD) candidate region to <100 kb. Am J Hum Genet 1996; 59: 1313–1320.

Toda T, Miyake M, Mizuno K, Kobayashi C, Matsushita I, Hirai M, Tokunaga K, Nakahori Y. Positional cloning of the FCMD gene (in Japanese). In: Takagi A, ed. The 1995 annual report of the research committee on pathogenesis and treatment of progressive muscular dystrophy and related disorders, sponsored by the Ministry of Health and Welfare of Japan. Tokyo, 1996: 77–79.

Toda T. Toward identification of the Fukuyama-type congenital muscular dystrophy (FCMD) gene. In: Ozawa E, Takeda S, eds. Molecular biology of muscular dystrophy. Proceedings of International Workshop between Japan and France held at Toranomon Pastoral, Tokyo, 1996. Kodaira: NCNP, 1997: 113–118.

Tokuomi H, Hirase T, Kawasaki S, Yamada T, Hamazaki Y, Ikeya Y, Yamanaga Y, Antoku T. A study on CSF proteins in muscular dystrophies (in Japanese). In: Sobue I, ed. The 1981 annual report of the research committee on clinics, epidemiology and management of progressive muscular dystrophy, sponsored by the Ministry of Health and Welfare of Japan. Nagoya, 1982: 247–250.

Tomé FMS, Evangelista T, Leclerc A, Sunada Y, Manole E, Estournet B, Barois A, Campbell KP, Fardeau M. Congenital muscular dystrophy with merosin deficiency. C R Acad Sci Paris/Sci Vie, 1994; 317: 351–357.

Tomé FMS, Helbling-Leclerc A, Guicheney P, Fardeau M. Abnormal proteins in congenital muscular dystrophies (abstract). Neuromusc Disord 1996; 6(2): S17.

Tomé FMS. Merosinopathies. In: Ozawa E, Takeda S, eds. Molecular biology of muscular dystrophy. Proceedings of International Workshop between Japan and France held at Toranomon Pastoral, Tokyo, 1996. Kodaira: NCNP, 1997: 119–129.

Topaloğlu H, Yalaz K, Renda Y, Kale G, Çağlar M, Göğüs S. Congenital muscular dystrophy (non-Fukuyama type) in Turkey: a clinical and pathological evaluation. Brain Dev (Tokyo) 1989; 11: 341–344.

Topaloğlu H, Renda Y, Yalaz K, Gücüyener K, Çağlar M, Göğüs S, Kale G. Classification of congenital muscular dystrophy (correspondence). J Pediatr 1990; 117: 116.

Topaloğlu H, Yalaz K, Kale G, Ergin M. Congenital muscular dystrophy with cerebral involvement – report of a case of "occidental-type cerebromuscular dystrophy"? Neuropediatrics 1990; 21: 53–54.

Topaloğlu H, Yalaz K, Renda Y, Çağlar M, Göğüs S, Kale G, Gücüyener K, Nurlu G. Occidental type cerebromuscular dystrophy: a report of eleven cases. J Neurol Neurosurg Psychiatry 1991; 54: 226–229.

428

Topaloğlu H, Gücüyener K, Yalaz K, Renda Y, Topçu M, Aysun S, Özdirim E, Anlar B. Selective involvement of the quadriceps muscle in congenital muscular dystrophy: an ultrasonographic study. Brain Dev (Tokyo) 1992; 14: 84–87.

Topaloğlu H, Kale G, Yalnizoğlu D, Tasdemir AB, Karaduman A, Topçu M, Kotiloğlu E. Analysis of "pure" congenital muscular dystrophies in thirty-eight cases. How different is the classical type I from the occidental type cerebromuscular dystrophy? Neuropediatrics 1994; 25(2): 94–100.

Topaloğlu H, Cila A, Tasdemir AB, Saatçi I. Congenital muscular dystrophy with eye and brain involvement. The Turkish experience in two cases. Brain Dev 1995; 17(4): 271–275.

Topaloğlu H. Congenital muscular dystrophy (abstract). Abstracts of the 5th Asian and Oceanian Congress of Child Neurology, Istanbul, Turkey, 1996: 22.

Topaloğlu H, Akcoren Z, Gücüyener K, Kale G. Merosin-positive congenital muscular dystrophy (abstract). Abstracts of the 5th Asian and Oceanian Congress of Child Neurology, Istanbul, Turkey, 1996: 54.

Topçu M, Topaloğlu H, Gücüyener K, Aysun S, Serdaroglu A, Renda Y, Yalaz K. Visual and auditory evoked potential studies of occidental type cerebromuscular dystrophy (abstract). Abstract No. 266, 6th Congress of the International Child Neurology Association, Buenos Aires, 1992.

Toscano A, Monici MC, Rodolico C, Parano E, Falsaperla R, Fiumara A, Vita G. Congenital muscular dystrophy: clinical, histological and immunohistochemical features in a group of Sicilian patients (abstract). Neuromusc Disord 1996; Suppl: S27.

Toshimori K, Inoue K, Tsuruda K, Kurihara T. A study of short latency SEP in muscular dystrophies (abstract in Japanese). Rinsho Shinkeigaku (Clin Neurol) (Tokyo) 1983; 23: 1193.

Toti P, De Felice C, Malandrini A, Megha T, Cardone C, Villanova M. Localisation of laminin chains in the human retina: possible implications for congenital muscular dystrophy associated with α2- chain of laminin deficiency. Neuromusc Disord 1997; 7(1):21-25.

Towfighi J, Sassani JW, Suzuki K, Ladda RL. Cerebro-ocular dysplasia-muscular dystrophy (COD-MD) syndrome. Acta Neuropathol (Berlin) 1984; 65: 110–123.

Toyokura Y, Iwata M, Kurisaki H, Iida M. Cerebral cortex in Fukuyama type muscular dystrophy. Angioarchitectonic study of verrucose dysplasia. In: Miyoshi K, ed. The 1978 annual report of the research committee on clinical study on pathogenesis of progressive muscular dystrophy, sponsored by the Ministry of Health and Welfare of Japan. Tokushima, 1979: 117–118.

Trevisan C, Carollo C, Massocchi P, Laverda AM, Giordano R, Angelini C. Central nervous system involvement in congenital muscular dystrophy (abstract). Acta Neurologica (Napoli) 1984; 6: 364.

Trevisan CP, Segalla P, Angelini C, et al. Alterations of central nervous system in the occidental form of congenital muscular dystrophy. India Neurol 1989; 37(Suppl 1): 511D02.

Trevisan CP, Segalla P, Angelini C, Drigo P, Carollo C. Subclinical brain involvement in typical congenital muscular dystrophy (abstract). J Neurol Sci 1990; 98(supplement): 435–436.

Trevisan CP, Carollo C, Segalla P, Angelini C, Drigo P, Giordano R. Congenital muscular dystrophy: brain alterations in an unselected series of Western patients. J Neurol Neurosurg Psychiatry 1991; 54: 330–334.

Trevisan CP, Carollo C, Martinello F, et al. Neuroradiological alterations in classical congenital muscular dystrophy (in Italian). Riv Neuroradiol 1992; 5: 39–42.

Trevisan CP, Martinello F, Ferruzza E, Angelini C. Divergence of central nervous system involvement in 2 Italian sisters with congenital muscular dystrophy: a clinical and neuroradiological follow-up. Eur Neurol 1995; 35(4): 230–235.

Trevisan CP, Martinello F, Fanin M, Pastorello E, Angelini C, Javicoli R. Merosin expression in muscle of Western cases with Fukuyama-like congenital muscular dystrophy (abstract). Neuromusc Disord 1996; Suppl: S21–S22.

Trevisan CP, Martinello F, Fanin M, et al. Merosin expression in muscle of Western cases with Fukuyama-like congenital muscular dystrophy. Basic Appl Myol 1996; 6: 101–106.

Trevisan CP, Martinello F, Ferruzza E, Fanin M, Chevallay M, Tomé FMS. Brain alterations in the classical form of congenital muscular dystrophy. Clinical and neuroimaging follow-up of 12 cases and correlation with the expression of merosin in muscle. Childs Nerv Syst 1996; 12: 604–610.

Tsubura H, Kubo S, Yamashina M, and 8 collaborators. Care of congenital muscular dystrophy children. In: Aoyagi A, ed. The 1984 annual report of the research committee on clinical and psychological study of care and nursing of progressive muscular dystrophy, sponsored by the Ministry of Health and Welfare of Japan. 1985: 28–32.

Tsuji S. A study of myelin deficiency in the central nervous system of mice with genetic muscular dystrophy. In: Tsukada Y, ed. Genetic approaches to developmental neurobiology. Proceedings of the International Symposium on Genetic Approaches to Developmental Neurobiology, Tokyo, 1981. Tokyo: University of Tokyo Press, 1982: 139–152.

Tsukagoshi H, Toyokura M, Sugita H, Murakami S. An autopsy case of Fukuyama type congenital muscular dystrophy. In: Okinaka S, ed. Cumulative articles of the research committee on progressive muscular dystrophy, sponsored by the Ministry of Health and Welfare, (II). Tokyo, 1974: 25–30.

Tsukamoto H, Tanaka J, Okada S. A case of dystrophinopathy clinically resembling Fukuyama type congenital muscular dystrophy (in Japanese). Shonika Rinsho (Jpn J Pediatr) (Tokyo) 1994; 47: 1715–1719.

Tsutsui S, Mizutani A, Nagahara M, Kawamura N, Kumagai T, Natsume K. Four autopsy cases of Fukuyama type congenital muscular dystrophy at Aichi Prefectural Colony for Physical/Mental Handicapped. Annual Report No. 18 of the Institute for Developmental Research, Aichi Prefectural Colony. Kasugai, 1989: 57.

Tsutsumi A, Kameyama K, Uchida Y, Osawa M, Hara M, Fukuyama Y. Ocular fundi findings in congenital muscular dystrophy of the Fukuyama type (in Japanese). Ganka Rinsho Iho (Jpn Rev Clin Ophthalmol) (Tokyo) 1983; 77: 1438–1442.

Tsutsumi A, Uchida Y, Osawa M, Fukuyama Y. Ocular findings in Fukuyama type congenital muscular dystrophy. Brain Dev (Tokyo) 1989; 11: 413–419.

Turner JWA. The relationship between amyotonia congenita and congenital myopathy. Brain 1940; 63: 163–177.

Turner JWA. On amyotonia congenita. Brain 1949; 72: 25–34.

Turner JWA, Lee F. Congenital myopathy, a fifty-year follow-up. Brain 1962; 85: 733–740.

Ueda K. An enzyme-chemical study of myopathies (in Japanese). In: The Japanese Medicine, 1967. Lectures at the 17th General Assembly of the Japanese Association of Medical Sciences, Vol 4. Tokyo: Kanehara Shuppan, 1967: 1044–1053.

Ueda K, Ito T, Matsumoto K, Nakada S, Ohara T, Kishino B, Shimoji T, Inoue A, Nishikawa M. Hypotonic infant. Nihon Rinsho (Jpn J Clin Med) (Osaka) 1968; 26: 3231–3256.

Ueda K. Heredity in congenital muscular dystrophy (genetic diseases on picture series) (in Japanese). Pharmaceutical Review (Tokyo) 1970; 21: 8–9.

Ueda S, Hirakata Y, Tajima Y, Fukuyama Y, Segawa M. A study on rehabilitation of congenital muscular dystrophy. Report 1. Characteristic features of motor disturbances and physical therapy (abstract in Japanese). Rehabilitation Igaku (Rehabilitation Med) (Tokyo) 1970; 7: 53–54.

Ueda S, Eto F. Rehabilitation of the children with neuromuscular disorders (in Japanese). No To Hattatsu (Brain Dev) (Tokyo) 1975; 7: 469–478.

Ueda S, Eto F, Kikuchi N. Rehabilitation of the children with congenital muscular dystrophy (Fukuyama type) (in Japanese). Sogo Rehabilitation (Sogo Rehab) (Tokyo) 1975; 3: 51–64.

Ullrich O. Kongenitale, atonisch-sklerotische Muskeldystrophie. Monatsschr Kinderheilk 1930; 47: 502–510.

Ullrich O. Kongenitale, atonisch-sklerotische Muskeldystrophie, ein weiterer Typus der heredodegenerativen Erkrankungen des neuromuskulären Systems. Z gesamt Neurol Psychiatr 1930; 126: 171–201.

Une K, Nonaka I, Nakashima T. A histological and histochemical study on the biopsied muscle from Ullrich disease (Kongenitale atonisch-sklerotische Muskeldystrophie) (in Japanese). Shonika Shinryo (J Pediatr Pract) (Tokyo) 1979;42: 1415–1418.

Une K, Haraguchi H, Sato C. Two cases of congenital muscular dystrophy (Fukuyama type) with atypical clinical features (in Japanese). Shonika Shinryo (J Pediatr Pract) (Tokyo) 1981; 44: 1919–1923.

Vajsar J, Jay V, Babyn P. Infantile myositis presenting in the neonatal period. Brain Dev 1996; 18(5): 415–419.

Vajsar J, Jay V, Siegel-Bartelt J, Momen A. Heterogeneity in severe form of congenital muscular dystrophy (abstract). Neuromusc Disord 1996; Suppl: S23–S24.

Valanne L, Pihko H, Katevuo K, Karttunen P, Somer H, Santavuori P. MRI of the brain in muscle-eye-brain (MEB) disease. Neuroradiology 1994; 36: 473–476.

Vallat J-M, Vital C, Le Blanc M. Les myopathies congénitales. Bordeaux Méd 1972; 5: 2439–2451.

Van Bogaert L, Bessa JS, Nunes Vicente A. Sur une affection musculaire congénitale à évolution lentement favorable caractérisée par une <cirrhose> musculaire à dépôts protéinique (réticulose musculaire?). Acta Neurol Psychiatr Belg 1962; 62: 973–983.

Van Engelen BGM, Leyten QH, Bernsen PLJA, Gabrëels FJM, Barkhof F, Joosten EMG, Hamel BCJ, Ter Laak HJ, Ruijs MBM, Cruysberg JRM, Valk J. Familial adult onset of muscular dystrophy with leukoencephalopathy. Ann Neurol 1992; 32: 577–580.

Vassella F, Mumenthaler M, Rossi E, Moser H, Wiesmann U. Die kongenitale Muskeldystrophie. Dtsch Z Nervenheilk 1967; 190: 349–374.

Vassella F, Mumenthaler M, Rossi E. Congenital muscular dystrophy. In: Walton JN, Canal N, Scarlato G, eds. Muscle diseases. Proceedings of an International Congress, Milan, 1969. Amsterdam: Excerpta Medica ICS, 1970; 199: 620–623.

Veneselli E, Biancheri R, Celle ME, Guzzetta F. Ferriere G. Congenital muscular dystrophy and epileptic syndromes in infancy and childhood. Gaslini 1995; 27(Suppl 1 al N2): 85–86.

Velin P, Dupont D, Lods F, Gambini L. Le syndrome de Walker–Warburg. Une nouvelle observation. Pédiatrie 1987; 42: 597–601.

Villanova M, Malandrini A, Sabatelli P, Toti P, Squarzoni S, Maraldi NM, Guazzi GC. Localization of merosin in the human skeletal muscle and peripheral nerve by immunogold labelling and electron microscopy (abstract). Neuromusc Disord 1996; Suppl: S22–S23.

Villanova M, Malandrini A, Toti P, Salvestroni R, Six J, Martin JJ, Guazzi GC. Localisation of merosin in the normal human brain: implications for congenital muscular dystrophy with merosin deficiency. J Submicroscop Cytol Pathol 1996; 28: 1–4.

Vilquin J-T, Roy B, Goulet M, Engvall E, Tóme FMS, Fardeau M, Tremblay JP. *In vivo* laminin-2 α2 chain restoration by muscle cell transplantations in dystrophic (*dy/dy*) mouse (abstract). Neuromusc Disord 1996; Suppl: S29.

Vles JSH, de Krom MCTF, Visser R, Höweler CJ. Two Dutch siblings with congenital muscular dystrophy (Fukuyama type). Clin Neurol Neurosurg 1983; 85: 175–180.

Vohra N, Ghidini A, Alvarez M, Lockwood C. Walker–Warburg syndrome: prenatal ultrasound findings. Prenat Diagn 1993; 13: 575–579.

Voit T, Fardeau M, Tomé FMS. Prenatal detection of merosin expression in human placenta. Neuropediatrics 1994; 25: 332–333.

Voit T, Sewry CA, Meyer K, Hermann R, Straub V, Muntoni F, Kahn T, Unsold R, Helliwell TR, Appleton R, Lenard RG. Preserved merosin M-chain (or laminin-α2) expression in skeletal muscle distinguishes Walker–Warburg syndrome from Fukuyama muscular dystrophy and merosin-deficient congenital muscular dystrophy. Neuropediatrics 1995; 26(3): 148–155.

Voit T. Recent advances in the classification of congenital muscular dystrophies (abstract). Neuromusc Disord 1996; 6(2): S17.

Vuolteenaha R, Nissinen M, Sainio K, Byers M, Eddy R, Hirvonen H, Shows TB, Sariola H, Engvall E, Tryggvason K. Human laminin M chain (merosin): complete primary structure: chromosomal assignment and expression of the M and A chain in human fetal tissue. J Cell Biol 1994; 124: 381–394.

Wada S, Masuda K, Hiraki Y, Sasaki C, Iku K, Koide S, Hatano E, Yoshida M. The 1979 survey of autopsy registry for progressive muscular dystrophy. Particularly on heart findings in congenital muscular dystrophy (in Japanese). In: Sobue I, ed. The 1979 annual report of the research committee on clinics, epidemiology and management of progressive muscular dystrophy, sponsored by the Ministry of Health and Welfare of Japan. Nagoya, 1980: 317–322.

Wakayama Y, Kumagai T, Shibuya S. Freeze fracture studies of muscle plasma membrane in Fukuyama-type congenital muscular dystrophy. Neurology 1985; 35: 1587–1593.

Wakayama Y, Kumagai T, Jimi T. Small size of orthogonal array in muscle plasma membrane of Fukuyama type congenital muscular dystrophy. Acta Neuropathol 1986; 72: 130–133.

Wakayama Y, Kumagai T, Jimi T, Shibuya S. Freeze-fracture analysis of cholesterol in muscle plasma membrane of Fukuyama-type congenital muscular dystrophy. Acta Neuropathol 1987; 75: 46–50.

Wakayama Y, Shibuya S, Onishi H, Eto T, Saito M, Nonaka I. Ultrastructural analysis of skeletal muscle membrane in *dy* mice – a comparison with that in *mdx* mice. In: Takagi A, chairman. Abstract for the 1995 annual meeting of the research committee on pathogenesis and treatment of progressive muscular dystrophy and related disorders, sponsored by the Ministry of Health and Welfare of Japan, Tokyo, 1995: 45.

Wakayama Y, Murahashi M, Jimi T, Kojima H, Shibuya S, Oniki H. Immunogold and freeze etch electron microscopic studies of merosin localization in basal lamina of human skeletal muscle fibers. Acta Neuropathol 1997; 93: 34-42.

Walker AE. Lissencephaly. Arch Neurol Psychiatry 1942; 48: 13–29.

Walter JM, Marescaux CHR, Coquillat G, Walter P, Micheletti G, Rohmer F. Syndrome autosomique recessif associant myopathie et atteinte du système nerveux central et périphérique. J Neurol Sci 1981; 49: 135–151.

Walton JN, Nattrass FJ. On the classification, natural history and treatment of the myopathies. Brain 1954; 77: 169–231.

Walton JN. Amyotonia congenita: a follow-up study. Lancet 1956; 1: 1023–1027.

Walton JN, Geschwind N, Simpson JA. Benign congenital myopathy with myasthenic features. J Neurol Neurosurg Psychiatry 1956; 19: 224–231.

Walton JN. "The limp child". J Neurol Neurosurg Psychiatry 1957; 20: 144–154.

Walton JN. The amyotonia congenita syndrome. Proc R Soc Med 1957; 50: 301–308.

Wang Z-P, Osawa M, Fukuyama Y. Morphometric study of the corpus callosum in Fukuyama type congenital muscular dystrophy by magnetic resonance imaging. Brain Dev (Tokyo) 1995; 17: 104–110.

Warburg M. The heterogeneity of microphthalmia in the mentally retarded. Birth Defects 1971; 7: 136–154.

Warburg M. Heterogeneity of congenital retinal non-attachment, falciform fold and retinal dysplasia. Hum Hered 1976; 26: 137–148.

Warburg M. Hydrocephaly, congenital retinal non-attachment, and congenital falciform fold. Am J Ophthalmol 1978; 85: 192–197.

Warburg M. Ocular malformations and lissencephaly. Eur J Pediatr 1987; 146: 450–452.

Warburg M. Muscle-eye-brain disease and Walker–Warburg syndrome: phenotype-genotype speculations. Commentary to Pihko's paper (pp. 57–61). Brain Dev 1995; 17(l): 62–63.

Wargowaski DS, Chitayat D, Wes Tyson R, Norman MG, Friedman JM. Lethal congenital muscular dystrophy with cataracts and a minor brain anomaly – new entity or variant of Walker–Warburg syndrome. Am J Med Genet 1991; 39: 19–24.

Watanabe A, Konishi T. Amyotonia congenita syndrome: probably autosomal recessively inherited Duchenne muscular dystrophy – a case report (in Japanese). Rinsho Shoni Igaku (Jpn J Clin Pediatr) (Sapporo) 1966; 14: 91–94.

Watanabe K, Kumagai T, Wakayama Y, Hara K, Yamada H. Congenital myopathy and communicating hydrocephalus. A possible pathogenetic combination. Brain Dev (Tokyo) 1982; 4: 455–462.

Watanabe T. Congenital muscular dystrophy in two siblings (in Japanese). Shonika Shinryo (J Pediatr Pract) (Tokyo) 1961; 24: 1620–1629.

Weinberg AG. Case 1: Walker–Warburg syndrome. Pediatr Pathol 1989; 9: 749–755.

Werneck LC, Shiebler E, Minetti C, Bonilla E. Immunohistochemical alterations of dystrophin in congenital muscular dystrophy (abstract). Neurology 1991; 41(Suppl 1): 136.

Wewer UM, Durkin ME, Zhang X, Laursen H, Nielsen NH, Towfighi J, Engvall E, Albrechtsen R. Laminin $\beta 2$ chain and adhalin deficiency in the skeletal muscle of Walker–Warburg syndrome (cerebro-ocular dysplasia – muscular dystrophy). Neurology 1995; 45: 2099–2101.

Wewer UM, Engvall E. Merosin/laminin 2 and muscular dystrophy. Neuromusc Disord 1996; 6: 409–418.

Wharton BA. An unusual variety of muscular dystrophy. Lancet 1965; i: 248–249.

Whitley CB, Thompson TR, Mastri AR, Gorlin RJ. Warburg syndrome; lethal neurodysplasia with autosomal recessive inheritance. J Pediatr 1983; 102: 547–551.

Williams RS, Swisher CN, Jennings M, Ambler M, Caviness VS Jr. Cerebro-ocular dysgenesis (Walker–Warburg syndrome); neuropathologic and etiologic analysis. Neurology 1984; 34: 1531–1541.

Winter RM, Garner A. Hydrocephalus, agyria, pseudoencephalocele, retinal dysplasia and anterior chamber anomalies. J Med Genet 1981; 18: 314–317.

Winter RM, Baraitser M. Congenital muscular dystrophy, type Fukuyama. In: Winter RM, Baraitser M, eds. Multiple congenital anomalies. A diagnostic compendium. London: Chapman and Hall, 1991: 129.

Wolburg H, Schlote W, Langohr HD, Peiffer J, Reither KH, Hecki RW. Slowly progressive congenital myopathy with cytoplasmic bodies. Clin Neuropathol (Tokyo) 1982; 2: 55–66.

Wu L, Oguni H, Osawa M, Fukuyama Y. Fukuyama type congenital muscular dystrophy with centrotemporal EEG foci. Tokyo Joshi Ikadaigaku Zasshi (J Tokyo Wom Med Coll) (Tokyo) 1993; 63: S345–S352.

Wu L, Oguni H, Osawa M, Fukuyama Y. Fukuyama type congenital muscular dystrophy with central-temporal EEG foci (Rolandic spikes). Chin Med Sci J 1993; 8(3): 162–166.

Wu M, Sasaki T, Nishida N, Sugimoto T, Kobayashi O, Nonaka I. A case of merosin-negative congenital muscular dystrophy associated with numerous nemaline bodies (abstract in Japanese). No To Hattatsu (Brain Dev) (Tokyo) 1996; 28S: S215.

Xu H, Christmas P, Wu X-R, Wewer UM, Engvall E. Defective muscle basement membrane and lack of M laminin in the dystrophic *dy/dy* mouse. Proc Natl Acad Sci USA 1994; 91: 5572–5576.

Xu H, Wu X-R, Werner UM, Engvall E. Murine muscular dystrophy. Defect of laminin M in skeletal and cardiac muscles and peripheral nerves of the homozygous dystrophic *dy/dy* mice. Nat Genet 1995; 8: 297–302.

Yagishita A, Aida N, Tamagawa K. Fukuyama type congenital muscular dystrophy – correlation between cranial MRI and neuropathological findings (in Japanese). Byori To Rinsho (Pathol Clin) (Tokyo) 1994; 12(4): 469–474.

Yamada H, Oi S. Follow-up of the hydrocephalic state in a case of congenital muscular dystrophy (Fukuyama type). Discussion of the change in white matter and functional prognosis after shunt procedure (in Japanese). CT Kenkyu (Prog Comput Tomogr) (Tokyo) 1985; 7(1): 88–93.

Yamada H, Komiyama J, Suzuki Y, Misugi N, Hasegawa O. A case of non-Fukuyama type congenital muscular dystrophy with progression in early adulthood, ocular involvement and sensorineural deafness (in Japanese). Rinsho Shinkeigaku (Clin Neurol) (Tokyo) 1993; 33(4): 405–410.

Yamada H, Shimizu T, Tanaka T, Campbell KP, Matsumura K. Dystroglycan is binding protein of laminin and merosin in peripheral nerve. FEBS Lett 1994; 352: 49–53.

Yamada H, Hori H, Tanaka T, Fujita S, Fukuta-Ohi H, Hojo S, Tamura A, Shimizu T, Matsumura K. Secretion of laminin α2 chain in cerebrospinal fluid. FEBS Lett 1995; 376: 37–40.

Yamada H, Tomé FMS, Higuchi I, Kawai H, Azibi K, Chaouch N, Roberds SI, Tanaka T, Fujita S, Mitsui T, Fukunaga H, Miyoshi K, Osame M, Fardeau M, Kaplan J-C, Shimizu

T, Campbell KP, Matsumura K. Laminin abnormality in severe childhood autosomal recessive muscular dystrophy. Lab Invest 1995; 72: 715–722.

Yamada H, Chiba A, Endo T, Kobata A, Anderson LVB, Hori H, Fukuta-Ohi H, Kanazawa I, Campbell KP, Shimizu T, Matsumura K. Characterization of dystroglycan-laminin interaction in peripheral nerve. J Neurochem 1996; 66: 1518–1524.

Yamada H, Denzer A, Hori H, Tanaka T, Anderson LVB, Fujita S, Fukuta-Ohi H, Simizu T, Ruegg MA, Matsumura K. Dystroglycan is a dual receptor of agrin and laminin-2 in Schwann cell membrane. J Biol Chem 1996; 271: 23418-23423.

Yamada S, Nishimura M. Muscle CT findings in lower extremities of progressive muscular dystrophy patients (in Japanese). In: Nishitani H, ed. The 1985 annual report of the research committee on genetics, epidemiology, clinics and treatment of progressive muscular dystrophy, sponsored by the Ministry of Health and Welfare of Japan. Kyoto, 1986: 26–30.

Yamada S, Nishimura M, Nishimura S. A comparative study between muscle CT findings and ultrasound scanning of thigh and calf muscles in progressive muscular dystrophy patients (in Japanese). In: Nishitani H, ed. The 1986 annual report of the research committee on genetics, epidemiology, clinics and treatment of progressive muscular dystrophy, sponsored by the Ministry of Health and Welfare of Japan. Kyoto, 1987: 5–9.

Yamada S, Nishimura M, Nishimura S, Yamauchi K. Ultrasound cross-sectional scannings of skeletal muscles in neuromuscular disorders (in Japanese). In: Nishitani H, ed. The 1988 annual report of the research committee on genetics, epidemiology, clinics and treatment of progressive muscular dystrophy, sponsored by the Ministry of Health and Welfare of Japan. Kyoto, 1989: 134–137.

Yamagata K, Fujimoto T, Misawa M, Amimoto S, Sekiya N. Rehabilitation of Fukuyama type congenital muscular dystrophy (in Japanese). Tokyo Joshi Ikadaigaku Zasshi (J Tokyo Wom Med Coll) (Tokyo) 1983; 53: 215–223.

Yamagata K, Fujimoto T. Effect of rehabilitation on Fukuyama-congenital muscular dystrophy (in Japanese). Tokyo Joshi Ikadaigaku Zasshi (J Tokyo Wom Med Coll) (Tokyo) 1993; 63(Suppl): S440–S445.

Yamagata Y. A case of congenital muscular dystrophy (in Japanese). Shonika Shinryo (J Pediatr Pract) (Tokyo) 1967; 30: 792–795.

Yamaguchi E, Hayashi T, Kondoh H, Tashiro N, Tsukahara M, Nagamitsu T, Eguchi Y. A case of Walker–Warburg syndrome with uncommon findings. Double cortical layer, temporal cyst and increased serum IgM. Brain Dev (Tokyo) 1993; 15: 61–66.

Yamamoto T, Komori T, Shibata N, Kobayashi M, Kondo E, Saito K, Osawa M, Toda T. Fukuyama congenital muscular dystrophy: cortical dysplasia of the cerebrum in a 20 week fetus. Neuropathology (Tokyo) 1996; 16(3): 184–189.

Yamamoto T, Toyoda C, Kobayashi M, Kondo E, Saito K, Osawa M. Pial-glial barrier abnormalities in fetuses with Fukuyama congenital muscular dystrophy. Brain Dev 1997; 19(1): 35–42.

Yamashita S, Misugi N, Shimazaki Y, Higashi K, Miyake S, Yamada M, Iwamoto H, Tanaka Y, Kobayashi T. Problems associated with Japanese non-Fukuyama type congenital muscular dystrophy (abstract). Muscle Nerve 1994; Suppl 1: S181.

Yamashita Y, Ohtaki E, Matsuishi T, Osari S, Kobayashi O, Nonaka I. Merosin-negative non-Fukuyama type congenital muscular dystrophy: a case report. Brain Dev 1996; 18: 131-134.

Yasutake T, Morikita M, Gocho M, Takagi N. An experience of nursing for congenital muscular dystrophy babies (in Japanese). In: Aoyagi A, ed. The 1986 annual report of the research committee on clinical and psychological study of care and nursing of progressive muscular dystrophy, sponsored by the Ministry of Health and Welfare of Japan. 1987; 183–185.

Yokochi K, Tanaka T, Nonaka I. Congenital muscular dystrophy with severe infantile scoliosis. Brain Dev (Tokyo) 1985; 7: 492–495.

Yoneda M. Myatonia congenita Oppenheim (in Japanese). Nyujigaku Zasshi (J Pedol) (Tokyo) 1928; 3: 359–380.

Yoshida M, Yoshida R, Izumi T, Shishikura K, Suzuki H, Osawa M, Fukuyama Y. A case of porencephaly associated with hyper-CK-emia, West syndrome and ocular anomalies. In: Fukuyama Y, Osawa M, eds. Program and abstracts of the International Symposium on Congenital Muscular Dystrophies, Tokyo. Tokyo: Tokyo Women's Medical College, 1994: 42.

Yoshikawa H, Hirayama Y, Kurokawa T, Houdo S. A case of Fukuyama type congenital muscular dystrophy presenting with rapidly progressive heart failure (in Japanese). Iryo (Tokyo) 1991; 45: 898–902.

Yoshioka M. Cranial CT findings in congenital muscular dystrophy (in Japanese). Shoni Naika (Jpn J Pediatr Med) (Tokyo) 1979; 11: 829–834.

Yoshioka M, Okuno T, Honda Y, Nakano Y. Central nervous system involvement in progressive muscular dystrophy. Arch Dis Child 1980; 55: 589–594.

Yoshioka M, Okuno T, Nakano Y, Honda K. Cranial CT findings in Fukuyama type congenital muscular dystrophy (in Japanese). CT Kenkyu (Prog Comp Tomogr) (Tokyo) 1980; 2: 341–348.

Yoshioka M, Okuno T, Itoh M, Konishi Y, Itagaki Y, Sakamoto Y. Congenital muscular dystrophy (Fukuyama type). Repeated CT studies in 19 children. Comp Tomogr 1981; 5: 81–88.

Yoshioka M, Mikawa H. Follow-up study of EEG in patients with congenital muscular dystrophy (Fukuyama type). Ann Paediatr Jpn (Kyoto) 1982; 28: 136–143.

Yoshioka M, Kuroki S, Mizue H, Itagaki Y, Kataoka K, Nakano S, Okuno T. Clinical studies of congenital muscular dystrophy of severe type in comparison to Fukuyama type (abstract). Brain Dev (Tokyo) 1987; 9: 239.

Yoshioka M, Kuroki S, Mizue H. Congenital muscular dystrophy of non-Fukuyama type with characteristic CT image. Brain Dev (Tokyo) 1987; 9: 316–318.

Yoshioka M, Saiwai S. Congenital muscular dystrophy (Fukuyama type): changes in the white matter low density on CT. Brain Dev (Tokyo) 1988; 10: 41–44.

Yoshioka M. Congenital muscular dystrophy of a non-Fukuyama type with characteristic CT images (letter). Brain Dev (Tokyo) 1988; 10: 60.

Yoshioka M, Kuroki S, Kondo T. Ocular manifestations in Fukuyama type congenital muscular dystrophy. Brain Dev (Tokyo) 1990; 12: 423–426.

Yoshioka M, Saiwai S, Kuroki S, Nigami H. MR imaging of the brain in Fukuyama type congenital muscular dystrophy. Am J Neuroradiol 1991; 12: 63–65.

Yoshioka M. Fukuyama type congenital muscular dystrophy (in Japanese). Shoni Naika (Jpn J Pediatr Med) (Tokyo) 1991; 23: 1129–1133.

Yoshioka M, Kuroki S, Nigami H, Kawai T, Nakamura H. Clinical variation within sibships in Fukuyama-type congenital muscular dystrophy. Brain Dev (Tokyo) 1992; 14: 334–337.

Yoshioka M, Kuroki S. Clinical manifestations of congenital muscular dystrophy. Complications or associations not relating to muscle, eye, or brain, and the prognosis (in Japanese). In: Takahashi K, ed. The 1992 annual report of the research committee on clinics, genetic counselling and epidemiology of progressive muscular dystrophy, sponsored by the Ministry of Health and Welfare of Japan. Hyogo, 1993: 256–258.

Yoshioka M, Kuroki S, Saiwai S. Re-evaluation of cranial CT/MRI findings in Fukuyama type congenital muscular dystrophy – evolution of cerebral white matter low density (in Japanese). In: Takahashi K, ed. The 1993 annual report of the research committee on clinics, genetic counselling and epidemiology of progressive muscular dystrophy, sponsored by the Ministry of Health and Welfare of Japan. Hyogo, 1994: 185–187.

Yoshioka M, Kuroki S. Clinical spectrum and genetic studies of Fukuyama congenital muscular dystrophy. Am J Med Genet 1994; 53: 245–250.

Yoshioka M, Kuroki S. Reevaluation of cranial CT/MRI findings in Fukuyama type congenital muscular dystrophy – evolution of cerebral white matter low density (abstract in Japanese). No To Hattatsu (Brain Dev) (Tokyo) 1994; 26 Suppl: S282.

Yoshioka M. Neuroimaging findings in non-Fukuyama type and other types of congenital muscular dystrophy (in Japanese). Shoni Naika (Jpn J Pediatr Med) (Tokyo) 1995; 27 Suppl: 1027–1030.

Yoshioka M. Fukuyama type congenital muscular dystrophy (in Japanese). Shoni Naika (Jpn J Pediatr Med) (Tokyo) 1996; 28 Suppl: 904–908.

Yoshitake S, Hoshi C, Sekine M, Sakamoto S, Masuo S, Suzuki T, Sasaki Y, Kurosu M, Kondo H. Problems involved in the electronic wheelchair for the use of Fukuyama type congenital muscular dystrophy (in Japanese). In: Aoyagi A, ed. The 1986 annual report of the research committee on clinical and psychological study of care and nursing of progressive muscular dystrophy, sponsored by the Ministry of Health and Welfare of Japan. 1987: 49–52.

Zeidler U. Über den Verlauf der infantilen progressiven spinalen Muskelatrophie der Typen Werdnig–Hoffmann und Oppenheim. Z Kinderheilk 1958; 81: 315–329.

Zellweger H. Congenital myopathies and their differential diagnoses. Paediatr Fortbildungskurse Prax 1966; 18: 105–138.

Zellweger H, Afifi A, McCormick WF, Mergner W. Severe congenital muscular dystrophy. Am J Dis Child 1967; 114: 591–602.

Zellweger H, Afifi A, McCormick WF, Mergner W. Benign congenital muscular dystrophy; a special form of congenital hypotonia. Clin Pediatr 1967; 6: 655–663.

Zellweger H, Afifi AK, McCormick WF, Mergner W. Congenital muscular dystrophy. In: Barbeau A, Brunette J-R, eds. Progress in neurogenetics, Proceedings of the 2nd International Congress of Neurogenetics and Neuro-ophthalmology of the WFN, Montreal, 1967, Vol 1. Amsterdam: Excerpta Medica, 1969: 235–236.

Zhao J, Yoshioka M, Miike T, Kageshita T, Arao T. Nerve growth factor receptor immunoreactivity on the tunica adventitia of intramuscular blood vessels in childhood muscular dystrophies. Neuromusc Disord 1991; 1: 135–141.

Subject index

α-actinin, 286
α-dystroglycan, 295
β-dystroglycan, 287
β-thalassemia, 148
δ lesion
    in FCMD myofiber, 215

aberrant myelinated nerve fibers, 82, 192, 239
absent corpus callosum, 93, 94
acridine orange-RNA fluorescence (AO), 254
adhalin, 267
agyria, 92
Alzheimer's neurofibrillary tangles, 193
    in FCMD, 190
amyotonia congenita syndrome, 9
animal models, 28, 291
arthrogryposis multiplex congenita, 180, 334

basal lamina, 72, 259
basement membranes, 79, 80
Batten, Frederick E., 1
benign congenital hypotonia, 9
brain malformation
    in FCMD, 231
    in WWS, 231
    muscle-eye-brain disease, 102
brainstem hypoplasia, 91, 93

C9, 254
caveolae density, 221
cerebellar hypoplasia, 91, 93, 236
cerebellar polymicrogyria, 58, 93, 191
cerebral cortical gyration abnormality, 329
cerebral dysplasia, 335
cerebro-oculo-muscular dystrophies, 171
chromosome 3p21, 306
chromosome 6, 26
chromosome 6q22–23, 79, 306
chromosome 9q, 24
chromosome 9q31, 302, 309
classical congenital muscular dystrophy (CMD),
    26, 137, 150, 297, 342
classical lissencephaly, 180, 201
classification
    congenital muscular dystrophies, 17, 63, 149
classification of muscular dystrophy
    ICD-10NA, 11

World Federation of Neurology Research
    Committee, 1991, 12
clinical features of FCMD
    cardiac involvement, 50
    facial muscle involvement, 39, 43
    growth, 49
    hyperextensibility of the joints, 36
    joint contractures, 39
    mental retardation, 45
    muscle atrophy, 36
    muscle weakness, 36
    non-neurologic congenital anomalies, 49,
        109
    pseudohypertrophy, 36
    round lesions, 38
    scoliosis, 42
    seizures, 45, 85, 108
    skin changes, 49
clinical spectrum
    of FCMD, 106
CMD plus, 171, 177, 182
CMD pure, 24, 171, 337
cobblestone lissencephaly, 89, 95, 147
collagen IV, 292
    in DMD, 262
    in FCMD, 262
    in non-FCMD, 262
congenital muscular dystrophy
    classical, 26, 137, 150, 297, 342
    classification of, 17, 63, 149
    in Sicilian patients, 147
    merosin-deficient, 16, 70, 83, 155, 174, 263,
        285, 297
    merosin-positive, 16, 64, 70, 73, 84, 155
    with leukodystrophy, 177
congenital myasthenic syndromes, 324
corpus callosum, 57, 235
cortical angioarchitecture in FCMD, 205
cortical dysplasia, 178, 189, 335, 346, 385
    in FCMD, 52, 200, 231
    in WWS, 231
corticospinal tracts, 178
costamere, 286
cramps, 322
craniosynostosis
    cobblestone lissencephaly, with, 95
C-terminal domains, 287

Dandy–Walker malformation, 93
denervation muscular atrophy, 329
desmin, 254
diagnostic criteria, 100
digitonin-cholesterol complexes, 227
double cortex, 339
Duchenne muscular dystrophy (DMD), 119, 221
    rehabilitation, 160
dy/dy mouse, 28, 291
dystroglycan
    peripheral nerve, 267
dystrophin, 155, 254, 262, 267
dystrophin costameres, 286
dystrophin-associated membrane protein complex
    (DAP), 297, 306
dystrophin-glycoprotein complex (DGC), 267, 275
dystrophinopathy, congenital, 175

Eichsfeld-type CMD, 175
electroretinograms (ERG), 93, 101
    in muscle-eye-brain disease, 94
Emery–Dreifuss muscular dystrophy (EDMD), 181
ENMC-sponsored International Workshop on
    CMD, 22, 26, 80, 91
epilepsy, 138
epileptic seizures, 45, 85, 100, 232
European Neuromuscular Centre (ENMC), 22, 26
exercise intolerance, 322
extracellular matrix (ECM), 79, 286, 295
eye abnormalities, 89, 147, 346, 348
    in muscle-eye-brain disease, 94, 101
    in Walker-Warburg syndrome, 93, 184
eye lesions, 47, 108, 232
eye pathology, 180

familial lethal cardiomyopathy, 177
FCMD fetal brain, 203, 315
FCMD locus, 302
female DMD carriers, 280
fetal cortical cytoarchitecture
    in FCMD, 203, 315
fetal muscle
    in DMD, 263
    in FCMD, 263
fetal phenotype probability calculation, 313
fetus muscles, 209
fibroglial bands, 92
Finnish muscle-eye-brain disease, 89
flash VEPs, 101
foot equinovarus deformity, 165
freeze fracture electron microscopy, 213
Fukuyama congenital muscular dystrophy
    (FCMD), 9, 69, 79, 95, 103, 105, 119, 141, 173,
    203, 231, 309, 334, 345
    ages at death, 108
    average CT numbers of muscles, 133

brain malformation, 52, 200, 231
    cause of death, 59
    cerebellar cysts, 58
    cerebellar polymicrogyria, 58, 93, 191
    clinical course, 31
    clinical spectrum, 106
    concept of FCMD, 31
    corpus callosum, 57
    delayed myelination, 54
    discovery of, 9
    educational status, 169
    EEG, 46
    epidemiological aspects, 34, 71
    genetic counseling, 61
    initial symptoms and signs, 35
    intrafamilial variability, 59
    laboratory findings, 51
    linkage analysis, 113, 310
    management, 60
    motor function level scale, 165
    motor function levels, 32, 33
    muscle CT scans, 51, 119
    muscle histopathology in, 51, 215, 232
    natural history, 162
    neuroimaging in, 109
    non-neurologic congenital anomalies, 109
    ophthalmological findings, 47, 108
    polymicrogyria, 52, 231
    prognosis, 59
    rehabilitation, 159, 168
    seizures, 108, 232
    serum CK, 51, 232
    subclassification system, 33
    white matter changes, 53, 71, 93, 102, 137
Fukuyama-like CMD, 138

genetic linkage analysis, 113, 302
GFAP-immunohistochemistry, 204
Golgi stain, 202

homozygosity mapping method, 302
Howard, Russel, 1
hydrocephalus, 53, 91, 94, 232
hypoplasia, 178
hypoplasia of the corpus callosum
    in WWS, 237

immunocytochemistry of muscle, 155
immunostaining
    spectrin, for, 254
incidence
    of classical form of CMD, 71
    of congenital muscular dystrophies, 70
    of FCMD, 71
    of merosin-positive CMD in Japan, 76
infantile spinal muscular atrophy (SMA), 2, 334

inflammatory myopathy, 325
International Workshop on Congenital Muscular
    Dystrophies, 22, 26, 80, 91
intramembranous particles, 214

laminin, 79
laminin α2, 140, 275, 291, 292
    in DMD, 260
    in FCMD, 260
    in non-FCMD, 260
laminin α2-chain deficiency, 16, 70, 83, 155, 174,
    263, 285, 297
laminin β1, 155, 260
    in DMD, 260
    in FCMD, 260
    in non-FCMD, 260
laminin A-chain, 155
laminin M chain, 153, 155, 270
leukoencephalopathy, 137, 177
    in FCMD, 53
    in MEB, 102
limb-girdle muscular dystrophy (LGMD), 181
linkage analysis
    of FCMD families, 113, 310
linkage disequilibrium, 305
lissencephaly, 52, 139
    cobblestone, 89, 94, 95, 147
    in FCMD, 231
    in WWS, 231
    type I, 180, 201
    type II, 91, 178, 190, 204
low affinity nerve growth factor receptor, 207

macrocephaly, 91
magnetic resonance imaging (MRI)
    aberrant cortico-spinal pathways, 237
    brain stem, 236
    in FCMD, 232
    in WWS, 232
    small dysplastic cerebellum, 236
membrane abnormality
    in DMD, 255
    in FCMD, 253
membrane-associated cytoskeleton, 255
meningeal gliomesenchymal overgrowth, 92, 192,
    239
mental retardation, 45, 100, 139
merosin, 140, 153, 155, 270
merosin deficiency, 64, 80, 263, 276
    dy mouse, 28
merosin-deficient (negative) CMD, 16, 70, 83, 155,
    174, 263, 285, 297
merosin-diminished CMD, 155
merosin-positive CMD, 16, 64, 70, 73, 84, 155
mfd220, 303, 313
muscle abnormalities

in Walker-Warburg syndrome, 94, 232
muscle basal lamina, 259
muscle CT scans, 119
    average CT numbers, 124
    comparison between DMD and FCMD, 134
    correlation between average CT number and
        age, 124
    macroscopic findings, 122, 132
muscle histopathology, 172
    dystrophin, 51
    dystrophin-associated glycoprotein, 51
    in FCMD, 51, 232
    in MEB, 100
    in merosin-negative CMD, 71
    in merosin-positive CMD, 74
    in WWS, 232
    merosin, 51
muscle plasma membrane, 213
muscle-eye-brain disease (MEB), 16, 22, 47, 64,
    94, 99, 105, 150, 177, 307, 345
    brain malformation in, 94, 102
    diagnostic criteria, 96
    electroencephalogram, 103
    genetic studies, 103
    mental retardation, 100
    muscsle histopathology, 96
    neuroimaging, 102
    ocular findings in, 94, 101
    seizures, 100
    VEP, 94
muscular dystrophy
    Batten-Turner type, 1
myalgia, 322
myelin basic protein, 199
myotendinous junctions, 276
myotonic dystrophy (MtD), 182

nemaline bodies, 174
neonatal hypotonia, 85
nerve growth factor, 207
neurofilament, 199
neuroimaging, 52, 139, 140, 232
    in FCMD, 109, 232
    in MEB, 102
neuromuscular junction (NMJ), 275
neuromuscular junctions of FCMD muscles, 219
neurotrophin-3, 207
non-Fukuyama muscular dystrophy (non-FCMD),
    10, 22, 254

occidental type cerebromuscular dystrophy
    (OMCD), 153
occipital cephaloceles, 91
oculo-pharyngeal muscular dystrophy (OPMD),
    181
ophthalmological findings, 89

in FCMD, 47, 108
in WWS, 232
round lesions, 47
Oppenheim
amyotonia congenita, 2
orthogonal array density, 226

pachygyria, 52, 92, 190, 329, 339
in FCMD, 237
in muscle-eye-brain disease, 94
Pena–Shokeir syndrome, 334
peripheral nerve
in *dy* mice, 28, 270
in FCMD, 270, 297
in merosin deficiency, 270
in WWS, 239
peripheral neuropathy
plasmalemmal undercoat, 214
in FCMD myofiber, 216
polymicrogyria, 92, 190, 334, 351
in FCMD, 52, 231
in muscle-eye brain disease, 94
in WWS, 231
polymorphism analysis, 313
prenatal diagnosis
in FCMD, 310
pure CMD, 24, 337
with merosin deficiency and brain
malformations, 342

recombination mapping, 304
regenerating muscle fibers, 207
rehabilitation
long leg braces, 163
psycho-social education, 167
sliding cart, 162
stabilizer-type standing braces, 161
research diagnostic criteria
MEB syndromes, 96
retina
in WWS, 184
retinal abnormality, 147
retinal detachment, 93, 180
retinal dysplasia, 346, 348

Santavuori disease, 47
sarcoglycan complex, 276
seizures, 45, 100, 232

in FCMD, 108
septum pellucidum agenesis
in FCMD, 237
severe childhood autosomal recessive muscular
dystophy (SCARMD), 270
single teased muscle fibers, 277
sympathetic nervous system
in FCMD, 210
synaptophysin immunohistochemistry, 200
syringomyelia, 148

tubular aggregates, 321
tumor necrotic factor, 207
tunica adventitia of blood vessels
in FCMD, 208
Turkish CMD patients, 157
type-I fiber predominance, 174

Ullrich's congenital atonic sclerotic syndrome, 79
utrophin, 267, 275, 287
utrophin costameres, 281
utrophin-glycoprotein complex, 267

ventriculomegaly, 93
visual evoked potential (VEP), 93
in muscle-eye-brain disease, 94
verrucous dysplasia, 190

Walker–Warburg syndrome (WWS), 16, 22, 47,
64, 89, 99, 103, 105, 137, 150, 177, 201, 307
a milder form, 345
clinical course, 91
cobblestone lissencephaly, 91
eye abnormalities, 93, 184
in Japan, 231
manifestations of, 90
muscle histopathology in, 94, 232
ophthalmological findings, 232, 346
previous diagnostic criteria, 91
retina in, 184
Werdnig–Hoffmann disease, 2, 334
white matter changes, 53, 85, 93, 102, 137
white matter dysmyelination, 91
white matter lucency, 71, 73, 346

xeroderma pigmentosum, 24

Zellweger disease, 182